CUMMINGS

Review of
OTOLARYNGOLOGY

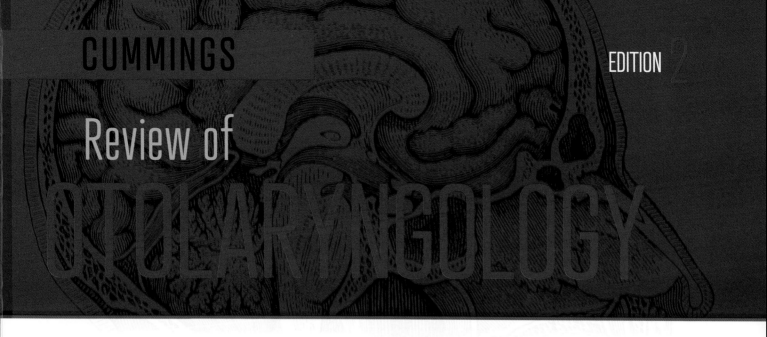

CUMMINGS

EDITION 2

Review of
OTOLARYNGOLOGY

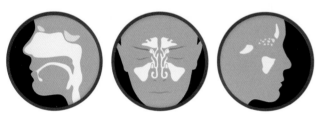

Harrison W. Lin, MD

Associate Professor of Otolaryngology—Head and Neck Surgery
University of California
Irvine, California
United States

Daniel S. Roberts, MD, PhD

Associate Professor
Otolaryngology
University of Connecticut
Farmington, Connecticut
United States

Jeffrey P. Harris, MD, PhD

Chair and Distinguished Professor
Department of Otolaryngology—Head and Neck Surgery
University of California
San Diego, California
United States

ELSEVIER

Elsevier
1600 John F. Kennedy Blvd.
Ste 1800
Philadelphia, PA 19103-2899

CUMMINGS REVIEW OF OTOLARYNGOLOGY, SECOND EDITION   ISBN: 978-0-323-77610-3

Notice

Practitioners and researchers must always rely on their own experience and knowledge in evaluating and using any information, methods, compounds or experiments described herein. Because of rapid advances in the medical sciences, in particular, independent verification of diagnoses and drug dosages should be made. To the fullest extent of the law, no responsibility is assumed by Elsevier, authors, editors or contributors for any injury and/or damage to persons or property as a matter of products liability, negligence or otherwise, or from any use or operation of any methods, products, instructions, or ideas contained in the material herein.

Previous edition copyrighted 2017.

Content Strategist: Jessica L. McCool
Senior Content Development Manager: Somodatta Roy Choudhury
Publishing Services Manager: Shereen Jameel
Project Manager: Gayathri S
Design Direction: Renee Duenow

Printed in India

Last digit is the print number: 9 8 7 6 5 4 3 2 1

Working together
to grow libraries in
developing countries

www.elsevier.com • www.bookaid.org

Contributors

Amir Afrogheh, BChD, MSc, MChD, PhD
Associate Professor and Head
Department of Oral and Maxillofacial Pathology
University of the Western Cape and National Health Laboratory Service;
Extraordinary Senior Lecturer
Division of Anatomical Pathology
University of Stellenbosch
Stellenbosch, South Africa

Sarah N. Bowe, MD, EdM
Associate Professor
Department of Otolaryngology—Head and Neck Surgery
San Antonio Uniformed Services Health Education Consortium, JBSA;
Vice Chair
Department of Surgery
Brooke Army Medical Center, JBSA
Fort Sam Houston, Texas
United States

Divya Chari, MD
Physician
Department of Otolaryngology—Head and Neck Surgery
Massachusetts Eye and Ear
Boston, Massachusetts
United States

Brian S. Chen, MD
Otology, Neurotology and Skull Base Surgery
Tripler Army Medical Center, TAMC
Honolulu, Hawaii;
Assistant Professor
Department of Surgery
Uniformed Services University of the Health Sciences
Bethesda, Maryland
United States

Kevin C. Coughlin, MD
Resident Physician
Department of Otolaryngology—Head and Neck Surgery
University of Tennessee Health Science Center
Memphis, Tennessee
United States

M. Jennifer Derebery, MD
Associate
Department of Neurotology
House Ear Clinic;
Clinical Professor
Department of Otolaryngology
University of Southern California
Los Angeles, California
United States

Jayme Rose Dowdall, MD
Associate Professor
Department of Otolaryngology—Head and Neck Surgery
University of Nebraska Medical Center
Omaha, Nebraska
United States

William C. Faquin, MD, PhD
Director
Department of Head and Neck Pathology
Massachusetts Eye and Ear;
Professor of Pathology
Harvard Medical School
Boston, Massachusetts
United States

Daniel Fink, MD
Assistant Professor, Laryngology and Voice Disorders
Department of Otolaryngology—Head and Neck Surgery
University of Colorado School of Medicine
Aurora, Colorado
United States

M. Boyd Gillespie, MD, MSc
Professor and Chair
Department of Otolaryngology—Head and Neck Surgery
University of Tennessee Health Science Center
Memphis, Tennessee
United States

John L. Go, MD, FACR
Director of Head and Neck Imaging
Associate Professor of Radiology and Otolaryngology
Keck School of Medicine
University of Southern California
Los Angeles, California
United States

Sachin Gupta, MD
Physician
Department of Neurotology
Swedish Medical Center
Seattle, Washington
United States

Corbett A. Haas, DDS, MD, FACS
Partner
Prairie Oral Surgery
Fargo, North Dakota
United States

Jeffrey P. Harris, MD, PhD
Chair and Distinguished Professor
Department of Otolaryngology—Head and Neck Surgery
University of California
San Diego, California
United States

Karen Hawley, MD
Assistant Professor
Department of Surgery
University of New Mexico
Albuquerque, New Mexico
United States

Allen S. Ho, MD
Associate Professor of Surgery
Division of Otolaryngology—Head and Neck Surgery, Department of Surgery
Cedars-Sinai Medical Center;
Director, Head and Neck Cancer Program
Samuel Oschin Comprehensive Cancer Institute
Cedars-Sinai Medical Center
Los Angeles, California
United States

Marc H. Hohman, MD, FACS
Facial Plastic and Reconstructive Surgeon
Director, Otolaryngology Residency Program
Madigan Army Medical Center
Tacoma, Washington;
Associate Professor
Department of Surgery
Uniformed Services University of the Health Sciences
Bethesda, Maryland
United States

Charissa Kahue, MD
Assistant Professor
Department of Otolaryngology—Head and Neck Surgery
University of Tennessee Health Science Center
Memphis, Tennessee
United States

Kiran Kakarala, MD
Associate Professor
Department of Otolaryngology—Head and Neck Surgery
University of Kansas School of Medicine
Kansas City, Kansas
United States

Elliott D. Kozin, MD
Attending
Harvard Department of Otolaryngology
Massachusetts Eye and Ear
Boston, Massachusetts
United States

Shelby Leuin, MD, FACS
Associate Clinical Professor of Surgery
Pediatric Otolaryngology
Rady Children's Hospital, University of
    California
San Diego, California
United States

Aaron Lin, MD, MA
Pediatric Otolaryngologist
Head and Neck Surgery
Kaiser Permanente
Downey, California
United States

Harrison W. Lin, MD
Associate Professor of Otolaryngology—
    Head and Neck Surgery
University of California
Irvine, California
United States

James Lin, MD, FACS
Professor
Department of Otolaryngology—Head
    and Neck Surgery
University of Kansas Medical Center
Kansas City, Kansas
United States

Theodore R. McRackan, MD, MSCR
Associate Professor and Director of Skull
    Base Center
Department of Otolaryngology—Head
    and Neck Surgery
Medical University of South Carolina
Charleston, South Carolina
United States

Lauren Miller, MD, MBA
Clinical Resident
Department of Otolaryngology—Head
    and Neck Surgery
Massachusetts Eye and Ear
Boston, Massachusetts
United States

James G. Naples, MD
Assistant Professor in Otolaryngology
Department of Otolaryngology
Harvard Medical School, Beth Israel
    Deaconess Medical Center
Boston, Massachusetts
United States

Anandh G. Rajamohan, MD
Director of MR Imaging
Division of Neuroradiology
Southern California Permanente Medical
    Group
Kaiser Permanente Los Angeles Medical
    Center
Los Angeles, California
United States

Douglas Reh, MD
Director of Clinical Research
ENT Associates at GBMC Division
Centers for Advanced ENT Care
Baltimore, Maryland
United States

Daniel Stewart Roberts, MD, PhD
Assistant Professor
Department of Otolaryngology
University of Connecticut
Farmington, Connecticut
United States

Peter M. Sadow, MD, PhD
Director
Department of Head and Neck Pathology
Massachusetts General Hospital;
Associate Professor
Department of Pathology
Harvard Medical School
Boston, Massachusetts
United States

Ryan J. Smart, DMD, MD, FACS
Assistant Clinical Professor of Surgery
University of North Dakota School of
    Medicine and Health Sciences
Grand Forks, North Dakota;
Partner
Prairie Oral Surgery
Fargo, North Dakota
United States

Srinivas M. Susarla, MD, DMD, MPH
Associate Professor
Division of Plastic Surgery and
    Department of Surgery, Division of
    Plastic Surgery and Department of
    Oral and Maxillofacial Surgery
University of Washington Medical
    Center;
Attending Surgeon
Craniofacial Center
Seattle Children's Hospital
Seattle, Washington
United States

Jonathan Ting, MD
Professor & Chair
Department of Otolaryngology
Indiana University School of Medicine
Indianapolis, Indiana
United States

Aurora G. Vincent, MD, FACS
Assistant Professor
Department of Surgery
Uniformed Services University
Bethesda, Maryland
United States

Preface

Cummings Review of Otolaryngology is a review book designed for physicians taking the otolaryngology written and oral board, recertification, and in-service examinations; the otolaryngology intern, resident, and fellow trainees looking to augment their knowledge base; and medical students preparing for subinternships and residency training. If you are reading this book, you likely have performed at a high level on written examinations for most of your life. Although *Cummings Review of Otolaryngology* and other texts will prepare you for written examinations in the field of otolaryngology in a systematic and logical way, excelling on clinical rounds and on oral board examinations is a skill that improves with familiarity of oral testing formats and compartmentalizing your fund of knowledge in an organized, easily accessible manner.

We believe that this book is the primary and go-to resource that a medical student or resident will read before clinical rounds with the attending surgeon, a complex surgical case, a mock oral board examination, or the American Board of Otolaryngology examinations. The learning and information conveyed through the book will allow readers to have the most important clinical information—such as a differential diagnosis, clinical algorithm, treatment options, or a how-to list—instantly accessible in their memory to respond quickly to questions in a clinical or testing situation, to facilitate teaching of other residents and medical students, and to assist in patient management. This organized and structured way of thinking is central to success in the oral board format as well as in clinical rotations and patient care.

For this second edition, our authors have refined their chapters to incorporate new data, trends, and algorithms that have been developed since the first edition was published. We are confident that these additions will again enable you to perform at the highest level as a trainee or practicing otolaryngologist.

Harrison W. Lin, Daniel S. Roberts, Jeffrey P. Harris

Acknowledgments

For this second edition, we would like to once again acknowledge all of our teachers and mentors, who have dedicated their lives to both the highest level of patient care and passing on their craft to subsequent generations of surgeons. They serve as continued inspiration toward our academic pursuits. In addition, we wish to thank the students and trainees whose probing questions constantly push us to stay current and to serve as a stimulus for our own creativity.

Harrison W. Lin, Daniel S. Roberts, Jeffrey P. Harris

Contents

1 Preparing for Clinical Rounds and Board Examinations

Harrison W. Lin, Daniel S. Roberts, and Divya Chari

INTRODUCTION

We wrote the *Cummings Review of Otolaryngology* to provide high-yield information and clinical pearls to otolaryngology trainees. This book provides a comprehensive review of the field of otolaryngology and offers readers the foundation upon which they can build and expand their fund of knowledge with articles, textbooks, and discussions with colleagues. Although this text aims to augment the knowledge base of the reader in a systematic and organized manner, success on clinical rounds and in-service and board examinations is optimized with better understanding of how to prepare for attending rounds and improved familiarity with the testing formats. This chapter provides a systematic approach to these tasks. Indeed, incorporating learning strategies to help *organize* and *compartmentalize* information into digestible pieces is essential for trainees, particularly when there is limited time and a large breadth of material to cover.

WRITTEN EXAMS

As an otolaryngology resident, you likely have performed well on numerous written exams in undergraduate and medical school. You may have your own test strategies and study techniques. During residency, you will be expected to complete an annual in-service examination. This test serves two primary purposes: (1) to ensure that you are accruing an adequate fund of knowledge that is comparable to your peers and (2) to prepare you for the American Board of Otolaryngology examination (board exam). The pass rate for the written exam is generally around 90%. Failure to pass the board exam precludes board certification and may limit one's ability to work at certain hospitals or health care settings. While it is important to study every year for the in-service exam, you should consider additional time during your PGY4 and PGY5 years as data suggests that this correlates the most with performance on board examinations. Performing well during your senior years of residency will decrease stress and unpredictability during the board examination.

Most eligible trainees will prepare for and take the board exam in the year following completion of otolaryngology residency. The test is administered on a computer at a local testing center and consists of eight 50-minute sections. A whiteboard and marker are provided for notes during the test. While you can modify question answers within an active section, you cannot change answers to completed sections. You generally need to bring your own food and beverages for break period. Consider taking at least 1 or 2 breaks to give your mind a rest and be sure to eat. The board exam is nearly identical in style and difficulty of questions as the in-service exams, so if you generally did well on in-service exams, you should be well prepared for the written board exam.

Pearls for Success on Written Exams

- Preparation and repetition are the keys to success.
- Consider participating in study groups. Teaching a concept to someone else is the best way to learn the topic yourself. Study with your fellow residents by teaching one another.
- Mental endurance is critical. Given the length of the exam, prepare your mental stamina as the test date approaches by studying for 3- to 4-hour stretches at a time. Remember that those final questions are worth just as much as the first set of questions.
- Do not perseverate on one or a handful of questions. Remember that some questions are "experimental" and will not be counted toward your final score.
- Read the question stem carefully. For example, if the question stem asks for the "best answer" or the "next course of action" involving an unvaccinated child presenting with drooling and stridor, the correct answer may be to intubate the child rather than establish the diagnosis.
- During your clinical rotations, try to think through differential diagnoses for different presenting symptoms.
- Remember your patients. Success on written exams is facilitated by correlating clinical experiences with medical knowledge.
- The radiology and pathology images in *Cummings Review of Otolaryngology* are arranged in a high-yield format for exams in otolaryngology. Review these images before your in-service, written, and oral board exams. These images represent some of the most frequently encountered pathologies in our field, and you may find many on your exams.

ORAL EXAMINATIONS

Familiarity with the format of oral exams will help ensure success. For most residents and medical students, written exams have been the mainstay of testing, with far less training in the oral exam format. Historically, American Board of Otolaryngology oral examination took place in Chicago, Illinois over a 2-day period in a hotel near the O'Hare International Airport. During the COVID-19 pandemic, however, the board exam was conducted virtually over video conference. It remains to be seen whether the American Board of Otolaryngology will choose to retain the virtual format or revert to the in-person format. There are five subspecialty topics: (1) Head and Neck Surgery, (2) Otology and Neurotology, (3) Facial Plastic and Reconstructive Surgery, (4) General Otolaryngology (Allergy/Rhinology/Sleep Medicine and Surgery), and (5) General Otolaryngology (Laryngology and Pediatric Otolaryngology). Examiners will assess the test taker's ability to discuss appropriate diagnostic workup, differential diagnosis, and management options.

Success on the oral board exam depends on one's ability to communicate an organized and structured thought process. Oral board formats are similar to the workup of a patient in a clinic. Points are attained by starting with the chief complaint and obtaining a thorough history of the present illness, past medical history, past surgical history, family history, social history, list of medications and allergies, and review of systems. After completing the full history, the examinee should ask to perform a physical exam, first asking for the patient's vital signs. If there is an emergency, you will be expected to discuss basic life support and assess the patient's *airway*, *breathing*, and *circulation.* A brief summary statement with pertinent information from the history and physical, along with a comprehensive differential diagnosis, should be provided at some point after the initial assessment is completed. Asking for additional information—such as laboratory tests, imaging, and audiograms—will also be necessary in many cases. Pathology is typically incorporated into several cases during the testing day. Imaging, pathological slides, and test results will give you an opportunity to refine your differential diagnosis as needed.

As you discuss the case with your examiner, the examiner may focus, narrow, expedite, or redirect your questioning if necessary. When medical treatment or surgery is indicated, you should be able to recite the various options in management, the risks and benefits of each, and the postoperative care protocols. You may need to recognize and manage complications in the postoperative setting.

Finally, while demonstrating fund of knowledge is important, arguably more critical is (1) demonstrating safe clinical care and (2) being organized. For example, if someone has hearing loss, you would want to trial hearing aids prior to going to the operating room for cochlear implantation. You also want to demonstrate your critical thinking skills. Thus, it is important to "think aloud" to demonstrate to the examiner that you are considering different options in an organized fashion.

Pearls for Success on Oral Exams

- Stay organized. You are provided a pencil and paper and should take notes.
- Each case has a different aim. Some cases have a complex and involved differential diagnosis. In others, the purpose of the clinical vignette is to discuss management strategies for a diagnosis. Even if you miss a diagnosis or are incorrect in treatment, you may still be able to obtain points by logically moving through the workup of a patient just as you would in the clinical setting.
- Remember that the examiner cannot read your mind. It is important to verbally state all history questions you would ask, studies you would obtain, diagnoses you would consider, and treatment options you would offer. Demonstrate an organized and linear thought process.
- Stay calm throughout the test. It is difficult for the examiner to assess your fund of knowledge if you become flustered.
- This review textbook discusses the key points that can be helpful in your workup and management of otolaryngology patients not only in the board exam setting but also when evaluating patients in the clinical setting. For example, if a patient presents with hoarseness, you should be able to ask specific questions in your history to narrow the differential diagnosis. When performing parotid surgery, you should know which key landmarks can help in the identification of the facial nerve. If you believe that a rhinoplasty patient could benefit from an increase in tip projection, you should be able to mention the three ways you could accomplish that.
- When providing a differential diagnosis use a mnemonic to stay organized. It can be an effective way to systematically go through a differential diagnosis. Any of the examples below can be helpful. Note, however, that you may have limited time during the oral exam and it may not always be appropriate to go through a complete differential if the clinical vignette does not call for it.
  - KITTENS (K—congenital; I—infectious, iatrogenic; TT—toxins, trauma; E—endocrine; N—neoplastic; S—systemic)
  - VITAMIN-C (V—vascular; I—infectious, inflammatory; T—toxins, trauma; A—autoimmune; M—metabolic; I—iatrogenic; N—neoplastic; C—congenital)
  - VINDICATE (V—vascular; I—infectious, inflammatory; N—neoplastic; D—drugs; I—iatrogenic; C—congenital; A—autoimmune; T—trauma, toxins; E—endocrine)
- For pathology questions, describe the finding you see on the image, even if you are unable to provide the correct diagnosis. Partial credit may be obtained for an accurate description of the pathological specimen.
- Ask for one test or imaging study at a time. If you are correct in asking for the study, you will be presented the results and will need to interpret them accurately in an organized fashion that demonstrates to your examiner your knowledge and abilities.
- Review computed tomography (CT) scans and magnetic resonance imaging (MRI) by stating (1) the type of imaging, (2) the view, (3) the type of sequences if applicable, and (4) roughly where the slice is within the series. For example, you could state, "this is an axial CT of the neck, soft-tissue windows, with contrast, at the level of the larynx," or "this is an MRI of the temporal bone, coronal cuts, T1 imaging with contrast, at the level of the internal auditory canal." You may be provided with and asked to interpret a stack of images from the same scan, and not just one isolated image. Be systematic and help yourself by stating the normal anatomy, which both demonstrates to your examiner your familiarity with the anatomy and helps build a mental image in your brain of where you are. Recognition and familiarity with *normal* will help you identify *abnormal*. Partial credit can be given for an accurate radiological description of the abnormal findings whether the correct diagnosis is obtained or not.
- Take advantage of any opportunity to take mock examinations. Do not miss formal mock exams that may be provided by your residency programs during your chief year and, if doing a fellowship, consider practicing with your co-fellows in other subspecialties. If you take the time to prepare mock exam case files with radiology and pathology images from your own files, publications, or Google searches, and practice going through the formal routine of taking an oral board exam, the actual exam will seem much more familiar and easier.
- Bringing other viewpoints, standards of care, and opinions is another benefit of talking to and studying with co-fellows or residents of other programs. This is especially true for graduates of smaller residency programs who may have been exposed to only a limited number of subspecialty-trained attending physicians. Discussing the "board answers," that is, what you should say in the board exam, rather than your local surgeon's independent viewpoint, would serve you well. For instance, your otology-attending physician may have gone forward with a stapedectomy in the setting of a persistent stapedial artery or overhanging facial nerve, but the "board answer" may be to abort. It would be appropriate to bring up the fact that you may have witnessed a successful completion of this case by a more experienced surgeon, but you would abort the case and refer it to a more seasoned otologist.
- Your examiner is not trying to trick you. Usually, it is just the opposite. Most examiners are trying to get you through the questions appropriately. If they indicate that there are no further answers in a given section and that you should move on to the next part of the vignette, you should do so.

CLINICAL ROUNDS

Cummings Review of Otolaryngology is a powerful tool for rapid learning and review for medical students and residents both in the clinical setting and when studying for oral and written in-service and board exams. This book provides a logical, systematic approach that can be applied to any oral exam format; to frequently asked questions by chief residents, fellows, and attending physicians; and to address any clinical situation: *what questions should you ask in the history, what findings are you looking for on physical exam, what is the differential diagnosis, what are the critical findings on radiology and pathology studies, what are the treatment options, what is your best option, what are ways to perform this, and what is your postoperative management?* Once these lists are reviewed and memorized, the reader will have an armamentarium of knowledge that can be instinctively accessed and effectively used in any clinical or examination scenario.

You will often need to go to the reference books and other texts to get more detail for many of the key buzzwords that are in this review book. Repetition is key: the more times you review these concepts, the more likely you are to remember them. We wish you success on your written and oral examinations and congratulate you in your choice of a career in Otolaryngology—Head and Neck Surgery.

2 Otology and Neurotology

Brian S. Chen, Theodore R. McRackan, James Lin, Sachin Gupta, James G. Naples, and Jeffrey P. Harris

AUDITORY ANATOMY AND PHYSIOLOGY

1. External Ear
   a. Outer ear resonance frequency 3000 to 5000 Hz
      i. Concha resonant frequency 5000 Hz
      ii. Ear canal resonance frequency 2500 Hz
   b. Provides cues to brain for localization via
      i. Interaural time difference
      ii. Interaural intensity difference
2. Eardrum/Ossicular Chain (Fig. 2.1)
   a. Eardrum: Footplate ratio 20:1 (26 dB advantage)
   b. Ossicular chain lever ratio 1.3:1 (2.3 dB advantage)
   c. *Theoretical* gain of eardrum/ossicular chain: 28 dB
   d. *Actual* gain or eardrum/ossicular chain: 20 dB
3. Resonance frequency of ossicular chain 2000 Hz (Carhart's notch, otosclerosis)
4. Cochlea (Fig. 2.2)
   a. Pressure wave: Oval window → scala vestibuli (perilymph filled) → helicotrema → scala tympani (perilymph filled) → round window
   b. Basilar membrane (Fig. 2.3) is
      i. Tonotopic: High frequencies at basal region (stiffer)
      ii. Lower frequencies at apical region (more flexible)
      iii. Stiffness difference allows it to be a frequency filter and is basis for traveling wave
   c. Outer hair cells (see Fig. 2.3) sensory cells containing muscle proteins
      i. Actively contract cycle-by-cycle amplifying traveling wave for low/moderate input levels → basis for otoacoustic emission
   d. Inner hair cells (see Fig. 2.3) transduce vibrations into neural impulse
      i. Vibratory wave → deflection of hair cell stereocilia → potassium influx → depolarization (resting potential in endolymph +60 to 100 mV relative to perilymph) → action potential at first-level neurons of spiral ganglion (Fig. 2.4)
   e. Potassium recirculated back through supporting cells and back into the perilymph via the stria vascularis
5. Central Auditory Pathways (Fig. 2.5)
   a. Auditory nerve (CN VIII, auditory portion of CN VIII)
   b. Cochlear nuclei
      i. Dorsal cochlear nucleus
      ii. Anterior ventral cochlear nucleus
      iii. Posterior ventral cochlear nucleus (the majority of auditory fibers cross the midline)
   c. Superior olivary complex
   d. Lateral lemniscus
   e. Inferior colliculus
   f. Medial geniculate body
   g. Auditory cortex
   h. This pathway is the physiological basis of the auditory brainstem response (ABR), middle latency response (MLR) and auditory late response (ALR)
6. Stapedius Reflex
   a. Reflex pathway: Auditory nerve → cochlear nucleus → interneurons → bilateral facial motor nuclei → facial nerve → bilateral stapedius tendons
   b. Absent with conductive hearing loss (CHL), severe/profound sensorineural hearing loss (SNHL), CN VIII disorders and auditory neuropathy
   c. Measures: Reflex threshold (70–95 dB HL [decibel hearing level]) and reflex decay (50% amplitude reduction in 10 seconds)

VESTIBULAR ANATOMY AND PHYSIOLOGY

1. Coplanar Semicircular Canals (Paired Angular Accelerometers) (Fig. 2.6)
   a. Left and right horizontal (lateral) canals
   b. Left anterior (superior), right posterior (inferior)
   c. Right anterior (superior), left posterior (inferior)
   d. Resting firing rate from each ampulla
      i. Excitatory with angular acceleration in the direction of the leading canal, and inhibitory in the coplanar, lagging canal; therefore,
         (1) Ampullopetal flow of the perilymph in the lateral canals is excitatory
         (2) Ampullofugal flow of the perilymph in the superior and posterior canals is excitatory (see Ewald's Laws)
   e. Otolithic organs (linear accelerometers)
   f. Saccule: Vertical acceleration
   g. Utricle: Horizontal acceleration, head tilt
   h. Innervation (CN VIII, vestibular portion)
      i. Superior vestibular nerve
         (1) Utricle
         (2) Superior semicircular canal
         (3) Lateral semicircular canal
      ii. Inferior vestibular nerve
         (1) Saccule
         (2) Posterior semicircular canal

Eustachian Tube

1. Medial two-thirds is cartilaginous; lateral one-third is bony
2. Tensor veli palatini is the primary dilator
3. Normal development infancy to adulthood leads to increased slope of the tube as well as increased length, diameter, and efficiency of the opening
4. *Ostmann fat pad*: Metabolically sensitive adipose in the lateral wall of the Eustachian tube medially (rapid weight loss can cause atrophy of the fat pad, which results in patulous Eustachian tube syndrome)

AUDIOLOGIC TESTING

Behavioral Measures of the Auditory System
   a. Audiogram (Fig. 2.7): Sensitivity to pure tones (dB HL) plotted as a function of frequency (Hz).
   b. 125–8000 Hz typical frequency range for human speech, typical audiogram range
   c. 9000–20,000 Hz used to monitor effects of ototoxicity and tinnitus assessments

d. Symbols indicate side of head where transducer is placed
    i. O = right-ear air conduction
    ii. X = left-ear air conduction
    iii. Δ = right-ear air masked

    iv. □ = left-ear air masked
    v. < = right unmasked bone
    vi. > = left unmasked bone
    vii. [= right masked bone
    viii.] = left masked bone

Audiogram Terminology

1. *Air-bone gap*: Difference between air- and bone-conducted threshold, measure of loss of air-conducted signal compared with bone-conducted signal
2. *Crossover* (air or bone sound presented to one ear is heard by opposite ear)

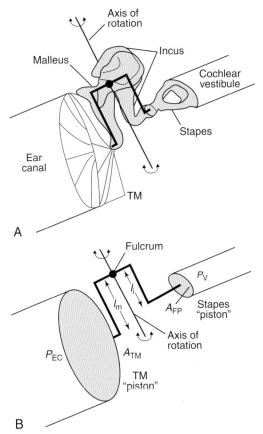

Fig. 2.1 Schematic of the middle ear system. (A) Motion of the ossicular chain along its axis of rotation is illustrated. **(B)** Area of the TM (A_{TM}) divided by area of the footplate (A_{FP}) represents the *area ratio* (A_{TM}/A_{FP}). The length of the manubrium (l_m) divided by the length of the incus long process (l_i) is the *lever ratio* (l_m/l_i). P_{EC}, External canal sound pressure; P_V, sound pressure of the vestibule. (From Merchant SN, Rosowski JJ. Auditory physiology. In: Glasscock ME, Gulya AJ, eds. *Glasscock-Shambaugh Surgery of the Ear.* 5th ed. Hamilton, ON: Decker; 2003:64, Fig. 129.2.)

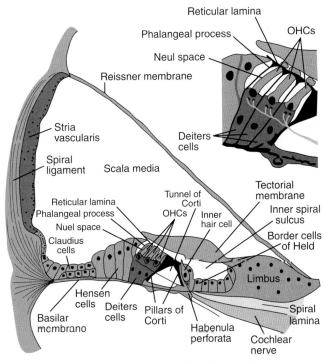

Fig. 2.3 Cross-section of the organ of Corti showing the major cellular structures. *OHC,* Outer hair cell. (From Flint PW, Haughey BH, Lund VJ, et al. *Cummings Otolaryngology—Head and Neck Surgery.* 6th ed. Philadelphia, PA: Saunders; 2015, Fig. 128.2.)

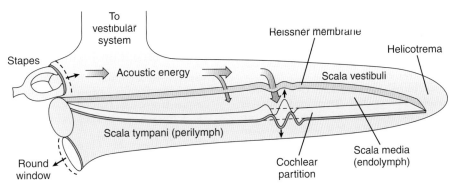

Fig. 2.2 Schematic showing sound propagation in the cochlea. As sound energy travels through the external and middle ears, it causes the stapes footplate to vibrate. The vibration of this footplate results in a compressional wave on the inner ear fluid. Because the pressure in the scala vestibuli is higher than that in the scala tympani, this sets up a pressure gradient that causes the cochlear partition to vibrate as a traveling wave. Because the basilar membrane varies in its stiffness and mass along its length, it is able to act as a series of filters that respond to specific sound frequencies at specific locations along its length. (From Geisler CD. *From Sound to Synapse: Physiology of the Mammalian Ear.* New York, NY: Oxford University Press; 1998:51 and Flint PW, Haughey BH, Lund VJ, et al. *Cummings Otolaryngology—Head and Neck Surgery.* 6th ed. Philadelphia, PA: Saunders; 2015, Fig. 129.6.)

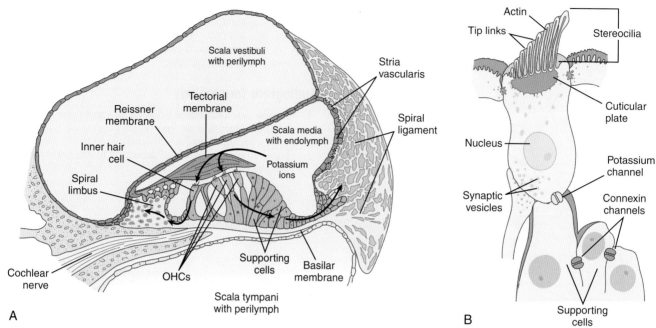

Fig. 2.4 Mechanoelectrical transduction of the auditory signal depends on the recycling of potassium ions in the organ of Corti. (**A**) Schematic cross-sectional view of the human cochlea. The scala media (cochlear duct) is filled with endolymph; the scala vestibuli and tympani are filled with perilymph. The endolymph of the scala media bathes the organ of Corti, located between the basilar and tectorial membranes and containing the inner and outer hair cells. A relatively high concentration of potassium in the endolymph of the scala media relative to the hair cell creates a cation gradient maintained by the activity of the epithelial supporting cells, spiral ligament, and stria vascularis. (**B**) Cells contain stereocilia along the apical surface and are connected by tip links. The potassium gradient is essential to enable depolarization of the hair cell following influx of potassium ions in response to mechanical vibration of the basilar membrane, deflection of stereocilia, displacement of tip links, and opening of gated potassium channels. Depolarization results in calcium influx through channels along the basolateral membrane of the hair cell, which causes degranulation of neurotransmitter vesicles into the synaptic terminal and propagates an action potential along the auditory nerve. Gap junction proteins between the hair cells (potassium channel, *yellow*) and epithelial supporting cells (connexin channels, *red*) allow for the flow of potassium ions back to the stria vascularis, where they are pumped back into the endolymph. *OHC,* Outer hair cell. (From Willems PJ. Genetic causes of hearing loss. *N Engl J Med.* 2000;342(15):1101–1109 and Flint PW, Haughey BH, Lund VJ, et al. *Cummings Otolaryngology—Head and Neck Surgery.* 6th ed. Philadelphia, PA: Saunders; 2015, Fig. 129.4.)

3. *Interaural attenuation* (amount of dB loss with crossover, transducer and frequency dependent)
4. Bone: 0–10 dB
5. Air (headphones on pinna [TDH]): 40 to 65 dB
6. Air (foam insert phones in ear canal): 55 to 100 dB
7. Air (circumaural headphones)
8. Crossover is the basis for masking
9. Crossover occurs for all sounds (pure tones, speech, masking noise, etc.)
   a. Masking: Noise used to "cover up" crossed-over signal, allows isolation of test ear
   b. Overmasking: When the masker level crosses over to the test ear, which masks (raises threshold) in the test ear, precludes accurate threshold measure
   c. Masking dilemma: Initial masking level causing overmasking; threshold cannot be determined. Masker presented to contralateral ear crosses over to test ear, causing masking of test ear. Result is poorer apparent threshold in test ear.
      i. Commonly encountered with bilateral CHL exceeding 40 dB HL
      ii. Insert earphones less likely to encounter dilemma due to larger interaural attenuation than TDH headphones (standard on-the-ear audiometer headsets)
10. *Pure tone average* (PTA): Average of 500, 1000, 2000 Hz thresholds
11. *Most comfortable level* (MCL): Preferred listening level based on comfort
12. *Uncomfortable loudness level* (UCL): Maximum loudness tolerable
13. *Dynamic range* (DR): Difference between threshold of hearing and UCL
14. *Signal-to-noise ratio* (SNR): dB difference of a sound stimulus and background noise
15. *Recruitment*: Abnormal growth of loudness, occurs with cochlear hair cell loss
16. *Adaptation*: Abnormally long neural recovery time, occurs with retrocochlear lesions

Speech Perception Testing

1. Speech Recognition Threshold (SRT): Threshold for recognizing familiar two-part words (spondees; two-syllable equal-stress; e.g., hotdog, downtown, shoelace, goldfish)
   a. Cross-check for PTA, within ±10 dB of 500, 1000, 2000 Hz
2. Speech Awareness Threshold/Speech Detection Threshold (SAT/SDT): Lowest dB HL to detect speech
   a. Cross-check for best (lowest) threshold at 125 to 8000 Hz
3. Word Recognition Score (WRS): % of 25 one-syllable words repeated correctly presented in quiet
   a. Phonetically balanced (PB) lists of words (consonant-vowel-consonant); common recordings: NU-6, W-22
   b. Excellent (90%–100%), Good (80%–88%), Fair (60%–76%); Poor (50%–59%); Very poor (<50%)
   c. Poorer scores related to greater hearing loss

d. One or more levels chosen at or above MCL to estimate best (max) score
e. PI-PB function: % correct as a function of presentation level from threshold to max tolerable (UCL)
f. Rollover: Measure for WRS decrement using very high presentation levels
   i. % using maximum dB HL tolerable (UCL-5), compare to standard level %. PBmax-PBmin

ii. Retrocochlear lesions "rollover" by 35%, cochlear/conductive rollover by <35%
4. Speech in noise: Statistically meaningful real-life ability to recognize speech in noise (static, adaptive, broadband noise, multitalker-babble noise)
   a. Word-in-noise test (WINT), Speech-in-noise (SPIN), Speech recognition in noise test (SPRINT; used by the US Army for active duty personnel)
   b. Sentence-in-noise tests: QuickSIN, AzBio, Bamford-Kowal-Bench (BKB-SIN), Hearing-in-noise test (HINT)

Objective Measures of the Auditory Pathway

1. Tympanometry (acoustic admittance [mmhos] from –400 to +200 daPa pressure sweep using 226 Hz probe tone)
   a. Ear canal volume (mL): Adult (0.6–2.0), children (0.3–0.9)

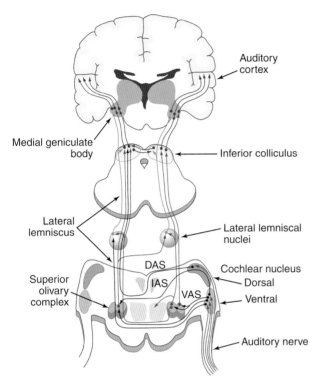

Fig. 2.5 Illustration of the major central ascending auditory pathways for sound entering via the right cochlea. Commissural pathways and descending feedback projections from higher centers are not depicted. *DAS,* Dorsal acoustic stria; *IAS,* intermediate acoustic stria; *VAS,* ventral acoustic stria. (From Flint PW, Haughey BH, Lund VJ, et al. *Cummings Otolaryngology—Head and Neck Surgery.* 6th ed. Philadelphia, PA: Saunders; 2015, Fig. 128.6.)

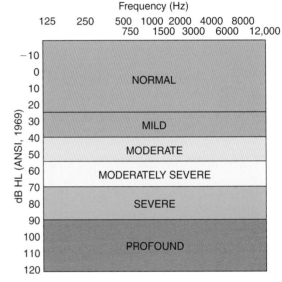

Fig. 2.7 Audiogram showing a range of hearing loss. *ANSI,* American National Standards Institute; *dB HL,* decibel hearing level. (From Flint PW, Haughey BH, Lund VJ, et al. *Cummings Otolaryngology—Head and Neck Surgery.* 6th ed. Philadelphia, PA: Saunders; 2015, Fig. 133.1.)

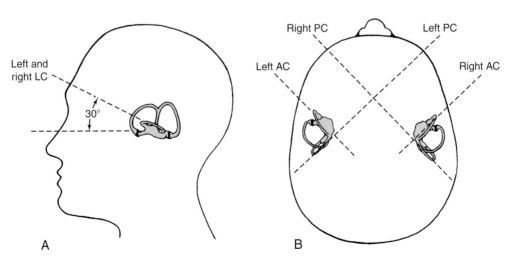

Fig. 2.6 Orientation of semicircular canals. (**A**) The horizontal canal is tilted 30 degrees upward from a horizontal plane at its anterior end. (**B**) Vertical canals are oriented at roughly 45 degrees from the midsagittal plane. *AC,* Anterior canal; *LC,* lateral canal; *PC,* posterior canal. (Modified from Barber HO, Stockwell CW. *Manual of Electronystagmography.* St. Louis, MO: Mosby-Year Book; 1976 and Flint PW, Haughey BH, Lund VJ, et al. *Cummings Otolaryngology—Head and Neck Surgery.* 6th ed. Philadelphia, PA: Saunders; 2015, Fig. 130.2.)

b. Static compliance (mmhos): Adult (0.3–170), children (0.25–1.05)

c. Peak pressure (daPa): Adults and children (–100 to +50)

d. Tympanogram types:

  i. Type A (normal)

  ii. Type As (reduced compliance)

    (1) Tympanosclerosis

    (2) Otosclerosis

  iii. Type Ad (excessive compliance)

    (1) Disarticulation of ossicles (wide tympanogram)

    (2) Tympanic membrane (TM) dimere or monomere (narrow tympanogram)

  iv. Type B (no compliance/flat)

    (1) Middle ear effusion (normal canal volume)

    (2) Perforation (large canal volume)

  v. Type C (negative peak pressure, normal compliance)

    (1) Eustachian tube dysfunction

    (2) Excessive sniffling

e. Stapedial reflex: Bilateral reflex named for stimulated ear

  i. Ipsilateral (e.g., left ipsilateral: stimulus left/probe left)

  ii. Contralateral (e.g., right contralateral: stimulus right/probe left)

  iii. Normal ≤95 dB HL, elevated 100-110 dBHL, absent >110 dB HL

  iv. Acoustic reflex decay: Positive for retrocochlear > 50% amplitude decay in 10 seconds

  v. Absent for conductive and severe/profound sensorineural loss, auditory neuropathy

2. Wideband tympanometry (acoustic admittance using sweep of pressure –400 to +200 daPa and frequency (250–8000 Hz)

3. Multifrequency tympanometry (MFT) use of more than one probe frequency (e.g., 660, 1000, 2000 Hz) measures:

  a. Resonant frequency

  b. Conductance (G, mmho); resistance, real component of impedance

  c. Susceptance (B, mmho); reactance, imaginary component of impedance

4. Otoacoustic emissions (OAEs): Natural by-product of normal outer hair cell (OHC) function

  a. Assesses OHC function on a frequency-specific basis

    i. Type of OAE determined by stimulus

    ii. All sounds create emissions, different methods needed to separate stimulus from emission

    iii. Good measure of OHC/cochlear function by frequency, poor measure to estimate threshold

  b. Pure tone stimuli used for distortion products (DPOAE)

    i. Stimulus is a two-tone pair (f1 and f2) separated by multiple of 1.22 Hz

    ii. Traveling wave overlap creates distortions, best human distortion at 2f1-f2

    iii. DPgram: 2f1-f2 amplitude plotted across frequency ~1000–8000 Hz

  c. Broadband click stimuli used for transiently evoked emissions (TEOAE)

    i. Emission energy recorded after click stimulus, averaged over 260 clicks to improve OAE detection from physiological noise in ear canal

    ii. TEOAE amplitude shown for 5 to 8 frequency bands.

  d. Spontaneous OAE

    i. Emissions present in the absence of stimulus

    ii. Not clinically useful

5. Electrocochleography (ECoG) measured at ~1.2 to 2.5 msec, amplitude ratio of cochlear summating potential (SP) and eighth nerve action potential (SP/AP ratio); AP = wave I auditory brainstem response (ABR); ratio >0.35 is abnormal (hydrops or inner ear third window via fistula or semicircular canal dehiscence)

6. Auditory Brainstem Response (ABR), a.k.a. Brainstem Auditory Evoked Response (BAER)- Five waves occurring at approximately 1.5 to 6 msec associated with:

  a. Distal eighth nerve (I)

  b. Proximal eighth nerve (II)

  c. Cochlear nuclei (III)

  d. Superior olivary complex (IV)

  e. Lateral lemniscus (V)

    i. Threshold assessment

     (1) Frequency-specific tone bursts (500, 1000, 2000, 4000 Hz)

     (2) Within 10 to 20 dB of behavioral thresholds

    ii. Eighth nerve assessment (90 dB nHL 100-μsec click stimulus)

     (1) No wave V

     (2) Prolongation I–III

     (3) Prolongation I–V

     (4) Wave V interaural difference should be <0.2 msec

     (5) <1 cm tumor only 60% sensitive

     (6) Stacked ABR increases sensitivity

    iii. Auditory neuropathy/dyssynchrony

     (1) Abnormal or absent ABR

     (2) Present OAEs

7. Auditory MLR (10–80 msec)

  a. Derived from medial geniculate body, inferior colliculus, primary auditory cortex

  b. Used for auditory threshold detection, better amplitude while awake

  c. Negative peak (Na) 12 to 18 msec, positive peak (Pa) 25 to 30 msec, positive peak (Pb) 50 msec

8. Auditory Late Evoked Response (ALR; 60–250 msec)

9. P300: Late-late auditory evoked response at 300 m sec

  a. Generated at hippocampus

  b. Two stimuli (rare and frequent) presented in oddball paradigm, response dependent on internal thought process attention to rarely occurring stimulus

10. Vestibular Evoked Myogenic Potential (VEMP):

  a. Descending vestibular cervical pathway (cVEMP): Air/bone conducted energy → saccule → inferior vestibular nerve → vestibular nuclei → ipsilateral spinal accessory nucleus → relaxation of ipsilateral sternocleidomastoid (SCM)

  b. Ascending vestibular ocular pathway (oVEMP): Air/bone conducted energy → utricle → superior vestibular nerve → vestibular nuclei → contraction of contralateral inferior oblique muscle

Newborn Hearing Screening: Important Points

1. *1-3-6 Rule*: **Screen** all by 1 month, **identify** by 3 months, **intervene** by 6 months

2. 2 to 3 per 1000 have hearing loss at birth, old "High-Risk Register" has high miss rate

3. Screen all well babies by 1 month with OAE or ABR

4. *Neonatal intensive care unit (NICU) babies must have ABR* to catch higher incidence of auditory neuropathy

Treatments/Aids for Hearing Loss

- Hearing aids (HAs)
- Assistive listening devices (ALDs)
- Osseointegrated hearing system (OIHS)
- Active middle ear implants (AMEIs)
- Cochlear implants (CIs)
- Auditory brainstem implants (ABIs)

1. Hearing Aid Amplification

  a. Refer for hearing aids when patient reports difficulty hearing/understanding speech

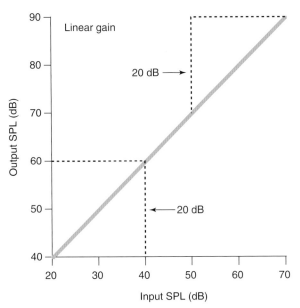

Fig. 2.8 Schematic representation of the components of a hearing aid. (From Flint PW, Haughey BH, Lund VJ, et al. *Cummings Otolaryngology—Head and Neck Surgery*. 6th ed. Philadelphia, PA: Saunders; 2015, Fig. 162.3.)

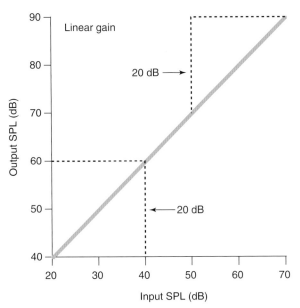

Fig. 2.9 The relationship of sound input to output in a linear hearing aid circuit. Gain remains at a constant 20 dB regardless of input level. (From Flint PW, Haughey BH, Lund VJ, et al. *Cummings Otolaryngology—Head and Neck Surgery*. 6th ed. Philadelphia, PA: Saunders; 2015, Fig. 162.4.)

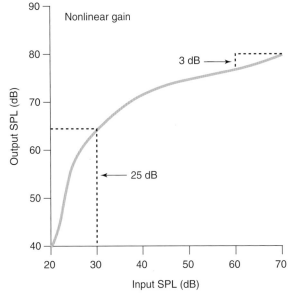

Fig. 2.10 The relationship of sound input to output in a nonlinear hearing aid circuit. The amount of gain changes as a function of input level. (From Flint PW, Haughey BH, Lund VJ, et al. *Cummings Otolaryngology—Head and Neck Surgery*. 6th ed. Philadelphia, PA: Saunders; 2015, Fig. 162.5.)

b. Types
  i. BTE: Behind the ear (with tubing and earmold)
  ii. RIC: Receiver in the ear (behind the ear with electrical wire to receiver in ear canal)
  iii. Natural sound quality/no tubing or earmold resonances
  iv. ITE: In the ear (molded shell fills concha)
  v. ITC: In the canal (molded shell fills canal and canal aperture)
  vi. CIC: Completely in the canal (molded shell fills canal)
  vii. CROS/BiCROS: Unaidable ear wears microphone, radio transmitted to better ear wearing a hearing aid. Better ear receives input from both sides. Overcomes head shadow effect.
c. Components (Fig. 2.8)
  i. The basic components of hearing aids are a microphone, transducer, amplifier, and a receiver (speaker). All hearing aids are now digital.
  ii. *Transducers* (convert one form of energy into electrical energy)
  iii. Microphone (acoustic to electrical)
  iv. Receiver/speaker (electrical to acoustic)
  v. Telecoil (t-coil, electromagnetic energy to electrical)
  vi. Wireless transducer (e.g., frequency modulation, radio, or Bluetooth)

d. Terminology/Concepts
  i. *Gain*: The amount of energy added to the input signal
  ii. *Linear* gain (Fig. 2.9)
  iii. *Compression*, nonlinear gain (Fig. 2.10), more gain for low-level signals, less gain for high-level signals
  iv. *Dynamic range*: An individual's threshold of sound perception to discomfort
    (1) Compression allows a hearing aid to amplify into a smaller dynamic range (Fig. 2.11)
  v. *Feedback*: When amplified signal in ear canal reaches microphone; controlled by closing ear canal, reducing high-frequency gain, and software-controlled feedback suppression
    (1) BTE/RIC: Better microphone/receiver separation than ITE, ITC, and CIC
    (2) *Venting* increases likelihood of feedback
  vi. *Occlusion*
    (1) Reduction of natural acoustic energy by the aid plugging the ear
    (2) Own voice resonance of lower frequencies is worsened
    (3) Helped by venting
  vii. *Maximum power output* (MPO): Highest hearing aid output across frequency
  viii. *Frequency Response*: Graphical representation of hearing aid output across frequency

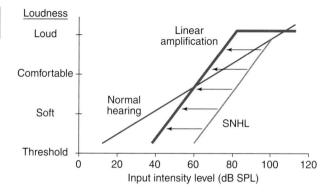

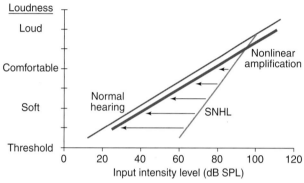

Fig. 2.11 Representation of the difference between linear and nonlinear amplification in an ear with sensorineural hearing loss and nonlinear loudness growth. (From Stach B. *Clinical Audiology: An Introduction.* San Diego, CA: Singular Publishing; 1998:486 and Flint PW, Haughey BH, Lund VJ, et al. *Cummings Otolaryngology—Head and Neck Surgery.* 6th ed. Philadelphia, PA: Saunders; 2015, Fig. 162.6.)

      ix. *Speechmapping*: Verification tool for hearing aid fitting; microphone near TM measures hearing aid output using a live speech signal, displays frequency response of hearing aid in relation to scientific-driven target values for individual audiogram; verifies audibility of soft to loud speech across frequency

2. Assistive Listening Devices (ALDs): Devices to augment hearing aids—wireless microphone, TV streamer, vibrating alarm clocks, flashing lights, and so on
3. Osseointegrated Hearing System (OIHS)
   a. Conductive/mixed losses >30 dB ABG, single-sided deafness
   b. External processor delivers signals to osseointegrated implant
   c. Direct bone drive
      i. Percutaneous vibration: External processor → abutment → bone-anchored passive implant
        (1) Oticon Ponto, Cochlear Baha
      ii. Transcutaneous induction: External processor → induction link → active implant
        (1) MedEl Bonebridge, Cochlear Osia
   d. Over skin drive
      i. Transcutaneous vibration to bone (no implant)
        (1) MedEl ADHEAR: Processor attached postauricularly with strong sticker
        (2) Cochlear Baha Soundarc: Pressure-attached processor with headband
      ii. Transcutaneous vibration to passive implant (retention with magnet)
        (1) Cochlear Baha Attract
        (2) Medtronic Sophono

4. Active Middle Ear Implant (AMEI) devices, approved by the US Food and Drug Administration (FDA)
   a. Fully implanted Envoy Esteem (piezoelectric transducers)
   b. Acoustic sound → TM → malleus → incus head → sensor converts vibrations to electrical → underscalp processor amplifies, filters, converts to mechanical → driver vibrates stapes head. Disarticulation at lenticular process prevents feedback.
   c. Partially implanted MedEl Vibrant Soundbridge (electro-magnetic transducer)
   d. External processor picks up acoustic sound → transmitter coil → internal receiver processes signal → wire to floating mass transducer delivers amplified vibrations directly to incus
   e. Conductive, mixed and SNHLs
5. Cochlear Implants
   a. External speech processor → transmitting coil → internal receiver stimulator → multichannel array in scala vestibuli (typical)
   b. FDA-approved devices: Advanced Bionics, Cochlear Americas, MedEl
   c. Audiologic indications vary: Manufacturers' FDA labeling, and insurance-specific criteria based on best aided sentence perception scores (best of left, right, and binaural aided conditions)
   d. Refer for audiologic CI evaluation when:
      i. Adult—60/60 rule: WRS <60% or PTA >60 dB HL, and little benefit from hearing aids
      ii. Pediatric—moderately severe to profound SNHL and failure to meet auditory developmental milestones
   e. Adult candidacy
      i. Standard: ≤60% on open-set recorded sentences in the best aided condition for most private insurance, ≤ 40% for Medicare and Medicaid
      ii. Hybrid (low-frequency acoustic hearing aid, high-frequency electric hearing)
        (1) Ear to be implanted ≤60% aided monosyllabic words
        (2) Contralateral ear ≤80% (for MedEl) or ≤60% (for Cochlear)
        (3) Only for adults ≤18 years
      iii. Single-sided deafness and asymmetric SNHL
        (1) Ear to be implanted profound SNHL, <5% aided monosyllabic words, ≤10 years' duration deafness, functional nerve, experience with CROS/OIHS.
        (2) Contralateral ear can have anywhere from normal hearing sensitivity to moderately severe SNHL
        (3) Only for ≥5 years or older
   f. Pediatric candidacy
      i. Bilateral profound SNHL (severe to profound if ages 2–17)
      ii. Lack of progress despite proper amplification
      iii. ≤30% on open-set speech recognition in the best aided condition
   g. Additional considerations:
      i. Surgical/medical considerations
      ii. Realistic goals, expectations, and motivation
      iii. Duration of hearing loss, duration of amplification use
      iv. Vestibular function: Caloric testing may clarify side to implant
      v. Tinnitus severity: Electrical stimulation may alleviate tinnitus perception
      vi. Vision, cognitive status, and family/caretaker support system
6. Auditory Brainstem Implant (ABI)
   a. FDA-approved device: Cochlear Americas

b. Uses: NF2, cochlear dysplasia/aplasia, cochlear nerve aplasia
c. External speech processor> → transmitter coil → internal receiver-stimulator → multichannel implant array on cochlear nucleus
d. Provides hearing sensations/awareness of sound/poor speech perception results

Other Auditory Disorders

1. Tinnitus (subjective/objective causes)
   a. Assessment: Tinnitus pitch and loudness matching, residual inhibition
2. Decreased Sound Tolerance
   a. Hyperacusis: Decreased tolerance of everyday sounds
3. Misophonia: Dislike of certain sound(s) (e.g., chewing, pen tapping)
4. Auditory processing disorder
   a. Generalized or specific neurological disorder causing functional deficits, often exacerbated in noisy environments; leads to language, memory, behavioral, auditory and learning deficits; unique to auditory system or cross modality
   b. Disruption in the efficiency and effectiveness of the ascending auditory pathway to decode and use auditory stimuli for recognizing patterns, discriminating between sounds, localizing sound sources, deciphering degraded signals, and hearing in noise.
   c. Common causes/influencing disorders: Disease, damage, degeneration, delayed maturation, for example, delayed auditory development, auditory deprivation (chronic middle ear effusion), head/blast injury, stroke, extreme fever, Alzheimer disease, multiple sclerosis

IMAGING OF THE SKULL BASE AND TEMPORAL BONE

1. Computed Tomography: The Study of Choice for Bony Anatomy
   a. Atresia
   b. Canal cholesteatoma
   c. Exostoses
   d. Osteoma
   e. Glomus tympanicum
   f. Aberrant carotid artery
   g. Cholesteatoma, uncomplicated
   h. Uncomplicated chronic otitis media (OM)
   i. Coalescent mastoiditis
   j. Glomus tympanicum versus jugulare if visible lesion is below the annulus (examine the jugular plate)
   k. Inner ear malformations
      i. Lateral canal dysplasia
      ii. Enlarged vestibular aqueduct
      iii. Cochlear dysplasia
   l. Labyrinthitis ossificans
   m. Superior canal dehiscence/inner ear third windows
2. Magnetic Resonance Imaging (MRI) is Better for Soft-Tissue Anatomy: The Study of Choice for Intracranial Pathology
   a. Cerebellopontine angle (CPA) lesions
      i. Vestibular schwannoma
      ii. Meningioma
      iii. Epidermoid
      iv. Eighth nerve deficiency (highly weighted T2 images: FIESTA or CISS sequences)
      v. Early cochlear fibrosis (i.e., early labyrinthitis ossificans before calcification)
3. When MRI and Computed Tomography (CT) Are Complementary
   a. Complicated OM/cholesteatoma
   b. Glomus jugulare tumors
   c. Endolymphatic sac tumors
   d. Cholesterol granuloma
   e. Facial nerve lesions (schwannoma/hemangioma)
   f. Cerebrospinal fluid (CSF) leak/meningoencephalocele
4. Imaging Characteristics of Petrous Apex Lesions (Table 2.1)
   a. The most common petrous apex lesions encountered are asymmetric pneumatization, retained secretions, cholesterol granuloma, mucoceles, and cholesteatomas. Please refer to Table 2.1 for the CT and MRI characteristics of ear entity.
5. Imaging Characteristics of Cerebellopontine Angle Lesions (Table 2.2)
   a. The most common CPA lesions are acoustic neuromas, meningiomas, arachnoid cysts, epidermoids and lipomas. Table 2.2 provides the characteristics for CT and MRI of each entity.

TABLE 2.1 Imaging Characteristics of Petrous Apex Lesions

Lesion	CT	T1	T2	T1+ Contrast	Notes
Asymmetric pneumatization	Bone marrow filled, no air cells	Hyperintense to intermediate intensity	Hyperintense	No enhancement	T1 signal disappears with fat suppression
Retained secretions	Air cell trabecular preservation, nonexpansile	Hypointense	Hyperintense	No enhancement	
Cholesterol granuloma	Air cell trabecular breakdown, expansile	Hyperintense	Hyperintense	No enhancement	T2 hyperintensity unchanged with fat saturation
Mucocele	Air cell trabecular breakdown, expansile	Hypointense	Hyperintense	Rim enhancement	
Cholesteatoma	Air cell trabecular breakdown, expansile	Hypointense	Hyperintense	May have rim enhancement if granulation tissue is present	DWI restriction (bright signal)

CT, Computed tomography; *DWI,* diffusion-weighted imaging.
From Flint PW, Haughey BH, Lund VJ, et al. *Cummings Otolaryngology—Head and Neck Surgery.* 6th ed. Philadelphia, PA: Saunders; 2015, Table 135.1.

TABLE 2.2 Imaging Characteristics of Cerebellopontine Angle Lesions

Lesion	T1	T2	T1+ Contrast	Notes
Vestibular schwannoma	Isointense to brain	Slightly hyperintense	Enhances	
Meningioma	Isointense to brain	Hypointense/hyper-intense	Enhances	T2 signal depends on calcium content
Arachnoid cyst	Hypointense	Hyperintense	No enhance-ment	Signal characteristics mirror those of CSF
Epidermoid	Hypointense	Hyperintense	No enhance-ment	T2 signal is slightly more dense than CSF is; DWI shows restriction (bright signal)
Lipoma	Hyperintense	Hyperintense	No enhance-ment	T1 signal disappears with fat suppression

CSF, Cerebrospinal fluid; *DWI,* diffusion-weighted imaging.

From Flint PW, Haughey BH, Lund VJ, et al. *Cummings Otolaryngology—Head and Neck Surgery.* 6th ed. Philadelphia, PA: Saunders; 2015, Table 135.2.

OTITIS EXTERNA

1. External Auditory Canal Defense
   a. Acidic pH 6.0 to 6.5
   b. Migratory nature of keratin debris (drum is centrifugally out)
2. Normal Flora
   a. *Staphylococcus auricularis*
   b. *Staphylococcus epidermidis*
   c. *Corynebacterium*
   d. *Streptococcus*
   e. *Enterococcus*
   f. Rarely *Pseudomonas*
   g. Rarely fungus
3. Acute Otitis Externa
   a. 90% bacterial
      i. *Pseudomonas*
      ii. *S. epidermidis*
      iii. *Staphylococcus aureus*
   b. 2% to 10% fungus/other
      i. *Aspergillus*
      ii. *Candida*
   c. Treatment: Always remove debris ("bacterial/fungal potato chips")
      i. Mild otitis externa (OE): Acidify ½ white vinegar/distilled water ± rubbing alcohol
      ii. Moderate OE (with more edema and purulence): Add antibiotic topical drop ± steroid; wick may be necessary if drum is not visible
      iii. Severe OE (extension to periauricular and auricular tissues): Antibiotic topical drop ± steroid; wick may be necessary; add systemic antibiotic with pseudomonal coverage (quinolone likely)
      iv. Fungal OE: Antibiotics may precipitate and steroids worsen; debride and antifungal (nystatin cream, ampho B powder/cream, and clotrimazole powder/cream)
   d. Complications
      i. Chondritis (*Pseudomonas*)
      ii. Perichondritis
      iii. Cellulitis
      iv. Malignant OE: *Pseudomonas* is the most common at 90% (*S. aureus* is second)
   e. Other acute OE causes
      i. Herpes zoster virus (HZV) (Ramsay Hunt)
      ii. Erysipelas (β-hemolytic strep)
      iii. Furuncle (*S. aureus*)
      iv. Bullous myringitis (viral vs. mycoplasma vs. *Streptococcus*)
         (1) Can have SNHL component 65%, resolution with infection resolution 60%
4. Malignant OE buzzwords
   a. Diabetic, immunosuppressed; facial paralysis
   b. *Pseudomonas* #1; fungal less likely
   c. Granulation at the bony-cartilaginous junction or tympanomastoid suture line
   d. Biopsy needed: Rule out malignancy
   e. Imaging
      i. CT scan: Bony erosion
      ii. MRI: Soft-tissue involvement (likely study of choice)
      iii. Technetium scan: Can diagnose bony activity and will show long-term change, even after resolution
      iv. Follow with gallium scan or indium scan with tagged white blood cells
   f. Labs
      i. Erythrocyte sedimentation rate: Follow disease
      ii. C-reactive protein
   g. Treatment: Intravenous antibiotics, surgery only for definitive biopsy; let infectious disease follow

CHRONIC OTITIS MEDIA, MASTOIDITIS, PETROUS APICITIS, AND COMPLICATIONS OF OTITIS MEDIA

1. Acquired Cholesteatoma Development Theories
   a. Invagination (retraction pocket)
   b. Basal cell hyperplasia (a defect in the basal membrane allows ingrowth of epithelial cells)
   c. Migration theory (through a perforation without contact inhibition into the middle ear)
   d. Squamous metaplasia of middle ear mucosa
2. Petrous Apex Drainage Tracts
3. Posterior Petrous Apex (30% of them pneumatized in temporal bones)
   a. Subarcuate
   b. Sinodural
4. Anterior Petrous Apex (10% pneumatized in temporal bones)
   a. Peritubal
   b. Retrofacial
   c. Infralabyrinthine
   d. Infracochlear
   e. Glenoid fossa (Ramandier and Lempert)
5. Gradenigo Syndrome (Triad): Due to petrous apicitis; rare
   a. Draining ear
   b. Retro-orbital pain
   c. Ipsilateral abducens palsy (due to compression of CN VI through Dorello's canal)
6. Complications of Acute and Chronic Otitis Media: Suggestion that complications are more common with pneumococcal vaccine and microbial resistance; complications are more common in pediatric population

7. Extracranial
   a. Acute mastoiditis
   b. Coalescent mastoiditis (erosion of mastoid air cell septations)
   c. Chronic mastoiditis
   d. Masked mastoiditis (partially treated with antibiotics but still painful)
   e. Subperiosteal abscess
      i. Postauricular (through the cribriform area, with direct extension through bone, and/or thrombophlebitic)
      ii. Bezold's (medial wall of mastoid tip medial to SCM muscle into the neck)
      iii. Luc's (zygomatic root)
   f. Petrous apicitis (Gradinego syndrome)
   g. Labyrinthine fistula
   h. Facial paralysis
   i. Suppurative labyrinthitis
   j. Encephalocele
   k. CSF leakage
8. Intracranial
   a. Meningitis
   b. Epidural abscess
   c. Subdural empyema
   d. Brain abscess
   e. Lateral/sigmoid sinus thrombosis
   f. Otitic hydrocephalus

TEMPORAL BONE TRAUMA

1. What You Should Care About
   a. Facial motion present/not present on initial evaluation
   b. Otorrhea—that is, CSF
   c. Potential carotid canal injury
   d. Dizziness
   e. SNHL (tuning fork can help)
2. Types of Fractures
   a. Old system
      i. Longitudinal fracture (80%)
         (1) CHL > SNHL
         (2) TM tears/EAC lacerations
         (3) Less facial weakness
      ii. Transverse (20%): More force and blow to occiput
         (1) SNHL is more likely
         (2) Facial weakness is more likely
      iii. Oblique: A mixture of fracture types
   b. New system
      i. Otic capsule sparing
         (1) CHL/mixed hearing loss (HL) > SNHL
         (2) Less facial weakness (6%–14%)
         (3) Less risk of CSF leakage
      ii. Otic capsule disrupting
         (1) SNHL likely
         (2) Facial weakness (30%–50%)
         (3) Increased risk of CSF leak (8× otic capsule sparing)

Facial Nerve Trauma (Fig. 2.12): Use ENoG to Guide Surgical Decision Making (see Electrophysiological Tests of Facial Nerve)

1. Sunderland Classification
   a. First degree: Neuropraxia (conduction block)
   b. Second degree: Axonotmesis (axons cut, but their endoneurium stays intact; no synkinesis)
   c. Third degree: Neurotmesis (endoneurium disrupted; synkinesis possible on regeneration)
   d. Fourth degree: Neurotmesis transects entire trunk (endoneurium and perineurium); epineurium intact

   e. Fifth degree: Neurotmesis (all three layers cut; endo-, peri-, and epineurium)
2. Cerebrospinal Fluid Otorhinorrhea (Fig. 2.13)
   a. Very rarely will traumatic CSF otorhinorrhea require surgery
   b. The use of antibiotics prophylaxis for meningitis is controversial
3. Hearing Loss From Temporal Bone Trauma
   a. Ossicular injuries
      i. Incudostapedial joint separation (82%)
      ii. Dislocation incus (57%)
      iii. Fracture stapes crura (30%)
      iv. Fixation ossicles in epitympanum (25%)
      v. Malleus fracture (11%)
   b. Otic capsule violating fractures can cause SNHL
4. Bottom-line evaluation of temporal bone fractures
   a. Any facial function on admission? If not documented, assume there was no facial function
   b. Otorrhea? Observe and put on bed rest and conservative measures to avoid drops; can become confused with "CSF otorrhea"
   c. Dizzy/HL? Take supportive measures and observe CHL for at least 6 months because subluxations can resolve; for SNHL, can try steroids if allowable given other injuries
   d. Get a CT scan of temporal bones: At the very least, ensure that there are no carotid canal injuries/sphenoid sinus fluid (the latter may be more indicative of carotid injury than carotid canal fracture); if either is noted, perform CT angiography (CTA) versus true angiogram

HEARING LOSS IN ADULTS

1. History
   a. Tinnitus
   b. Vertigo
   c. Disequilibrium
   d. Otalgia
   e. Otorrhea
   f. Headaches
   g. Ophthalmological symptoms
   h. Neurological complaints
   i. History of surgery
   j. Trauma
   k. Noise exposure
   l. Family history of HL/syndromes
   m. Cardiovascular disorders
   n. Rheumatological disorders
   o. Endocrine disorders
   p. Neurological disorders
2. Exam
   a. Speech
   b. Gross hearing
   c. Communication type
   d. Auricles, ear canals, and eardrums
   e. Tuning forks
      i. Weber
      ii. Rinne
   f. Cranial nerves
   g. Remainder head and neck
3. Potential Causes
   a. Genetic
      i. Too numerous to count
   b. Infectious
      i. HZV (Ramsay Hunt)
      ii. Measles
      iii. Mumps
      iv. *Cytomegalovirus* (CMV)
      v. Syphilis

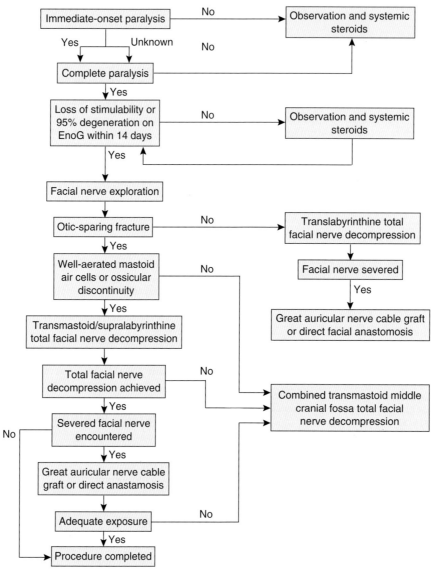

Fig. 2.12 Management of traumatic facial paralysis. Of note, some otologists may offer decompression surgery for traumatic delayed-onset, complete paralysis with >95% degeneration on ENoG and absent electromyography potentials. *EnoG,* Electroneuronography. (From Flint PW, Haughey BH, Lund VJ, et al. *Cummings Otolaryngology—Head and Neck Surgery.* 6th ed. Philadelphia, PA: Saunders; 2015, Fig. 145.11.)

vi. Rocky Mountain spotted fever
vii. Lyme disease
c. Vascular
d. Neoplastic
e. Traumatic
  i. Physical trauma
  ii. Noise
    (1) Transient threshold shift (TTS) recovers 24 to 48 hours
    (2) Permanent threshold shift does not recover
    (3) The Occupational Safety and Health Administration Act (OSHA Act; noise intensity doubles every 3 dB; OSHA Act rounded to 5 dB)
      (a) 90-dB exposure 8-hour limit
      (b) 95-dB exposure 4-hour limit
      (c) 100-dB exposure 2-hour limit
      (d) 105-dB exposure 1-hour limit
      (e) 110-dB exposure 0.5-hour limit
f. Toxic agents damage outer and inner hair cells
  i. Aminoglycosides (permanent damage)

    (1) Vestibulotoxicity is greater than cochleotoxicity for streptomycin and gentamicin
    (2) Cochleotoxicity is greater than vestibulotoxicity for kanamycin, tobramycin, amikacin, neomycin, and dihydrostreptomycin
  ii. Chemotherapeutics (permanent damage)
    (1) Cisplatin and carboplatin
  iii. Salicylates (temporary)
  iv. Loop diuretics (temporary)
  v. Quinine (temporary)
g. Iatrogenic
h. Degenerative
i. Immunological
  i. Cogan syndrome (eye/ear disorder)
  ii. Polyarteritis nodosa
  iii. Relapsing polychondritis
  iv. Wegener granulomatosis
  v. Scleroderma
  vi. Temporal arteritis
  vii. Systemic lupus erythematosus

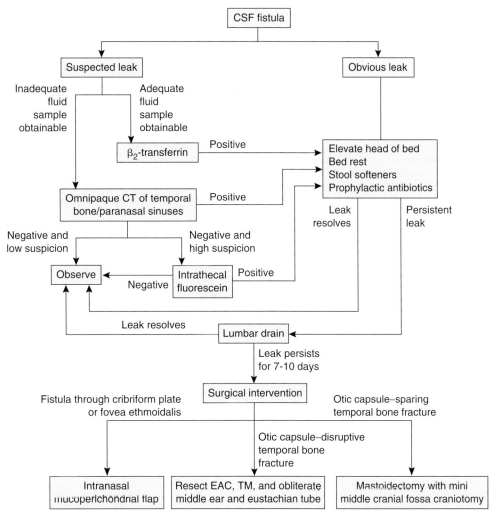

Fig. 2.13 Management of traumatic cerebrospinal fluid fistula. *CT*, Computed tomography; *EAC*, external auditory canal; *TM*, tympanic membrane (From Flint PW, Haughey BH, Lund VJ, et al. *Cummings Otolaryngology—Head and Neck Surgery.* 6th ed. Philadelphia, PA: Saunders; 2015, Fig. 145.13.)

viii. Sarcoidosis
    ix. Vogt-Koyanagi-Harada (can be seen in melanoma patients)
    x. Primary autoimmune inner ear disease
    xi. Antibodies to 68 kDa protein in 50% to 70%
4. Sudden SNHL
  a. Etiology is mostly idiopathic; thought to be either a viral or vascular insult
  b. Must rule out retrocochlear lesion with MRI
  c. Treat with oral prednisone as soon as possible
  d. If it fails, can offer intratympanic dexamethasone injection
  e. No advantage for antivirals in placebo-controlled studies

Tinnitus

- Differentiate tinnitus versus bothersome tinnitus
- 40% comorbidity with hyperacusis
- Subjective versus objective tinnitus
- Unilateral versus bilateral (or midline)
1. Pulse Synchronous
  a. Arteriovenous fistula/arteriovenous malformation
  b. Paraganglioma
  c. Carotid artery stenosis
  d. Other atherosclerotic disease
  e. Arterial dissection

  f. Persistent stapedial artery
  g. Intratympanic carotid artery
  h. Vascular compression of CN VIII
  i. Hypermetabolic state (pregnancy and thyrotoxicosis)
  j. Intraosseous hypervascularity (Paget and otosclerosis)
  k. Pseudotumor cerebri
  l. Venous hum
  m. Dural venous sinus abnormalities, jugular bulb high riding, and diverticulae
  n. Superior semicircular canal dehiscence
2. Pulse Asynchronous
  a. Palatalmyoclonus
  b. Middle ear spasm
3. Nonpulsatile
  a. Spontaneous otoacoustic emission
  b. Abnormally patulous Eustachian tube
4. Subjective Tinnitus Types
  a. From HL (e.g., noise-induced hearing loss and presbycusis)
5. Somatic tinnitus
  a. Temporomandibular joint (TMJ)
  b. Neck disorder
  c. Gaze evoked
  d. Cutaneous evoked
6. Typewriter tinnitus
  a. Fatigue induced
  b. Musical/complex

c. Intrusive
d. Associated affective disorder
7. Treatments for Tinnitus
  a. Ambient sound stimulation
  b. Personal listening software
  c. Hearing aid when appropriate for hearing loss
  d. Masking (ear level masking device or feature of hearing aid)
  e. Tinnitus retraining therapy (specific program of acoustic stimulation with education and counseling)
  f. Acoustic desensitization protocol (neuromonics)
  g. Cognitive behavioral therapy
  h. Transcranial magnetic stimulation
  i. Transcutaneous electrical nerve stimulation (on mastoid)
  j. Electrical stimulation
  k. Cochlear implantation
  l. Pharmacological (note, however: *nothing* is proven)
    i. Studies on gabapentin
    ii. Sertraline, tricyclic antidepressants
  m. Supplements (not proven)
    i. Lipoflavanoids

Noise-Induced Hearing Loss

1. Definition
  a. Permanent SNHL with damage to cochlear hair cells, primarily OHCs
  b. History of long-term exposure to dangerous noise levels >85 dB/sound-pressure level (SPL) for 8 hours/day on average
  c. Gradual loss of hearing over the first 5 to 10 years of exposure
  d. Blast injury, sudden loss
  e. HL initially involves high frequencies (3–8 kHz)
  f. Word-recognition scores initially consistent with audiometric loss
  g. HL continues after noise exposure is terminated
2. Random Noise-Induced Hearing Loss Facts
  a. 3- or 4-kHz notch a result of resonant frequency external auditory canal (EAC)
  b. TTS: Causes buckling of pillar cells (24–48 hours)
  c. Medial olivocochlear bundle and OHCs may have protective effect by "conditioning" cochlea to noise exposure and changes of basilar membrane stiffness

INFECTIONS OF THE LABYRINTH

1. Congenital Viral
  a. CMV: Number 1 nongenetic cause of HL
  b. Rubella: Worldwide important cause
  c. Herpes simplex virus
2. Congenital Nonviral
  a. Syphilis
  b. Toxoplasmosis
3. Acquired Labyrinthine Infections
  a. Mumps
  b. Measles
  c. Syphilis
  d. Bacterial meningogenic labyrinthine infections
  e. Cryptococcal
  f. Varicella zoster
  g. No strong correlation with other viral meningitis

OTOTOXIC AND VESTIBULOTOXIC MEDICATIONS

1. Aminoglycosides (likely from reactive oxygen species injuring the outer hair cells—consider OAEs)
2. Cisplatin: High frequencies affected more often, likely from reactive oxygen species injuring the stria vascularis and the outer hair cells; consider OAEs
3. Carboplatin (less ototoxic compared with cisplatinum)
4. Difluoromethylornithine (antitumor agent also used to treat West African sleeping sickness)
5. Loop diuretics (affect the stria vascularis)
  a. Lasix
  b. Ethacrynic acid
  c. Less so, bumetanide
  d. Less so, torsemide
6. Macrolides
  a. Erythromycin: Possibly reversible
  b. Azithromycin: Likely reversible
7. Desferoxamine: Possibly reversible SNHL and a chelating agent
8. Hydrocodone: From mostly abuse/recreational use
  a. Rapidly progressive, bilateral
  b. Not responsive to corticosteroids
  c. Cochlear implants work and typically help
9. Methadone: Possibly reversible according to case report(s)
10. Vancomycin: Questionable ototoxicity
11. Quinines: Possibly permanent but has a reversible component
12. Acetylsalicylic acid: Typically reversible, and it affects the motor protein prestin in OHCs

CENTRAL NEURAL AUDITORY PROSTHESES

1. Auditory Brainstem Implant
  a. Two manufacturers
    i. Cochlear ABI (approved in the United States)
    ii. Med-El ABI (not approved in the United States)
  b. Two indications
    i. Neurofibromatosis II (NF2) (only indication in the United States): Does not do as well with ABI as indication #2 does
    ii. Cannot perform a cochlear implant (Michel deformity, cochlear nerve agenesis, and ossified cochlea): Not yet an indication in the United States
  c. Two types
    i. Surface paddle electrode on the cochlear nucleus
    ii. Penetrating ABI (theoretically should be better but is not better than surface)
  d. Two approaches
    i. Translabyrinthine (especially when removing a vestibular schwannoma)
    ii. Retrosigmoid
2. Auditory Midbrain Implant
  a. Stimulates the inferior colliculus

APPLIED VESTIBULAR PHYSIOLOGY

1. Balance: Integration of vestibular, visual, and proprioceptive input to facilitate orientation and navigation, plus maintain upright posture and visual focus on the world while static or in motion
2. The vestibular system has basal firing rates from the end organs on both sides
  a. Irritative lesion increases firing rates (Ménière disease in 30%, early labyrinthitis)
  b. Destructive lesion decreases firing rates
  c. Unequal firing rates due to a peripheral lesion cause the sensation of movement toward the side with relatively higher firing rate
3. Nystagmus is named by direction of fast phase
  a. Slow phase generated by peripheral system, fast phase controlled by central system

4. Important to differentiate central from peripheral nystagmus
   a. Central: Continuous, does not fatigue, does not suppress with fixation
   b. Peripheral: Delayed in onset, fatigable, suppresses with fixation
   c. Note: Vertical nystagmus is considered central and requires MRI
5. Ewald's Laws
   a. A stimulation of the semicircular canal causes a movement of the eyes in the plane of the stimulated canal (*relative to the head, not the orbit!*); basis of vestibular-ocular reflex (VOR) test
      i. A semicircular canal is excited by head rotation about the axis of that canal, which brings the forehead toward the ipsilateral side
   b. In the horizontal semicircular canals, an ampullopetal endolymph movement causes a greater stimulation than an ampullofugal one does (ampullofugal actually suppresses from the baseline firing rate); acceleration to excitation of the ipsilateral canal is stronger than inhibition is
   c. In the vertical (superior and posterior canals) semicircular canals, the reverse is true; the difference between rule 2 and rule 3 is due to the orientation of the ampullae themselves; turning your head to the right leads to ampullopetal flow, and turning your head down to the right (stimulating the right superior canal) leads to ampullofugal flow
6. Other Key Points
   a. Central vestibular nuclei store velocity information (i.e., velocity storage mechanism—nystagmus from rotation will continue after the endolymph and cupula reach the same speed and the cupula is no longer deflected)
      i. Damage to peripheral vestibular input weakens the storage system
7. Alexander's law: Nystagmus from a *peripheral* vestibular lesion is **worsened** with gaze in the direction of the **fast** phase
8. Central compensation
   a. Brain increases firing rate on lesioned side acutely
   b. Fine tuning of firing rate under stress (head movement) occurs over time and with activity

EVALUATION OF THE PATIENT WITH DIZZINESS (FIG. 2.14)

1. History
   a. Onset of dizziness
   b. Vertigo (spinning or nautical), lightheadedness, or "foggy sensation"
   c. Episodic or continuous
      i. Length of episodes
      ii. Remitting and exacerbating factors
   d. Lifestyle (stress, sleep, and diet)
   e. Environment (pressure changes, lights, and noise-induced)
   f. Headache
   g. Head trauma
   h. Hearing loss
   i. Accompanying symptoms (with episodic dizziness)/triggers
   j. Medications (polypharmacy is common in elderly population)

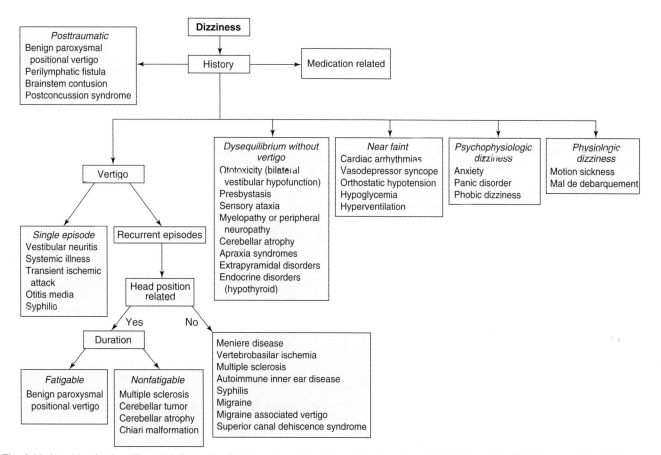

Fig. 2.14 Algorithm for the differential diagnosis of dizziness based on information from the patient's history. (Modified from Baloh RW, Fife TD, Furman JM, Zee DS. The approach to the patient with dizziness. In: Mancall EL, ed. *Continuum: Lifelong Learning in Neurology.* Cleveland, OH: Advanstar Communication; 1996:25–36 and Flint PW, Haughey BH, Lund VJ, et al. *Cummings Otolaryngology—Head and Neck Surgery.* 6th ed. Philadelphia, PA: Saunders; 2015, Fig. 164.4.)

2. Exam
   a. Otoscopy with insufflation (check for fistula)
   b. Cranial nerves, especially extraocular muscle
   c. Remaining head and neck
   d. Tuning forks (CHL or pseudoconductive in third windows): Check tuning fork on medial malleolus for sickle cell disease
   e. Cerebellar function (finger to nose, rapid alternating movements, heal/shin tests
   f. Head thrust (check VOR)
   g. Romberg, tandem
   h. Fukuda step test
   i. Hallpike
3. Ancillary Testing
   a. Audiogram asymmetric HL, pseudoconductive loss, and reflexes?
   b. Videonystagmography (VNG): Video goggles (or electronystagmography [ENG] using electrodes around eyes to measure eye movements via corneal retinal potential)
      i. Spontaneous nystagmus
      ii. Gaze nystagmus
      iii. Saccades
      iv. Smooth pursuit
      v. Optokinetic nystagmus
      vi. Positional
         (1) Lateral head right, left, and center
         (2) Lateral body
         (3) Tests for benign paroxysmal positional vertigo (BPPV) of horizontal canals
      vii. Positioning: Hallpike
         (1) Test for vertical canal BPPV
      viii. Caloric (lateral canal/superior vestibular nerve test only)
         (1) Stimulation of individual canal with warm/cool air or water normally induces nystagmus
         (2) Assesses only vestibular response to slow/low-frequency input
         (3) Compare velocity of nystagmus slow phase between ears to symmetry
      ix. Fistula test with pressure
   c. Video head impulse testing (vHIT) (All canals, inferior/superior vestibular nerve tested)
      i. Complementary test to VNG
      ii. Measures VOR in all planes (right anterior–left posterior [RALP]/left anterior–right posterior [LARP]/horizontal, i.e., each of 6 canals assessed)
      iii. Test ability to maintain focus on a target while head is quickly moved away from center
      iv. Normal response: Eyes remain fixed on target
      v. Overt saccades: Examiner can see eyes make slow corrective movement back to target
      vi. Covert saccades: Video measurable fast corrective eye movement back to target
   d. Rotary chair
      i. VOR: Elicited by head movement (stimulation of both horizontal canals simultaneously), allows for visual focus while head is in motion
      ii. Measured features of reflex: Phase, gain, and symmetry across large range of frequency input
      iii. Visual fixation test: Ability to suppress VOR with a fixed visual stimulus
      iv. Visually enhanced VOR: Enhanced VOR by including optokinetic nystagmus
   e. Vestibular evoked myogenic potential (VEMP)
      i. Independent of hearing status
      ii. Used to confirm third window pathology

iii. cVEMP: Acoustic sound → saccule → inferior vestibular nerve → spinal accessory, ipsilateral → **relaxation** of **ipsilateral** SCM
      iv. oVEMP: Acoustic sound or bone oscillation → utricular stimulation → superior vestibular nerve → contralateral oculomotor nucleus → **contraction** of **contralateral** inferior oblique
   f. Posturography: Isolates **functional** contributions of vision, proprioception, and vestibular systems for balance
      i. Analysis of amount of sway when visual and/or proprioceptive cues are removed
      ii. Helps identify malingerers, monitor disease, and rehabilitation progress
      iii. Commonly used in physical therapy

PERIPHERAL VESTIBULAR DISORDERS

1. Benign Paroxysmal Positional Vertigo (BPPV)
   a. Posterior canal most common, 85% to 90%
      i. Canalithiasis: Rx, Epley/Brandt Daroff
      ii. Cupulolithiasis: Rx, possibly Semont liberatory maneuver
   b. Lateral canal second most common
      i. Canalothiasis: Geotropic nystagmus; Rx, log roll
      ii. Cupulothiasis: Ageotropic nystagmus; Rx is not well determined
   c. Superior canal: Very uncommon; can have pure downbeat nystagmus; Rx, deep head hang
2. Ménière Disease
   a. Low-salt diet, no caffeine and diuretics
   b. Vasodilators (betahistine)
   c. Low intermittent pressure therapy to affected ear
   d. Transtympanic steroids
   e. Transtympanic gentamicin
   f. Oral steroids for exacerbations
   g. Supportive care for acute attacks
3. Vestibular Neuronitis: Rx, supportive care, possibly steroids in early onset, vestibular exercises, or therapy to speed up compensation
4. Superior Canal Dehiscence Syndrome
   a. Dehiscence of the superior canal along the floor of the middle cranial fossa creates a "third window affect"
   b. *Hennebert's sign*: Pressure-induced vertigo caused by straining or external pressure applied on examination
   c. *Tullio's phenomenon*: Sound-induced vertigo
   d. Diagnose by history, CT of temporal bones, low-frequency mild CHL, VEMP (increased amplitude and decreased thresholds)
   e. Treat with surgery (see "Surgery for Vertigo" section)
5. Perilymphatic Fistula: Rx, fistula repair for dizziness that does not respond to bed rest and conservative measures
6. Cogan's: Rx, steroids and immunosuppressants
7. Otosyphilis: Rx, antibiotics (penicillin) and corticosteroids
8. Labyrinthine Concussion: Rx, supportive care
9. Enlarged Vestibular Aqueduct: Rx, supportive care for attacks
10. Familial Vestibulopathy Autosomal-Dominant Migraine Headaches: Rx, acetazolamide and supportive care
11. Bilateral Vestibulopathy (Dandy/oscillopsia): Rx, vestibular therapy; substitution exercises

CENTRAL VESTIBULAR DISORDERS

1. Vestibular migraine
   a. Comorbid with
      i. Ménière disease
      ii. BPPV
      iii. Anxiety

b. Treatment
  i. Diet changes, stress modification, and sleep hygiene
  ii. Tricyclic antidepressants
    (1) Amitryptiline
    (2) Nortryptiline
  iii. Calcium channel blockers
    (1) Verapamil
  iv. Antiseizure medications
    (1) Topiramate
    (2) Gabapentin
  v. β-Blockers
    (1) Propranolol
    (2) Atenolol (off label)
  vi. Other antidepressants
    (1) Venlafaxine
  vii. Supportive measures for acute attacks
c. Benign paroxysmal vertigo of childhood likely a migraine equivalent
2. Persistent postural perceptual dizziness (PPPD)
  a. Treat with selective serotonin reuptake inhibitors
  b. Physical therapy
3. Vertebrobasilar insufficiency; likely has other neurological findings
  a. HINTS test: *h*ead *i*mpulse *n*ystagmus, *t*est of *s*kew (helps to differentiate central from peripheral)
    i. Head impulse usually normal if central
    ii. Nystagmus vertical, direction changing, purely torsional, and/or independent of gaze direction if central
    iii. Skew deviation/abnormal vertical smooth pursuit is central (may require experienced examiner)
4. Lateral medullary syndrome (Wallenberg) (ipsilateral vertebral artery; rarely, posterior inferior cerebellar artery occlusion)
5. Lateral pontomedullary syndrome (anterior inferior cerebellar artery occlusion and, therefore, labyrinthine artery occlusion)
6. Cerebellar infarction
  a. Nodular infarction (central paroxysmal positional vertigo)
    i. Short latency nystagmus, atypical direction, no fatigability, and no response to Epley
  b. Cerebellar hemorrhage: Emergency!
  c. Vertebral artery dissection
7. Tumors of posterior fossa
8. Cervical vertigo: Controversial; Rx, neck PT
9. Disorders of the craniovertebral junction
  a. Basilar impression (clivus compresses medulla)
  b. Assimilation of the atlas
  c. Atlantoaxial dislocation
  d. Chiari malformation
    i. Upper-extremity weakness, sensory loss, and pain
    ii. Occipital headaches with straining
    iii. Ataxia and nystagmus
    iv. Lower cranial nerve dysfunction
10. Multiple sclerosis (can involve medial longitudinal fasciculus [MLF])
11. Cerebellar ataxia syndromes
  a. Friedreich (#1), autosomal recessive
  b. Spinocerebellar atrophy
  c. Cerebellar atrophy
  d. Familial episodic ataxia (Rx, acetazolamide)
  e. Paraneoplastic cerebellar degeneration
    i. Anti-Purkinje cell antibodies: Small cell cancer of lung, breast, ovary, and Hodgkin
12. Focal seizures
13. Normal pressure hydrocephalus
  a. Dementia, gait disturbance, and urinary incontinence
  b. Rx: shunt
14. Motion intolerance
15. Mal de Debarquement syndrome

SURGERY FOR VERTIGO

1. BPPV treatment
  a. Singular neurectomy (rarely done)
  b. Posterior canal occlusion
2. Superior canal dehiscence
  a. Middle fossa plugging or resurfacing
  b. Transmastoid plugging or resurfacing
  c. Round window reinforcement (controversial)
3. Perilymphatic fistula
  a. Support oval and round windows with tissue (not loose, areolar tissue)
4. Ménière disease
  a. Nonablative
    i. Middle ear tenotomy (cut tendons in the middle ear; allow lateral expansion of the oval window; done in Europe)
    ii. Endolymphatic sac surgery
      (1) Decompression
      (2) Shunting (endolymphatic to mastoid)
      (3) Duct plugging (a relatively new procedure)
  b. Ablative
    i. Cochleosacculotomy (can be done under local anesthetic, utilized in older patients who cannot tolerate general anesthesia)
      (1) 3-mm hook into the round window toward the oval window
    ii. Labyrinthectomy (sacrifice hearing)
      (1) Transcanal: Increased possibility of leaving behind neuroepithelium
      (2) Transmastoid: Greater exposure of five organs (saccule, utricle, and ampullae of superior, lateral, and posterior canal)
        (a) Failure possibly because of traumatic neuromas of vestibular nerve branches
        (b) Posterior canal ampulla is most commonly left behind because the facial nerve is located lateral to it
    iii. Vestibular nerve section
      (1) Retrolabyrinthine
      (2) Retrosigmoid
      (3) Middle fossa
      (4) Translabyrinthine

VESTIBULAR REHABILITATION THERAPY

1. Peripheral vestibular insult leads to static compensation (central response to decreased asymmetric vestibular input) followed by dynamic compensation (compensates for asymmetric responses with head movement)
2. How dynamic compensation occurs (best to have a static insult to the vestibular system):
  a. Adaptation: Central neuronal compensation for insult to the vestibular system
  b. Habituation: Repeated maneuvers to decrease noxious response/symptoms from maneuvers
  c. Sensory substitution: Use of vision and proprioception to compensate for a decrease in vestibular function
3. Other terms
  a. Gait exercises: Improve ambulation
  b. Canalith repositioning (for BPPV)
  c. General conditioning: Improve fitness overall and decrease fatigability
  d. Maintenance: Maintain gains in posture and gait stability

TESTS OF FACIAL NERVE FUNCTION (FIG. 2.15; TABLE 2.3)

1. Topodiagnostic Tests (Historical Value Only)
   a. Schirmer test
   b. Taste test
   c. Salivary pH
   d. Salivary flow (via the submandibular gland)
   e. Acoustic reflex
2. Electrophysiological Tests
   a. Nerve excitability test: Thresholds for facial nerve stimulation at the stylomastoid foramen are compared (normal to abnormal)
   b. Maximal stimulation test: Test unaffected side for threshold that stimulates the facial nerve maximally, apply that stimulus level to the affected side, and measure percent response
   c. Electroneurography (evoked electromyography [EMG]): Uses surface electrodes maximally to stimulate both sides and measure resulting EMG bilaterally; compare percentage of response as a percentage (affected/unaffected); best between 3 and 21 days (Wallerian degeneration needs to occur because stimulation is at the stylomastoid foramen, distal to the site of injury in the temporal bone; at more than 21 days, dyssynchrony may occur and, therefore, degeneration may be overestimated)
   d. EMG is useful for prognosis
      i. Best after 14 days
      ii. Fibrillation potentials: Degeneration
      iii. Polyphasic potentials: Nerve regrowth
      iv. Determination of return of nerve function months after insult to nerve is useful in deciding on transposition surgery

CLINICAL DISORDERS OF THE FACIAL NERVE

1. Acute Facial Palsy (Fig. 2.16)
   a. Bell palsy: "Idiopathic" but likely secondary to herpes simplex viral activation 85% regeneration to HB 1-2
   b. Herpes Zoster (Ramsay Hunt): Worse prognosis (70% regeneration to HB 1-2); typically not decompressed; treat with steroids and antivirals

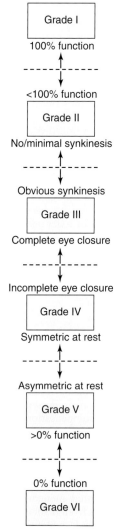

Fig. 2.15 Schematic diagram of a modified House-Brackmann grading scale using the major functional criteria of absolute movement, synkinesis, eye closure, asymmetry at rest, and absolute paralysis in assigning unambiguous and nonoverlapping degrees of facial paralysis. (From Flint PW, Haughey BH, Lund VJ, et al. *Cummings Otolaryngology—Head and Neck Surgery*. 6th ed. Philadelphia, PA: Saunders; 2015, Fig. 169.1.)

TABLE 2.3 House-Brackmann Facial Nerve Grading System

Grade	Description	Characteristics
I	Normal	Normal facial function in all areas
II	Mild dysfunction	Gross: Slight weakness noticeable on close inspection; may have very slight synkinesis
		At rest: Normal symmetry and tone
		Forehead motion: Moderate to good function
		Eye motion: Complete closure with minimum effort
		Mouth motion: Slight asymmetry
III	Moderate dysfunction	Gross: Obvious but not disfiguring difference between two sides; noticeable but not severe synkinesis, contracture, or hemifacial spasm
		At rest: Normal symmetry and tone
		Forehead motion: Slight to moderate movement
		Eye motion: Complete closure with effort
		Mouth motion: Slightly weak with maximum effort
IV	Moderately severe dysfunction	Gross: Obvious weakness and/or disfiguring asymmetry
		At rest: Normal symmetry and tone
		Forehead motion: None
		Eye motion: Incomplete closure
		Mouth motion: Asymmetric with maximum effort
V	Severe dysfunction	Gross: Only barely perceptible motion
		At rest: Asymmetry
		Forehead motion: None
		Eye motion: Incomplete closure
		Mouth motion: Slight movement
VI	Total paralysis	No movement

From Flint PW, Haughey BH, Lund VJ, et al. *Cummings Otolaryngology—Head and Neck Surgery*. 6th ed. Philadelphia, PA: Saunders; 2015, Table 169.1.

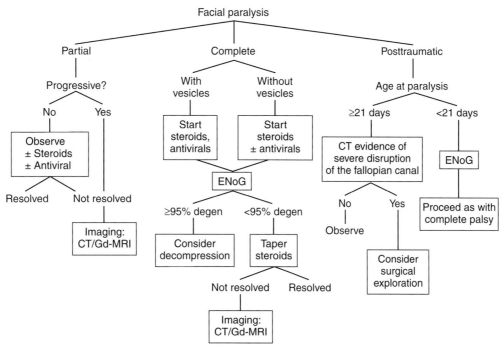

Fig. 2.16 Management algorithm for facial paralysis. *CT*, Computed tomography; *degen*, degeneration; *ENoG*, electroneuronography; *Gd*, gadolinium enhanced; *MRI*, magnetic resonance imaging. (Modified from Flint PW, Haughey BH, Lund VJ, et al. *Cummings Otolaryngology—Head and Neck Surgery*. 6th ed. Philadelphia, PA: Saunders; 2015, Fig. 170.1.)

c. Guillain-Barré
d. Autoimmune
e. Lyme (especially if bilateral, bilateral 10%)
f. Human immunodeficiency virus
g. Sarcoidosis
h. Melkersson-Rosenthal
i. Kawasaki
j. Trauma
k. OM, acute or chronic
l. Cerebrovascular disorders
2. Chronic Facial Palsy
a. Neoplasm: Parotid, temporal bone, cutaneous/facial, CPA, and brainstem
b. Cholesteatoma
3. Congenital Palsy
a. Mobius: Bilateral sixth and seventh nerve palsy
b. Congenital unilateral lower-lip paralysis (CULLP)
c. Oculoauriculovertebral
d. Mononeural agenesis
e. Hemifacial microsomia
f. Teratogens: Thalidomide and rubella
g. CHARGE syndrome (*c*oloboma, *h*eart disease, *a*tresia of the choanae, *r*etarded growth and mental development, *g*enital anomalies, and *e*ar abnormalities)
h. Poland syndrome: Agenesis of pectoralis major muscle
4. Other Notable Types of Facial Paralysis
a. Familial
b. Recurrent (check for tumor)
c. Bilateral: Lumbar puncture, lyme titer, complete blood count, fluorescent treponemal antibody, and MRI for workup

LATERAL SKULL-BASE SURGERY

1. Most Common
a. Temporal bone tumor: Paraganglioma
b. Adult temporal bone malignancy: Squamous cell carcinoma

c. Childhood temporal bone malignancy: Rhabdomyosarcoma
2. More Entities Lists
a. Primary Benign
i. Paraganglioma
ii. Meningioma
iii. Schwannoma/neurofibroma
(1) If bilateral, consider NF-2 (chromosome-22)
(2) Needs spinal MRI, evaluation by neurology, ophthalmology, genetics
iv. Adnexal tumors
(1) Ceruminous adenoma
(2) Eccrine cylindroma
(3) Pleomorphic adenoma
3. Mesenchymal Neoplasms
a. Chondroma
b. Chondroblastoma
c. Chondromyxoid fibroma
d. Lipoma
e. Myxoma
f. Fibro-osseous lesions
i. Fibrous dysplasia
ii. Ossifying fibroma
g. Giant cell granuloma
h. Aneurysmal bone cyst
i. Osteoblastoma
j. Osteoma/exostosis
k. Unicameral bone cyst
l. Teratoma
4. Dysontogenic Tissue
a. Choristoma
b. Inverting papilloma
c. Glioma
5. Metastatic Disease (can be bilateral, need to rule out in NF-2)
a. Prostate
b. Breast
c. Lung
d. Gastrointestinal

e. Renal cell
f. Myeloma
g. Lymphoma
h. Leukemia (granulocytic sarcoma/chloroma)
i. Melanoma
6. Primary Malignant Tumor
a. Epidermal
i. Squamous cell carcinoma
ii. Verrucous carcinoma
iii. Basal cell carcinoma
iv. Melanoma
v. Ceruminous adenocarcinoma
vi. Adenoid cystic
vii. Mucoepidermoid carcinoma
viii. Sebaceous cell carcinoma
ix. Papillary cystadenocarcinoma (endolymphatic sac tumor)
b. Mesenchymal malignancies
i. Rhabdomyosarcoma
ii. Fibrosarcoma
iii. Osteosarcoma
iv. Chondrosarcoma
v. Liposarcoma
vi. Dermatofibrosarcoma protuberans
vii. Fibrohistiosarcoma
viii. Angiosarcoma
ix. Osteoclastoma
x. Chordoma
xi. Plasmacytoma (extramedullary, solitary)
c. Contiguous tumor invasion
i. Neuroma
ii. Glioma
iii. Meningioma
iv. Choroid plexus papilloma
v. Primary parotid malignancy
vi. Primary cutaneous malignancy
vii. Pituitary
viii. Craniopharyngioma
ix. Nasopharyngeal carcinoma
7. Idiopathic
a. Langerhans cell histiocytosis
b. Inflammatory myofibroblastic tumor

Quantitative Cerebral Blood Flow Analysis

1. Xenon CT (most studied)
2. Positron emission tomography
3. MRI perfusion study
4. Cerebral perfusion CT

Approaches to the Internal Auditory Canal and Cerebellopontine Angle Tumors

1. Middle fossa craniotomy
a. Utilized for internal auditory canal (IAC) tumors with minimal CPA extension, age <65 years and serviceable hearing (PTA <50 and SDS >50%)
2. Translabyrinthine craniotomy
a. Utilized when hearing is not serviceable or for large CPA tumors for which hearing preservation is less likely
3. Suboccipital/retrosigmoid craniotomy
a. Utilized when hearing is serviceable and the tumor is primarily in the CPA with minimal IAC extension
4. Far lateral craniotomy
a. Utilized for tumors that extend inferiorly to the foramen magnum

Skull-Base Approaches

The carotid artery is always an important consideration (Fig. 2.17).
1. Temporal Bone Resections: Definitions May Vary!
Algorithm for EAC carcinoma (Fig. 2.18): Sleeve resection is controversial
a. Lateral temporal bone resection (primary tumor in the ear canal without involvement of the mucosa in the middle ear and mastoid)
i. With or without a parotidectomy
ii. With or without neck dissection
iii. If postoperative radiation therapy is required: Do not leave an open cavity; obliterate with vascular tissue (temporalis flap)
b. Subtotal temporal bone resection (for mucosal extension, perform a labyrinthectomy using middle and posterior fossa bony plates as margins, removing the cochlea and skeletonizing the petrous carotid)
i. Neck dissection with or without a parotidectomy
ii. With or without facial nerve rerouting or sacrifice
c. Total temporal bone resection (rarely indicated, involves carotid artery sacrifice)
2. Infratemporal Fossa Approaches (for Paraganglioma)
a. Paraganglioma Buzzwords
i. Brown's sign: Blanching with pneumatic otoscopy
ii. Aquino signs: Blanching with ipsilateral carotid compression MRI: "salt and pepper" appearance, representing vascularity and flow voids
iii. Pathology: Nests of "zellballen"
iv. Secreting tumors: Check serum and urine catecholamines, endocrine evaluation
v. Genetic tumors: SDH-B (succinyl dehydrogenase)
b. Transcanal: For glomus tympanicum in the mesotympanum not beyond the annulus
c. Mastoid extended facial recess: Glomus tympanicum beyond the annulus
d. Mastoid/extended facial recess/neck: Glomus tumor with extension into the jugular bulb; extracranial and not involving the carotid artery (leaves ear canal intact); identify internal carotid artery (ICA) jugular vein, CN 9–12 in neck; with or without "fallopian bridge"
e. Fisch A: Glomus jugulare in the middle ear, jugular bulb (same as letter d except for the closed-off ear canal; *classically* reroute facial nerve out of the descending fallopian bridge = facial weakness because of devascularization; sigmoid is packed off proximally and the jugular vein is taken inferiorly; jugular bulb is removed with the tumor, off of the vertical carotid if necessary; the Eustachian tube, middle ear, mastoid are obliterated)
i. With or without fallopian bridge
ii. With or without drilling out the inner ear
iii. With or without temporal craniotomy to better isolate the middle fossa floor/skull base
iv. Bleeding along the medial wall of the jugular vein via the inferior petrosal sinus and condylar vein
v. Lower cranial nerves through the pars nervosa along the medial wall of the jugular bulb
vi. Can also get out through the intracranial extension with ligation of the sigmoid and dural opening
f. Fisch B: Same as letter e, but for more anterior lesions typically (subtemporal region); *classically*, does not require transposition of the facial nerve. Add detachment of the zygomatic arch and temporalis origin with reflection downward, as well as downward displacement of the condyle; also typically includes downward reflection of the skull-base periosteum
i. With or without skeletonizing the horizontal carotid and possible transposition

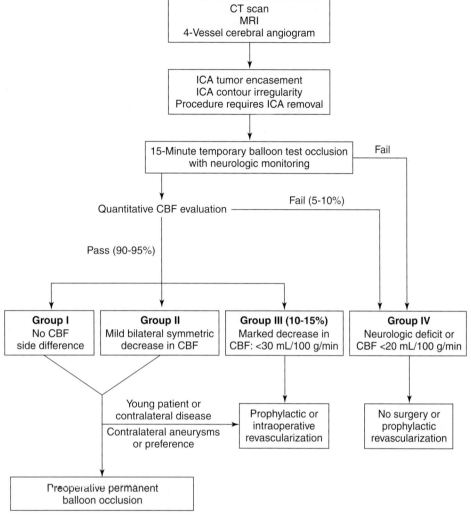

Fig. 2.17 Algorithm for preoperative internal carotid artery/cerebral blood flow evaluation. *CBF,* Cerebral blood flow; *CT,* computed tomography; *ICA,* internal carotid artery; *MRI,* magnetic resonance imaging. (From Flint PW, Haughey BH, Lund VJ, et al. *Cummings Otolaryngology—Head and Neck Surgery.* 6th ed. Philadelphia, PA: Saunders; 2015, Fig. 176.1.)

ii. With or without drilling away the middle cranial fossa floor

iii. With or without sacrificing the middle meningeal and transection of V3 at the foramen ovale

g. Fisch C: Same as letter f, but for further anterior exposure to the nasopharynx, sphenoid sinus, pterygoids, and posterior maxillary sinus

h. Fisch D: Preauricular infratemporal fossa; middle ear and ear canal are not entered; the Eustachian tube is obliterated (serous OM); the condyle is resected; typically, the temporalis and zygomatic arch are swung inferiorly

3. Approaches to the Jugular Foramen

a. Retrosigmoid craniotomy (no sacrifice of hearing or venous drainage)

b. Petro-occipital transsigmoid (sacrifices the sigmoid sinus, presumably for already occluded drainage): Retrolabyrinthine and retrosigmoid craniotomy with opening of the posterior fossa dura across the sigmoid with skeletonizing facial nerve; posteriorly based, therefore, can work medially to facial nerve; does not provide good exposure of the ICA; is better suited for jugular foramen schwannomas and meningiomas

c. Fisch type A approach: More laterally based; involves working around or transposing the facial nerve; provides better exposure of the ICA; better suited for glomus tumors

4. Fisch Classification of Glomus Tumors

a. Type A tumor: Limited to the middle ear cleft (glomus tympanicum)

b. Type B tumor: Limited to the tympanomastoid area with no infralabyrinthine compartment involvement

c. Type C tumor: Involves the infralabyrinthine compartment of the temporal bone and extends into the petrous apex

i. Type C1 tumor: With limited involvement of the vertical portion of the carotid canal

ii. Type C2 tumor: Invasion of the vertical portion of the carotid canal

iii. Type C3 tumor: Invasion of the horizontal portion of the carotid canal

d. Type D1 tumor: With an intracranial extension <2 cm in diameter

e. Type D2 tumor: With an intracranial extension >2 cm in diameter

5. Staging Tumors of the External Auditory Canal (Pittsburgh System)

a. *T Status*

i. T_1: Limited to the EAC without bony erosion or evidence of soft-tissue extension

ii. T_2: With limited EAC bony erosion (not full thickness) or radiographic finding consistent with limited (<0.5 cm) soft-tissue involvement

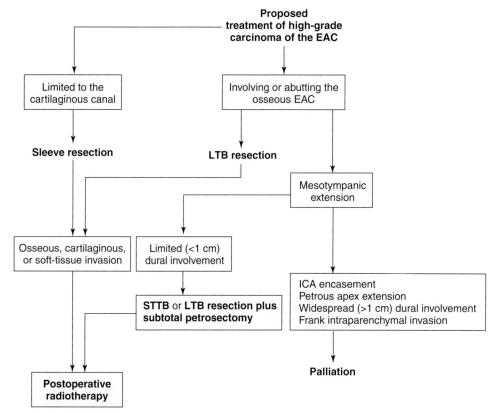

Fig. 2.18 Algorithm for management of high-grade malignancies of the external auditory canal (EAC) and temporal bone. *ICA*, Internal carotid artery; *LTB*, lateral temporal bone; *STTB*, subtotal temporal bone. (From Flint PW, Haughey BH, Lund VJ, et al. *Cummings Otolaryngology—Head and Neck Surgery.* 6th ed. Philadelphia, PA: Saunders; 2015, Fig. 176.25.)

iii. T_3: Tumor erodes the osseous EAC (full thickness) with limited (<0.5 cm) soft-tissue involvement or tumor involves the middle ear or mastoid

iv. T_4: Tumor erodes the cochlea, petrous apex, medial wall of the middle ear, carotid canal, jugular foramen, or dura or shows extensive (>0.5 cm) soft-tissue involvement or evidence of facial paralysis

v. Nodal status

   (1) Involvement of lymph nodes is a poor prognostic finding, automatically placing the patient in an advanced stage: stage III ($T_1 N_1$) or stage IV (T_2, T_3, and $T_4 N_1$) disease

vi. Metastatic status

   (1) Distant metastasis indicates a poor prognosis, immediately placing the patient in the stage IV category

STEREOTACTIC RADIATION FOR BENIGN SKULL-BASE LESIONS

Goal: Devascularize the tumor and decrease growth; *control rates 74% to 100%* (typically at least 90%) and studies have variable follow-up

1. Definitions
   a. Stereotactic radiation: Image-guided focus of radiation therapy with high precision to a lesion and a minimal dose to the adjacent tissues
   b. Stereotactic radiosurgery: Not surgery but rather stereotactically applied radiation in one to five shots

   c. Fractionated stereotactic radiation (FSR): As its name implies, goal is to fractionate to allow normal tissue recovery and possibly improve hearing preservation

2. Modalities
   a. Gamma knife: Typical "radiosurgical tool" (201 cobalt-60 sources pointing to center of the tumor; a rigid frame is applied to the patient's head and adjusted to keep the center of the sphere aimed at the tumor)
      i. Requires brief anesthetic to pin the frame into the head (rigid frame likely increases accuracy/precision)
      ii. 50% isodose levels currently 14 Gy: Has been lowered (typically, 12.5 Gy) to decrease the complication rate (below), and likely will lose some degree of tumor control in doing so
   b. Linear accelerator based can be used for FSR or radiosurgery
      i. Mask is applied to the patient; radiation source is moved in arcs around the patient
      ii. More comfortable in general, but may lose accuracy

3. Complications
   a. Hearing loss
   b. Worse vestibulopathy
   c. Facial weakness
   d. Trigeminal weakness
   e. Hydrocephalus
   f. Malignant transformation of tumor (1/1000)
   g. Failure of control may make surgical salvage more difficult

3 Facial Plastic Surgery

Marc H. Hohman, Srinivas M. Susarla, and Aurora G. Vincent

AESTHETIC SURGERY
Evaluation (See *Cummings Otolaryngology*, 7th ed., Chapter 16)

History Questions for Facial Plastic Surgery Patients

- Motivations
- Expectations
- Sun exposure, blistering sunburns
- Skin cancer
- Radiation
- Previous facial procedures (surgery, resurfacing, and injections)
- Facial trauma
- Poor wound healing, hypertrophic scarring or keloid formation
- Connective tissue disorders
- Bleeding or easy bruising/anticoagulant use
- Vitamin or herbal supplement use
- Tobacco, alcohol, or recreational drug use

Facial Analysis

- Quality of photographs
  - Intensity and symmetry of lighting
  - Focus
  - Exposure
  - Orientation in the Frankfort horizontal plane: line from the porion (superiormost aspect of the external auditory canal) to the orbitale (inferiormost aspect of the orbital rim) should be parallel to the floor
- Skin assessment
  - Thickness
  - Sebaceous quality
  - Glogau classification
  - Fitzpatrick classification
- Frontal view
  - Overall symmetry
  - Brow-dorsum-tip aesthetic line (best assessed in three-fourth view)
  - Facial fifths
  - Facial thirds
- Lateral view
  - Nasofrontal angle (115–135 degrees)
  - Nasion position/radix depth
  - Straightness of dorsum
  - Nasal length
  - Nasal projection
  - Nasolabial angle/nasal rotation (90–110 degrees)
  - Columella-alar relationship: 2 to 4 mm of columellar show
  - Tip to ala ratio of 1:1
  - Nasofacial angle (30–40 degrees)
  - Nasomental angle (120–132 degrees)
  - Chin projection
  - Cervicomental angle (90–105 degrees)
- Base view
  - Base shape
  - Tip bulbosity
  - Base width
  - Columella-lobule ratio of 2:1

Facial Fifths (Fig. 3.1)

- Horizontal width of the face divided evenly into five vertical segments, each the width of one eye
- Helix to lateral canthus, lateral canthus to medial canthus, medial canthus to medial canthus, medial canthus to lateral canthus, and lateral canthus to helix

Facial Thirds

- Vertical height of the face divided evenly into three horizontal segments
- Trichion (midpoint of the frontal hairline) to the glabella (midpoint between the brows), glabella to the subnasale (point where the nasal septum and upper lip meet), and subnasale to the menton (inferiormost point of chin; Fig. 3.2)
- When measured from the nasion (frontonasal suture) to subnasale, midface should account for 43% of height when compared to 57% for lower face.

Aesthetic Units of the Face

1. Forehead
2. Eyes
3. Nose
4. Lips
5. Chin
6. Ears
7. Neck

Glogau Photoaging Classification

- Type 1: No wrinkles, mild pigmentary changes, no keratoses, minimal wrinkles, and age in the 20s and 30s
- Type 2: Hyperkinetic wrinkles, early solar lentigines and palpable keratoses, parallel smile lines, and age in the 40s
- Type 3: Static wrinkles, dyschromia, telangiectasias, visible keratosis, and age in the 50s
- Type 4: Only wrinkles, yellow-gray skin with neoplasia, and age in the 60s and older

Fitzpatrick Skin Pigmentation Classification

- Based on first 60-minute unprotected exposure to midday sun at the beginning of spring
- Type 1: White, always burns, and never tans (typically red-headed or blonde with blue eyes)
- Type 2: White, usually burns, and tans with difficulty (typically blonde or brunette with blue eyes)
- Type 3: White, sometimes mildly burns, and, on average, tans (typically brunette with brown eyes)
- Type 4: Brown, rarely burns and tans with ease (Mediterranean, Hispanic, East Asian)
- Type 5: Dark brown, very rarely burns, tans very easily (South Asian)
- Type 6: Black, never burns, tans very easily (African, Caribbean)

Skin Lesions (See *Cummings Otolaryngology*, 7th ed., Chapter 17)

Benign Skin Lesions

- Seborrheic keratosis
- Dermatosis papulosa nigra
- Epidermal nevus
- Verruca vulgaris

Cysts and Subcutaneous Lesions

- Epidermal inclusion cyst
- Pilar cyst
- Milia
- Dermoid cyst

Melanotic Lesions

- Benign nevus
- Lentigo
- Ephelid

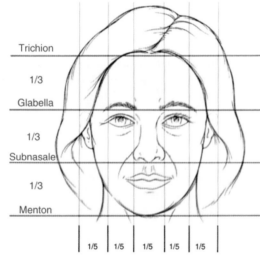

Fig. 3.1 Horizontal facial thirds and vertical facial fifths. (From Flint PW, Haughey BH, Lund VJ, et al. *Cummings Otolaryngology—Head and Neck Surgery.* 7th ed. Philadelphia, PA: Elsevier; 2020, Figs. 16.7 and 16.8.)

Fibroadnexal Lesions

- Nevus sebaceous
- Acrochordon
- Keloid and hypertrophic scars
- Neurofibroma
- Angiofibroma
- Dermatofibroma
- Sebaceous hyperplasia
- Xanthelasma
- Chondrodermatitis nodularis helicis
  - Eroded papules along the helical rim or crus from chronic trauma and vasculitis
  - Unilateral
  - Due to pressure from sleeping or phone use
  - Tender to touch
  - Treat with behavior change to avoid pressure, cryotherapy, excision abnormal tissue.

Malignant and Premalignant

- Melanoma
- Basal cell carcinoma
- Squamous cell carcinoma
- Merkel cell carcinoma
- Actinic keratosis
- Keratoacanthoma
- Dermatofibrosarcoma protuberans

Treatment of Skin Lesions

- Wide-local excision for melanoma, margins dependent on depth of tumor
- Cryosurgery, photodynamic therapy, laser resurfacing for benign skin lesions
- Staged excision of wide lesions on the face (to avoid long scar)
- Mohs micrographic surgery for nonmelanomatous skin cancers

Indications for Mohs Micrographic Surgery

- Aggressive histologic type or features
- Positive margins on recent excision
- Recurrent tumor or high risk of recurrence
- Need for tissue sparing

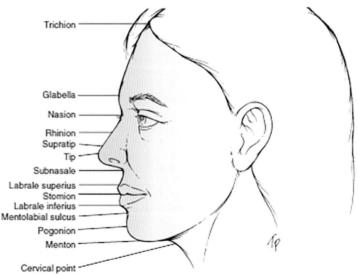

Fig. 3.2 Facial landmarks. (From Flint PW, Haughey BH, Lund VJ, et al. *Cummings Otolaryngology—Head and Neck Surgery.* 7th ed. Philadelphia, PA: Elsevier; 2020, Fig. 16.3B.)

- Location in H area of face
- Immunocompromised patient
- Patient with genetic skin syndrome
- Prior radiation to area

Facial Resurfacing (See *Cummings Otolaryngology*, 7th ed., Chapter 26)

History Questions for Facial Resurfacing

- Topical medications
- Isotretinoin use in last 12 months
- Cold sores

Indications for Facial Resurfacing

- Advanced-to-severe skin damage with wrinkles at rest
- Fine and deep rhytides
- Uncontrollable acne
- Acne scars
- Ephelides
- Lentigines
- Actinic keratosis
- Superficial basal cell carcinomas
- Lentigo maligna lentigenes
- Melasma (ensure that any hormonal changes have stabilized before treatment)

Absolute Contraindications for Facial Resurfacing

- Significant hepatorenal disease
- Human immunodeficiency virus (HIV)
- Immunosuppression
- Emotional instability or mental illness
- Ehlers-Danlos syndrome
- Scleroderma or collagen vascular diseases
- Recent isotretinoin treatment (within 6–12 months before)

Relative Contraindications for Facial Resurfacing

- Darker skin type (Fitzpatrick 4–6)
- History of keloid formation
- History of cold sores
- Cardiac abnormalities
- History of previous facial irradiation
- Unrealistic expectations
- Physical inability to perform quality postoperative care
- Anticipation of inadequate photo protection because of job, vocation, or recreation

Chemical Peels

Herpes Simplex Virus (HSV) Prophylaxis Before Perioral or Full-Face Resurfacing

- Valacyclovir 500 mg orally twice a day for 14 days, starting the day before the procedure

Sequelae of Facial Resurfacing

- Pigmentary changes
  - Hyperpigmentation with darker-skinned patients, usually temporary (give 4%–8% hydroquinone gel before surgery and sun protection factor [SPF] 30 sunblock after surgery, withhold systemic estrogens for prevention; hydroquinone to treat hyperpigmentation as well)
  - Hypopigmentation is less common; can be permanent (treat with topical steroids, sun exposure, blue light laser or broadband light/intense pulsed light, fractionated CO_2 laser)
  - Depigmentation (rarely, and in isolated areas)
- Persistence of rhytides
- Prolonged erythema
- Persistent texture change of skin
- Hypertrophic subepidermal healing
- Milia
- Skin pore prominence
- Increased prominence of telangiectasias
- Darkening and growth of preexisting nevi

Complications of Facial Resurfacing

- Skin infection
  - HSV outbreak
  - *Pseudomonas*, *Staphylococcus*, and *Streptococcus*
  - *Candida*
- Lower-eyelid ectropion
- Cardiac arrhythmias
- Renal failure
- Laryngeal edema
- Toxic shock syndrome
- Facial scarring
- Telangiectasias

Topical Adjuncts for Facial Resurfacing

- Retinoids (tretinoin)
- Bleaching agents (hydroquinone)
- Sunscreen
- Moisturizers
- Pretreat skin with these products before resurfacing, which may improve resurfacing results; some patients will not need resurfacing after the topical regimen

Peel Type	Indications	Examples	Application and Healing
Superficial: stratum granulosum + papillary dermis	Photoaging, melasma, comedonal acne, postinflammatory erythema	• Salicylic acid 5%–15% • Glycolic acid 40%–70%; must be rinsed off w/ H_2O or neutralized w/$NaHCO_3$ • Jessner solution (resorcinol, salicylic acid, lactic acid, and EtOH) • Trichloroacetic acid (TCA) 10%–25%	• Level 1 frosting (erythema with streaky whitening) • Healing: 1–4 days • Can repeat weekly or as desired

Medium: superficial reticular dermis	Fine rhytides, superficial scars, acne scars	• TCA 50% alone, can cause scarring
		• TCA 35% + dry ice pretreatment with Jessner solution and glycolic acid 70%
		• Phenol 88%
			• Level 2 or 3 frosting during treatment
			  • Level 2 frosting: white coat frosting with background of erythema
			  • Level 3 frosting: solid white enamel frosting with no background of erythema
			• Healing: 10 days
			• Do not repeat medium peel for at least 1 year

(continued)

Peel Type	Indications	Examples	Application and Healing

Deep: mid-reticular dermis	Glogau 3–4 rhytides	• Baker solution (3 mL phenol 88%, 8 drops septisol, 3 drops croton oil, and 2 mL distilled water); phenol penetrates farther with decreasing concentrations
		  • Phenol toxicity: central nervous system (CNS) excitation (tremors, hyperreflexia, hypertension) followed by CNS depression (respiratory failure, hypotension, cardiac arrhythmias)
		  • Affects cardiac, hepatic, and renal systems
		• Prevent and treat with IV fluids > 50% TCA (high risk of scarring and pigmentation problems)
			• Healing: 10 days (re-epithelization), redness can persist for weeks
			• Do not repeat deep peel for at least 1 year

Dermabrasion

- Addresses deep scarring, deep rhytides, and acne-related pits/scars
- Variable depth of resurfacing, often epidermis and papillary dermis
- Stimulates production of collagens I and III
- Pinpoint bleeding in chamois-colored tissue indicates level of papillary dermis
- Use freezing spray before mechanical abrasion to decrease tissue spatter
- Good for decreasing height of thick scars and treating rhinophyma

- Microdermabrasion is more superficial and requires no anesthesia or physician

Laser Resurfacing

- LASER: Light Amplified by the Stimulated Emission of Radiation

Laser Wave Characteristics
1. Collimated (parallel)
2. Monochromatic (same wavelength)
3. Coherent (in phase)

Lasers in Facial Plastic Surgery

Type		Wavelength (nm)	Chromophore	Indications
Ablative	Er:YAG (erbium-doped yttrium-aluminum-garnet)	2940; near-infrared	Water, collagen	• Resurfacing • Fractionated treatment: safer for patients with darker skin • Can be used in sequence: Er:YAG removes thermally necrotic tissue after CO_2 treatment • Ablative depth can be varied, typically deeper in fractionated treatments (150–300 μm)
	CO_2 (carbon dioxide)	10,600; far-infrared		
Nonablative	KTP (potassium-titanyl-phosphate)	532 (green)	Oxyhemoglobin, red pigment	• Colored tattoos • Telangiectasias • Port wine stains • Red lesions
	Pulsed-dye	585–595 (yellow)	Oxyhemoglobin	• Red lesions • Telangiectasias • Scar revision
	Alexandrite	755 (red)	Melanin, blue, green, black pigments	• Tattoo removal • Hair removal in fair-haired patients
	Nd:YAG (neodymium-doped yttrium-aluminum garnet)	1064 (near-infrared)	Oxyhemoglobin, melanin (in hair follicles), blue, black	• Hair removal (affects only hairs in anagen, takes several treatments separated by 4–6 weeks, works best on fair-skinned patients with dark hair) • Deepest penetration
	Nd:YAG	1320 (near-infrared)	Water	• Collagen remodeling without epidermal ablation
	Diode	1450 (near-infrared)	Water	• Collagen remodeling without epidermal ablation • Active acne
	Er:Glass	1540 (near-infrared)	Water	• Resurfacing • Low melanin absorption, less liable to cause eye damage
	Intense pulsed light/broadband light	500–1200 (not a true laser)	Dependent on wavelength filter used	• Melasma/dyspigmentation • Erythema • Hair removal • Acne control • Skin tightening • Requires multiple treatments, maintenance therapy

Scar Revision (See *Cummings Otolaryngology,* 7th ed., Chapter 18)

Scar Revision Considerations

- Scars take ~12 months to mature but may continue to improve spontaneously for 1 to 3 years
- Important to protect from sun exposure for the first 12 months
- Can revise as early as 2 months if poor healing is obvious
- Early pulsed-dye laser treatment will help decrease erythema as early as 3 weeks after injury/surgery

Scar Management Options

- Massage
- Topical therapy: Vitamin E oil, over-the-counter and prescription scar creams with moisturizer, and steroids
- Silicone sheeting: Apply 12 hours/day for 6 months
- Resurfacing
- Laser or dermabrasion, as discussed in the skin resurfacing section
- Surgical revision

Relaxed Skin Tension Lines (Fig. 3.3)

- Relaxed skin tension lines (RSTLs) follow furrows formed when the skin is relaxed
- RSTLs run perpendicular to the direction of underlying muscle contraction
- Incisions made parallel to tension lines heal better than those made tangentially to tension lines
- Lines of maximum extensibility run perpendicular to RSTLs

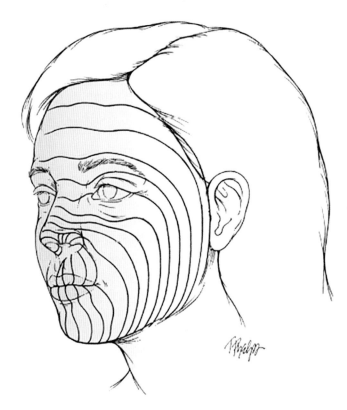

Fig. 3.3 Relaxed skin tension lines run perpendicular to the direction of the underlying facial muscles' contraction. (From Flint PW, Haughey BH, Lund VJ, et al. *Cummings Otolaryngology—Head and Neck Surgery.* 7th ed. Philadelphia, PA: Elsevier; 2020, Fig. 16.11.)

Operative Revision

- Z-plasty
- W-plasty
- Geometric broken line closure: a series of geometric shapes to break up the line of a scar
  - Shapes should be 3 to 6 mm in size to avoid contracting away during healing
- V to Y advancement: Lengthens the scar without changing orientation
- M-plasty: allows shortening of the long axis of fusiform excisions

Z-Plasty (Fig. 3.4)

- Combine serial Z-plasties along the scar to interdigitate wound edges and camouflage the scar better
- Z-plasties with angles <30 degrees may have skin necrosis at the tip
- Z-plasties with angles >60 degrees may result in standing cutaneous cone deformities
- If a Z-plasty of >60 degrees is necessary, two 60-degree Z-plasties may be compounded to achieve the effect of 120 degrees without standing cutaneous deformities
- Z-plasties may have asymmetric angles if necessary

Z-Plasty Effects

Angle (degrees)	Scar Lengthening (%)	Angle Change (degrees)
30	25	30
45	50	60
60	75	90

W-Plasty

- Zigzag excision provides an erratic scar that diffuses light
- Best for scars >2 cm in length
- Allows oblique or curvilinear scars to be broken down into small segments, parallel to RSTLs
- Each limb should not exceed 6 mm
  - <3 mm per limb will cause loss of irregularization as the scar contracts into a straight line
  - ≤90-degree angles

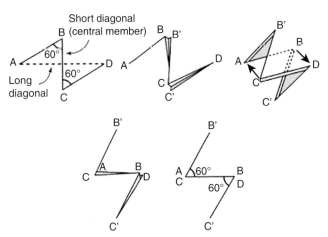

Fig. 3.4 Z-plasty. (From Flint PW, Haughey BH, Lund VJ, et al. *Cummings Otolaryngology—Head and Neck Surgery.* 7th ed. Philadelphia, PA: Saunders; 2020, Fig. 18.6.)

Keloid Treatment Considerations

- Multimodality treatment is preferred
- Preoperative intralesional steroid injection 3 times, separated by 6 weeks
- Subtotal resection with primary closure
  - Subtotal resection with positive margins all around prevents violation of virgin tissue
  - Elevation of overlying skin flaps away from the keloid, rather than resection of the skin and keloid en bloc, allows primary closure and obviates need for and risk associated with skin graft harvest
- Postoperative pressure therapy, particularly in ear lobule keloids, may help
- Silicone sheeting

Adjunctive Keloid Treatment

- Immediate postoperative electron-beam radiation therapy
- Laser treatment, such as fractionated Er:YAG

- Cryotherapy
- Intralesional injection of 5-fluorouracil, bleomycin, interferon-α2b
  - Often mix with steroid to prevent inflammation from chemotherapeutic agents
- Topical mitomycin C application, imiquimod

Injectables (See *Cummings Otolaryngology*, 7th ed., Chapter 25)

Dermal Filler Indications

- Static rhytides
- May help fill in dynamic rhytides after chemodenervation
- Restoration of lost volume in orbits, temples, midface, and lower face
- Augmentation of lips
- Augmentation of nasal dorsum
- Restoration of resting symmetry in facial paralysis

Dermal Fillers

Generic Filler	Brand Names	Duration	Use
Hyaluronic acid	Restylane PerlaneJuvederm	6–12 months	• Inject into dermis or subdermis • Hyaluronidase for excess or misplaced injection
Calcium hydroxylapatite	Radiesse	>12 months	• Inject into dermis or subdermis • Not for injection into lips
Poly-L-lactic acid	Sculptra	>12 months, semi-permanent	• Inject subdermally • HIV lipoatrophy • Results may take 4 weeks to appear
Autologous fat	—	80% of patients keep 80%–100%, 20% of patients resorb nearly all	• Harvest from abdomen/thigh • Centrifuge to concentrate adipocytes • Inject subdermally and deeper • Transferred fat will retain characteristics of harvest site (will gain and lose volume accordingly)
Collagen	ZydermZyplast	Permanent, may require touch-up at 6–18 months	• Inject into superficial papillary dermis • Rarely used anymore • Allergy to bovine collagen testing before injection

Dermal Filler Complications

- Injection site reaction, bruising
- Contour irregularities and nodularity
- Tyndall effect: visible blue hue from hyaluronic acid injected too superficially
- Skin necrosis due to arterial occlusion
  - Treat with injected hyaluronidase, warm compresses, topical nitroglycerin paste, aspirin, steroids, phosphodiesterase inhibitors, hyperbaric oxygen
- Blindness due to occlusion of central retinal artery via embolization from injection, typically during glabellar injections

Chemodenervation Characteristics

- Takes 1 to 2 weeks to reach maximum effect
- Lasts 3 to 4 months
- Shorter duration of action and smaller effect may result from development of antibodies
- With repeated facial cosmetic doses, patients often require less toxin or have a longer period between injections with the same effect

- Acts by preventing release of acetylcholine in the neuromuscular junction
- Recovery occurs first by development of new synapses, followed by recovery of function at the original synapse

Common Chemodenervation Indications

- Dynamic rhytides of the upper face: frown lines, crow's feet, bunny lines, forehead wrinkles
- Lip eversion ("lip flip")
- Decrease a gummy smile by weakening the levator labii superioris
- Elevate the corners of the mouth by weakening the depressor anguli oris
- Rejuvenate the neck by reducing platysmal banding
- Decreasing facial spasms and tension in post-paralytic synkinesis, blepharospasm, and hemifacial spasm
- Frey syndrome
- Bogorad syndrome ("crocodile tears")
- Hyperhidrosis
- Ptyalism or reduction of sialocele
- Weakening facial muscles may also help decrease scar widening from surgery

Chemodenervation Agents

- Botulinum toxin comes in seven varieties: A to G
  - A and E cleave SNAP-25
  - B, D, and F cleave synaptobrevin (VAMP)
  - C cleaves syntaxin

BOTULINUM TOXIN CONVERSION FACTORS

Generic Filler	Brand Name	Conversion to Botox
Onabotulinumtoxin A	Botox	—
Abobotulinumtoxin A	Dysport	3:1
Incobotulinumtoxin A	Xeomin	1:1
Rimabotulinumtoxin B	Myobloc	50:1

Chemodenervation Complications

- Injection site reaction, bruising
- Facial asymmetry: brow ptosis, oral commissure droop, asymmetric smile, lower lip asymmetry
- Blepharoptosis: Treat with apraclonidine drops
- Diplopia

Deoxycholic Acid (Kybella)

- Used predominantly for reduction of submental fat
- Requires four to six treatments, 4 to 6 weeks apart
- Induration and edema are common side effects
- May reveal platysmal banding after reduction of fat

Hair Restoration (See *Cummings Otolaryngology*, 7th ed., Chapter 22)

Hair Anatomy and Growth Cycle

- Scalp contains 100,000 to 150,000 hairs
- ~90% of follicles are in the growth (anagen) phase
- Next stage is involutional (catagen); <1% of the hair follicles arc in this phase
- 5% to 10% of hair follicles are in the resting (telogen) phase

Male Pattern Baldness (Androgenic Alopecia)

- Mediated by increased 5α-reductase activity and by lack of aromatase enzyme in specific regions of the scalp, thereby resulting in higher levels of dihydrotestosterone (DHT)
- Most common in Whites, then Asians, and then Blacks
- Incidence increases with age, ~30% at 30 years of age in White males; 50% to 60% at 50 years of age
- Bitemporal recession occurs first and then balding of the vertex

Norwood Male Hair-Loss Classification (Fig. 3.5)

- Type 1: Adolescent or juvenile hairline with no recession; rests at upper brow crease
- Type 2: Minimal frontotemporal recession, ≤1.5 cm above the upper brow crease
  - Type 2A: Additional recession in the central anterior region
- Type 3: Deepening temporal recession, the first stage of balding
  - Type 3A: Additional recession in the central anterior region
  - Type 3V: Additional hair loss at the vertex
- Type 4: Further frontotemporal recession with hair loss from the vertex; areas of recession are separated by a solid band of hair
  - Type 4A: Frontotemporal hair loss beyond type 3A, but without loss at vertex
- Type 5: Vertex loss is separated from the frontotemporal hairline by a narrow band of hair
  - Type 5A: Severe thinning of the central anterior hairline in continuity with thinning at the vertex
  - Type 5V: Additional loss at the vertex further thins the band separating it from the frontotemporal hairline
- Type 6: Frontal and vertex regions of hair loss are joined, and hairline is relatively high temporally
- Type 7: A narrow band of hair remains in a horseshoe shape, connecting the sides and back of the scalp

Ludwig Female Androgenic Hair-Loss Classification (See Fig. 3.6)

- Grade I: Perceptible thinning of the hair on the crown, limited in the front by a line situated 1 to 3 cm behind the frontal hair line
- Grade II: Pronounced rarefaction of the hair on the crown within the area seen in Grade I
- Grade III: Full baldness within the area seen in Grades I and II

Medical Management of Alopecia

- Minoxidil (Rogaine)
  - Causes vellus hairs to develop into terminal hairs; miniaturized hair follicles revert to normal morphology, and the number of hair follicles in anagen increases
  - Mechanism of action unknown, likely linked to vasodilation and opening of potassium channels
  - Increases follicle size and percentage of follicles in anagen phase
- Finasteride (Propecia)
  - Inhibits action of 5α-reductase type 2, blocking conversion of testosterone to DHT
  - Cannot be safely used in women of reproductive age because 5α-reductase inhibition during pregnancy may lead to genital abnormalities in male fetus
- Platelet-Rich Plasma (PRP) Injections
  - Drawn from patient's own blood
  - Platelets contain several growth factors
  - PRP is injected into tissue where hair growth is desired; multiple treatments are often required
- Results are seen only after several months of therapy and are rapidly reversed upon discontinuing therapy

Surgical Hair Replacement

- Goals of surgery are to create a natural-appearing hairline and to increase scalp coverage
- Prediction of future hair loss needs to be factored into the surgical planning
- Frontal hairline is most important
- Patient must have adequate donor hair available

Punch Method

- 4- to 5-mm, sharp, round punches to harvest from the parietal and occipital scalp with 10 to 20 hairs per punch
- Recipient sites are slightly smaller than donor site and are spaced so as not to compromise blood supply
- 6 weeks between sessions; usually at least four sessions are required

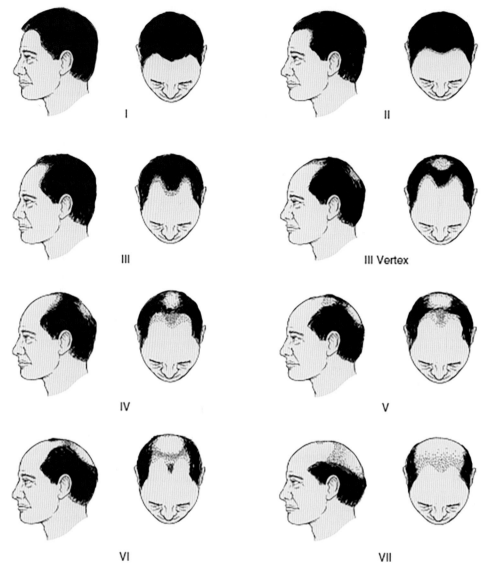

Fig. 3.5 Norwood male hair-loss classification. (From Flint PW, Haughey BH, Lund VJ, et al. *Cummings Otolaryngology—Head and Neck Surgery*. 7th ed. Philadelphia, PA: Saunders; 2020, Fig. 22.5.)

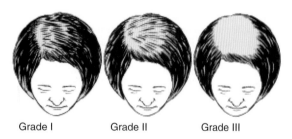

Grade I   Grade II   Grade III

Fig. 3.6 Ludwig female androgenic hair-loss classification. (From Flint PW, Haughey BH, Lund VJ, et al. *Cummings Otolaryngology—Head and Neck Surgery*. 7th ed. Philadelphia, PA: Saunders; 2020, Fig. 22.6.)

Strip Grafting

- 5 to 8 mm in width, typically in two sessions to recreate frontal hairline
- Donor site incised to the galea level and then elevated and closed primarily
- Graft inset to angle hairs anteriorly

Follicular-Unit Transplantation

- Most commonly used method
- Multiple minigrafts (3–4 hairs per graft) and micrografts (1–2 hairs per graft) are used
- Donor hair is harvested from the occipital scalp in a large ellipse
- Donor tissue is first cut into 2-mm segments, aligning all incisions in the direction of follicle growth and then further dissected into micro- and minigrafts, taking care to preserve natural groupings of hair follicles
- Slits are created in the recipient scalp 4 to 5 mm apart; a second and sometimes third pass over the area may be performed to obtain the desired density
- Telogen effluvium "shock loss" can occur at donor and recipient regions due to anagen hairs suddenly transitioning to a telogen phase
  - Hairs will regrow 3 months after stressor event; reassure patient

Scalp Reduction

- Serial excisions to remove bald areas
- Limited by amount of available hair-bearing scalp and wound tension

- Can use tissue expanders to increase hair-bearing area or use silastic sutures to support incision closure and decrease tension
- Juri temporoparietal transposition flaps based on superficial temporal arteries can be rotated to address frontal baldness

Brow Lift (See *Cummings Otolaryngology*, 7th ed., Chapter 25)

Ideal Brow Position (See Fig. 3.7)

- Women: Begins medially at a vertical line from the medial canthus; terminates at an oblique line drawn through the ala of the nose and extending past the lateral canthus; apex of brow arc between the lateral limbus and lateral canthus
- Men: Lies at the supraorbital rim and does not arch as high as in women

History Questions for Brow Lift and Blepharoplasty

- Prior periorbital trauma or surgery
- Xerophthalmia
- Ocular disorders or visual acuity/field deficits
- Graves disease

Brow Lift Considerations

- Glabellar creases
  - Transverse creases caused by procerus, most superficial muscle of the glabella, also depresses medial brow (lateral brow is depressed by depressor supercilii, a superolateral segment of the orbicularis oculi)
  - Vertical creases caused by corrugator supercilii, superficial to frontalis and deep to procerus
  - Division of the corrugator has a similar effect as permanent chemodenervation but may lateralize the medial brows
- Frontal branch of the facial nerve
  - Within 2 mm of zygomaticotemporal "sentinel" vein between the temporoparietal fascia (TPF/superficial temporal fascia) above and the temporalis muscle fascia (deep temporal fascia) below

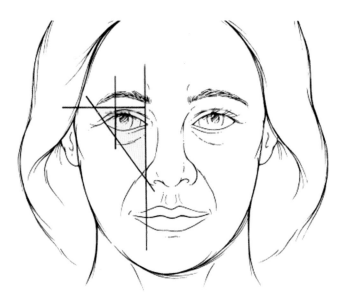

Fig. 3.7 Ideal female brow position. (From Flint PW, Haughey BH, Lund VJ, et al. *Cummings Otolaryngology—Head and Neck Surgery.* 7th ed. Philadelphia, PA: Saunders; 2020, Fig. 25.4 A.)

Indications for Brow Lift

- Brow ptosis, especially when it contributes to an upper visual field deficit with dermatochalasis
- Corrugator and procerus hyperactivity are indications for endoscopic forehead lift
- Baldness is not a contraindication

Endoscopic Brow Lift

- Patients with short, flat foreheads (<6 cm from brow to hairline), brow ptosis, or corrugator and procerus hyperactivity
- Subperiosteal dissection
- Avoid supratrochlear and supraorbital neurovascular bundles when releasing the periosteum from the supraorbital rim
- Release the periosteum all along the lateral orbital rim (arcus marginalis) to permit temporal lifting and relief of lateral periocular hooding
- 1.5-cm longitudinal incisions placed behind the hairline in median and paramedian positions (superior to the lateral limbus), and longer incisions placed behind the temporal hair tufts
- Periosteum secured in the elevated position with absorbable anchors, or sutures through bone bridges placed under paramedian incisions, or screws and staples
- Decreased scarring, alopecia, and numbness of the scalp compared with an open procedure

Coronal and Pretrichial/Trichophytic Brow Lift

- Subgaleal dissection
- Coronal approach may elevate hairline
- Pretrichial (just in front of hairline) and trichophytic (just behind hairline) approaches minimize hairline elevation
- Scar may become visible with time as hair thins, particularly in male patients; avoid in bald patients

Midforehead Brow Lift

- Excise and elevate via an incision in a transverse forehead rhytid
- More often used in men
- Tends to leave noticeable scar
- Not commonly used

Direct Brow Lift

- Incisions made along the superior margin of brows
- Most effective for correcting lateral brow ptosis and hooding
- Lateral excisions without medial extension are called a "temporal brow lift"
- Skin of lower forehead is more sebaceous and more likely to scar over medial brow

Transblepharoplasty Browpexy

- Frontal bone is accessed via upper blepharoplasty incision
- Fixation with suture between dermis of brow and periosteum or with absorbable anchors similar to endoscopic brow lift
- Best for lateral brow lift because medial dissection risks damage to supraorbital and supratrochlear neurovascular bundles
- Good for preventing post-blepharoplasty brow ptosis

Brow Lift Complications

- Forehead itching (25%)
- Diffuse alopecia (5%)
- Patchy areas of permanent numbness (1%)

EXCESSIVE BROW ELEVATION (0.3%)

Blepharoplasty and Blepharoptosis Repair (See *Cummings Otolaryngology*, 7th ed., Chapter 26)

Eyelid Anatomy (Fig. 3.8)

- Orbicularis oculi forms the transition from the brow into the upper eyelid and surrounds the eye
  - Orbital portion overlies the bony orbit
  - Palpebral portion overlies the eyelid: pretarsal and preseptal portions
  - Tarsal plate and orbital septum lie deep to palpebral orbicularis
- Orbital septum divides the lid into the anterior and posterior lamellae
  - Anterior lamella: skin and orbicularis oculi
  - Posterior lamella: conjunctiva, eyelid retractor, and upper or lower tarsal plate
  - Orbital septum and tarsal plate constitute "middle lamella"
  - Septum originates at the arcus marginalis, a confluence of the periosteum of the facial skeleton and the periorbita at the bony orbital rims
  - In the upper lid, the septum does not extend over the upper surface of the tarsal plate, but is found as a thin membrane 10 mm or more above the lid margin, inserting on the upper lid retractors
  - In the lower lid, the septum is attached to the inferior edge of the tarsal plate
  - Tarsal plate is 10 to 12 mm tall in the upper lid
  - Tarsal plate is 3 to 5 mm tall in the lower lid

Preaponeurotic Fat

- Deep to the septum, superficial to the levator aponeurosis
- Dissection through the septum more superiorly avoids injury to the levator aponeurosis and Müller's muscle, which will result in ptosis
- Upper lid has two fat pads
  - Nasal (medial) and middle (largest), with the temporal (lateral) compartment being occupied by the lacrimal gland, which may be prominent or ptotic
- Lower lid has three fat pads
  - Medial (nasal), central, and lateral (temporal)
  - Inferior oblique muscle separates the medial and central compartments
- Medial compartment in both the upper and lower lids contains denser, whiter fat

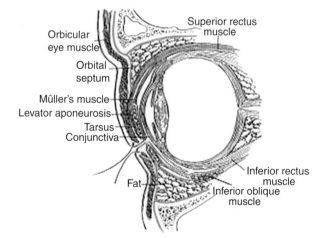

Orbicular eye muscle
Orbital septum
Mûller's muscle
Levator aponeurosis
Tarsus
Conjunctiva
Superior rectus muscle
Fat
Inferior rectus muscle
Inferior oblique muscle

Fig. 3.8 Cross-section of globe and eyelids. (From Flint PW, Haughey BH, Lund VJ, et al. *Cummings Otolaryngology—Head and Neck Surgery.* 7th ed. Philadelphia, PA: Saunders; 2020, Fig. 26.9.)

Lid Retractors

- Upper eyelid
  - Retracted by levator palpebrae superioris and Müller's muscle
  - Primary retractor is the levator muscle, originating in the orbital apex; lies immediately superior to the superior rectus; at the orbital aperture, it is supported by Whitnall's ligament
  - Levator palpebrae superioris splits into the levator aponeurosis anteriorly and Müller's muscle posteriorly
  - Müller's muscle travels inferiorly, closely adherent to the conjunctiva, and inserts on top of the tarsal plate
  - Levator aponeurosis inserts laterally and medially into the canthal tendons, and fuses with the orbital septum and dermis at the upper-eyelid crease; inferiorly, fibers travel anteriorly and posteriorly, attaching to the orbicularis oculi and tarsal plate, respectively
- Lower eyelid
  - Capsulopalpebral fascia of the lower eyelid is analogous to the levator aponeurosis of the upper lid, an extension of the inferior rectus muscle, which depresses the lower lid on downward gaze
  - Densely adherent to the conjunctiva and is routinely transected in lower-lid transconjunctival approaches

Eyelid Proportions

- Palpebral fissure width/intercanthal distance
  - Males: 26.5 to 38.7 mm
  - Females: 25.5 to 37.5 mm
- Palpebral fissure height
  - 10 to 12 mm
- Margin-reflex distance (MRD)
  - MRD1 from light reflex to upper-lid margin: 4 to 5 mm
  - MRD2 from light reflex to lower-lid margin: 5 to 6 mm
- Brow fat span (BFS): Distance from upper lid crease to the inferior margin of brow
- Tarsal platform show (TPS): Distance from lash line to upper eyelid crease
  - Youthful TPS:BFS ratio should be 1:1.5 medially and 1:3 laterally in a female
- Tarsal crease 10 to 12 mm above the lash line in females, 7 to 8 mm in males
- Upper lid should cover a small portion of the iris; inferior limbus should be within 1 to 2 mm of the lower lid
- Lateral canthus should be ~2 mm higher than the medial canthus

Blepharoplasty Tests

- Schirmer test: Strip of filter paper is inserted at the lower-eyelid margin (both eyes are measured at once) and left in place for 5 minutes with eyes closed; degree of wetting read as a linear measurement on the filter paper (normal ≥10 mm)
- Snap test: Measures how quickly the lid margin snaps back against the globe after being distracted; longer than 1 to 2 seconds indicates lid margin laxity

Blepharochalasis

- Rare variant of angioedema
- Recurrent, painless periorbital edema leads to chronic changes in eyelid skin elasticity, atrophy, hyperpigmentation, and upper lid ptosis
- Can lead to lacrimal gland and fat prolapse

Dermatochalasis

- Redundancy and draping of the eyelid skin in the aged face
- Called "pseudoptosis" when it progresses to the point that skin drapes over the upper eyelashes and causes visual field defects

Festoons

- Redundant folds of lax skin and orbicularis muscle
- Usually on the lower lid

Blepharoptosis

- Aponeurotic
  - Levator dehiscence is the most common cause of blepharoptosis, especially in the elderly; patients often have a high supratarsal crease
- Myogenic
  - Myositis
  - Muscular dystrophy
- Neurogenic
  - Myasthenia gravis
  - Multiple sclerosis
  - Horner syndrome
- Mechanical
  - Trauma/iatrogenic injury
  - Mass effect from tumor
- Congenital

Upper-Lid Incision Considerations

- When deciding how much skin to take, pinch with forceps until slight lid eversion is evident; this will lead to slight postoperative lagophthalmos, which will resolve
- Plan to leave ≥15 mm of skin between the lash margin and the inferior aspect of the brow
- Do not carry the incision medial to the medial canthus as this may cause webbing
- Orbicularis oculi muscle excision in patients with history of dry eyes should be conservative or not performed

Lower Lid Blepharoplasty Approaches

- Transconjunctival
- Subciliary skin-muscle flap
- Subciliary skin pinch excision

Transconjunctival Approach to Lower-Lid Blepharoplasty

- For older patients with pseudoherniation of orbital fat, limited amount of skin excess
- Young patients with familial hereditary pseudoherniation of orbital fat and no excess skin
- Revision blepharoplasty patients, patients who do not want to have an external scar or have a history of keloid, or dark-skinned individuals because of the possibility of hypopigmentation of an external scar
- Does not disrupt the orbicularis oculi, minimizing the incidence of ectropion
- Avoid damage to the inferior oblique muscle
- Do not pull fat out of the orbit; coax it out gently and cauterize carefully to avoid intraorbital hematoma

Preseptal Approach to Transconjunctival Blepharoplasty
- Conjunctival incision made 2 mm posterior to the inferior border of the inferior tarsal plate
- Dissect along the anterior face of the septum and then open the septum to access orbital fat
- Good approach for orbital floor fractures; allows elevation of the orbital floor periosteum without entering fat

Postseptal Approach to Transconjunctival Blepharoplasty
- Conjunctival incision made 4 mm posterior to the inferior border of the inferior tarsal plate in the inferior fornix

- Accesses orbital fat compartments directly
- Septum remains intact; decreased risk of ectropion

Subciliary Approach to Lower-Lid Blepharoplasty

- For large amounts of excess skin and orbicularis oculi
- Safely and easily dissect in a relatively avascular submuscular plane
- Ability to remove redundant lower-eyelid skin
- Can achieve additional tightening of skin and muscle with lateral suspension sutures
- Do not carry incision past the inferior punctum
- Leave at least 5 mm of intact skin between upper lid incision and subciliary lower lid incision at lateral canthus
- Skin-muscle flap procedure: subciliary incision with elevation of skin over the preseptal portion of the orbicularis oculi, then dissection dives under the remainder of the muscle inferiorly; fat resection can be performed transseptally and excess skin trimmed before closure
- May be combined with transconjunctival approach to address skin, muscle, and fat

Blepharoptosis Repair

- Evaluate for occult, asymmetric ptosis by elevating the brow on the ptotic side and looking for appearance of ptosis contralaterally (Hering phenomenon)
- Examine levator function by observing range of motion of upper eyelid by having patient look all the way down and then all the way up; there should be ≥12 mm of movement
  - If the levator function is insufficient, patient may need a frontalis sling
- Advancement of a properly functioning levator palpebrae superioris muscle is performed via an upper blepharoplasty incision
- Resection and shortening of Müller's muscle is performed transconjunctivally

Asian Eyelid Considerations

- Defined by the epicanthal fold and absence of upper-eyelid tarsal crease
- 50% of Asians have a tarsal crease ("double eyelid")
- If the crease is absent, the orbital septum and levator aponeurosis attach to the skin farther inferiorly, anterior to tarsal plate
- Orbital fat prolapses anteriorly, preventing the formation of a prominent upper-eyelid crease and creating fullness of the upper eyelid

Blepharoplasty Complications

- Asymmetry
- Milia
- Hematoma/blindness
  - If intraocular pressure (IOP) >40 mm Hg, lateral canthotomy and inferior cantholysis can reduce IOP by 30 mm Hg
  - Also consider steroids, mannitol, topical β-blockers, raise the head of bed
  - After 90 minutes of ischemia, the retina will suffer irreversible damage
- Lagophthalmos
- Ectropion: Eversion from excessive lower-lid skin or muscle excision, lid contracture, or lateral laxity
- Ptosis
- Epiphora
- Diplopia
- Conjunctival chemosis/ecchymosis

Ectropion Management

- Lower-lip tape splinting or forceful eye closure
- Gentle massage + corneal protection
- Surgical correction after 3 months
  - Full-thickness skin graft (FTSG) from the upper lid
  - If from lateral lid laxity
    - Horizontal lid shortening (lateral tarsal strip)
      - Tarsal strip may also be performed at the time of the lower lid blepharoplasty as prophylaxis against postoperative ectropion
  - Z-plasty

MUSCLE SUSPENSION

Face Lift (See *Cummings Otolaryngology*, 7th ed., Chapter 24)

Rhytidectomy Anatomy by Layers (Fig. 3.9)

- Skin
- Subcutaneous fat and hair follicles
- Galea aponeurotica/frontalis muscle/TPF superior to zygomatic arch, contiguous with superficial musculoaponeurotic system (SMAS) in the mid- and lower face, and then platysma in the lower face and neck
- Parotidomasseteric fascia surrounds the parotid posteriorly and the masseter anteriorly, contiguous with the periosteum of zygomatic arch and temporalis fascia
  - Temporalis fascia (deep temporal fascia) splits into superficial and deep layers to invest the superficial temporal fat pad just superior to the zygomatic arch
  - Deep temporal fat pad lies between the deep layer of the deep temporal fascia/zygomatic arch superficially and the temporalis muscle deeply

Dedo Aging Neck Classification

- Type 1: Normal cervicomental angle, good muscle tone, and no submental fat
- Type 2: Cervical skin laxity and obtuse cervicomental angle
- Type 3: Submental adiposity; rejuvenation will require submental lipectomy
- Type 4: Platysmal banding; rejuvenation will require imbrication or plication
- Type 5: Retrognathia/microgenia; rejuvenation will require genioplasty or orthognathic surgery
- Type 6: Low-lying hyoid; manage by setting appropriate expectations

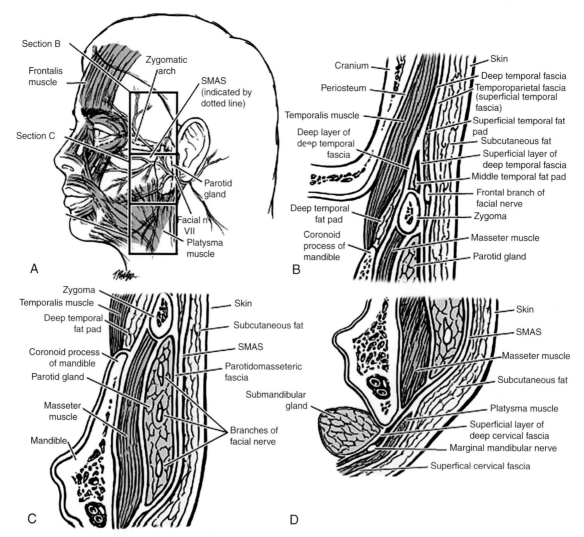

Fig. 3.9 Facial fascial planes. (A) The superficial musculoaponeurotic system (SMAS) is always superficial to the facial nerve. The relationship of the SMAS and facial nerve branches is shown in cross-section in the temporal (**B**), lateral cheek (**C**), and neck areas (**D**). (From Flint PW, Haughey BH, Lund VJ, et al. *Cummings Otolaryngology—Head and Neck Surgery.* 7th ed. Philadelphia, PA: Saunders; 2020, Fig. 24.3.)

Rhytidectomy Incisions

- Female: Typically posttragal to break up the scar
- Male: Typically preauricular to avoid pulling hair-bearing beard skin closer to the auricle or onto the tragus; there is usually a <1-cm wide vertical band of non–hair-bearing skin anterior to the auricle that should remain intact

Subcutaneous Face Lift

- Original facelift operation
- Short-lived results
- No longer performed

SMAS Face Lift

- Subcutaneous flap raised in the face and neck
- SMAS incised overlying parotid and plicated or imbricated to bear tension of the lift
  - Plication: Folding over and suturing
  - Imbrication: Excising a strip and suturing the edges together
- Facial nerve branches are not ordinarily visualized

Deep-Plane Face Lift

- Subcutaneous flap raised until the line between the lateral canthus and the angle of mandible is reached; SMAS is incised and dissection carried anteriorly along the plane of the zygomaticus major muscle, elevating the malar fat pad into the flap
- Facial nerve branches visualized and avoided
- Entire flap bears tension; excellent vascularity medially because of the thickness of the flap
- Neck is addressed as for SMAS flap rhytidectomy, leaving face and neck dissections in different planes, separated by the platysmal insertion at the level of the mandible
- Helps efface nasolabial folds by suspending malar fat pads

Composite Face Lift

- Deep-plane lift with repositioning of suborbicularis oculi fat (SOOF) via transconjunctival lower-lid blepharoplasty

Minimal-Access Cranial-Suspension (MACS) Lift

- Purse-string loops of suture plicate SMAS to elevate the face in a vertical vector
  1. Vertical loop elevates the neck
  2. Oblique loop elevates the jowl
  3. Malar loop elevates the midface
- Short incision with no postauricular component

Midface Lift Considerations

- Elevates malar fat pad and SOOF
- Effaces deep nasolabial folds
- Often combined with lower-lid blepharoplasty to avoid redundant lower-lid skin after lift
  - SOOF may be transferred inferiorly to augment malar eminence
  - May augment effect with fillers and/or cheek implants

Midface Lift Approaches

- Endoscopic access
  - Similar to the lateral aspect of the endoscopic brow lift but periosteal elevation and release are carried around the infraorbital rim
  - Periosteum suture is suspended to the temporalis fascia
- Intraoral access
  - Subperiosteal dissection of midface via a gingivobuccal sulcus incision
  - Absorbable implant suspends the midface periosteum to the temporalis fascia
  - Implant anchored to the temporalis fascia via a temporal hair-tuft incision
- Lower lid blepharoplasty approach
  - Via transconjunctival incision with lateral canthotomy and inferior cantholysis or subciliary incision
  - Suture or absorbable anchors suspend SMAS to temporalis fascia or lateral orbit
- Deep plane facelift
  - Addresses midface by repositioning malar fat pad superolaterally
- MACS lift
  - Malar loop suspends malar fat pad

Platysmaplasty

- Addresses platysmal banding
- Often performed with submental liposuction and/or direct lipectomy
- Medial borders of the platysma are sutured together down to the hyoid level or lower
- May also divide platysma transversely at the level of the hyoid bone
- Provides additional cervical soft-tissue support before lateral suspension
- Aims to restore normal cervicomental angle of 90 to 105 degrees

Rhytidectomy Complications

- Great auricular nerve injury: Most common nerve to be injured
- Frontal branch and marginal mandibular branch injury: Most common facial nerve branches injured
- Hematoma: Generally within 24 hours of surgery, and more common in males because of increased blood flow to hair follicles
- Pixie (satyr) ear lobe: Because of tension on the lobule of the auricle at the closure secondary to excessive skin resection
- Cobra neck deformity: Because of excessive central neck adipose tissue removal with insufficient removal laterally
- Parotid injury, sialocele
- Alopecia
- Widened scar
- Pigment changes
- First bite syndrome

Rhinoplasty and Septoturbinoplasty (See *Cummings Otolaryngology*, 7th ed., Chapters 29–34)

History Questions for Nasal Surgery

- Nasal trauma or surgery: Use of auricular/costal cartilage or implant
- Nasal sprays
- Effect of Breathe Right strips or nose cones
- Fixed versus variable obstruction
- Unilateral versus bilateral obstruction
- NOSE score to evaluate nasal obstruction

Nasal Subunits

1. Tip
2. Columella

3. Dorsum
4. Sidewalls ×2
5. Alae ×2
6. Soft-tissue facets/triangles ×2

Nasal Landmarks

- Tip defining points: Light reflection from the skin overlying the domes of alar cartilages; excessive distance between points causes boxy/trapezoidal tip
  - Rhinion: Junction of bone and cartilage in the midline of the dorsum, where the skin is thinnest
  - Thin skin at the rhinion means that hump reduction must consider skin thickness and not completely remove the hump or the appearance of a saddle will result once the skin and soft tissue are replaced
  - Skin is thickest in the tip/lower one-third and glabellar region/upper one-third
- Nasion: Midpoint of the nasofrontal suture, which marks the midpoint of the radix, where the upper nose meets the glabella
- Gull-in-flight: Ideal appearance of the nasal tip on frontal view, with columella hanging just inferior to the alar rims
- Supratip break: Just superior to the domal region; helps distinguish the dorsum from the tip; absent in "polly beak" deformity
- Double-break: First break where the tip turns posteroinferiorly onto the infratip lobule; second break at the midcolumella, where the columella takes a more horizontal course and extends posteriorly to the subnasale
- Non-White nose: Thicker and more sebaceous skin, short nasal bones, flatter and broader dorsum, less resilient lateral cartilages, less tip projection, wider alar base that may extend from lacrimal caruncle to lacrimal caruncle, greater alar flare, larger inferior turbinates
  - Classical White nose: Leptorrhine
  - Intermediate nose: Mesorrhine
  - Flatter/broader nose, found in many sub-Saharan Africans: Platyrrhine

Nasal Surgery Considerations

- Thickness of skin soft-tissue envelope
- Straightness of dorsum, smooth brow-dorsum-tip aesthetic line
- Tip support
- Tip projection
- Tip light reflex/symmetry of the nasal tip defining points
- Tip tension with smile
- Dynamic alar/sidewall collapse
- Modified Cottle maneuver to assess obstruction at the internal and external valves
- Columellar show: 2 to 4 mm; differentiate hanging columella from alar retraction
- Ala-to-tip ratio 1:1 when viewed from the side
- Basal view should be triangular, not trapezoid; ratio of the infratip lobule length to the nostril length should be 1:2

Nasofacial Relationships (Fig. 3.10)

- Nasofrontal angle: 115 to 135 degrees
- Nasofacial angle: 30 to 40 degrees, ideally 36 degrees
- Nasolabial angle
  - Males: 90 to 95 degrees
  - Females: 95 to 110 degrees; greater rotation acceptable in shorter women
- Nasomental angle: 120 to 132 degrees

Tip Projection Analysis Methods

1. Simons method: Tip projection to upper-lip length 1:1 ratio
2. Goode method: Tip projection to nasal length 0.55 to 0.6:1 ratio
3. Crumley method: Tip projection, nasal height, and nasal length make a 3-4-5 triangle

Nasal Anatomy

- Three, occasionally four, pairs of turbinates: Erectile tissue wrapped around bony shelves that regulate and humidify airflow
  - Inferior turbinate: Inferior conchal bone separate from the others, nasolacrimal duct drains into inferior meatus
  - Middle turbinate: Part of ethmoid bone; frontal, anterior ethmoid, and maxillary sinuses drain into middle meatus
  - Superior turbinate: Part of ethmoid bone; sphenoid and posterior ethmoid sinuses drain into sphenoethmoidal recess
  - Supreme turbinate: Part of ethmoid bone, not found in all patients
- Septum composed predominantly of cartilage anteriorly, bone posteriorly (Fig. 3.11)
  - Quadrangular cartilage anteriorly (supports the external nose), overlaps bony septum with a long "tail" on one side posteriorly
  - Perpendicular plate of ethmoid bone superoposteriorly, contiguous with skull base at cribiform plate superiorly, occasionally dehiscent
  - Vomer bone posteroinferiorly, often very thin
  - Maxillary crest, a ridge of bone with a trough in it that supports the cartilaginous septum; runs from the anterior to posterior nasal spines
- Lateral cartilages (Fig. 3.12)
  - Upper lateral cartilages (ULCs) articulate with the dorsal quadrangular cartilage medially and the piriform rim laterally, run up underneath the nasal bones for several millimeters, and support the sidewalls of the middle one-third of the external nose
  - Lower lateral cartilages (LLCs) articulate with the ULCs at the "scroll" region, usually overlapping them
    - Lateral crura support the sidewall superior to the alae, which are themselves supported by fibrofatty tissue only
    - Medial crura form the columella
    - Region between medial and lateral crura referred to as "domes" or "intermediate crura," which form the nasal tip
- Tripod model of nasal tip
  - Conjoined medial crura of the LLCs act as the central leg of the tripod and the lateral crura act as the other two legs
  - Manipulating one leg of the tripod will affect the other two legs
- Major nasal tip support elements
  1. Size, shape, and resiliency of the medial/lateral crura of the LLCs
  2. Attachment of medial crural footplates to the caudal margin of the cartilaginous septum
  3. Attachment of the cephalic margins of the LLCs to the caudal borders of the ULCs
- Minor nasal tip support elements
  1. Interdomal ligaments
  2. Dorsal cartilaginous septum
  3. Membranous septum
  4. Skin and subcutaneous tissue
  5. Sesamoid cartilages
  6. Nasal spine

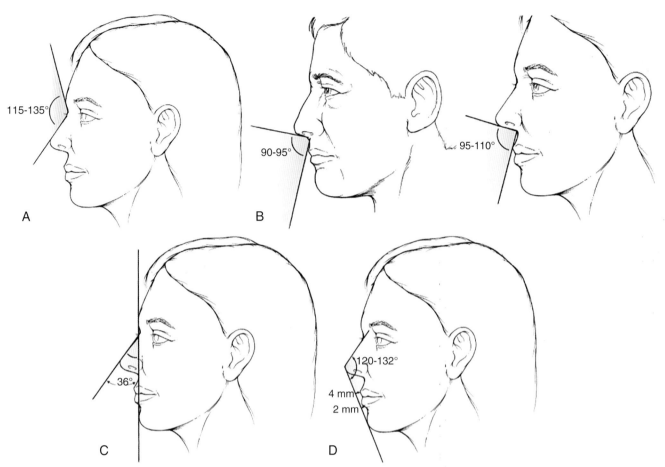

Fig. 3.10 Nasofacial relationships. (**A**) Nasofrontal angle, (**B**) nasolabial angle in men and women, (**C**) nasofacial angle, and (**D**) nasomental angle. (From Flint PW, Haughey BH, Lund VJ, et al. *Cummings Otolaryngology—Head and Neck Surgery.* 7th ed. Philadelphia, PA: Saunders; 2020, Fig. 16.17.)

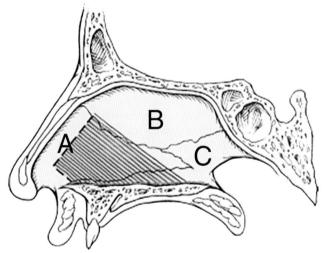

Fig. 3.11 Nasal septal anatomy. (**A**) Quadragular cartilage, (**B**) perpendicular plate of ethmoid, (**C**) vomer. The shaded area indicates the portion of the septum commonly removed during septoplasty; the L-strut remains intact to the left of the dashed line. (From Flint PW, Haughey BH, Lund VJ, et al. *Cummings Otolaryngology—Head and Neck Surgery.* 7th ed. Philadelphia, PA: Saunders; 2020, Fig. 29.17.)

- Nasal valves (Fig. 3.13)
  - Internal nasal valve
    - Bordered by the nasal septum, caudal margin of the ULC, piriform aperture, and face of the inferior turbinate

- Angle of the internal nasal valve is ~15 degrees when septal swell body present; otherwise, 30 to 40 degrees
- Swell body present in ~50% of noses: Thickening under mucosa at dorsal septum due to presence of glandular tissue
- Evaluate with modified Cottle maneuver, using a thin probe, cerumen loop, or similar to stent open the nasal airway gently at different levels to determine location of collapse
- External nasal valve
- Bordered by the caudal edge of the lateral crus of the alar cartilage, the soft-tissue alae, the membranous septum, and the sill of the nostril
- Evaluate by looking for dynamic alar collapse with inspiration

Turbinoplasty Techniques

- Microdebrider debulking of submucosal soft tissue
- Radiofrequency ablation of submucosal soft tissue
- Electrocautery ablation of submucosal soft tissue
- Resection of inferior conchal bone and/or redundant soft tissue
- Partial turbinectomy

Septoplasty Approaches

- Hemitransfixion incision: Made unilaterally through membranous septum at caudal border of quandrangular cartilage

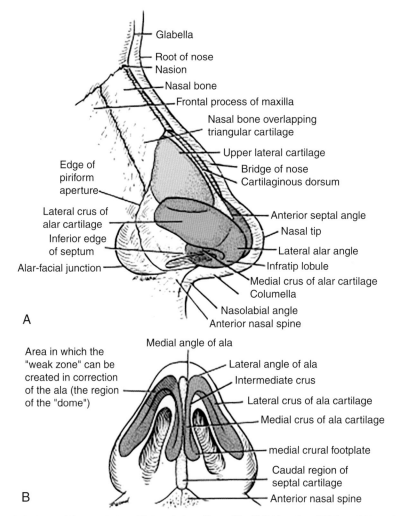

Fig. 3.12 Anatomy of the nasal skeleton. (**A**) Lateral view, (**B**) basal view. (From Flint PW, Haughey BH, Lund VJ, et al. *Cummings Otolaryngology—Head and Neck Surgery.* 7th ed. Philadelphia, PA: Saunders; 2020, Fig. 31.1.)

- Full transfixion incision: Same as hemitransfixion, but through-and-through the septum, often part of tip delivery rhinoplasty or midfacial degloving approaches
- Killian incision: Made posteriorly, just anterior to a spur or other septal deflection that needs to be addressed in the absence of complete septal exposure, often performed endoscopically for improved access for sinus surgery
- Open rhinoplasty approach (see Open Structure Rhinoplasty section)

Septoplasty Considerations

- Critical to leave 10- to 15-mm L-shaped strut of dorsal and caudal quadrangular cartilage intact to maintain support of external nose
- Critical to leave the bony-cartilaginous junction of the dorsal L-strut and perpendicular plate of ethmoid ("keystone area") intact in order to prevent saddle nose deformity
  - Osteotomy of the perpendicular plate of ethmoid inferior to this region may also destabilize the keystone area
- Preferable to leave the bony-cartilaginous junction of the caudal L-strut and the anterior nasal spine/maxillary crest intact to maintain tip support

- Substantial deviations or fractures in the L-strut may require batten grafting (spreader grafts also function as dorsal septal batten grafts)
  - Often best addressed via open rhinoplasty approach
- Cases of severe septal trauma or multiple revision cases may require extracorporeal septoplasty
  - Reconstruct L-strut with extended spreader grafts and caudal septal replacement graft
  - Often requires additional graft material, such as auricular or costal cartilage
- Additional improvement in nasal airway may be obtained by reducing the septal swell body, a collection of submucosal glandular tissue in the area of the internal valve

Septoturbinoplasty Complications

- Recurrent deviation
- Synechiae
- Change in sense of smell
- Hematoma
- Infection
- Septal perforation
- Saddle nose deformity

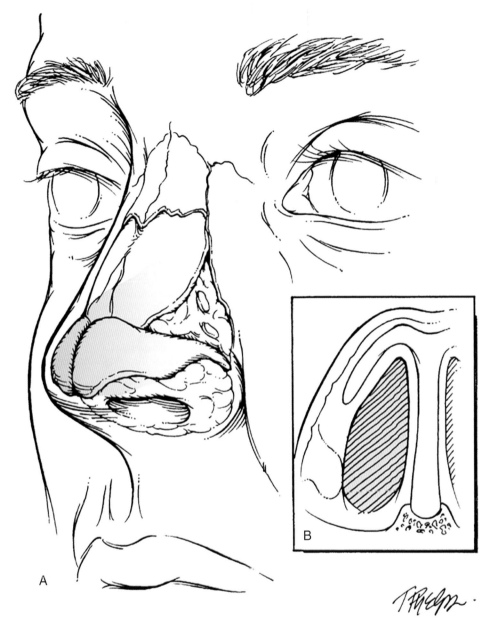

Fig. 3.13 Nasal valves. (A) External, **(B)** internal. (From Flint PW, Haughey BH, Lund VJ, et al. *Cummings Otolaryngology—Head and Neck Surgery*. 7th ed. Philadelphia, PA: Saunders; 2020, Fig. 29.8.)

- Empty nose syndrome, particularly with overly aggressive or repeated turbinoplasty
- Cerebrospinal fluid (CSF) leak

Surgical Techniques for Correction of the Narrow Internal Nasal Valve

- Spreader grafts (Fig. 3.14)
- Flaring sutures
- Butterfly grafts (horizontal spreader grafts)
- Orbital suspension suture
- Lateral batten grafts
- Lateral crural "flip-flop"

Surgical Technique for Correction of External Nasal Valve Collapse

- Alar batten grafts
- Lateral crural strut grafts

- Articulating rim grafts
- Columellar narrowing sutures
- Septoplasty
- Spreading sutures
- Nasal-floor cartilage graft

Functional Nasal Outcome

- In appropriately selected patients:
  - Septal swell body ablation should reduce the NOSE score by ~21 points
  - Turbinoplasty should reduce the NOSE score by ~39 points
  - Septoturbinoplasty should reduce the NOSE score by ~44 points
  - Open septoturbinoplasty with spreader grafts (functional rhinoplasty) should reduce the NOSE score by ~51 points

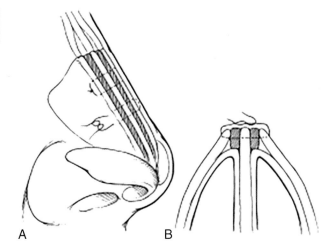

Fig. 3.14 Spreader grafting. (A) Oblique view, (**B**) basal view. (From Flint PW, Haughey BH, Lund VJ, et al. *Cummings Otolaryngology—Head and Neck Surgery*. 7th ed. Philadelphia, PA: Saunders; 2020, Fig. 32.24.)

Methods to Increase Nasal Tip Projection

- Transdomal suturing: Mild increase in projection and no increase to tip support
- Lateral crural steal: Recruits medial aspect of lateral crura into the domes; greater increase in projection and no added tip support
- Tip grafting: onlay graft of autologous cartilage adds more tip definition
- Columellar strut: cartilage graft placed in a pocket between the medial crura; gives the most tip support of all techniques and is often used in combination with other techniques for support; does not need to contact the nasal spine
- Septocolumellar suture: Suspend the medial crura high on the caudal septum, best performed with either a columellar strut or a septal extension graft

Methods to Decrease Nasal Tip Projection

- Full transfixion incision
- Division of interdomal ligaments during open approach rhinoplasty
- Shortening of the medial crura
- Dome division
- Medial crural steal
- Shaving of the dorsal and caudal septum if the cartilaginous septum is excessive on physical examination
- Septocolumellar suture: suspend medial crura low on the caudal septum
- Genioplasty, with implant or osteotomy, can decrease apparent tip projection

Methods to Increase Nasal Tip Rotation

- Cephalic trims of the LLCs
  - Excise a portion of the bilateral cephalic margins of the lateral crura of the alar cartilages
  - 6- to 8-mm residual strip should be left for tip and alar support
  - Incomplete remaining strips of the lateral crura will further increase tip rotation
- Tongue-in-groove suture the caudal septum between medial crura
- Suspend the cephalic margins of the lateral crura of the LLCs onto the ULCs in a more cephalad position than that of the natural scroll region

Methods to Decrease Nasal Tip Rotation

- Septal extension graft
- Extended spreader grafts

Methods to Refine the Nasal Tip

- Transdomal sutures
- Dome division
- Excision of subcutaneous tissue
- Shield and cap grafting
- Cephalic trim, leaving 7- to 9-mm width of intact lateral crura
- Cephalic turn-in flaps (cephalic trim but with folding cephalic aspect of the lateral crura underneath the remaining strip rather than removing it; this helps to reinforce the lateral crura and remove irregular curvatures)

Methods to Address Asymmetric Tip

- Asymmetric interdomal sutures may recreate symmetry
- Asymmetric intradomal sutures may help
- Shield grafting or crushed-cartilage camouflage grafting
- Lateral crural strut grafting (on deep surface of the lateral crura of the LLCs)
- Cephalic turn-in flaps
- Lateral crural "flip-flop" division and reversal of lateral crura

Methods to Correct Wide Nasal Base

- Weir excisions: Wedge excisions in alar-facial grooves
- Nasal sill excisions: Maintain the natural curvature of nostrils, avoid alar-facial webbing, and may cause step-off deformity in the nasal sill
- Cinching stitch: Permanent suture placed via the gingivobuccal sulcus

Methods to Correct Caudal Septal Deflection

- Excise deviated portion if quadrangular cartilage is too long
- Replace the caudal septum with a septal extension graft
- Tongue-in-groove suture with or without cartilage scoring
- Swinging-door technique
- Extended spreader grafts/septal batten grafts

Methods to Address Crooked Nose

- Septoplasty
- Spreader grafts if midvault/internal valve obstruction is present
- Onlay camouflage graft for solely cosmetic purposes
- Osteotomies to straighten or narrow the upper one-third
- Dorsal septotomy of perpendicular plate of ethmoid when standard osteotomies are insufficient

Osteotomy Considerations

- To alter width of upper vault, begin with lateral osteotomy on the concave side and then ipsilateral medial osteotomy, contralateral medial osteotomy, and contralateral lateral osteotomy
- If the dorsal hump has been removed, shorter medial osteotomies will suffice
- To mobilize bones back toward midline with the upper vault intact (no narrowing or widening required), perform lateral osteotomies and transverse root osteotomy
- Intermediate osteotomy may be required if nasal bone widths are significantly asymmetric (often the case if the nose is deviated)—perform before lateral osteotomy on that side

- Intranasal approach requires no external incisions and can be used to push out concave bone segments but causes continuous osteotomies, which may lead to less stable bone fragments
- Percutaneous osteotomies
  - 2-mm osteotome through one to two stab incisions per side permits "postage stamp" lateral, transverse, and intermediate osteotomies that cause minimal periosteal and mucosal trauma, and have an irregular osteotomy line, which helps prevent flail bone fragments

Endonasal Approaches to Rhinoplasty

- Nondelivery
  - Good for minor irregularities, revisions with camouflage grafting
  - Addresses dorsal irregularities, such as a hump
  - Less tip support disruption, more control of healing/scarring
  - Permits osteotomies and spreader grafting in the absence of major asymmetries
  - Via intercartilaginous incisions, disrupts scroll region
- Delivery
  - Additionally allows for manipulation of the tip
  - Less edema than occurs with an open approach
  - Via intercartilaginous-full transfixion and marginal-lateral columellar incisions

Open Structure Rhinoplasty

- Maximal exposure
- Significant postoperative edema
- Disrupts tip support with violation of interdomal ligaments
- Provides access to correct deviations/fractures of L-strut and major asymmetry of tip
- Common approach in major revision and reconstruction cases
- Via transcolumellar and marginal incisions

Rhinoplasty Incisions

- Intercartilaginous: Made at the internal nasal valve between the upper cartilages and LLCs; suboptimal healing may lead to nasal obstruction
- Intracartilaginous: Parallel to the lateral crus cephalic border, 2 to 6 mm closer to the nostril opening, incising through the LLC and removing a 3- to 5-mm strip of cartilage as a cephalic trim; lowers the risk of nasal valve stenosis
- Marginal: Follows the caudal border of the LLC, not the alar rim
- Transcolumellar: For open approach, use an inverted-V incision and make sure to connect with the marginal incisions at right angles

Graft Material Options

- Septal cartilage
- Auricular cartilage
- Autologous rib cartilage (sixth or seventh rib): May be calcified in adults and tends to warp; must soak the graft to allow warping to occur before placement; consider cutting the graft into layers and laminating it before placement or cutting the grafts obliquely across the cartilage to reduce warping
- Split calvarial bone: Outer table harvested from nearly flat parietal skull ipsilateral to the dominant hand; inner table is left intact
- Cadaveric rib cartilage and bone: May have a higher potential for resorption than autologous materials
- Gore-Tex: Allows tissue ingrowth and provides support

- Silicone: Forms a capsule, does not allow tissue ingrowth, high rate of extrusion and chronic infection
- For nonstructural grafts, temporalis fascia and acellular dermis (Alloderm) work well to camouflage contour irregularities

Methods to Address Septal Perforation

- Silastic button
- Local flaps, bipedicled with cartilage or Alloderm graft interposed between mucoperichondrial flaps
  - Releasing incisions may be made superior and inferior, taking care not to oppose the releasing incisions
  - Tissue expander placement may increase available tissue for advancement
- Regional flaps, including the inferior turbinate (usually anteriorly pedicled), pericranium, gingivobuccal sulcus mucosa, and facial artery musculomucosal flap; may require a second stage to divide the interpolated pedicle
- Free flap, such as fascia-only radial forearm: Access via an external rhinoplasty approach or midfacial degloving

Rhinoplasty Complications of the Upper Third of the Nose

- Rocker deformity: Phenomenon in which depressing the nasal bones to narrow the upper vault results in lateral displacement of the superior aspect of the bony fragments because the osteotomies continued too high into the radix, past the nasion, where the bone begins to flare laterally
- Step deformity: Step-off between the nasal bones and maxilla after osteotomy usually due to overly medial placement of a lateral osteotomy rather than in the nasofacial junction
- Open-roof deformity: Midline defect of nasal bones, commonly caused by dorsal hump reduction in the absence of subsequent osteotomies or onlay grafting to close the defect

Rhinoplasty Complications of the Middle Third of the Nose

- Inverted-V deformity: The caudal margins of the nasal bones become visible due to collapse of the ULCs, commonly caused by disarticulation of the ULCs from the dorsal septum or the nasal bones
- Saddle nose: Concave bowing of the midvault because of insufficient strength of the dorsal septal strut (often due to fractures or failure to leave adequate L-strut width intact) or disarticulation of the keystone region
- Parenthesis deformity: Visible caudal margins of cephalically malpositioned lateral crura of the LLCs
- Polly beak deformity: Excessive supratip fullness associated with tip deprojection and ptosis

Saddle Nose Deformity Characteristics

- Surgical correction for patients without obstruction: Onlay grafting
- With obstruction: Replace part or all of septal L-strut with extended spreader grafts and caudal septal replacement graft; may require rib or split calvarial bone
- Aim to restore middle vault function, reverse internal valve narrowing, reinforce nasal tip and dorsal support mechanisms

Causes of Saddle Nose Deformities

- Traumatic
- Iatrogenic
- Granulomatosis with polyangiitis (Wegener granulomatosis)
- Relapsing polychondritis
- Leprosy (Hansen disease)

- Syphilis
- Ectodermal dysplasia
- Intranasal cocaine

Causes of Polly Beak Deformity

- Over-resection of the bony dorsum
- Under-resection of the cartilaginous dorsum
- High cartilaginous hump at the anterior septal angle
- Over-resection of alar cartilages, leading to loss of tip support and ptosis
- Dead space between the dorsal nasal skin and the nasal skeleton; scar tissue will fill this space and produce supratip fullness

Rhinoplasty Complications of the Lower Third of the Nose

- Malrotation
- Malprojection
- Bossae: Knuckling at the domes, showing through skin
- Pinched tip: Overtightening of interdomal sutures distorts domes and eliminates natural tip bifidity
- Alar retraction due to excessive cephalic trimming

HANGING COLUMELLA RESULTS FROM FAILURE TO REDUCE OVERLY LONG CAUDAL SEPTAL CARTILAGE

Otoplasty (See *Cummings Otolaryngology*, 7th ed., Chapter 28, Fig. 28.1)

Auricular Subunits (Fig. 3.15)

- Helix
  - Crus helicis (root of helix) divides the cymba and the cavum conchae
- Antihelix
  - Superior/posterior crus
  - Anterior/inferior crus
- Darwin's tubercle
- Fossa triangularis (bounded by the antihelical crura and the helix)
- Tragus
- Antitragus
- Intertragal incisura (divides the tragus and the antitragus)
- Scapha (scaphoid fossa)

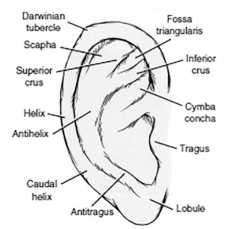

Fig. 3.15 Auricular surface anatomy. (From Flint PW, Haughey BH, Lund VJ, et al. *Cummings Otolaryngology—Head and Neck Surgery.* 7th ed. Philadelphia, PA: Saunders; 2020, Fig. 28.1.p.)

- Conchal bowl
  - Cymba concha; superior to the crus helicis
  - Cavum concha; inferior to the crus helicis, contiguous with the external auditory meatus
- Lobule

Auricular Embryology: Hillocks of His

- Hillocks of first pharyngeal arch:
  1. Tragus
  2. Root of helix
  3. Helix
- Hillocks of second pharyngeal arch:
  1. Superior antihelix
  2. Inferior antihelix
  3. Lobule
- This concept has been reinvestigated numerous times over the years with varying results relating hillocks to terminal structures and questioning the validity of the hillock model itself
- Interruption of development at week 6 leads to microtia

Auricular Proportions

- Ratio of auricular width to height: 1:2
- Auricular height 60 to 65 mm
  - Height roughly equal to nasal height
- Superior margin of the helical rim at the brow level
- Inferior margin of the lobule at the nasal ala level
- Superior pole rotated posteriorly 15 degrees
- Auriculocephalic angle, 20 to 30 degrees
  - 10 to 12 mm from the helix to the mastoid at the superior pole
  - 16 to 18 mm from the helix to the mastoid at the midauricle
  - 20 mm from the lobule to the mastoid at the superior lobule

Indications for Otoplasty

- Prominauris
  - "Lop ear" deformity resulting from antihelical-fold deficiency
  - "Cup ear" deformity because of conchal bowl excess
- Stahl's ear
  - Third, more superoposterior antihelical crus causes pointed, unfurled superior helix
  - Difficult to correct
  - May require wedge or star-shaped resection
- Outstanding lobule
  - Prominent cauda helicis
  - Often exacerbated by placement of Mustardé and Furnas sutures
  - Addressed with resection or weakening of the cauda helicis
  - Posterior suture fixation to the conchal bowl may help rotate the lobule inferomedially
- Cryptotia
  - Superior aspect of auricular cartilage buried under skin
- Ear Molding
  - In neonates with sufficient cartilage, auricular molding initiated before 3 to 6 weeks of life can provide a normal contour
- Typically, three visits separated by 2 weeks are required to place and adjust the apparatus, with end result at 6 weeks

Mustardé Sutures

- Used to create an antihelical fold

- Horizontal mattress sutures 15 mm anteroposteriorly × 10 mm superoinferiorly
- 2 mm between sutures, usually three or four sutures in total
- May be placed percutaneously without a postauricular incision

Furnas Sutures

- Shaving or resection of cartilage in the conchal bowl and resection of postauricular soft tissue allows retrodisplacement of the auricle and suspension to the mastoid periosteum, usually three sutures

Otoplasty Complications

- Hematoma: Typically within 24 hours of surgery
- Perichondritis
- Infection
- Asymmetry: >3 mm of difference
- Telephone ear deformity or reverse telephone ear caused by overtightening of the central Furnas suture relative to the superior and inferior sutures, or the reverse
- External auditory meatus stenosis: Caused by medialization of the auricle with Furnas sutures without retrodisplacement
- Hidden helix: Overtightening of the Mustardé sutures such that the antihelix becomes the most prominent and lateral feature of the auricle in the frontal view rather than the helical rim
- Outstanding lobule: Occurs when the cauda helicis is prominent but the antihelix and concha are addressed by Mustardé and Furnas sutures, medializing the rest of the auricle but leaving the lobule in a lateral position
- Hypesthesia
- Cold sensitivity
- Prolonged pain: Auricles are often tender and sore for several months after otoplasty
- Suture extrusion or granuloma: Late complication

Microtia Repair Considerations (See *Cummings Otolaryngology*, 7th ed., Chapter 195)

- 85% of auricular growth is complete by age 3 to 4 years
- Repair best undertaken at age 10 years or older so that the patient can participate in care and has sufficient costal cartilage to construct an auricular skeleton
- Canal atresia repair undertaken after microtia repair to avoid disruption of blood supply before auricular reconstructive surgery

Marx Classification of Microtia

- Grade 1: Most subunits present, although decreased in size
- Grade 2 (conchal type): Lobule and helical remnant is present
- Grade 3 (lobular type): "Peanut ear," with lobule and cartilage remnant present (most common)
- Grade 4: Anotia, no external structures present
- Microtia more common on the right side
  - May be associated with hemifacial microsomia, Goldenhar syndrome

Brent Microtia Repair Technique (4 Stages)

1. Construction and placement of costal cartilage construct: Taken from synchondrosis of the contralateral ribs six and seven, with the eighth rib cartilage used for the helical rim
2. Lobule transposition: Modified Z-plasty used to transfer the "peanut" remnant from the anterior vertical position to the

inferior horizontal position; cartilage is removed from the remnant at this time
3. Elevation of auricle: a split-thickness skin graft (STSG) from the groin is used to create the postauricular sulcus and a previously harvest piece of ninth rib cartilage is used as a wedge for elevation
4. Tragal reconstruction: Contralateral conchal bowl composite graft and postauricular skin graft taken to create tragus and line conchal bowl

Nagata Microtia Repair Technique (2 Stages)

1. Construction and placement of costal cartilage construct, from ipsilateral ribs six to nine, which includes a tragus carved from costal cartilage, and simultaneous lobule transposition
2. Elevation of the auricle and placement of a pedicled TPF flap along with STSG, which may be harvested from the shaved parietal scalp, in continuity with the full-thickness skin overlying the costal cartilage construct

Microtia Repair With Porous Polyethylene Implantation

- Implant use avoids costal cartilage harvesting and carving; higher rate of extrusion
- Requires a two-stage procedure: placement and elevation
- TPF flap may be used to improve vascularity

Auricular Prostheses for Microtia

- May be secured with adhesive or via osseointegrated implants and magnets
- May require two prostheses if patients have fair skin that changes color significantly between spring/summer and fall/winter
- Wear out over time
- Adhesive attachment good for poor surgical candidates

Complications of Microtia Repair

- Skin breakdown and cartilage erosion
  - Typically at the superior helical rim
  - May require multiple revisions
  - TPF flap and STSG coverage of exposed cartilage as soon as possible
- Migration of implant or costal cartilage, particularly anteroinferiorly onto the cheek
- Hairy ear because of low hairline and placement of an implant or construct under hair-bearing scalp; treat with laser hair removal

RECONSTRUCTIVE SURGERY

Reconstructive Options (See *Cummings Otolaryngology*, 7th ed., Chapter 77)

The Reconstructive Ladder

1. Wound healing by secondary intention: allows granulation tissue to fill a defect, may require prosthesis later
2. Primary closure
3. Delayed primary closure: allows granulation tissue to progress until the area is sufficiently well vascularized to permit operative closure
4. Skin graft
5. Tissue expansion
6. Local flap
7. Regional flap
8. Free flap
9. Composite tissue allograft (face transplantation)

Phases of Primary Wound Healing

Phase	Duration	Activity
Hemostatic	0–2 hours	• Vasoconstriction • Coagulation
Inflammatory	0–4 days	• Infiltration of neutrophils, macrophages, fibroblasts
Proliferative	4 days–2 weeks	• Re-epithelialization • Neovascularization • Collagen deposition (type III) • Wound contraction by myofibroblasts
Maturation	2 weeks–2 years	• Type I collagen replaces type III • Increase in tensile strength
		• 3 weeks: 15% of original tensile strength • 6 weeks: 60% of original tensile strength • ≥6 months: maximum tensile strength = 70%–80% of original

Factors That Compromise Wound Healing

- Local factors
  - Infection, desiccation, hematoma, neoplasm, contamination, and radiation
  - Vascular insufficiency
    - No-reflow phenomenon: Flow within macroscopic vessels has been established, but capillary and interstitial flow is blocked, leading to flap compromise
    - Reperfusion injury: Histologic injury due to circulating inflammatory mediators and reactive oxygen species after periods of ischemia
- Systemic factors
  - Malnutrition, metabolic derangement, vasculopathy, smoking, connective tissue disorders, and immunodeficiency
- Medications
  - Steroids, nonsteroidal antiinflammatory drugs, chemotherapy, and immunosuppressive agents
- Technical errors
  - Traumatic technique, closure under tension, and poor hemostasis

Factors That Improve Wound Healing

- Hyperbaric oxygen (increases oxygen-carrying capacity by 20%)
- Nutritional supplementation
- Metabolic optimization, for example, management of hypothyroidism or diabetes
- Debridement of contaminants and nonviable tissue
- Appropriate dressings

Phases of Skin Graft Healing

1. Plasmatic imbibition
2. Capillary inosculation
3. Neovascularization

Split-Thickness Skin Grafting

- Epidermis and partial-thickness dermis
- Poor color and texture match
- Significant contracture
- More reliable healing than FTSG
- May remain insensate and dry
- Harvested with dermatome, often from thigh, upper arm, back, or scalp

Full-Thickness Skin Grafting

- Epidermis and full-thickness dermis
- Better color and texture match
- Less contracture
- Lower success rate compared with STSG
- Likely to develop sensory innervation and sebaceous function, possibly hair growth
- Harvested with scalpel, often from groin, post/preauricular, and supraclavicular

Composite Grafting

- Full-thickness skin and cartilage
- Graft size >1.5 cm leads to vascular compromise and poor healing
- Often harvested from helical root or cymba concha

Histological Changes From Tissue Expansion

- Increased vascularity leads to potential for increased flap length-to-width ratio
- Epidermis thickens
- Dermis thins
- Subcutaneous fat thins
- Muscle thins
- Fibrous capsule with vascular network develops (adds tensile strength to wound)
- Underlying bone may resorb and scallop

Internal Tissue Expansion

- Silastic balloon with resealable injection port for normal saline; use before tissue is resected
- May be used briefly during surgery (for 20 minutes) to augment skin creep
- Make incisions for expander placement along the margins of the planned excision
  - Avoid disrupting major blood vessels or cutaneous nerves
  - May leave sutures in place for the duration of the expansion
- Fill 10% of the expander's volume at time of surgery
- Add volume as tolerated 1 to 2 times/week for 6 to 8 weeks
  1. Pain level and stress relaxation determine frequency of expansion
  2. Begin expansion 10 to 14 days after surgery
  3. Wound dehiscence is not an absolute contraindication to further expansion; however, further expansion may serve only to widen the dehiscence
  4. Plan to produce 10% more expanded tissue than needed to cover the base of the defect

External Tissue Expansion

- Skin anchors, purse-string line, and tension controller reels apply tension to approximate the wound edge

- Use after tissue is resected and the wound is open
- Tension controller does not require additional patient visits to increase tension
- Serial excision is another example of external tissue expansion

Biological Principles of Tissue Expansion

- Skin creep: When a constant tension is applied, skin lengthens by stretching collagen fibers and displacing interstitial fluid
- Stress relaxation: When stretched to a constant length, tensile force on skin required to maintain that length decreases over time

Local Flaps (See *Cummings Otolaryngology*, 7th ed., Chapter 21; Fig. 3.16)

- Random
- Blood supplied via the subdermal plexus
- Length depends on the intravascular resistance of the supplying vessels and the perfusion pressure
- Axial
  - Perfusion comes from a named vessel
  - Length-to-width ratio of the flap may exceed 4:1

Advancement Flaps

- Tissue slides to close the defect
- Undermining >4 cm will not further decrease closing tension
- Length-to-width ratio should not exceed 4:1 in order to preserve perfusion
- May align incisions in RSTLs
- Unipedicle
- Bipedicle
- V to Y and Y to V (see Scar Revision section)
- O to H: Bilateral advancement to close a defect using back cuts to recruit tissue from the sides in order to avoid extending the defect vertically to reduce standing cutaneous deformities, often used superior to eyebrow
- A to T: Bilateral advancement–rotation advancement that aids restoration of facial subunit boundaries, such as the vermilion border or temporal hairline
- Subcutaneously pedicled island

Rotation Flap

- Tissue pivots around a point
- Increasing arc of rotation to >90 degrees will not further decrease closing tension
- Flap rotation decreases the effective length
  - Rotating a flap by 45 degrees reduces length by 5%
  - Rotating a flap by 90 degrees reduces length by 15%
  - Rotating a flap by 180 degrees reduces length by 40%
- Standing cutaneous deformity will occur at the base of the flap: Burow's triangle excision is required
- Difficult to align in RSTLs
- O to Z
  - Dual advancement–rotation flaps allow closure of a circular defect, usually scalp
  - Three flaps may be used if necessary
- Rieger dorsal nasal flap: For reconstruction of midnasal dorsal defects up to 2 cm
- Tenzel semicircular flap: For reconstruction of eyelid defects up to 50% of eyelid width; may require periosteal release for larger defects

Transposition Flaps

- Also pivots around a point and creates a standing cutaneous cone
- Length of random transposition flap should not exceed 3 times its width
- Difficult to align in RSTLs
  - Rhombic (Fig. 3.17)
  - Limberg described the classic rhombic flap
  - Uses a rhombus with 120-degree and 60-degree angles
  - Rotates flap through 60 degrees
- Dufourmentel modification
  - Variable angles within a rhombus
  - Variable arc of rotation
  - Spares more tissue
- Note flap
  - Variant of rhombic flap to close a circular defect
- Bilobe (Fig. 3.18)
  - Zitelli modification
    - Rotation through 90 degrees instead of 180 degrees
    - First lobe is equal to the size of the defect or slightly smaller if the skin is sufficiently elastic
    - Second lobe is smaller than the first
    - Good for repair of nasal defects <1.5 cm; base flap laterally on nose when possible
    - Also good for lateral cheek defects up to 6 cm
- Z-plasty (see Scar Revision section)

Interpolated Flaps

- Flap is advanced and/or rotated over normal tissue
- Requires a second stage to divide the pedicle and complete the inset of the flap
- Melolabial flap: Good for reconstruction of the medial cheek and nasal alar defects
- Hughes tarsoconjunctival flap
  - Tarsal plate and conjunctiva of the upper eyelid are used to reconstruct 50% to 100% of the defect in the lower lid
  - Requires advancement of skin from cheek
- Cutler-Beard flap: Full-thickness advancement of the lower eyelid into 50% to 100% of an upper eyelid defect
- Many interpolated flaps can also be characterized as regional or axial

Hinge Flap

- Trapdoor, turn-in, turn-down flaps
- Flap is flipped, turned over, so that epithelial surface provides internal lining of a facial defect, most commonly the nose
- Requires coverage of exposed subcutaneous surface by a second flap

Local Axial Flap Examples

- Temporoparietal fascia flap
  - Based on the superficial temporal artery
  - Good for providing bulk or a barrier in the face or auricle: Used for temporal wasting, microtia, and Frey syndrome
- Karapandzic flap
  - Based on labial arteries
  - May reconstruct up to two-third of the lip width
  - Oral sphincter function is preserved
  - Produces microstomia
- Gillies fan and McGregor flaps
  - Based on labial arteries
  - May reconstruct full lip defects of the lower (Gillies) and upper (McGregor) lips

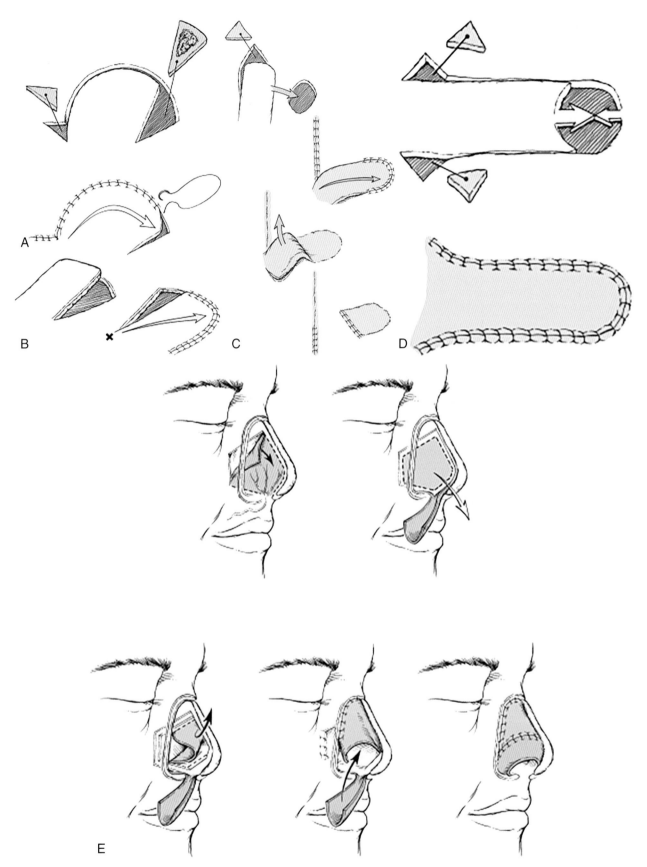

Fig. 3.16 Types of local flaps. (**A**) Rotation flap, (**B**) transposition flap, (**C**) interpolated flap, (**D**) advancement flap, and (**E**) hinge flap. (From Flint PW, Haughey BH, Lund VJ, et al. *Cummings Otolaryngology—Head and Neck Surgery*. 7th ed. Philadelphia, PA: Saunders; 2020, Figs. 21.3, 21.4, 21.5, 21.6, and 21.13.)

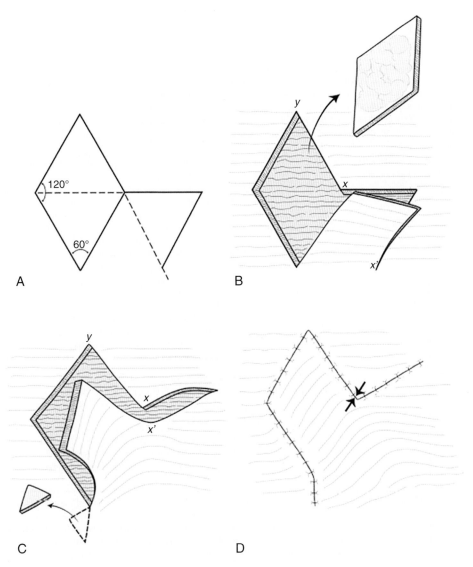

Fig. 3.17 (**A**) Limberg rhombic flap design; (**B**) defect is modified, thus configuration is 60- to 120-degree rhombus; (**C**) flap transposed, standing cutaneous deformity excised; (**D**) primary vector of tension is approximately parallel to the original border of the defect adjacent to the flap (*opposing arrows*); standing cutaneous deformity excised at base of flap. (From *Baker SR. Local Flaps in Facial Reconstruction*. 4th ed. Philadelphia, PA: Saunders Elsevier; 2022, Fig. 11.2.)

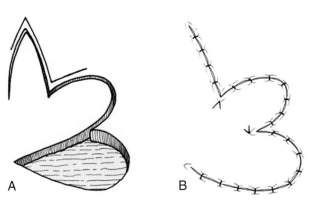

Fig. 3.18 Bilobe flap. (**A**) Bilobe flap incisions. Note the acute angle at the left of the defect; this is where the standing cutaneous deformity would occur. (**B**) Flap transposed and defect closed. (From *Baker SR. Local Flaps in Facial Reconstruction*. 4th ed. Philadelphia, PA: Saunders Elsevier; 2022, Fig. 10.1.)

Regional Flap Examples

Regional Flap	Arterial Supply	Indications
Deltopectoral	Second, third, fourth perforators of internal mammary	• Anterior and lower neck cutaneous defects • Distal tip can have random-pattern supply, be higher risk for necrosis
Facial artery musculomucosal (FAMM)	Facial artery branches (anterograde or retrograde flow)	• Intraoral defects • Intranasal defects
Latissimus dorsi	Thoracodorsal	• Myofascial or myocutaneous • Defects of neck and lower face • Preferable in women to avoid breast deformation from pectoralis flap harvest
Lip switch	Labial	• Abbé flap • Reconstruction of full-thickness lip defects not involving commissure • Flap width 50% of defect width • Rotates through 180 degrees • May reconstruct up to 50% of lip width • Requires second procedure at 3+ weeks to divide pedicle
		Estlander flap • For defects involving oral commissure • Blunts oral commissure • Does not require a procedure to divide the pedicle • Secondary commissuroplasty may be performed
Paramedian forehead	Supratrochlear (located 15–20 mm lateral to midline)	• Nasal tip defects >1.5 cm Supratrochlear artery can perfuse a similarly oriented pericranial flap for internal nasal use for septal perforation or mucosal reconstruction
Pectoralis major myocutaneous	Thoracoacromial	• Myofascial or myocutaneous • Muscle coverage of neck, vessels • Epithelial reconstruction of pharynx, esophagus, defects of anterior neck
Submental island	Submental	• May be harvested with anterograde or retrograde flow, or as a free flap • May include platysma or just skin and subcutaneous tissue • Floor-of-mouth and intra-oral defects
Supraclavicular island	Supraclavicular	• Fascia-only or fasciocutaneous • Pharyngeal/esophageal defects • Cutaneous defects of neck and lower face • Tissue coverage of neck structures

Free Flap Examples (See *Cummings Otolaryngology*, 7th ed., Chapter 78)

Flap	Vascular Supply	Nerve	Indications
Anterolateral thigh (ALT)	Septocutaneous/musculocutaneous perforators of lateral circumflex femoral artery, venae comitantes	Lateral femoral cutaneous	• Fasciocutaneous /myocutaneous • Skin (up to 20 × 30 cm) and subcutaneous tissue + varying amounts of vastus lateralis muscle
Deep inferior epigastric perforator (DIEP)	Deep inferior epigastric artery perforators, deep and superior epigastric veins	Sensory branches of 10th/11th intercostals	• Fasciocutaneous • No muscle
Fibula	Peroneal artery, venae comitantes	Lateral sural cutaneous	• Osseous/osteocutaneous • Mandible/maxilla reconstruction • Can include up to 30 cm of bone depending on patient height • Leave 6 cm of bone intact distally to stabilize ankle and proximally to protect common peroneal nerve (injury causes foot drop) • Preoperative angiography to confirm "3-vessel runoff" perfusion of foot • Bone stock suitable for dental implants

Flap	Vascular Supply	Nerve	Indications
Iliac crest	Deep circumflex iliac artery and vein	—	• Osseous/osteocutaneous/osteomyocutanous • Up to 8 × 18 cm of bone (suitable for dental implants) • Harvest can cause hernia and gait disturbance
Jejunum	Superior mesenteric artery and vein	—	• Esophagopharyngeal reconstruction • May never develop vascular independence from pedicle • Poor tolerance of ischemia (<2 hours) • Inherent peristalsis requires appropriate orientation during flap inset • Monitor paddle can help flap evaluation in early postoperative period
Latissimus dorsi	Thoracodorsal, vena comitans	Thoracodorsal	• Myocutaneous/myofascial • Long pedicle (up to 15 cm) • Significant amount of broad, pliable soft tissue • Full-scalp reconstruction
Radial forearm	Radial artery, vena comitantes and cephalic vein	Lateral antebrachial cutaneous	• Fasciocutaneous • May include all of forearm skin except that overlying the ulnar artery • May include up to 60% of the thickness of the radius (poor bone stock for dental implants) • May include palmaris longus tendon for facial suspension (e.g., lower lip) • Preoperative Allen's test (avoid devascularization of the hand)
Scapular/parascapular	Circumflex scapular artery and vein	—	• Osseous/osteocutaneous/fasciocutaneous • Can be harvested with latissimus dorsi as "mega flap" for greater soft-tissue coverage based on subscapular artery (above bifurcation of circumflex scapular and thoracodorsal arteries) • Usually cannot support dental implants

Complications of Free Tissue Transfer

- Venous congestion most common (8%–14% rate)
- 80% of flaps can be salvaged if compromise is recognized soon enough
  - If perfusion is restored within 6 hours, salvage rate is 75%
  - 80% of vessel compromise is venous, and 80% will occur in first 48 hours
    - Corresponds to timeline for re-endothelialization of vessels
    - Angioneogenesis generally sufficient to make flap independent of original pedicle by 2 to 3 weeks
  - 90% of arterial compromise will occur in first 24 hours
- Hematoma second most common, can apply pressure and compromise vessels (5.6%–11 7% rate)
- Infection
- Fistula

Composite Tissue Allografts (Facial Transplantation)

- Type I: Lower central face, including the nose, lips, and chin
- Type II: Midface, including the nose, upper lip, and cheeks (soft tissue with or without maxilla)
- Type III: Upper face, including the forehead, eyelids, and root of the nose
- Type IV: Total facial skin
- Type V: Full face, including complete soft tissue, with or without maxilla and/or mandible
- Most commonly performed for trauma in patients who have undergone multiple prior reconstructive procedures
- Entire graft may be perfused via a single facial artery

- Sensory function returns even without trigeminal neurorrhaphy
- Motor coordination is improved (less synkinesis) with distal facial branch neurorrhaphies rather than main trunk neurorrhaphy
  - Results are comparable to or better than homograft neural reconstruction, likely because of tacrolimus
- Full face transplant may provide a better aesthetic result than partial transplant, but if the graft fails, the consequences are worse
  - Acute rejection is very common (~100%), but generally manageable
  - Chronic rejection is less common, but may lead to transplant failure
- Risk of death from cancer and infection after transplantation high due to immunosuppression
  - Facial transplantation has been performed in 40 patients to date worldwide with 8 total deaths, although not all were directly attributable to transplantation
- Because the operation is uncommon and still being developed, it is nearly impossible to obtain true informed consent

Cleft Lip (See *Cummings Otolaryngology*, 7th ed., Chapter 188)

Upper Lip Subunits

1. Philtrum dimple
2. Philtral columns
3. Melolabial folds
4. Cupid's bow
5. Vermilion border

Perioral Proportions (Fig. 3.19)

- Upper to lower lip height 1:2
- Line drawn from the menton to the nasal tip: Upper lip lies 4 mm posterior; lower lip lies 2 mm posterior
- Zero meridian of Gonzalez-Ulloa (perpendicular to the Frankfort plane; runs from the nasion to the pogonion): the mentolabial sulcus lies 4 mm posterior

Perioral Abnormalities

- Types of lip clefts
  - Bilateral and unilateral
  - Complete: Through the nasal sill
    - Often associated with defect of alveolar ridge
  - Incomplete: Simonart's band remains intact
    - Incomplete clefts have a band of tissue bridging the gap across the cleft at the nasal sill; it contains only skin and mucosa, no functional muscle
- More common on the left than on the right, 2:1
- More common in males than in females
- Risk of second child with a cleft lip/palate after the first is affected: 4%
- Most common syndrome with cleft lip/palate: Van der Woude, characterized by lower-lip pits
- 70% of isolated cleft lips are nonsyndromic

Cleft Lip Anatomy and Embryology

- Paired medial nasal and maxillary prominences fuse to form the lip at 6 to 7 weeks of development
- Incomplete orbicularis oris sphincter: Muscle parallels cleft margin and inserts into the nasal sill
- Anterior septum deviated toward the noncleft side and posterior septum deviated toward the cleft

- Nasal tip and base of columella deviate away from the cleft
- Nostril on the cleft side is flattened and stretched inferiorly, posteriorly, and laterally
- LLCs are the same length, but medial crus on cleft side is relatively shorter and the dome is flatter

Cleft Lip Rule of 10 s

1. Repair when child weighs 10 lb
2. Child is 10 weeks old
3. Child has a hemoglobin of ≥10 mg/dL

Cleft Lip Surgical Considerations

- Preoperative care may improve surgical results
  - Lip adhesion of the superior aspect of the cleft may help narrow the soft-tissue defect
  - Lip taping also acts as a tissue expander to help narrow the cleft preoperatively
  - Presurgical nasoalveolar molding may also improve nasal morphology
- Millard advancement–rotation technique most common for unilateral cleft lip (Fig. 3.20)
  - Reconstructs the philtral column and Cupid's bow
  - Rotation of tissue from the noncleft side and advancement from the cleft side
  - Important to reconstruct the orbicularis oris
    - Insufficient approximation of the orbicularis sphincter causes a notch in the vermilion ("whistle deformity")

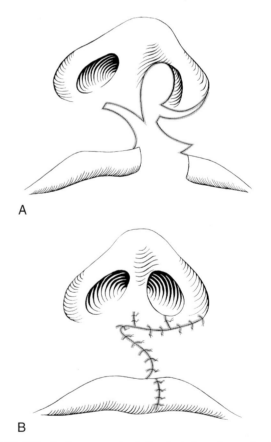

Fig. 3.20 Millard advancement-rotation technique for repair of unilateral cleft lip. (**A**) Rotation-advancement technique: flaps incised and elevated. (**B**) Rotation-advancement technique: final suturing. (From Flint PW, Haughey BH, Lund VJ, et al. *Cummings Otolaryngology—Head and Neck Surgery.* 7th ed. Philadelphia, PA: Saunders; 2016, Figs. 188.22 and 188.23.)

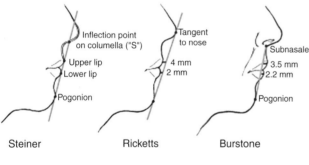

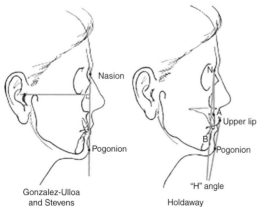

Fig. 3.19 Perioral proportions. (From Flint PW, Haughey BH, Lund VJ, et al. *Cummings Otolaryngology—Head and Neck Surgery.* 7th ed. Philadelphia, PA: Saunders; 2020, Fig. 27.5.)

- Other repairs include the Skoog, Noordhoff, and Fisher subunit repair techniques
- Repair of bilateral lip clefts results in better symmetry, but achieving columellar length and nasal tip projection is more difficult
- Primary rhinoplasty is often performed at time of lip repair
  - Improve tip projection, narrow the alar base, straighten the caudal septum, and reshape the cleft-side LLC
  - Definitive rhinoplasty may be performed during teenage years
    - Often requires V to Y advancement of medial crus and overlying skin with cleft lip scar to provide more columellar height and repositioning of cleft LLC with lateral crural strut graft
- Bilateral cleft lip repair
  - A narrow central prolabial flap is elevated, and the lateral lip elements are advanced medially
  - Primary rhinoplasty provides tip projection and support via interdomal sutures and suspension of the LLCs to the upper lateral cartilages
  - Restores complete orbicularis oris sphincter
  - Facial symmetry is easier to obtain with bilateral cleft lip repair than with unilateral, although nasal projection is more difficult

Facial Paralysis (See *Cummings Otolaryngology*, 7th ed., Chapters 173 and 174)

Anatomy of the Facial Nerve

- Exits the brainstem at the pontomedullary junction with the cochleovestibular nerve
- Intracanalicular (meatal) segment in the internal auditory canal (8–10 mm in length)
- Labyrinthine segment between the fundus of the internal auditory canal and geniculate ganglion
  - Narrowest portion of the facial nerve: diameter of the fallopian canal decreases from 1.2 to 0.7 mm
  - 2 to 4 mm in length
  - Segmented inflamed in Bell's palsy
  - Geniculate ganglion most commonly involved in temporal bone fracture
- Tympanic (horizontal) segment 11 mm in length
  - Passes over the oval window/stapes footplate
- Mastoid (vertical) segment 12 to 14 mm in length
  - Gives off chorda tympani
- Exits the temporal bone via the stylomastoid foramen
- Divides into five main branches at the pes anserinus within the parotid, separating deep and superficial lobes of the gland
- Frontal (temporal branch) exits the superior aspect of the parotid and traverses the zygomatic arch
  - Crosses over the junction of the posterior and middle one-third of the zygomatic arch and the travels on the deep surface of TPF
  - Passes across the brow from inferoposterior to superoanterior to innervate the frontalis muscle
    - Runs along Pitanguy's line from 5 mm inferior to the tragus to 15 mm above the lateral extent of the brow
- Midfacial branches (zygomatic and buccal) exit the anterior surface of the parotid, traveling on the superficial surface of the masseteric fascia
  - Significant redundancy because of neural anastomoses
  - Transverse facial vessels course superior to parotid duct, near buccal branches

- Mimetic muscles are innervated from the deep surface except for the mentalis, levator anguli oris, and buccinator
- Zuker's point marks location of primary buccal branch to zygomaticus major muscle
  - Halfway along line between root of helix and oral commissure
- Marginal mandibular and cervical branches exit the inferior aspect of the parotid
  - Marginal mandibular branch crosses into the submandibular space at the gonial notch, along with facial vessels, and follows them back toward the oral commissure anteriorly
  - Closely associated with and often wrapped around the facial vein
  - Innervates the depressor labii inferioris (DLI), depressor anguli oris (DAO), and mentalis
  - Nerve dips lower below the mandible in older patients
- Cervical branch innervates the platysma
  - Located roughly 1 cm below the angle of the mandible

Branches of the Facial Nerve

1. Greater superficial petrosal nerve
2. Nerve to the stapedius muscle
3. Sensory auricular branch of the facial nerve
4. Chorda tympani nerve
5. Branches to auricular muscles
6. Nerve to the posterior belly of the digastric muscle
7. Nerve to the stylohyoid muscle
8. Temporal/frontal branch
9. Zygomatic branch
10. Buccal branch
11. Marginal mandibular branch
12. Cervical branch

Surgical Methods to Find the Facial Nerve

1. 1-cm deep, 1-cm inferior, and 1-cm anterior to the tragal pointer
2. Just deep to the posterior belly of the digastric (use as a depth indicator with the tragal pointer as direction indicator)
3. 1-cm deep to the proximal end of the tympanomastoid suture line
4. Locate a vertical segment in the mastoid and follow it distally
5. Locate a distal branch in the midface and follow it proximally

Differential Diagnosis for Facial Paralysis

1. Bell's palsy
2. Iatrogenic injury
3. Ramsay Hunt syndrome
4. Temporal bone fracture
5. Facial trauma
6. Lyme disease
7. CNS lesion
8. Autoimmune disease (e.g., Melkersson-Rosenthal, Guillain-Barré, and sarcoidosis)
9. Otologic disease (acute otitis media and cholesteatoma)
10. Stroke
    - Brainstem stroke presents as hemifacial palsy ipsilateral to stroke because of involvement of the facial nucleus
    - Cortical stroke presents as mid- and lower facial palsy contralateral to stroke
    - Most strokes will present with other neurological signs beyond facial weakness
11. Neoplasm (usually presents with insidious onset but not always)

Evaluation Scales for Facial Paralysis

- Yanagihara
- House-Brackmann
- Facial Nerve Grading System 2.0 (House-Brackmann 2.0)
- Sunnybrook
- eFace

House-Brackmann Facial Nerve Grading System

1. House-Brackmann (HB) I: Normal
2. HB II: Mild asymmetry with movement, symmetric at rest, complete eye closure with gentle effort, and slight synkinesis
3. HB III: Obvious asymmetry with movement, symmetric at rest, complete eye closure with full effort, and noticeable synkinesis
4. HB IV: Obvious asymmetry with movement, grossly symmetric at rest, and incomplete eye closure
5. HB V: Minimal movement and grossly asymmetric at rest
6. HB VI: No movement

Sunderland (and Seddon) Classification of Peripheral Nerve Injuries

- Class I (neurapraxia): Conduction block with focal demyelination; anticipated complete recovery
- Class II (axonotmesis): Wallerian degeneration of axons with endoneurium, perineurium, and epineurium intact; anticipated complete recovery
- Class III (axonotmesis): Wallerian degeneration of axons and endoneurial disruption with perineurium and epineurium intact; anticipated synkinesis
- Class IV (axonotmesis): Wallerian degeneration of axons as well as endoneurial and perineurial disruption with epineurium intact; anticipated synkinesis
- Class V (neurotmesis): Nerve completely transected with Wallerian degeneration of axons and disruption of endoneurium, perineurium, and epineurium; will require neurorrhaphy and severe synkinesis is anticipated
- Class VI (mixed injury): Rush and transection components, with variable prognosis

Management of Acute Facial Paralysis (Fig. 3.21)

- Oral steroids (length, of course, dependent on etiology)
- Antivirals (dose and length, of course, dependent on etiology)
- Corneal protection
- Electrodiagnostic testing for HB VI paralysis, particularly in cases of Bell's palsy and temporal bone fracture

Facial Nerve Repair and Decompression

- Electrodiagnostic testing should be performed for complete hemifacial paralysis of sudden onset (immediate onset in case of trauma)
  - If electroneuronography (ENoG) shows ≥90% degeneration compared with the unaffected side, perform needle electromyography (EMG)
  - If EMG shows no voluntary motor units, consider exploration or decompression
  - ENoG: A form of EMG in which a transcutaneous current at the stylomastoid foramen causes facial muscle contractions (orbicularis oculi and zygomaticus major), which are measured and compared with the good side
    - Requires unilateral paralysis
  - ENoG will not show any decrease of conduction in Sunderland class I injuries due to lack of Wallerian degeneration

- ENoG cannot differentiate among Sunderland classes II to VI injuries
- EMG may show fibrillation potentials, positive sharp waves, or insertional activity during acute denervation
- Polyphasic potentials on EMG indicate regenerating axons, but ENoG may still show poor conduction due to early deblocking phenomenon (phase cancellation due to asynchronous signal transduction along the nerve)
- Absence of electrical activity occurs in muscles that are no longer receptive to reinnervation
- If the nerve is injured across >50% of its diameter, resect the injured segment and repair primarily
- If tension-free neurorrhaphy cannot be performed, place an interposition (cable) graft
  - Harvest from the greater auricular, sural, or medial antebrachial cutaneous nerve
  - Reverse the direction of the graft to minimize axonal loss through the branches

Facial Reinnervation

- Repair of facial nerve injuries must be accomplished early so that axons can regrow before muscle begins to atrophy
  - Axons grow at 1 mm/day
  - Facial muscles atrophy irreversibly after 12 to 18 months of denervation
- Coapting a donor nerve to the main trunk of the facial nerve will result in severe synkinesis, which may be worse than flaccid paralysis
  - Neural coaptation should be done with a specific muscle target in mind, such as the orbicularis oculi or zygomaticus major, to maximize functional recovery
- Cranial nerve transpositions
  - Hypoglossal-facial neurorrhaphy
    - Good for resting tone of the face due to high resting tone of tongue
    - Multiple options for hypoglossal-facial transfer
      - Coaptation of the entire hypoglossal nerve to the facial nerve main trunk
      - Coaptation of the facial nerve main trunk to the side of the hypoglossal nerve
      - Coaptation of a section of the hypoglossal nerve to the facial nerve main trunk
      - Interposition graft coapted end-to-side into both facial and hypoglossal nerves
    - The greater the number of axons taken from the hypoglossal nerve, the greater the facial reinnervation and the greater the tongue morbidity
  - Masseteric-facial neurorrhaphy
    - Good for voluntary movement but has low resting tone
    - Reliably provides strong movement
    - Requires jaw clenching to activate the reinnervated muscle initially, usually the zygomaticus major
      - Children often can achieve spontaneity
      - Many adults no longer need to clench the jaw to smile after a few months, but still have to think about smiling rather than achieve true spontaneity
    - Donor muscle morbidity well tolerated
    - Masseteric nerve located 3-cm anterior to tragus, 1-cm inferior to zygomatic arch, 1.5-cm deep to masseter fascia
  - Cross-face nerve grafting
    - Allows good side to control paralyzed side, which provides true spontaneity
    - Typically done as a buccal branch to buccal branch graft to rehabilitate smile or a zygomatic branch to zygomatic branch graft to rehabilitate eye closure

Acute Facial Palsy

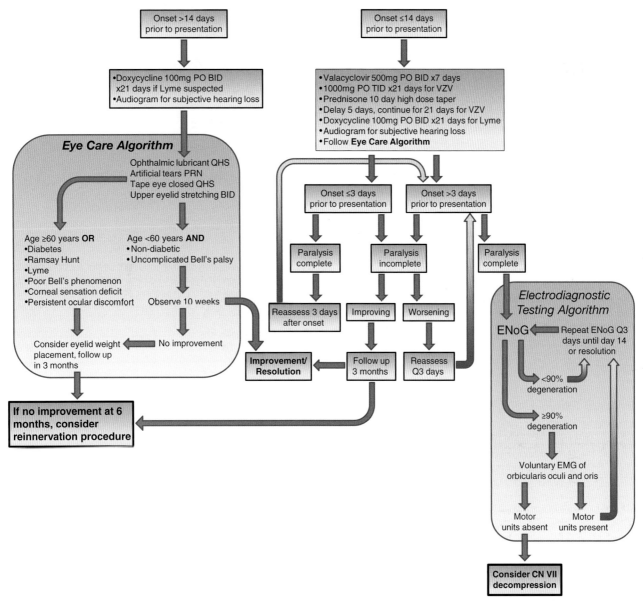

Fig. 3.21 Algorithm for management of acute facial paralysis. (Adapted with permission from Hohman MH, Hadlock TA. Etiology, diagnosis, and management of facial paralysis: 2000 patients at a facial nerve center. *Laryngoscope*. 2014;124(7):E283–E293, Fig. 1.)

- Long graft length and two neurorrhaphies make success inconsistent
  - More reliable in children
  - Cannot use if patient liable to develop facial paralysis on the other side, for example, neurofibromatosis type II
- Other nerve options
  - Spinal accessory and phrenic nerves can be used for reinnervation or to control free muscle flaps

Facial Reanimation

- First priority is corneal protection: drops, lubricant, nightly taping, eyelid stretching exercises
- May be performed at any time after onset of paralysis

Static Reanimation

- Brow lift
- Eyelid weight
- Tarsal strip, canthopexy, lateral tarsoconjunctival flap, and tarsorrhaphy
- Fascia lata/Gore-Tex sling
- Chemodenervation with botulinum toxin may improve symmetry by weakening overactive areas on the unaffected side or by releasing synkinetic muscle spasm on the ipsilateral side
  - Selective neurectomy may accomplish a similar goal but is often also temporary
  - Myomectomy of the platysma, depressor angulis oris (DAO), and DLI may provide longer-term effect

Dynamic Reanimation

- Free tissue transfer
  - Generally used for smile rehabilitation, may be used for restoration of blink
    - Classic smile rehabilitation has concentrated on imitating function of the zygomaticus major muscle to elevate and lateralize the oral commissure
    - Modern techniques aim to elevate the upper lip and potentially depress the lower lip as well through "multivector" reanimation
  - Recipient vessels are typically facial artery and vein, although superficial temporal vessels are occasionally used
  - Masseteric nerve most commonly used to control muscle flap in adults
  - Cross-face nerve grafting often used in children without Möbius syndrome
    - Bilateral facial paralysis obviates use of cross-face grafting
    - Often done as two-stage procedure with graft placed first and muscle transferred 6 to 9 months later, after axons have grown across the graft, in order to minimize chance of muscle atrophying before reinnervation
  - Many surgeons use both to achieve reliability and strength with spontaneity ("dual innervation")
  - Deep temporal nerve may also be used to control a free muscle flap but this nerve is short and filamentous, thus, is often employed after other more preferable options have been used

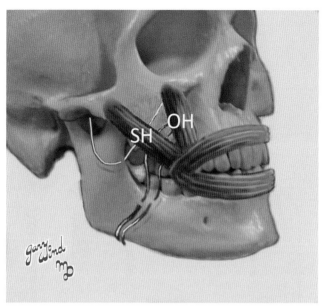

Fig. 3.22 Sterno-omohyoid free muscle transfer for dual-vector smile rehabilitation. The masseteric nerve, facial artery, and facial vein are depicted coapted to the ansa cervicalis, superior thyroid artery, and middle thyroid vein, respectively. The sternohyoid replaces the zygomaticus major muscle and the omohyoid replaces the levator labii superioris muscle. *OH*, Omohyoid; *SH*, sternohyoid. (Adapted with permission from Vincent AG, Bevans SE, Robitschek JM, Groom KL, Herr MW, Hohman MH. Sterno-omohyoid free flap for dual-vector dynamic facial reanimation. *Ann Otol Rhinol Laryngol.* 2020;129(2):195–200, Fig. 1.)

Free Muscle Transfer Examples

Flap	Vascular Supply	Nerve	Features
Gracilis	Adductor artery and venae comitantes	Obturator	• Adds moderate bulk to the face • May be split into several individual slips of muscle to provide multivector smile reanimation but requires more bulk in order to do so and dissection risks denervating the muscle • 94% success rate with masseteric nerve, 81% with cross-face graft • May include overlying skin
Latissimus dorsi	Thoracodorsal artery and vena comitans	Thoracodorsal	• Adds moderate bulk to the face • May also be dissected for multi-vector reanimation with similar risks to gracilis • May include overlying skin, if necessary
Pectoralis minor	Variable arterial supply (thoracoacromial, lateral thoracic, axillary), variable venous drainage (lateral thoracic vein/vena comitans)	Medial pectoral (20% innervated by lateral pectoral)	• Adds moderate bulk to face • May include overlying skin
Serratus anterior	Thoracodorsal artery and vena comitans	Long thoracic	• Natively has multiple individual slips of muscle, making it well-suited to multivector reanimation with minimal risk of slip denervation • Adds large amount of bulk to face
Strap muscle: sternohyoid, omohyoid, sterno-omohyoid (Fig. 3.22)	Superior thyroid artery, variable venous drainage: superior thyroid vein/middle thyroid vein/ranine veins	Ansa cervicalis (permits dual innervation, as both ends can be used)	• If both muscles are harvested, dual vector reanimation is straightforward, with the sternohyoid (the larger muscle) replacing zygomaticus major and the omohyoid replacing the levator labii superioris • If only the sternohyoid is harvested, the ansa cervicalis will reach the contralateral facial nerve for direct "cross-face" neurorrhaphy • Adds minimal bulk to face

Regional Muscle Transfer Examples

Flap	Vascular Supply	Features
Anterior digastric	Facial	• Restore lower lip depression
Masseter	Facial	• Smile reanimation (uncommonly used due to lateral vector orientation, unnatural smile)
Platysma	Facial	• Restore lower lip depression from isolated marginal mandibular palsy (iatrogenic injury, trauma)
Temporalis	Deep temporal	Rotational Flap • Superior muscle is reflected over zygomatic arch, secured to commissure • Can restore blink • Unnatural postoperative appearance due to bulk over the zygomatic arch and temporal hollowing
		Advancement Flap • Tendon detached from coronoid process and secured at commissure or coronoid process advanced with tendon • Technique can avoid external scar • No significant change in facial bulk • More reliable than free muscle transfer • Cannot provide multivector smile rehabilitation

Gender Dysphoria and Gender Affirmation Facial Surgery

History Questions for Transgender Patients

- Preferred pronoun
- Hormone therapy and duration
- Duration of "real-life experience" (living 24/7 in preferred gender)
- History of behavioral health issues
  - Depression
  - Anxiety
  - Suicidality
- Prior conservative treatments
  - Speech therapy
  - Counseling
  - Cosmetics, wigs, female grooming, etc.
- Prior surgical history
  - Prior vocal feminization surgery may require a smaller endotracheal tube
  - History of complications, particularly blood clots due to hormones
- Goals for surgery
  - Will cosmetic aging face procedures be performed concurrently?

Differences Between Ideal Male and Female Faces

Feature	Female	Male
Hairline	Round	M-shape
Forehead height	Lower hairline (5–6 cm)	Higher hairline (6–7 cm)
Forehead shape	Rounder	Flatter
Brow prominence	Less-pronounced bony brow ridges, thinner skin	Pronounced brow ridges, thicker skin
Eyebrow height	Above supraorbital ridge	At supraorbital ridge
Eyebrow shape	Arched	Flat
Upper eyelid crease	10–12 mm above lash line	7–8 mm above lash line
Zygomatic arches	Wider	Narrower
Buccal fat pads	Fuller	Less prominent
Radix	Shallower	Deeper
Nasal dorsum	Lower dorsum, slight scoop	Higher, straight
Nasal tip rotation	100–115 degrees	90–95 degrees
Nasal skin	Thinner	Thicker
Lips	Fuller, more red-lip show	Thinner, less red-lip show
Dental show	Greater maxillary dental show at rest	Minimal-to-no dental show at rest
Dental profile	Smaller with rounded edges	Larger and more square
Facial hair	None	Beard, Mustache
Mandibular angle	Obtuse	Acute/right angle, flared
Mandibular width	Narrow	Wider
Masseter volume	Less	More
Chin width	Narrower	Wider
Chin protrusion	Less projection of pogonion	More projection of pogonion

Surgical Options for Facial Feminization

- Upper third
  - Hairline adjustment via pretrichial approach
  - Hair transplantation
  - Brow lift
  - Frontal cranioplasty: Reduction of supraorbital ridge and prominence of superolateral orbit, often with removal and recession of the anterior table of the frontal sinus
    - Overcorrection is recommended to take into account thicker male brow skin

- Middle third
  - Cheek implants
  - Fat or filler injections into the malar fat pad and lips
  - Rhinoplasty
  - Lip lift via bullhorn subnasal incision
    - Open rhinoplasty may be performed through this incision
- Lower third
  - Genioplasty
  - Mandibular angle ostectomies
- Neck
  - Chondrolaryngoplasty ("tracheal shave")
- Nonsurgical modalities are important as well
  - Patients should try conservative and reversible medical therapies first, typically for several months or years, before proceeding with irreversible surgery
  - Speech therapy is more important than chondrolaryngoplasty
  - Wearing a wig
  - Learning to apply cosmetics
  - Laser facial hair removal, electrolysis
  - Growing out scalp hair
  - Grooming eyebrows
  - Bimatoprost drops for eyelashes

Facial Masculinization

- Buccal fat resection
- Fillers of implants to make the chin and mandibular angles more prominent
  Testosterone therapy typically provides the majority of required changes; surgical masculinization of the face is rare

MAXILLOFACIAL AND SOFT-TISSUE TRAUMA (SEE *CUMMINGS OTOLARYNGOLOGY*, 7TH ED., CHAPTER 20)

History Questions for Trauma Patients

- Mechanism of injury
- Other injuries, especially cervical spine
- Loss of consciousness
- Neurological symptoms, vision, and hearing
- Rhinorrhea or salty taste in the mouth
- Occlusion and loose or missing teeth
- Tetanus status

Craniomaxillofacial Trauma Primary Evaluation

- Airway, breathing, circulation, disability, exposure
  - Orotracheal versus nasotracheal intubation versus tracheostomy
- Vital signs
- Neurological exam
  - Cranial nerves with visual acuity and tuning forks
  - Assess for intracranial injury
  - Cervical spine injury occurs in 10% of maxillofacial trauma cases
- Inspect for lacerations, bleeding, and ecchymosis
  - Periorbital or postauricular ecchymosis may indicate skull-base fracture
- Evaluate ears for hemotympanum, canal step-offs, and clear or bloody otorrhea (CSF leak)
- Evaluate the neck for tracheal deviation, subcutaneous emphysema, and bulging veins (tension pneumothorax or cardiac tamponade)

Craniomaxillofacial Trauma Secondary Evaluation (Top Down)

Upper face

- Scalp lacerations
- Skull deformities
- Frontal sinus/nasofrontal outflow tract injury
- CSF leak

Midface

- Orbit
  - Periorbital edema and ecchymosis
  - Bony step-offs at orbital rim
  - Assess pupillary response to light
    - Marcus-Gunn pupil: Afferent pupillary defect
  - Assess extraocular muscle movement (forced ductions if patient is unresponsive)
    - Diplopia
  - Assess for eyelid and lacrimal system injuries
  - Ophthalmology consultation to rule out globe injury
  - Look for telecanthus
- Zygoma
  - Assess for widening of the midface, trismus, and malar depression
- Maxilla
  - Assess for bony step-offs and mobility of the palate or midface
  - Assess for midfacial hypesthesia/anesthsia
- Nasal
  - Most common facial fracture
  - Assess for mobility, crepitus, tenderness, and swelling
  - Check for clear or bloody rhinorrhea (CSF leak)
  - Check for septal hematoma
    - May cause septal necrosis and buckling or saddle deformity if untreated
    - Incise and leave a rubber band drain

Lower face

- Oral cavity: Assess for dental injuries, lacerations, ecchymosis, and trismus
- Occlusion: Assess for open bite, crossbite, inability to close mouth, and loose/missing teeth
- Angle dental occlusion classification:
  - Class 1: Mesiobuccal cusp of first maxillary molar fits in buccal groove of first mandibular molar
  - Class 2 (overjet): Mesiobuccal cusp of first maxillary molar contacts mesial to buccal groove of first mandibular molar
  - Class 3 (underjet): Mesiobuccal cusp of first maxillary molar contacts distal to buccal groove of first mandibular molar
- Mandible
  - Assess for step-offs and mobility of fractured segments
  - Evaluate maximal incisal opening
  - Assess for deviation of the mandible on opening, premature contact of the molars, loss of mandibular height, and anterior open bite
    - All are signs of ipsilateral subcondylar fracture
  - Look for floor-of-mouth hematoma
  - Assess sensation of the mental nerve

Radiography

- Pre- and postoperative computed tomography (CT) scanning without contrast is useful in evaluating fractures and their repair
- Can aid in producing patient-specific cutting guides and plates

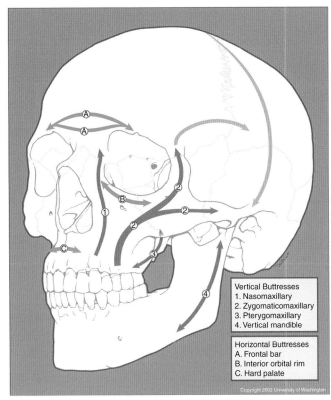

Fig. 3.23 Buttresses of the facial skeleton. (From Linnau KF, Stanley RB Jr, Hallam DK, et al. Imaging of high-energy midfacial trauma: what the surgeon needs to know. Eur J Radiol 2003;48:17–32.)

Facial Buttress Characteristics (See Fig. 3.23)

- Pillars of the maxillofacial skeleton that provide structural support
- Commonly recognized facial fracture patterns in the midface follow the buttresses

Vertical Buttresses of the Face

1. Nasomaxillary
2. Zygomaticomaxillary
3. Pterygomaxillary
4. Ramus/condyle unit of mandible

Horizontal Buttresses of the Face

1. Frontal bar
2. Infraorbital rims
3. Maxilla/hard palate
4. Mandibular body

Facial Skeletal Proportions

- Facial width determined by bizygomatic and intergonial distances
  - Inadequate reduction of zygomatic or mandibular fractures can result in a widened face
- Facial height is determined by vertical buttresses and the mandibular ramus/condyle unit
  - Inadequate reduction of Le Fort injuries and mandibular ramus/condyle fractures can result in abnormal height

Frontal Sinus Fractures

- Anterior and posterior tables
  - Nondisplaced: No treatment necessary
  - If displaced more than one table width, open reduction may be useful, but observation may suffice

- Fillers can camouflage a displaced anterior table; often, bone will remodel and minimize the deformity
  - Comminution or loss of part of the posterior table is an indication for cranialization
- Nasofrontal outflow tract injury
  - May be identified on sagittal or coronal slices on CT
  - If injured, obliterate the duct
  - Frontal sinus mucocele: May occur if the nasofrontal duct is not obliterated or if the sinus lining is not completely extirpated after injury
- CSF leak
  - Presents with rhinorrhea
  - Evaluate using halo test, glucose level, β-2 transferrin, or β-trace protein assay
  - Metrizamide CT detects other sources of CSF leak
  - Observe for 7 to 10 days with conservative interventions (head of bed elevated, no straining, no coughing) to see whether the leak resolves in the setting of a nondisplaced fracture
  - Consider a lumbar drain
  - Cranialization of the frontal sinus with galeal and pericranial flaps, repair of dural tear, and lumbar drain for displaced fracture

Naso-Orbito-Ethmoid Fracture Presenting Signs

- Telecanthus
  - Defined as intercanthal distance >35 to 40 mm
  - Distinguish from hypertelorism: Increased intraorbital distance
- Saddle nose deformity
- Epiphora

Markowitz-Manson Naso-Orbito-Ethmoid Fracture Classification (Fig. 3.24)

- Type I: Single central fragment with the medial canthal tendon attached—treatment is open reduction and internal fixation (ORIF) if displaced, via a coronal incision
- Type II: Comminuted central fragment, medial canthal tendon attached—treatment is ORIF if displaced
- Type III: Comminuted with disruption of medial canthal attachment—treatment is ORIF with an open transnasal medial canthoplasty

Orbital Injuries

- Globe injury
  - Anisocoria, ocular pain, visual acuity changes, and diplopia
- Traumatic optic neuropathy
  - From shear force on the optic nerve
  - Mild injury may present with diminished color perception and afferent pupillary defect
  - Severe injury may cause blindness
  - Steroids, possible orbital canal decompression
- Superior orbital fissure (SOF) versus orbital apex syndrome
  - SOF syndrome: Only cranial nerves III, IV, V1, and VI are affected
  - Orbital apex syndrome: The same nerves affected by SOF syndrome plus the optic nerve are affected

Absolute Indications for Orbital Floor Fracture Repair

1. Entrapment: Presents with diplopia, nausea, bradycardia, and pain
2. Loss of >50% of the orbital floor or fracture size >1.5 cm²
3. Persistent diplopia in the absence of other causes (>2 weeks)
4. Enophthalmos ≥2 mm

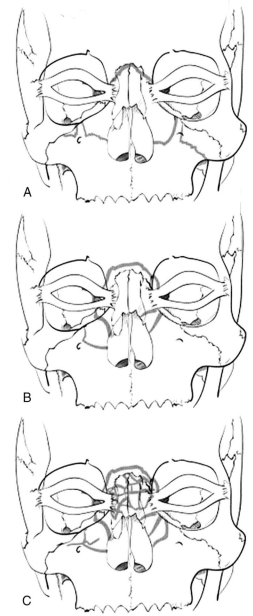

Fig. 3.24 Markowitz-Manson classification of naso-orbito-ethmoid fractures. (A) Type I, **(B)** Type II, **(C)** Type III. (From Flint PW, Haughey BH, Lund VJ, et al. *Cummings Otolaryngology—Head and Neck Surgery.* 7th ed. Philadelphia, PA: Saunders; 2020, Fig. 20.13. Modified from Markowitz BL, Manson PN, Sargent L, et al. Management of the medial canthal tendon in nasoethmoid orbital fractures: the importance of the central fragment in classification and treatment. *Plast Reconstr Surg.* 1991;87:843–853.)

Orbital Floor Fracture Considerations

- Relative indication for repair: Mild diplopia (within 20–30 degrees of primary gaze)
- Repair is best approached via a transconjunctival incision
  - Preseptal approach facilitates elevation of the floor periorbita
  - Endoscope may improve visualization
  - Reconstruct floor with titanium mesh, porous polyethylene sheet, porous polyethylene-covered titanium mesh, nylon sheet, or bone/cartilage grafts
- Medial wall fractures
  - Lamina papyracea of the ethmoid bone fractures easily because of its paper-like thinness

- Use a transcaruncular approach (superficial to the septum and deep to Horner's muscle) to access the medial orbit
- Intraoperative or postoperative CT scan will ensure appropriate placement of floor implant and avoid muscle entrapment

Nasal Fracture (See *Cummings Otolaryngology,* 7th ed., Chapter 30)

- Types: Unilateral, bilateral, comminuted, depressed, open-book, impacted, greenstick
- Management: Closed reduction, intranasal packing, and external casting; may require osteotomies with closed reduction if bones have begun to set
  - Reduce within a few hours of injury (before edema ensues) or 2 to 10 days afterward (before bones become immobile)
  - Can often reduce under local and topical anesthesia
    - Must block anterior and posterior ethmoid, sphenopalatine, nasopalatine, infraorbital, infratrochlear, and dorsal nasal nerves
- Septal fracture: Closed reduction with internal splints
  - Inadequate septal reduction most common reason for persistent nasal deformity
- If unsuccessful, will need definitive rhinoplasty 6 to 12 months later
  - 80% to 90% success rate with closed reduction

Zygomatic Fracture

- The zygomatic bone has four articulations
  1. Zygomaticofrontal
  2. Zygomaticosphenoid
  3. Zygomaticotemporal
  4. Zygomaticomaxillary
- Zygomaticomaxillary complex (ZMC) (tripod) fracture disrupts all four
- Reduction of a ZMC fracture requires restoration of all four articulations
  - Zygomaticosphenoid alignment is the most reliable method of ensuring adequate reduction
  - Inadequate reduction may cause inappropriate midfacial width, malar flattening, and vertical dystopia
  - Upper and lower eyelid and gingivobuccal sulcus incisions provide access for ORIF; coronal approach can be used to access the arch
  - Zygomatic arch fracture disrupts the zygomaticotemporal joint and may cause trismus from impingement on the temporalis tendon/coronoid process
  - Isolated arch fractures can be approached via an incision in the temporal scalp (Gillies) with placement of an elevator at the depth of the temporalis fascia to avoid frontal branch injury or by an intraoral approach (Keen)
  - Should explore orbital floor after ZMC reduction for possible second fracture

Le Fort Midfacial Fracture Classification (Fig. 3.25)

- Le Fort I: Separates the maxillary dentoalveolar segment and palate from the midface
- Le Fort II: Separates the maxilla and nasal complex from the facial skeleton
- Le Fort III: Separates the facial skeleton from the skull, and includes Naso-Orbito-Ethmoid (NOE) fracture

Le Fort Fracture Characteristics

- All patterns include pterygoid plate fractures
- Present with malocclusion, typically an open bite because of posterosuperior displacement of the maxilla

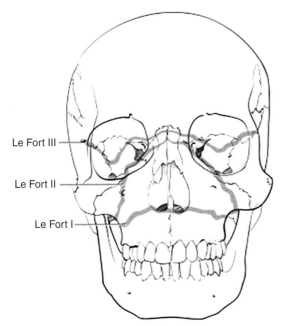

Fig. 3.25 Le Fort classification of midfacial fractures. (From Flint PW, Haughey BH, Lund VJ, et al. *Cummings Otolaryngology—Head and Neck Surgery.* 7th ed. Philadelphia, PA: Saunders; 2020, Fig. 20.12.)

- Displaced fractures with associated malocclusion should be managed with ORIF
- Incomplete fractures may require osteotomies to mobilize the midface and allow for adequate reduction
- Fractures with a palatal split should be managed with reestablishment of the transverse width and occlusion using a palatal plate or an acrylic dental splint

Mandible Fractures

- Often present with malocclusion (prematurity and open bite), wear facets do not align
- Bilateral mandible fractures could pose acute airway risk
- Management options are based on anticipated patient compliance and fracture type
- Nondisplaced fractures without malocclusion in a reliable patient are often managed with a soft diet
- Displaced fractures in the dentate mandible are managed with 4 to 6 weeks of maxillomandibular fixation (MMF) or ORIF
  - Rigid fixation requires an inferior border plate with bicortical screws and a tension band on the superior margin of the mandible (miniplate or arch bar)
- Displaced fractures of the mandibular angle are managed with ORIF: a semirigid fixation (Champy) involves a single miniplate along the oblique line, which requires a soft diet unless another plate is placed along the inferior border
- Teeth in the line of the fracture: Should be removed when they interfere with reduction or are fractured, loose, or do not have a functional use (i.e., no opposing tooth)
- Consider ORIF rather than MMF in patients with seizure disorders, high risk for vomiting, or poor likelihood of follow-up
- Edentulous fractures can be managed with Gunning splints (dentures that allow for MMF); displaced fractures of the atrophic, edentulous mandible may require ORIF with bone grafting
- Generally, consider the shortest possible interval for MMF to allow for adequate mobilization after surgery and avoid temporomandibular joint ankylosis
  - 7 to 10 days: Intracapsular condylar fractures
  - 2 to 4 weeks: After ORIF of an angle fracture with a Champy plate

- 4 to 6 weeks: Fractures managed by closed reduction
- No postoperative MMF is required if ORIF is performed
- Arch bars may be used for placement of guiding elastics and to assist with physical therapy (e.g., for subcondylar injuries)

Condylar Head Fractures

- Intracapsular injuries are managed with 7 to 10 days of MMF if there is malocclusion
- If no malocclusion, soft diet and early mobilization
- Condylar/subcondylar injuries are managed closed if minimally displaced

Absolute Indications for ORIF of Condylar/Subcondylar Fractures

1. Condylar displacement into the middle cranial fossa or external auditory canal
2. Inadequate occlusion with closed reduction
3. Lateral extracapsular condylar displacement
4. Intraarticular invasion with a foreign body (e.g., bullet)

Relative Indications for ORIF of Condylar/Subcondylar Fractures

1. Bilateral subcondylar fractures with comminuted midface, edentulous patient, or prior malocclusion
2. If splinting is not recommended, ORIF is indicated

Mandible Reconstruction

- Nonvascularized
  - Bone chips from iliac crest, anterior tibia
  - Can fill defect up to 6 cm in length
  - Requires healthy, well-vascularized surrounding tissue and titanium tray to hold bone in position
  - May not permit dental rehabilitation
- Vascularized free tissue transfer
  - Fibula, iliac crest, scapula, radial forearm
- Fibula and iliac crest readily allow dental implant placement
- Patient specific planning and models can improve accuracy and efficiency of intraoperative reconstruction

Panfacial Fractures

- Repair from "known to unknown," from stable toward unstable, from periphery toward center
- Reestablish occlusion first, if possible, before plating begins

Soft-Tissue Trauma (See *Cummings Otolaryngology*, 7th ed., Chapter 19)

Wound Classification

- Class 1: Clean (e.g., surgical incision on prepped skin)
- Class 2: Clean-contaminated (e.g., surgical incision in the pharynx)
- Class 3: Contaminated (e.g., gross spillage of gastrointestinal contents into the wound)
- Class 4: Dirty (e.g., infected wound)

Tetanus Guidelines

- If immunization history is unknown or series is incomplete, give vaccine
- If the wound is dirty, give tetanus immunoglobulin
- If the immunization series was completed or boosted <5 years ago, do nothing

- If the series was completed or boosted ≥5 years ago and the wound is dirty, give vaccine
- If series completed or boosted ≥5 but <10 years ago and wound clean, no vaccine required
- If series completed or boosted ≥10 years ago, give vaccine

Indications for Antibiotics

- Broad spectrum for class 3 and class 4 wounds, commonly human bite wounds
- Debatable for animal bites, but amoxicillin-clavulanate is often used
- Not required for most other lacerations unless debris or foreign bodies are in the wound

Wounds Not to Be Closed

- Puncture wounds: Wound is deeper than it is wide, and the depths are not visible
- Grossly contaminated wounds (e.g., gunshot wounds): Because of the introduction of debris and foreign bodies deep into the wound tract and high infection risk
- Delayed presentation: Up to 24 hours it is generally safe to close in the head and neck, because of blood supply

Local and Regional Anesthesia Characteristics

- Lidocaine
  - Aminoamide anesthetic
  - Maximum dose: 7 mg/kg with epinephrine, 4 mg/kg without epinephrine
  - Onset: Rapid (<1 minute) for lidocaine, 10 to 15 minutes for vasoconstrictive effect of epinephrine
  - Duration: 2 hours, up to 4 hours with epinephrine
  - Toxicity: CNS and cardiac
    - CNS excitation at lower doses: Anxiety, circumoral paresthesia, and seizures
    - CNS depression at higher doses: Lethargy, respiratory depression, and loss of consciousness
    - Cardiac: Hypotension, bradycardia, arrhythmia, and cardiac arrest
- Bupivicaine
  - Aminoamide anesthetic
  - Maximum dose: 4 mg/kg (1 mL/kg of 0.25% solution)
  - Onset: Slow
  - Duration: 4 hours; up to 8 hours with epinephrine
  - Toxicity: More cardiotoxic than other local anesthetics, but also CNS toxic
  - Overdose: Give intralipid for cardiotoxicity

Local Infiltration Versus Regional Blocks

- Large areas: Regional blocks are best
  - Avoids toxicity with large doses of locally infiltrated anesthetic
  - Avoids distortion from large volumes of infiltrated solution
  - Drawback: No hemostasis
- Small areas: Local infiltration best
  - Hemostasis from epinephrine in anesthetic solution
  - Rapid onset
  - Only anesthetizes area of concern

Suture Technique

- Irrigate copiously before beginning closure
- Remove all foreign bodies
- Debride nonviable tissue
- Reapproximate free margins and subunit borders first (e.g., vermilion border)

- Wound eversion to prevent depressed scars: Vertical mattress sutures if necessary

Parotid Injuries

- Injury to the buccal branch of the facial nerve is common with parotid-duct injury
  - Duct runs along the line from the tragus to the midpoint of the upper lip
- Suture repair over a stent if possible
  - Remove the stent in 2 to 3 weeks
  - If a large segment of the duct is avulsed, replant into the buccal mucosa
  - If unable to replant because of proximal injury, ligate the duct
- Consider pressure dressing, anticholinergics, botulinum toxin, and nothing by mouth for salivary fistula or sialocele

Lacrimal Apparatus and Eyelids

- Ophthalmological evaluation of globe
- Canalicular evaluation of lacrimal system, repair over silicone stent
- Assess for traumatic telecanthus (normal intercanthal distance is 30–35 mm), resuspend medial canthal tendon if necessary

Facial Nerve

- Assess facial function before injection of local anesthetic
- Lacerations with facial nerve injury lateral to the lateral canthus should be explored within 3 days of injury, primary repair of nerve ends attempted with 9-0 or 10-0 monofilament
- Lacerations medial to the lateral canthus do not require exploration (small nerves, redundant innervation)
- Missing segments of nerve can be replaced with a cable graft from the great auricular nerve or sural nerve
- Vigilant eye care

Ear

- Avulsion: Replant and sew the avulsed segment in its original position; a robust vascular supply to the ear allows survival of large segments of tissue on a relatively small pedicle
- Auricular hematoma: Require prompt drainage with bolster or quilting suture application to avoid cartilage resorption, necrosis, and cauliflower deformity
- Antibiotic therapy with fluoroquinolone (penetrates cartilage, covers *Pseudomonas aeruginosa*)

Penetrating Neck Trauma (See *Cummings Otolaryngology*, 7th ed., Chapter 120)

Zones of the Neck (Fig. 3.26)

- More recently, a "No Zone" approach to neck trauma has been adopted in some centers (Fig. 3.27)

	Area	Trauma Evaluation
Zone I	Clavicle to cricoid cartilage	• Lung apices, trachea, great vessels, esophagus, thoracic duct, cervical sympathetic trunks, cervical vertebrae, and spinal cord • Surgical exploration for the unstable patient; otherwise, consider studies and endoscopy (CT-angiography, bronchoscopy, and esophagoscopy) dictated by suspicion of injury

	Area	Trauma Evaluation
Zone II	Cricoid cartilage to mandibular angle	• Neck vasculature, trachea/esophagus, spinal cord, larynx • Role of invasive studies is debatable • Surgical exploration for the symptomatic or unstable patient; otherwise, consider radiographic studies
Zone III	Mandibular angle to skull base	• Neck vasculature, pharynx, and facial nerve • Surgical exploration for the unstable patient; otherwise, consider radiographic studies • Operative management may require mandibular disarticulation and skull-base access

Classification of Burns

Classification	Depth	Symptoms and Features
First degree (superficial)	Epidermis	• Pain, erythema • Heals with minimal to no scarring or permanent damage
Second degree (partial thickness)	Partial-thickness dermis	• Pain, erythema, blistering • Preserves adnexal structures • Heals with minimal scarring
Third degree (full thickness)	Full-thickness dermis	• Gray skin, numb • Destroys adnexal structures • Healing from secondary intention causes significant hypertrophic scarring
Fourth degree	Extends through skin into deeper structures (muscle, bone)	• Requires debridement and surgical reconstruction

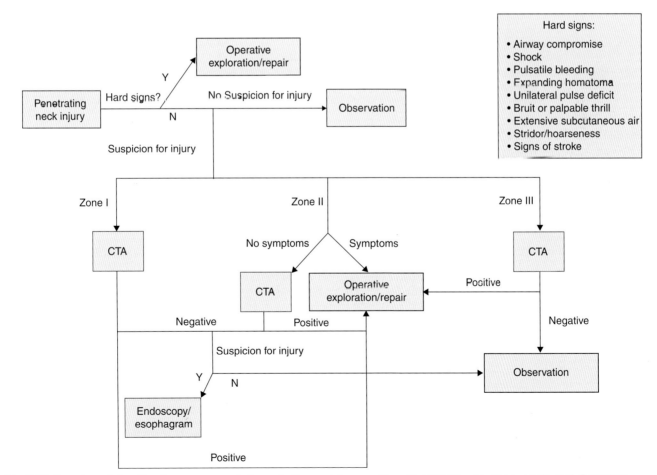

Fig. 3.26 Zone-based algorithm for management of penetrating neck trauma. (From Flint PW, Haughey BH, Lund VJ, et al. *Cummings Otolaryngology—Head and Neck Surgery*. 7th ed. Philadelphia, PA: Saunders; 2020, Fig. 120.5. Data from Sperry JL, Moore EE, Coimbra R, et al. Western Trauma Association critical decisions in trauma: penetrating neck trauma. *J Trauma Acute Care Surg*. 2013;75(6):936–940.)

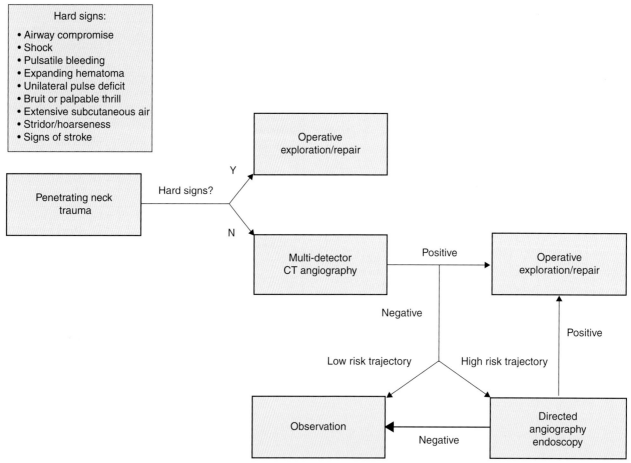

Fig. 3.27 No-zone algorithm for management of penetrating neck trauma. (From Flint PW, Haughey BH, Lund VJ, et al. *Cummings Otolaryngology—Head and Neck Surgery.* 7th ed. Philadelphia, PA: Saunders; 2020, Fig. 120.4. Modified from Shiroff AM, Gale SC, Martin ND, et al. Penetrating neck trauma: a review of management strategies and discussion of the "No Zone" approach. *Am Surg.* 2013;79(1):23–29.)

Assessment and Treatment of Burns

- Evaluate for inhalation injury, early airway intervention
- Nasotracheal/orotracheal intubation (avoid tracheostomy, if possible) for burns of anterior neck to avoid poor healing and pulmonary sepsis due to an infected eschar
- Parkland formula for fluid resuscitation
- Initial treatment with skin grafts; provide re-epithelialization by 14 days after injury
- Spontaneous healing or debridement/excision with or without skin grafting
- Secondary reconstruction with regional or free tissue transfer
- Systemic hyperinflammatory state may persist for several months after burn injury, resulting in abnormally exuberant scarring during reconstructive surgeries, particularly at graft harvest sites

Oral Commissure Burns

- Usually occur in small children because of biting electrical cords
- Manage conservatively
  - Minimize early debridement
  - Consider splinting to prevent microstomia

Frostbite

- Rapid rewarming is the most important treatment
- 40°C water bath for 15 to 30 minutes

FURTHER READINGS

Alam DS. The sternohyoid flap for facial reanimation. *Facial Plast Surg Clin North Am.* 2016;23(1):61–69.

Andrews JE, Jones NN, Moody MP, et al. Nasoseptal surgery outcomes in smokers and non-smokers. *Facial Plast Surg Aesthet Med.* doi:10.1089/fpsam.2020.0349.

Banks CA, Jowett N, Azizzadeh B, et al. Worldwide testing of the eFaCE facial nerve clinician-graded scale. *Plast Reconstr Surg.* 2017;139(2):491e–498e.

Bhama PK, Lindsay RW, Weinberg JS, et al. Objective outcomes analysis following microvascular gracilis transfer for facial reanimation: a review of 10 years' experience. *JAMA Facial Plastic Surgery.* 2014;16(2):85–92.

Boahene K. Omohyoid free flap for smile and blink restoration. Presented at the 13th International Facial Nerve Symposium, Los Angeles, CA, August, 2017.

Borschel GH, Kawamura DH, Kasukurthi R, et al. The motor nerve to the masseter muscle: an anatomic and histomorphometric study to facilitate its use in facial reanimation. *J Plast Reconstr Aesth Surg.* 2011;65(3):363–366.

Brent B. Auricular repair with autogenous rib cartilage grafts: two decades of experience with 600 cases. *Plast Reconstr Surg.* 1992;90(3):355–374, discussion 375–376.

Catalano P, Ashmead MG, Carlson D. Radiofrequency ablation of septal swell body. *Ann Otolaryngol Rhinol.* 2015;2(11):1069.

Champy M, Lodde JP, Muster D, et al. Osteosynthesis using miniaturized screw-on plates in facial and cranial surgery. Indications and results in 400 cases. *Ann Chir Plast.* 1977;22(4):261–264.

Crowther JA, O'Donoghue GM. The broken nose: does familiarity breed neglect? *Ann R Coll Surg Engl.* 1987;69(6):259–260.

Dedo DD. "How I do it"—plastic surgery: practical suggestions on facial plastic surgery: a preoperative classification of the neck for cervicofacial rhytidectomy. *Laryngoscope.* 1980;90(11, Pt 1):1894–1896.

Dorafshar AH, Borsuk DE, Bojovic B, et al. Surface anatomy of the middle division of the facial nerve: Zuker's point. *Plast Recontr Surg.* 2013;131(2):253–257.

Dufourmentel C. [The L-shaped flap for lozenge-shaped defects. Interview with Claude Dufourmentel by E. Achard]. *Ann Chir Plast.* 1979;24(4):397–399.

Fisher DM. Unilateral cleft lip repair: an anatomical subunit approximation technique. *Plast Reconstr Surg.* 2005;116(1):61–71.

Fitzpatrick TB. The validity and practicality of sun-reactive skin types I-VI. *Arch Dermatol.* 1988;124(6):869–871.

Friedman M, Ibrahim H, Ramakrishnan V. Inferior turbinate flap for repair of nasal septal perforation. *Laryngoscope.* 2003;113(8):1425–1428.

Fritsch MH. Incisionless otoplasty. *Laryngoscope.* 1995;105(5 Pt 3, suppl 70):1–11.

Furnas DW. Correction of prominent ears by conchamastoid sutures. *Plast Reconstr Surg.* 1968;42(3):189–193.

Gantz BJ, Rubinstein JT, Gidley P, Woodworth GG. Surgical management of Bell's palsy. *Laryngoscope.* 1999;109(8):1177–1188.

Gilbert S, McBurney E. Use of valacyclovir for herpes simplex virus-1 (HSV-1) prophylaxis after facial resurfacing: a randomized clinical trial of dosing regimens. *Dermatol Surg.* 2000;26(1):50–54.

Glogau RG. Aesthetic and anatomic analysis of the aging skin. *Semin Cutan Med Surg.* 1996;15(3):134–138.

Gunter AE, Llewellyn CM, Perez PI, et al. First bite syndrome following rhytidectomy: a case report. *Ann Otol Rhinol Laryngol.* doi:10.1177/0003489420936713.

Hamra ST. The deep-plane rhytidectomy. *Plast Reconstr Surg.* 1990;86(1):53–61.

His W. Die Formentwickelung des ausseren Ohres. *Anatomie Menschlicher Embryonen. Part III. Leipzig: Vogel.* 1885:211–221.

Hohman MH. Wound healing and optimization, including skin grafting, tissue expansion, and soft tissue techniques. In: Cheney ML, Hadlock TA, eds. *Facial Surgery: Plastic and Reconstructive.* 2nd ed. Boca Raton, FL: CRC Press; 2015:65–92.

Hohman MH, Hadlock TA. Etiology, diagnosis, and management of facial paralysis: 2000 patients at a facial nerve center. *Laryngoscope.* 2014;124(7):E283–E293.

House JW, Brackmann DE. Facial nerve grading system. *Otolaryngol Head Neck Surg.* 1985;93(2):146–147.

Isse NG. Endoscopic facial rejuvenation: endoforehead, the functional lift. Case reports. *Aesthetic Plast Surg.* 1994;18(1):21–29.

Karapandzic M. Reconstruction of lip defects by local arterial flaps. *Br J Plast Surg.* 1974;27(1):93–97.

Katz MI. Angle classification revisited 2: a modified angle classification. *Am J Orthod Dentofacial Orthop.* 1992;102(3):277–284.

Kridel RW, Appling WD, Wright WK. Septal perforation closure utilizing the external septorhinoplasty approach. *Arch Otolaryngol Head Neck Surg.* 1986;112(2):168–172.

Larrabee WF. A finite element model of skin deformation. *Laryngoscope.* 1986;96(4):399–405.

Lengelé BG. Current concepts and future challenges in facial transplantation. *Clin Plast Surg.* 2009;36(3):507–521.

Limberg AA. Design of local flaps. *Mod Trends Plast Surg.* 1966;2:38–61.

Ludwig E. Classification of the types of androgenetic alopecia (common baldness) occurring in the female sex. *Br J Dermatol.* 1977;97(3):247–254.

Markowitz BL, Manson PN, Sargent L, et al. Management of the medial canthal tendon in nasoethmoid orbital fractures: the importance of the central fragment in classification and treatment. *Plast Reconstruct Surg.* 1991;87(5):843–853.

Marx H. Die Missbildungen des ohres. In: Denker AK, ed. *Handbuch der Spez Path Anatomie Histologie.* Berlin: Springer; 1926:131.

Millard Jr. D.R. ***. *Cleft Craft.* Vols. 1–3. Boston, MA: Little Brown; 1976.

Miman MC, Deliktaş H, Özturan O, et al. Internal nasal valve: revisited with objective facts. *Otolaryngol Head Neck Surg.* 2006;134(1):41–47.

Mitz V, Peyronie M. The superficial musculo-aponeurotic system (SMAS) in the parotid and cheek area. *Plast Reconstr Surg.* 1976;58(1):80–88.

Murrell GL, Karakla DW, Messa A. Free flap repair of septal perforation. *Plast Reconstr Surg.* 1998;102(3):818–821.

Mustardé JC. The correction of prominent ears using simple mattress sutures. *Br J Plast Surg.* 1963;16:170–178.

Nagata S. A new method of total reconstruction of the auricle for microtia. *Plast Reconstr Surg.* 1993;92(2):187–201.

Noordhoff MS. Reconstruction of vermilion in unilateral and bilateral cleft lips. *Plast Reconstr Surg.* 1984;73(1):52–61.

Norwood OT. Male pattern baldness: classification and incidence. *South Med J.* 1975;68(11):1359–1365.

Pitanguy I, Ramos AS. The frontal branch of the facial nerve: the importance of its variations in face lifting. *Plast Reconstr Surg.* 1966;38(4):352–356.

Pomahac B, Pirbaz J, Eriksson E, et al. Three patients with full facial transplantation. *New Engl J Med.* 2012;366(8):715–722.

Qi Z, Liang W, Wang Y, et al. "X"-shaped incision and keloid skin-flap resurfacing: a new surgical method for auricle keloid excision and reconstruction. *Dermatol Surg.* 2012;38(8):1378–1382.

Remenschneider AK, Michalak A, Kozin ED, et al. Is serial electroneuronography indicated following temporal bone trauma? *Otol Neurotol.* 2017;38(4):572–576.

Ross BG, Fradet G, Nedzelski JM. Development of a sensitive clinical facial grading system. *Otolaryngol Head Neck Surg.* 1996;114(3):380–386.

Seddon H. *Surgical Disorders of the Peripheral Nerves.* Baltimore, MD: Williams and Wilkins; 1972.

Shan R. *Baker: Local Flaps in Facial Reconstruction.* 3rd ed. Philadelphia, PA: Saunders Elsevier; 2014.

Sheen JH. Spreader graft: a method of reconstructing the roof of the middle nasal vault following rhinoplasty. *Plast Reconstr Surg.* 1984;73(2):230–239.

Skoog T. Repair of unilateral cleft lip deformity: maxilla, nose and lip. *Scand J Plast Reconstr Surg.* 1969;3(2):109–133.

Spiegel JH. Facial feminization for the transgender patient. *J Craniofac Surg.* 2019;30(5):1399–1402.

Streeter G. Development of the auricle in the human embryo. *Contrib to Embryol Carnegie Inst.* 1922;69:111–138.

Sunderland S. *Nerves and Nerve Injuries.* 2nd ed. New York, NY: Churchill Livingstone; 1978.

Tardy ME. Practical suggestions on facial plastic surgery— how I do it. Sublabial mucosal flap: repair of septal perforations. *Laryngoscope.* 1977;87(2):275–278.

Tebbetts JB. *Primary Rhinoplasty.* 2nd ed. Philadelphia, PA: Mosby; 2008.

Tonnard P, Verpaele A. The MACS-lift short scar rhytidectomy. *Aesthet Surg J.* 2007;27(2):188–198.

Urken ML, Cheney ML, Blackwell KE, et al. *Regional and Free Flaps for Head and Neck Reconstruction.* 2nd ed. Philadelphia, PA: Lippincott Williams & Wilkins; 2012.

Veugen CCAFM, Dikkers FG, de Bakker BS. The developmental origin of the auricular revisited. *Laryngoscope.* 2020;130(10):2467–2474.

Vincent AG, Bevans SE, Robitschek JM, et al. Sterno-omohyoid free flap for dual-vector dynamic facial reanimation. *Ann Otol Rhinol Laryngol.* 2020;129(2):195–200.

Vincent AG, Sawhney R, Ducic Y. Perioperative care of free flap patients. *Semin Plast Surg.* 2019;33(1):5–12.

Vrabec JT, Backous DD, Djalilian HR, et al. Facial Nerve Grading System 2.0. *Otolaryngol Head Neck Surg.* 2009;140(4):445–450.

Waters CM, Zanation AM, Thorp BD. Repair of septal perforation with endoscopic-assisted pericranial flap harvest and open rhinoplasty approach. *Facial Plast Surg Aesthet Med.* 2020;22(3):225–226.

Yanagihara N. Grading of facial palsy. In: Fisch U, ed. *Proceedings of the Third International Symposium on Facial Nerve Surgery.* Zurich: Kugler Medical Publications; 1976:533–535.

Zide BM, Swift R. How to block and tackle the face. *Plast Reconstr Surg.* 1998;101(3):840–851.

Zide MF, Kent JN. Indications for open reduction of mandibular condyle fractures. *J Oral Maxillofac Surg.* 1983;41(2):89–98.

Zitelli JA. The bilobed flap for nasal reconstruction. *Arch Dermatol.* 1989;125(7):957–959.

4

Rhinology and Endoscopic Sinus Surgery

Douglas Reh and Jonathan Ting

HISTORY, PHYSICAL EXAMINATION, AND ANCILLARY TESTS IN THE RHINOLOGICAL PATIENT

History

- Nasal congestion/obstruction
  - Alternating cyclic engorgement of nasal turbinates is part of normal physiology, usually every 2 to 4 hours.
  - Increased obstruction when lying down or on dependent side with lateral recumbent position is normal.
- Purulent drainage
- Facial pain/pressure
- Loss of smell and taste
- History of environmental allergies (itchy, water eyes and nose and sneezing)
- Fever
- History of sinusitis
- History of sinonasal surgery
- Exposure to chemicals or metals
- Asthma
- Aspirin sensitivity
- Current medications
- Previous courses of antibiotics

Ancillary Tests

1. Nasal endoscopy
2. Culture
3. Biopsy
4. Outcome measure
5. Radiologic studies
6. Allergy evaluation
7. Beta-2-transferrin for cerebrospinal fluid (CSF) leak suspicion
8. Pulmonary function test for coexisting reactive airway disease
9. Evaluation of smell
10. Measures of mucociliary function
11. Measures of nasal resistance and airflow

Nasal Endoscopy

- Three passes
  1. Inferior pass: Floor of nose, inferior turbinate, septum, Eustachian tube orifice, and nasopharynx
  2. Superior pass: Nasal valve, septum, middle turbinate (MT), olfactory cleft, sphenoethmoid recess, and superior turbinate
  3. Middle pass: Middle meatus, basal lamella attachment, ostiomeatal complex, and uncinate process
- Culture using endoscopic-directed middle meatal swabs if presence of bacterial sinusitis is suspected
- Biopsy (be aware not to biopsy encephaloceles or juvenile nasopharyngeal angiofibroma [JNA])

Outcome Measures

- Nasal Obstruction Symptom Evaluation (NOSE) scale for obstructive nasal symptoms

- Rhinosinusitis Disability Index (RSDI) and Chronic Sinusitis Survey (CSS)
- Sinonasal Outcomes Test (SNOT-22) for chronic rhinosinusitis (CRS) symptoms

Radiological Workup

- Computed tomography (CT) of the paranasal sinuses (>4 weeks after treatment in most cases)
- Magnetic resonance imaging (MRI) for workup of tumors/masses, intracranial pathology, and assessment of soft tissue

Smell Tests for Evaluation of Anosmia/Hyposmia

- University of Pennsylvania Smell Identification Test (UPSIT)
- Sniffing sticks
- Alcohol pad

Objective Measures of Mucociliary Transport Function

- Saccharine ± color test in vivo (normal ~10 minutes; abnormal >30 minutes)
- Radioisotope transport testing in vivo
- Measuring ciliary activity in vitro
- Ciliary biopsy and electron microscopy for ciliary defect
- Nasal nitric oxide was found to be tenfold lower in primary ciliary dyskinesia (PCD) patients, but it cannot be used to exclude or to prove PCD

Objective Measures of Nasal Resistance and Airflow

- Rhinomanometry and the nasal peak flowmeter both measure transnasal flow.
- Rhinomanometry (usually anterior because of the ease of testing) also simultaneously measures transnasal pressure, which allows calculation of nasal resistance (pressure/flow).
- No population threshold has been established for the resistance at which symptomatic obstruction occurs, but individual changes in measures after surgery and medical therapy are used.
- Intranasal dimensions of the nose can be assessed by acoustic rhinometry, CT, and computational fluid dynamics, MRI, fiberoptic videoendoscopy, and rhinostereometry.

ANATOMY OF THE PARANASAL SINUSES

Components of Mucociliary Clearance

- Pseudostratified ciliated columnar epithelium: Anterior border begins at the limen nasi
- Ciliary activity causes the transport of mucus, an essential defense mechanism, at a frequency of 10 to 15 beats/min, and mucous blanket streams at a rate of 2.5 to 7.5 mL/min
- Double-layered mucous blanket: Deep, less viscous, serous periciliary fluid (sol phase) and superficial, more viscous, mucous fluid (gel phase)

- Mucus-producing glands: Goblet cells, seromucinous glands, and intraepithelial glands
- Inborn disorders of mucociliary transport (MCT) because of:
  - Ciliary dysfunction, as in PCD
  - Increased viscosity of the respiratory secretions, as in cystic fibrosis (CF)
- MCT is frequently impaired because of inflammation, infection, and exposure to ciliotoxic agents

Embryological Derivations of the Ethmoturbinals

1. First ethmoturbinal: Ascending portion is the agger nasi and descending portion is the uncinate process
2. Second ethmoturbinal: Ethmoid bulla
3. Third ethmoturbinal: Basal lamella and attachment of MT to the lateral nasal wall
4. Fourth ethmoturbinal: Attachment of the superior turbinate to the lateral nasal wall
5. Fifth and sixth: Usually degenerate but can form a supreme turbinate

Five Anterior-to-Posterior Bony Lamina Encountered in Endoscopic Sinus Surgery

1. Uncinate process
2. Ethmoid bulla
3. Vertical portion of the basal lamella
4. Vertical portion of the lamella of the superior turbinate
5. Anterior wall of the sphenoid sinus

Ostiomeatal Complex

- Functional concept: Final common pathway for drainage of anterior sinuses
- Structures within ostiomeatal complex (Fig. 4.1)
  - Uncinate process: Sickle-shaped bone running anterosuperior to posteroinferior, with attachments along the lateral nasal wall. First structure encountered when MT is medialized
  - Ethmoid bulla
  - Hiatus semilunaris: Two-dimensional slit that lies between the free edge of the uncinate process and the ethmoid bulla; connects the middle meatus into the infundibulum laterally
  - Infundibulum: Funnel-shaped three-dimensional space between the uncinate process medially and the lamina papyracea laterally
  - MT
  - Maxillary sinus ostium

Superior Attachment of the Uncinate Process (Fig. 4.2)

Variable Site of Attachment

- Laterally to lamina papyracea: Most commonly resulting in a recessus terminalis; frontal recess drains medially to the uncinate and directly into the middle meatus
- Superiorly onto the skull base: Frontal recess drains laterally into the infundibulum

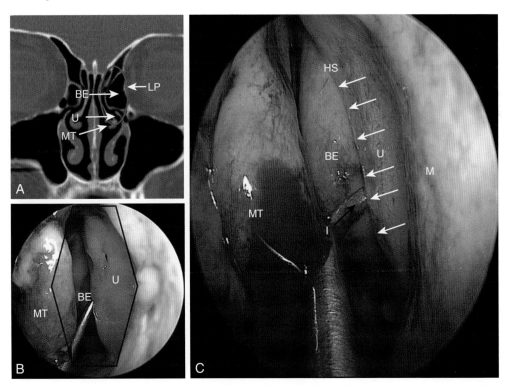

Fig. 4.1 Left ostiomeatal complex (enclosed by *blue line*) is bound laterally by the medial orbital wall or lamina papyracea (LP) and medially by the middle turbinate (MT). (**A**) Coronal computed tomography (CT) section outlining ostiomeatal complex boundaries. (**B**) Endoscopic view of the left nasal cavity with the MT being medialized. (**C**) Closer view of the left middle meatus. The uncinate process extends anteriorly to the anterior maxillary line (M). Its posterior free margin parallels the ethmoid bulla. The hiatus semilunaris (HS; *white arrows*) is a two-dimensional cleft between the posterior free edge of the uncinate and the ethmoid bulla. It is the gap through which the nasal cavity communicates with the ethmoid infundibulum (I). The infundibulum (*black arrow*) is a three-dimensional space between the uncinate process and lamina papyracea. This endoscopic figure shows the maxillary ball probe being passed through the linear hiatus semilunaris into the infundibulum. *BE*, Bulla ethmoidalis; *U*, uncinate process. (From Flint PW, Haughey BH, Lund VJ, et al. *Cummings Otolaryngology—Head and Neck Surgery*. 6th ed. Philadelphia, PA: Saunders; 2015, Fig. 49.1.)

- Medially to the MT: Frontal recess drains laterally into the infundibulum

Middle Turbinate

- Boomerang-shaped structure
- Basal lamella is the entire MT attachment to the lateral nasal wall and skull base
- Basal lamella can be conveniently thought of in three parts from the anterior to posterior aspects (Fig. 4.3)
  - Anterior part: Oriented in the sagittal plane (vertical) and attaches to the agger nasi region anteriorly and the cribriform plate superiorly
  - Middle: Oriented in the coronal plane obliquely and attached to the lamina papyracea

- Posterior: Oriented in the axial place (horizontal) and attached to the lateral nasal wall at the lamina papyracea, maxilla, and perpendicular process of the palatine bone
- Middle oblique part of the basal lamella is the only part of the MT that can be sacrificed without compromising the integrity of the turbinate: If the vertical or horizontal attachment is injured, the MT will lateralize the obstructing middle meatus and posterior ethmoid complex

Ethmoid Sinuses

- The ethmoid complex is divided by the basal lamella into the anterior and posterior ethmoid cells (Fig. 4.4)
- Anterior ethmoid cells
  - Drain into the middle meatus

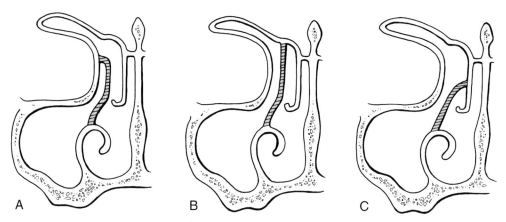

Fig. 4.2 Coronal schematic view of the ostiomeatal complex showing the superior attachments of the uncinate process to the lamina papyracea (LP) (**A**), the roof of the ethmoid (**B**), or the middle turbinate (MT) (**C**). If the uncinate process attaches to the roof of the ethmoid or to the MT, the frontal sinus drains into the infundibulum. If the uncinate attaches to the lamina papyracea, the frontal sinus drains medially, next to the MT. (From Flint PW, Haughey BH, Lund VJ, et al. *Cummings Otolaryngology—Head and Neck Surgery*. 6th ed. Philadelphia, PA: Saunders; 2015, Fig. 49.2.)

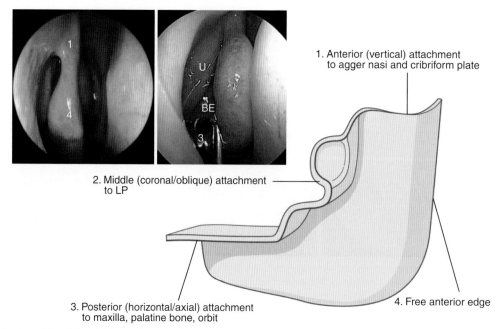

1. Anterior (vertical) attachment to agger nasi and cribriform plate

2. Middle (coronal/oblique) attachment to LP

3. Posterior (horizontal/axial) attachment to maxilla, palatine bone, orbit

4. Free anterior edge

Fig. 4.3 Schematic view of the right middle turbinate (MT) viewed from the lateral aspect illustrates the anterior vertical (*1*), middle oblique (*2*), and posterior horizontal (*3*) attachments. Inset, endoscopic views of the right MT show the free anterior edge (*4*) and the anterior (*1*) and posterior (*3*) attachments. *BE*, Bulla ethmoidalis; *LP*, lamina papyracea; *U*, uncinate. (From Flint PW, Haughey BH, Lund VJ, et al. *Cummings Otolaryngology—Head and Neck Surgery*. 6th ed. Philadelphia, PA: Saunders; 2015, Fig. 49.3.)

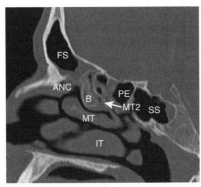 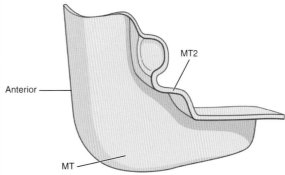

Fig. 4.4 The oblique, second part of the MT2 attaches to the lamina papyracea via the basal lamella, separating the anterior ethmoid (B) from the posterior ethmoid (PE) cells. This part lies in a coronal/frontal plane and is best viewed on a sagittal view computed tomography scan. *ANC,* Agger nasi cell; *FS,* frontal sinus; *IT,* inferior turbinate; *MT,* middle turbinate; *SS,* sphenoid sinus. (From Flint PW, Haughey BH, Lund VJ, et al. *Cummings Otolaryngology—Head and Neck Surgery.* 6th ed. Philadelphia, PA: Saunders; 2015, Fig. 49.4.)

- Ethmoid bulla: The largest and most prominent cell; it attaches laterally to the orbit
- May have a cleft behind the bulla (retrobullar recess) or above the bulla (suprabullar recess)
- Agger nasi at the attachment of the MT to the lateral wall is often pneumatized
  - Agger nasi cell is the most anterior of all ethmoid cells; it is present in >98% of CT scans
  - Key landmark in frontal sinus surgery
- Posterior ethmoid cells drain into the superior (or supreme) meatus
  - 1 to 5 cells
- Ethmoid cells may pneumatize into the adjacent sinuses and affect their drainage
  - Infraorbital or Haller cell into the maxillary sinus
  - Frontal, suprabullar, and supraorbital cells around the frontal sinus
  - Sphenoethmoid or Onodi cell over the sphenoid sinus, potentially placing the optic nerve and internal carotid artery (ICA) at risk if not recognized by surgeon

Maxillary Sinus

- Natural ostium
  - Drains into the inferior aspect (usually of the infundibulum) at a 45-degree angle
  - Elliptically shaped; accessory ostia are round and are present in the fontanelles in at least 10% of patients
  - Halfway between the anterior and posterior walls of the sinus
- Lateral nasal wall has two areas where bone is absent between the mucosa, called *fontanelles*
  - Anterior fontanelle is anterior to the uncinate bone
  - Posterior fontanelle

Sphenoid Sinus

- Natural os opens into the sphenoethmoidal recess
- Sphenoid os halfway to two-thirds up the anterior wall of the sinus
- Medial to the posterior end of the superior turbinate in the majority (83%) of cases
- Os is average of 7 cm from the nasal spine, at an angle of 30 degrees from the floor
- Walls of the sphenoid sinus contain several critical structures such as the ICA, optic nerve, and skull base
- Septations in the sphenoid frequently attach to the ICA

Frontal Sinus

- Originates embryologically from an anterior ethmoid cell
- Outflow tract has an hourglass shape, and the narrowest part is the internal frontal ostium
- Mucociliary flow is up the intersinus septum across the frontal sinus roof laterally and then medially along the floor of the frontal sinus down to the frontal recess
- Drains through the frontal recess into the middle meatus (commonly) or into the superior aspect of the infundibulum (less commonly) depending on the uncinated attachment
- Boundaries of the frontal recess
  - Medial: MT
  - Lateral: Lamina papyracea
  - Anterior: Posterior wall of the agger nasi
  - Posterior: Ethmoid bulla

Cells Related to the Frontal Sinus

- Frontal recess may contain anterior ethmoid cells (called *frontal recess cells*), which consequently narrow the frontal sinus drainage pathway (Fig. 4.5)
- Anterior to the frontal recess
  - Frontal cells
    - Type I: A single cell superior to the agger nasi cell
    - Type II: A tier of two or more cells above the agger nasi cell
    - Type III: A single cell that extends from the agger nasi cell into the frontal sinus, above the floor of the frontal sinus floor but <50% of the frontal sinus height
    - Type IV: An isolated cell within the frontal sinus (Kuhn) or a single cell that extends into the frontal sinus for >50% of the frontal sinus height (Wormald)
- Posterior to the frontal recess
  - Supraorbital ethmoid cell: Cells posterior to the frontal sinus, pneumatizing superiorly to the orbital roof
  - Interfrontal sinus cell: Pneumatizes intersinus septum and drains into one frontal sinus, medially to the frontal ostium
  - Suprabullar cell: Cell superior to the ethmoid bulla
  - Frontal bulla cell: Cell superior to the ethmoid bulla pneumatizing into the posterior frontal table (anterior skull base)

Bent and Kuhn Classification of Frontal Cells

1. Type I: A single frontal recess cell above the agger nasi
2. Type II: A tier of cells above the agger nasi projecting into the frontal recess

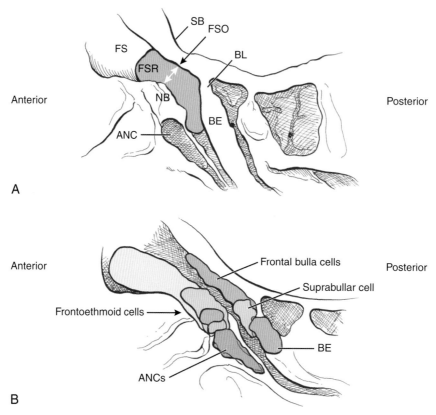

Fig. 4.5 (**A**) The frontal sinus recess (FSR) is an hourglass-shaped space (*shaded area*) with the waist at the frontal sinus ostium (FSO), which is its narrowest part. In the simplest configuration, the boundaries of the frontal recess are limited by the agger nasi cell (ANC) and nasal beak (NB) anteriorly, the bulla ethmoidalis (BE) and the bulla lamella (BL) posteriorly, the anterior skull base (SB) posterosuperiorly, the cribriform plate and middle turbinate (MT) medially, and the lamina papyracea laterally. (**B**) Frontoethmoid cells pneumatize around the frontal recess. Frontal cells lie anterior to the frontal recess; suprabullar, supraorbital ethmoid, and frontobullar cells lie posterior to the frontal recess. (From Flint PW, Haughey BH, Lund VJ, et al. *Cummings Otolaryngology—Head and Neck Surgery.* 6th ed. Philadelphia, PA: Saunders; 2015, Fig. 49.9.)

3. Type III: Single massive cell arising above the agger nasi, pneumatizing the cephalad into the frontal sinus
4. Type IV: Single isolated cell within the frontal sinus

Anatomical Variants (Fig. 4.6)

- Concha bullosa: Defined as aeration of the MT; cavity lines with the same epithelium as the rest of the nasal cavity
- Paradoxical MT: Curvature projecting laterally; may narrow or obstruct the nasal cavity, middle meatus, and infundibulum
- Atelectatic uncinate process: Free edge of the uncinate adheres to the orbital wall; associated with an occluded infundibulum and hypoplastic opacified ipsilateral maxillary sinus, possibly with a more inferior location of the orbit and increased risk of orbital complications during surgery
- Haller cell: An infraorbital ethmoid cell; pneumatizes into the maxilla
- Onodi cell: A sphenoethmoidal cell, a posterior ethmoid air cell pneumatizing over the sphenoid

Airspaces Within the Paranasal Sinuses

- Suprabullar recess: Air cell space left between the ethmoid bulla and the fovea ethmoidalis when the bulla does not extend up to the fovea
- Sinus lateralis/retrobullar recess: Air cell space found between the posterior surface of the ethmoid bulla and the vertical portion of the basal lamella

- Sinus terminalis: Uncinate process terminates in the lamina papyracea; frontal recess drains medially to the uncinate process; this sinus is essentially a superior ending of the infundibulum (blind pocket)
- Agger nasi cell: Remnant of the first ethmoturbinal, found superior, lateral, and anterior to the attachment of the MT; can also refer to ethmoid cells anterior to the frontal duct

Anterior Skull Base

- Formed by the cribriform medially and the fovea ethmodalis laterally
- Slopes downward posteriorly
- Skull base is thinner medially (0.1 mm) along the lateral lamella of the cribriform plate
- Inverse relationship between maxillary sinus height and the height of the ethmoid cavity (i.e., large maxillary sinus is related to lower-lying skull base)

Keros Classification of Lateral Lamella of Cribriform Height

1. Type 1: Cribriform plate 1 to 3 mm below the fovea
2. Type 2: Cribriform plate 4 to 7 mm below the fovea
3. Type 3: Cribriform plate 8 to 16 mm below the fovea (highest risk of skull-base penetration)

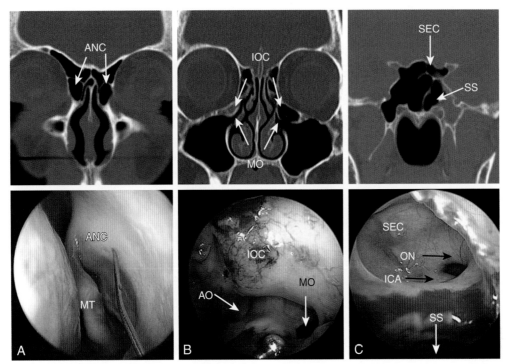

Fig. 4.6 Ethmoid cells. Top row shows a computed tomography (CT) scan with corresponding endoscopic view below. (**A**) The ANC is the most anterior cell seen on a coronal CT scan, anterior to the middle turbinate (MT). Endoscopically, it is seen as a bulge on the MT attachment and may narrow the superior ethmoid infundibulum. (**B**) Coronal CT section shows bilateral infraorbital ethmoid cells (IOC; Haller cells) narrowing the inferior ethmoid infundibulum and attaching laterally to the infraorbital canal. The maxillary sinus opens into the inferior part of the infundibulum at a 45-degree angle. Endoscopic view of the left infundibulum after uncinectomy shows the IOC narrowing the inferior infundibulum and potentially obstructing drainage of the natural maxillary ostium (MO). The natural MO is elliptically shaped and opens into the floor of the infundibulum at a 45-degree angle, not directly into the lateral wall. Accessory ostia (AO) are usually circular and are present here in the posterior fontanelle. (**C**) The sphenoethmoid cell (SEC), or Onodi cell, is a posterior ethmoid cell that is lateral and superior to the sphenoid sinus (SS), which is usually smaller, pushed medially and inferiorly. The figures show arrows pointing to a left SEC on coronal and sagittal CT cuts. The endoscopic image demonstrates the relationship of the SEC to the SS and shows the optic nerve (ON) and internal carotid artery lying in relation to the SEC lateral wall. (From Flint PW, Haughey BH, Lund VJ, et al. *Cummings Otolaryngology—Head and Neck Surgery.* 6th ed. Philadelphia, PA: Saunders; 2015, Fig. 49.5.)

RHINITIS

History and Physical

- Single most important factor in attaining a proper diagnosis is a complete history
- Symptoms: Nasal discharge, congestion/blockage, change in olfaction, postnasal drainage, episodes of sneezing, nasal itching, itchy eyes, and epiphora
- Symptom frequency: Intermittent or persistent?
- Medication history
- History of asthma and sensitivity to aspirin or nonsteroidal antiinflammatory drugs (NSAIDs)
- History of head trauma
- History of prior nasal/sinus surgery
- History of hay fever/seasonal allergies/allergy testing
- Other systemic disorders
- Inciting factors, including weather changes, certain odors or food, time of year, occupational history, chemical exposure at work, and improvement of symptoms on weekends/holidays (away from work)
- Examination should include nasal endoscopy

Workup

- Skin testing and/or serum testing for serum-specific immunoglobulin E (IgE) antibodies to relevant allergens
- Nasal cytology; scrapings from the inferior turbinate mucosa; high-power field of 5 to 25 eosinophils is compatible with a diagnosis of nonallergic rhinitis with eosinophilia syndrome (NARES) with negative allergy testing

Treatment Principles

1. Avoidance of triggers
2. Topical corticosteroids for allergic and nonallergic rhinitis
3. Consider topical nasal (and oral) antihistamines and anticholinergic sprays depending on etiology
4. Normal saline rinses as adjunct
5. In recalcitrant cases, may consider surgery, including turbinate reduction and potentially vidian neurectomy
6. Posterior nasal nerve ablation with either cryotherapy or radiofrequency can be done endoscopically in the office setting as alternative to vidian neurectomy

Causes of Rhinitis/Rhinorrhea

- Allergic rhinitis
- Churg-Strauss syndrome
- Infectious
- NARES
- Rhinitis sicca anterior
- Atrophic rhinitis

- Rhinitis medicamentosa
- Vasomotor rhinitis
- Hormonal rhinitis (e.g., pregnancy)
- Medication-induced rhinitis
- CSF rhinorrhea

Allergic Rhinitis

- Treat with avoidance of allergens, saline irrigations, oral and nasal antihistamines, nasal steroid sprays, oral decongestants, oral antileukotrienes, and nasal mast cell stabilizers
- Consider allergy testing and immunotherapy

Churg-Strauss Syndrome

- Asthma, eosinophilia (>10%), allergic rhinosinusitis, pulmonary infiltrates, vasculitis, and neuritis
- Treat with oral steroids, cyclophosphamide, and management of sinonasal symptoms

Infectious Rhinitis

- Viral (supportive Rx)
- Bacterial (commonly *Streptococcus pneumoniae*, *Haemophilus influenzae*, and *Moraxella catarrhalis*; treat with antibiotics)
- Rhinoscleroma (Mikulicz cells, Russell bodies on histopathology; treat with long-term ciprofloxacin or tertracycline)
- Rhinosporidiosis (*Rhinosporidium seeberi* is endemic in Africa and India): Painless, friable, "strawberry" lesion; pseudoepitheliomatous hyperplasia on histopathology; treat with excision, antifungals, and dapsone

Nonallergic Rhinitis With Eosinophilia Syndrome

- Nasal eosinophilia (10%–20% on smear) with negative allergy testing
- Symptoms and treatment are similar to allergic rhinitis

Rhinitis Sicca Anterior

- Dry, raw nasal mucosa caused by changes in temperature/humidity, nose picking, and dust
- Symptoms include dryness, crusting, and epistaxis
- Treat with saline irrigation, topical antibiotics, and oil-based nasal ointments

Atrophic Rhinitis

- Transition from functional, ciliated respiratory epithelium to a nonfunctional lining of nonciliated squamous metaplasia, with a loss of mucociliary clearance and squamous metaplasia
- Destroyed MCT and loss of mucosal glands
- Crusting, fetor, mucosal atrophy, and widely patent nasal cavities are seen in patients who complain of nasal congestion
- Causes include aggressive turbinectomy, excessive nasal surgery, nutritional deficiencies (iron or vitamin A or D deficiency), chronic bacterial infection (e.g., *Klebsiella ozaenae*, less common in antibiotic era), trauma, manifestations of granulomatous diseases, chronic cocaine abuse, and radiation therapy
- Symptoms include paradoxical nasal congestion/obstruction despite wide nasal cavity, nasal crusting, and odor
- Treatment options are limited: May include irrigations, humidification to provide moisture, and experimental surgical procedures

Rhinitis Medicamentosa

- Rebound congestion from decreased vasomotor tone or increased parasympathetic activity due to topical nasal decongestants or cocaine use
- Treat by discontinuing topical decongestants; consider short-term oral corticosteroids (for weaning)

Vasomotor Rhinitis

- Results from changes in vascular tone and permeability: Stimulation of afferent sensory nerves is the most likely pathophysiological mechanism, which activates the parasympathetic nerves that supply the nasal mucosal glands
- Symptoms include clear, watery rhinorrhea and occasionally sweating/epiphora
- More common in older adults
- Multiple triggers, including temperature change, eating (gustatory rhinitis, often with hot/spicy food), and anxiety
- Treat with anticholinergic nasal sprays (ipratropium bromide)
- Posterior nasal nerve ablation with either cryotherapy or radiofrequency can be done endoscopically in the office setting
- Vidian neurectomy is procedure under general anesthesia with a higher risk of chronic dry eye

Hormonal Rhinitis

- Fluctuating hormones with menstruation and puberty
- Rhinitis of pregnancy seen in >20%
- Increased in hypothyroidism and acromegaly

Medication-Induced Rhinitis (Box 4.1)

- Aspirin and NSAIDs in patients with aspirin-exacerbated respiratory disease (AERD)
- Multiple psychotropic agents (e.g., amitriptyline)
- Antihypertensives (e.g., beta-blockers and angiotensin-converting enzyme inhibitors)
- Hormonal replacement and oral contraceptives

Inhalant-Induced Rhinitis

- Proposed mechanism is the stimulation of chemical irritant receptors on sensory nerves (i.e., C fibers) to induce neuropeptide release, which produces the vasodilation and edema associated with inflammation independent of immune-mediated responses
- Chemical exposures classifications:
  - Immunological (high molecular-weight agents, e.g., wheat, latex, compounds in insecticides, adhesives, and auto-body spray paint)
  - Annoyant (perfumes, exhaust fumes, cleaning agents, room deodorizers, floral fragrances, and cosmetics)
  - Irritant (air pollution, smoke, tobacco smoke, paint fumes, formaldehyde, and volatile organic compounds) can lead to the synthesis of proinflammatory mediators and neuromediators
  - Corrosive (ammonium chloride, hydrochloric acid, vinyl chloride, organophosphates, and acrylamide exposures causing mucosal burns and ulcerations)

Cerebrospinal Fluid Rhinorrhea

- Clear, watery typically unilateral rhinorrhea; worse with lowering head
- Patients will often report that the watery drainage occurs when they bend; surgical therapy with high success rates of endoscopic closure (>90%)

BOX 4.1 Medications That Contribute to Rhinitis

INTRANASAL PREPARATIONS

Cocaine
Topical nasal decongestants

ANTIHYPERTENSIVES

α- and β-Adrenoceptor antagonists
Reserpine
Hydralazine
Felodipine
Angiotensin-converting enzyme inhibitors
β-Blockers
Methyldopa
Guanethidine
Phentolamine

AGENTS FOR PROSTATIC HYPERTROPHY

Doxazosin
Tamsulosin

HORMONES

Oral contraceptives

ANTIINFLAMMATORY AGENTS

Nonsteroidal antiinflammatory medications
Aspirin

ANTIPLATELET AGENTS

Clopidogrel

ANTIDEPRESSANTS

Selective serotonin reuptake inhibitors

NONBENZODIAZEPINE HYPNOTICS

Zolpidem

PHOSPHODIESTERASE TYPE-5 INHIBITORS

Sildenafil
Tadalafil
Vardenafil

PSYCHOTROPIC AGENTS

Thioridazine
Chlordiazepoxide
Chlorpromazine
Amitriptyline
Perphenazine
Alprazolam

From Flint PW, Haughey BH, Lund VJ, et al. *Cummings Otolaryngology—Head and Neck Surgery.* 6th ed. Philadelphia, PA: Saunders; 2015, Box 43.2.

NASAL OBSTRUCTION

Differential Diagnosis of Nasal Obstruction

- Rhinitis (inflammatory)
- Chronic sinusitis (with or without nasal polyps)
- Rhinitis medicamentosa (chronic use of nasal decongestants)
- Deviated nasal septum
- Inferior turbinate hypertrophy
- Nasal valve collapse
- Adenoid hypertrophy (children)
- Choanal atresia (infants, congenital)
- Empty-nose syndrome (prior total resection of inferior turbinates is the most likely cause)

Evaluation of Nasal Obstruction

- History and physical
  - Seasonal and/or daily variation of symptoms
  - History of nasal trauma

- History of past nasal surgery
- History and signs of allergic or nonallergic inflammation
- Examine external and internal nasal valves (modified Cottle maneuver to assess nasal valves)
- Nasal endoscopy
- Sinus CT
- Allergy testing

Treatment Options for Nasal Obstruction

- Trial of nasal steroids and antihistamines
- Oral steroids for chronic sinusitis
- Trial of Breathe Right® nasal strips if nasal valve collapse is suspected
- Inferior turbinoplasty (submucosal resection and outfracture)
  - Radiofrequency coblation
  - Submucosal debridement
  - Medial flap turbinoplasty with resection of bony turbinate
- Septoplasty
- Radiofrequency valve remodeling (in-office procedure)
- Nasal valve stent implant (in-office procedure)
- Functional rhinoplasty (closed or open)
  - Extracorporeal septoplasty (caudal deviations)
  - Nasal valve repair

NASAL SEPTAL PERFORATION

Causes of Nasal Septal Perforation

- Iatrogenic (septoplasty)
- Trauma and septal hematoma
- Drug use (cocaine, inhaled narcotics)
- Malignancy
- Granulomatous disease (granulomatosis with polyangiitis [GPA], sarcoidosis)
- Corticosteroid nasal spray (overuse)
- Infection (tertiary syphilis)

Treatment of Nasal Septal Perforation

- Consider workup for etiology in expanding perforations
- Nasal hygiene: Increase moisture (bactroban ointment); avoid digital manipulation
- Silastic buttons
- Surgical repair
- Extending perforation posteriorly

EPISTAXIS

Workup of Epistaxis

- Unilateral versus bilateral
- Duration
- Frequency
- Severity (trickle vs. high flow)
- Time of day (morning vs. nighttime)
- Anterior (tends to be unilateral, flows from nostril)
- Posterior (may be bilateral, with significant bleeding from the oropharynx/oral cavity as it runs posteriorly)
- Source (Keisselbach plexus, anterior ethmoid artery, posterior ethmoid artery, sphenopalatine artery, mucosal lesion, or neoplasm)
- Exacerbating factors (trauma, digital trauma, and temperature)
- Medical history (hypertension or coagulopathy)
- Family history
- Medications (aspirin, NSAIDs, and anticoagulants)

Causes of Epistaxis

- Bleeding from blood vessels in the Keisselbach plexus is the most common cause in 90% of cases (plexus in the anterior caudal septum is supplied by the anterior ethmoid artery, sphenopalatine artery, greater palatine artery, and superior labial artery)
- Mucosal trauma (digital manipulation)
- Toxic (inhaled drugs, including cocaine and heroin)
- Drugs (chemotherapy, anticoagulants, and alcoholism)
- Mucosal lesion (capillary hemangioma and telangiectasia)
- Neoplasm (JNA and malignant neoplasm)
- Congenital (hereditary hemorrhagic telangiectasias [HHT], hemophilia, and von Willebrand)
- Systemic (hypertension and coagulopathy)

Treatment Options for Epistaxis

- Nondissolvable packing (anterior pack: Kennedy Merocel vs. posterior pack)
- Dissolvable packing (hemostatic agents: Surgicel Gelfoam, and Floseal)
- In-office cauterization (silver nitrate or laser)
- Cauterization under anesthesia (coblation, bipolar cautery, monopolar cautery, or laser)
- Manage underlying condition or cause (neoplasm, hypertension, and coagulopathy)
- Endoscopic anterior ethmoid artery ligation
- Endoscopic sphenopalatine artery ligation (posterior epistaxis)
- Internal maxillary/sphenopalatine artery embolization

Hereditary Hemorrhagic Telangiectasias (Formerly Osler Weber Rendu)

- Diagnosis
  - Autosomal dominant (at least five genes identified)
  - Curacao criteria (definite if 3; suspected if 2; unlikely if <2)
    - Epistaxis
    - Mucosal telangiectasias (oral and sinonasal)
    - Visceral lesions (pulmonary arteriovenous malformation [AVM], cerebral AVM, hepatic AVM, and spinal AVM)
    - Family history (first-degree relative)
  - Medical management
    - Topical moisturizers (mupirocin and saline gel)
    - Topical rose geranium oil
    - Topical or oral estrogen agents (hormone replacement therapy and antiestrogen agents)
    - Topical timolol
    - Oral tranexamic acid
    - Topical or intravenous (IV) bevacizumab (Avastin)
    - In-office injected sclerotherapy
  - Surgical management
    - Cauterization (laser, bipolar, and radiofrequency)
    - Injected bevacizumab (Avastin)
    - Septodermoplasty
    - Young's procedure (surgical closure of nostril)

OLFACTORY PHYSIOLOGY AND DISORDERS

Airflow Through the Nasal Cavity (Fig. 4.7)

- Middle meatus (50%)
- Inferior meatus (35%)
- Olfactory cleft (15%)

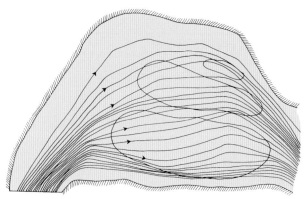

Fig. 4.7 Streamline patterns for resting inspiratory flow (250 mL/s) through an expanded (20× normal size) scale model of a healthy human adult-male nasal cavity (sagittal view). Lines show the paths taken by small dust particles entering at the external nares. (From Scherer PW, Scherer PW, Hahn II, Mozell MM. The biophysics of nasal airflow. *Otolaryngol Clin North Am*. 1989;22:265; and Flint PW, Haughey BH, Lund VJ, et al. *Cummings Otolaryngology—Head and Neck Surgery*. 6th ed. Philadelphia, PA: Saunders; 2015, Fig. 39.1.)

Olfactory Epithelium Basics

- Much thicker than normal respiratory mucosa and is intermixed with respiratory epithelium (which increases with age)
- Mucus of epithelium traps odorant molecules
- Club-shaped bipolar neurons extend into the olfactory epithelium and are exposed via dendrites and cilia
  - Traverses toward the cribriform plate and becomes encased by Schwann cells
  - Travels through 1 of 20 foramen in the cribriform and enters the central nervous system (CNS) and synapse to the olfactory bulbs at the base of the brain
  - Humans have about 6 million olfactory neurons bilaterally
  - Uniquely capable of regeneration
- There are also basal cells, sustentacular (supporting) cells, and microvilli cells, which may be specialized sensory cells

Olfactory Bulb Basics (Fig. 4.8)

- Lies at the base of the frontal cortex in the anterior fossa
- Serves as the first relay station in the olfactory pathway, where the primary olfactory neurons synapse with secondary neurons
- These synapses and their postsynaptic partners form dense aggregates of neuropil called *glomeruli*

Central Olfactory Connections

- Olfactory tubercle
- Prepiriform cortex
- Amygdaloid nuclei
- Nucleus of the terminal stria with further projections to a number of structures, including the hypothalamus

Common Chemical Sense Basics

- Added chemoreceptivity in the mucosa of the respiratory tract is provided by free nerve endings of three cranial nerves
  1. Trigeminal (most important)
  2. Glossopharyngeal
  3. Vagus
- The trigeminal nerves sense the burn of ammonia and the bite of hot pepper

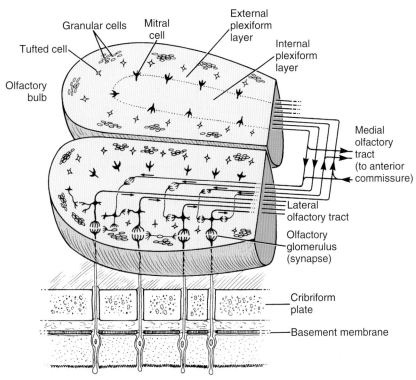

Fig. 4.8 Structure of olfactory bulbs and their neural connections to one another, the olfactory mucosa, and the brain. (From Flint PW, Haughey BH, Lund VJ, et al. *Cummings Otolaryngology—Head and Neck Surgery.* 6th ed. Philadelphia, PA: Saunders; 2015, Fig. 39.8.)

- In the nose, virtually all odorants stimulate olfactory and trigeminal nerves, even when no apparent pungency can be perceived

Smell Determinant Basics

- Theories range from odor binding proteins (OBPs) and olfactory receptors to tonotopic organization and receptor specialization
- Agreed-upon factors on what a molecule must have to illicit smell
  1. Water solubility
  2. Sufficient vapor pressure
  3. Low polarity
  4. Some ability to dissolve in fat (lipophilicity), which may be aided by OBP
  5. Size: No known odorants possess a molecular weight of > 294 kDa

Olfactory Tests

1. UPSIT: Most specific test; also Sniffin' Sticks
2. Gross perception
   - Odor sticks (e.g., marker-type pen)
   - 12-inch alcohol smell test
3. Threshold: Determine the threshold with serial dilutions of phenylethyl alcohol
4. Patient-reported questionnaires, for example, Self-reported Mini Olfactory Questionnaire (Self-MOQ)

Types of Olfactory Disorders

1. Transport or conductive
2. Sensory
3. Neural olfactory loss

Causes of Transport (Conductive) Olfactory Disorders

1. Nasal inflammation resulting from rhinitis, sinusitis, or upper-respiratory infection (URI)
2. Polyps
3. Neoplasm
4. Mass effect
5. Septal deviation or nasal obstruction

Causes of Sensory Olfactory Disorder

- From damage to the neuroepithelium caused by:
  1. Drugs
  2. Neoplasms
  3. External beam radiation therapy (XRT)
  4. Toxic-chemical exposure
  5. Viral URI:
     - Some patients never recover smell following URI
     - Overwhelming predominance of females in this group (80%)
     - Prognosis is poor, and etiology is not understood
     - Biopsy shows decreased or absence of receptors
     - COVID-19 (coronavirus disease 2019) causes temporary or long-term loss of smell; virus appears to damage olfactory support cells

Causes of Neural Olfactory Loss

1. Alcohol
2. Tobacco
3. Human immunodeficiency virus (HIV)
4. Age: Olfaction decreases in the sixth to seventh decade from olfactory neuron loss
   - Neurological: Parkinson, Huntington, and Alzheimer diseases

- Very high incidence of olfactory disorders in these dementia-related diseases
- May preferentially involve the olfactory system
5. Kallmann syndrome: X-linked disorder characterized by hypogonadism and anosmia
6. Korsakoff psychosis
7. Metabolic
   - B_{12} or zinc deficiency
   - Hypothyroidism
   - Diabetes mellitus
   - Malnutrition
8. Trauma
   - 5% to 10% incidence of anosmia following head trauma
   - Shearing of olfactory neurons is the predominating theory

Workup and Management of Decreased Olfaction

- May consider MRI in cases of idiopathic olfactory loss, but not cost-effective
- Consider olfactory training ± steroid rinses in documented olfactory loss

CEREBROSPINAL FLUID RHINORRHEA

Causes of Cerebrospinal Fluid Rhinorrhea (Box 4.2)

- Traumatic
  - Accidental (e.g., head trauma)
  - Iatrogenic (e.g., endoscopic sinus surgery [ESS])
- Spontaneous
  - Typically involves meningoencephalocele
  - Likely secondary to increased intracranial pressure (associated with obstructive sleep apnea [OSA], obesity, or pseudotumor cerebri)
  - 15% to 50% of CSF leak repairs
  - Highest repair-failure rate
- Neoplasm
- Congenital
- Infection

Options for Cerebrospinal Fluid Rhinorrhea Evaluation

- High-resolution CT scan (0.5 mm; Fig. 4.9) to evaluate bony skull base
- High-resolution MRI (Fig. 4.10) to evaluate for meningoencephalocele
- Presence of B-2 transferrin in nasal secretions is the gold standard (must collect 0.5 mL)
- CT cisternography (Fig. 4.11): thin section axial CT imaging in prone and supine positions before and after intrathecal contrast
- Radionuclide cisternography (technetium 99 m or indium 111-labeled diethylenetriaminepentaacetic acid): Identifies presence and side of leak
- Endoscopic and/or intraoperative evaluation with fluorescein (Fig. 4.12)

Treatment Options for Cerebrospinal Fluid Rhinorrhea

- Conservative management (particularly for traumatic leaks)
  - Bed rest with head of bed elevated
  - Stool softeners
  - Avoid Valsalva maneuver and nose blowing
  - Lumbar drain
- Craniotomy and repair

BOX 4.2 Cerebrospinal Fluid Rhinorrhea Classification

TRAUMATIC

Accidental
- Immediate
- Delayed

Surgical
- Complication of neurosurgical procedures:
  - Transsphenoidal hypophysectomy
  - Frontal craniotomy
  - Other skull-base procedures
- Complication of rhinological procedures:
  - Sinus surgery
  - Septoplasty
  - Other combined skull-base procedures

NONTRAUMATIC

Elevated Intracranial Pressure
- Intracranial neoplasm
- Hydrocephalus:
  - Noncommunicating
  - Obstructive
- Benign intracranial hypertension

Normal Intracranial Pressure
- Congenital anomaly
- Skull-base neoplasm:
  - Nasopharyngeal carcinoma
  - Sinonasal malignancy
- Skull-base erosive process:
  - Sinus mucocele
  - Osteomyelitis
- Idiopathic

From Flint PW, Haughey BH, Lund VJ, et al. *Cummings Otolaryngology—Head and Neck Surgery.* 6th ed. Philadelphia, PA: Saunders; 2015, Box 52.1.

- Endoscopic repair is the gold standard for amendable lesions
  - Grafts
    1. Bone: Mastoid cortex, septal, and turbinate
    2. Cartilage: Septal and pinna concha
    3. Fascia: Fascia lata and temporalis
    4. Mucosa free grafts: Septal, MT, and nasal floor
    5. Synthetic: Dural substitutes (DuraMatrix, DuraGen, and AlloDerm)
  - Pedicled flaps (overlay)
    1. Nasoseptal
    2. Turbinate
  - Spontaneous leaks: Must consider and treat increased intracranial pressure (e.g., acetazolamide and CSF shunt), evaluate for sleep apnea

RHINOSINUSITIS

Definitions of Rhinosinusitis

- Rhinosinusitis: Any inflammation of the nose and sinus mucosa
- Acute rhinosinusitis (ARS): Rhinosinusitis lasting 4 weeks or less
- Recurrent ARS: Four or more annual episodes of rhinosinusitis without persistent symptoms in between
- CRS: Rhinosinusitis lasting longer than 12 weeks

Etiologies of Acute Rhinosinusitis

- Viral (most common): Rhinovirus, parainfluenza virus, respiratory syncytial virus, influenza virus, and coronavirus

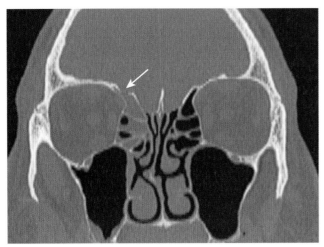

Fig. 4.9 High-resolution sinus computed tomography (CT) may be used to visualize even small bony defects of the skull base (SB). This coronal CT image was reconstructed from 1-mm direct axial CT image data using a robust image-processing software system. It should be noted that not all reformatted coronal images are of sufficient quality to permit this precise examination of the SB. A bony dehiscence (*arrow*) together with a positive β-2 transferrin study represents a likely site for an active cerebrospinal fluid (CSF) leak. However, in the absence of a positive β-2 transferrin study, the presence of a CSF leak should not be assumed from such a finding. (From Flint PW, Haughey BH, Lund VJ, et al. *Cummings Otolaryngology—Head and Neck Surgery*. 6th ed. Philadelphia, PA: Saunders; 2015, Fig. 52.6.)

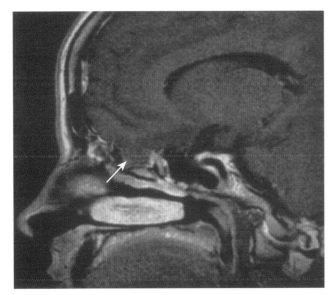

Fig. 4.10 Magnetic resonance provides excellent imaging of anterior skull base meningoencephaloceles. The arrow shows their characteristic appearance on this sagittal image. (From Flint PW, Haughey BH, Lund VJ, et al. *Cummings Otolaryngology—Head and Neck Surgery*. 6th ed. Philadelphia, PA: Saunders; 2015, Fig. 52.7.)

- Bacterial (acute bacterial sinusitis): *S. pneumoniae, H. influenzae, Moraxella catarrhalis, Staphylococcus aureus*, and *Streptococcus pyogenes*
- Fulminant fungal: *Aspergillus, Mucor*, and *Rhizopus*

Hallmark Symptoms of Acute Rhinosinusitis

1. Purulent rhinorrhea
2. Nasal obstruction/congestion

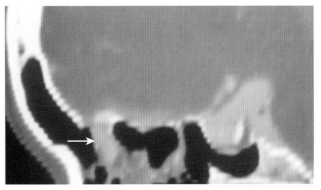

Fig. 4.11 A cerebrospinal fluid leak on computed tomography (CT) cisternography is characterized by the presence of contrast material within the pneumatized paranasal sinuses. The contrast should be in direct continuity so that a precise site of communication can be reliably demonstrated, as shown in this sagittal CT image reconstruction from a positive CT cisternogram. The arrow points to the area of the contrast within the ethmoid sinuses. (From Flint PW, Haughey BH, Lund VJ, et al. *Cummings Otolaryngology—Head and Neck Surgery*. 6th ed. Philadelphia, PA: Saunders; 2015, Fig. 52.3.)

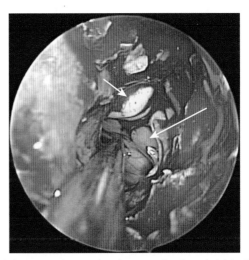

Fig. 4.12 Intraoperative nasal endoscopy after the administration of intrathecal fluorescein provides a way to confirm a cerebrospinal fluid (CSF) leak and precisely localize the corresponding skull-base defect. In this endoscopic image obtained after ethmoidectomy and sphenoidotomy, a meningocele arises from the superior (*short arrow*) and superolateral (*long arrow*) aspects of the left sphenoid sinus. The meningocele has a greenish hue because the fluorescein colors the CSF within it. (From Flint PW, Haughey BH, Lund VJ, et al. *Cummings Otolaryngology—Head and Neck Surgery*. 6th ed. Philadelphia, PA: Saunders; 2015, Fig. 52.5.)

3. Facial pain and/or pressure
4. Decreased sense of smell and taste

Workup and Diagnosis of Acute Bacterial Rhinosinusitis (Table 4.1)

- Acute bacterial rhinosinusitis (ABRS) must be distinguished from viral URIs and noninfectious etiologies such as allergic rhinitis
- Can be differentiated from these entities when:
  1. Symptoms or signs of ARS (hallmark symptoms) persist without evidence of improvement for at least 10 days or

TABLE 4.1 Rhinosinusitis Symptoms

Major	Minor
Facial pain/pressure	Headache
Facial congestion/fullness	Fever (nonacute)
Nasal obstruction/blockage	Halitosis
Nasal discharge/purulence with discolored posterior drainage	Fatigue
	Dental pain
Hyposmia/anosmia	Cough
Purulence on nasal exam	Ear pain, pressure, and/or fullness
Fever (acute rhinosinusitis only)	

Note: Diagnosis of rhinosinusitis requires two major or one major and two minor symptoms.

From Flint PW, Haughey BH, Lund VJ, et al. *Cummings Otolaryngology—Head and Neck Surgery*. 6th ed. Philadelphia, PA: Saunders; 2015, Table 46.1.

2. Symptoms of rhinosinusitis worsen within 10 days after an initial period of improvement ("double worsening")
- Only 0.5% to 2% of viral rhinosinusitis is complicated by ABRS
- Diagnosis is made on clinical grounds: Radiographical imaging should not be obtained for the diagnosis of ABRS unless complications are suspected

Treatment of Acute Bacterial Rhinosinusitis

- Observation (reliable patients with adequate follow-up); most patients improve within 2 weeks without antimicrobial therapy
- First-line antibiotic: Augmentin (amoxicillin 875 mg with clavulanate); shorter 5- to 7-day course appears to have similar response rates to longer duration of treatment
- First-line antibiotic in penicillin-allergic patients: Fluoroquinolone (levofloxacin and moxifloxacin) or doxycycline
- Symptomatic treatment: Saline irrigations, nasal steroids, and short-term decongestants for <3 consecutive days

Complications of Acute Bacterial Rhinosinusitis (Table 4.2)

- Chandler classification of orbital complications
  1. Preseptal cellulitis
  2. Orbital cellulitis
  3. Subperiosteal abscess
  4. Orbital abscess
  5. Cavernous sinus thrombosis
- Intracranial complications
  1. Meningitis
  2. Epidural abscess
  3. Subdural abscess
  4. Intracranial abscess

CHRONIC RHINOSINUSITIS

Pathophysiological Contributors to Chronic Rhinosinusitis

- Predominance of T helper 2 (Th2) cytokines
- Predominance of eosinophils
- Staphylococcal super-antigen
- Deficiency in innate immunity
- Impaired mucociliary clearance

TABLE 4.2 Signs and Symptoms of the Complications of Acute Rhinosinusitis

Complication	Clinical Findings
Preseptal cellulitis	Eyelid edema, erythema, and tenderness; unrestricted extraocular movement; normal visual acuity
Subperiosteal abscess	Proptosis and impaired extraocular muscle movement
Orbital cellulitis	Eyelid edema and erythema, proptosis, and chemosis; no limited impairment of extraocular movements; normal visual acuity
Orbital abscess	Significant exophthalmos, chemosis, ophthalmoplegia, and visual impairment
Cavernous sinus thrombosis	Bilateral orbital pain, chemosis, proptosis, and ophthalmoplegia
Meningitis	Headache, neck stiffness, and high fever
Epidural abscess	Headache, fever, altered mental status, and local tenderness; unenhanced CT reveals a hypodense or isodense crescent-shaped collection in the epidural space
Subdural abscess	Headache, fever, meningismus, focal neurological deficits, and lethargy with rapid deterioration; CT reveals a hypodense collection along a hemisphere or along the falx; MRI demonstrates low signal on T1 and high signal on T2 images with peripheral contrast enhancement
Intracerebral abscess	Fever, headache, vomiting, lethargy, seizures, and focal neurological deficits; frontal deficits can include changes in mood and behavior; MRI demonstrates a cystic lesion with a distinct hypointense, strongly enhancing capsule on T2 images
Frontal bone osteomyelitis (Pott's puffy tumor)	Fluctuant forehead swelling

CT, Computed tomography; *MRI*, magnetic resonance imaging.

From Flint PW, Haughey BH, Lund VJ, et al. *Cummings Otolaryngology—Head and Neck Surgery*. 6th ed. Philadelphia, PA: Saunders; 2015, Table 46.2.

- Biofilms
- Alterations in microbiome

Symptoms of Chronic Rhinosinusitis

- Nasal obstruction/congestion
- Hyposmia/anosmia
- Nasal discharge/postnasal drip
- Facial pressure
- Cough
- Wheeze (asthma)

Workup for Chronic Rhinosinusitis

- Examination: Nasal endoscopy reveals inflammation, with polyps in some cases
- Lab testing
  - Endoscopic-guided middle meatus cultures for concurrent bacterial infection (>80% accuracy)

TABLE 4.3 Summary of Recommendations for Medical Therapy in Chronic Rhinosinusitis

Medical Therapy	EPOS12[a]	EBRR[b]
Oral antibacterial • Nonmacrolide • <3–4 weeks	CRSsNP: B+ CRSwNP: C+	CRS: Option
Oral antibacterial • Macrolide • ≥12 weeks	CRSsNP: C+ CRSwNP: C+	CRS: Option
Intravenous antibacterial	CRSsNP: Did not review CRSwNP: Did not review	CRS: Recommend against
Topical antibacterial	CRSsNP: A– CRSwNP: No data	CRS: Recommend against
Oral antifungal	CRSsNP: A– CRSwNP: A–	CRS: Recommend against
Intravenous antifungal	CRSsNP: No data CRSwNP: No data	CRS: Recommend against
Topical antifungal	CRSsNP: A– CRSwNP: A–	CRS: Recommend against
Topical corticosteroid	CRSsNP: A+ CRSwNP: A+	CRSsNP: Recommend CRSwNP: Recommend
Systemic (oral) corticosteroid	CRSsNP: C+ CRSwNP: A+	CRSsNP: Option CRSwNP: Recommend
Saline irrigations	CRSsNP: A+ CRSwNP: D+	CRS: Recommend
Antihistamines (in allergic patients)	CRSsNP: No data CRSwNP: D+	—
Leukotriene antagonists	CRSsNP: No data CRSwNP: A–	—
Anti-IgE monoclonal antibodies	CRSwNP: A–	—
Anti-IL-5 monoclonal antibodies	CRSwNP: D+	—

[a]As reported in the European Position Paper on Rhinosinusitis and Nasal Polyps 2012.

[b]Published evidence-based reviews with recommendations.

A, Directly based on category-I evidence; *B*, directly based on category-II evidence or extrapolated from category-I evidence; *C*, directly based on category-III evidence or extrapolated from category-I or category-II evidence; *CRSsNP*, chronic rhinosinusitis without nasal polyps; *CRSwNP*, chronic rhinosinusitis with nasal polyps; *D*, directly based on category-IV evidence or extrapolated from category-I, category II, or category III evidence; *IgE*, immunoglobulin E; *IL-5*, interleukin 5; +, recommended; –, recommended against.

From Flint PW, Haughey BH, Lund VJ, et al. *Cummings Otolaryngology—Head and Neck Surgery.* 6th ed. Philadelphia, PA: Saunders; 2015, Table 44.3.

- Endoscopic biopsy for unilateral nasal mass/polyp or to differentiate from chronic granulomatous disease
- Sweat chloride test/genetic test if CF is suspected
- Allergy testing if concurrent allergic rhinitis is suspected
- Imaging studies
  - CT scan of paranasal sinuses without contrast is standard (conventional vs. in-office cone beam)
  - MRI if malignancy or other neoplasm is suspected

Treatment for Chronic Rhinosinusitis (Table 4.3)

- Medical treatment
  - Oral steroids (level-Ia evidence)
  - Topical steroids (level-Ia evidence): steroid sprays, or budesonide or other steroid irrigations
  - Saline irrigations (level-Ib evidence for symptomatic relief)
  - Short-term (<4 weeks) oral antibiotics (level-Ib evidence)
  - Long-term (>4 weeks) oral antibiotics (level-III evidence)
  - Proton pump inhibitors (level-II evidence)
  - Aspirin desensitization (level-II evidence for AERD)
  - Antileukotrienes (level-Ib evidence; treats concurrent asthma symptoms)
  - Antihistamines (topical or oral for concurrent allergic rhinitis)
  - Anti-IgE (omalizumab monoclonal antibody; injection)
  - Low-dose macrolides (antiinflammatory effect; 250 mg clarithromycin daily)
  - Antifungals (oral vs. topical, effective in some patients but not shown to have a significant effect on CRS patients in randomized controlled trials)
  - Consider monoclonal antibodies as biological therapy in patients with recalcitrant CRS with nasal polyps
- Surgical treatment of CRS
  - Functional endoscopic sinus surgery (FESS) is standard: Operating room under general anesthesia versus in-office procedures
  - Balloon dilation of paranasal sinuses may be an option in select cases

Etiologies of Chronic Rhinosinusitis

1. Eosinophilic chronic sinusitis
2. Allergic fungal sinusitis
3. AERD (also known as *Samter triad*)
4. CF

5. Chronic granulomatous disease (GPA, sarcoidosis)
6. Churg-Strauss

Eosinophilic Chronic Sinusitis Basics

- Chronic sinusitis with or without polyps
- Presence of thick mucin and eosinophils in tissue
- Concurrent asthma present in 50% to 70% of patients

Allergic Fungal Sinusitis Basics

- Bent Kuhn criteria
  - Major criteria
    1. Type 1 hypersensitivity
    2. Nasal polyposis
    3. Characteristic CT scan signs: Expansion of sinuses, asymmetry, and heterogeneously dense material in sinuses
    4. Positive fungal smear
    5. Eosinophilic mucin without tissue invasion
  - Minor criteria
    1. Asthma
    2. Unilateral predominance
    3. Serum eosinophilia
    4. Radiographical bone erosion
    5. Fungal culture
    6. Charcot-Leyden crystals
- Treatment
  - FESS to open sinuses and remove all fungal debris
  - Oral and topical steroids
  - Immunotherapy

Aspirin-Exacerbated Respiratory Disease (Samter Triad) Basics

- Presence of polyps, asthma, and asthma exacerbated by cyclooxygenase-1 (Cox-1) inhibitors (aspirin, NSAIDs)
- Caused by abnormality of arachidonic acid cascade that leads to increased production of proinflammatory leukotrienes
- Cox-1 inhibitors will exacerbate increased production of leukotrienes, leading to severe worsening of asthma symptoms and/or allergy-like symptoms
- Treatment
  - Similar to treatment for CRS
  - Aspirin desensitization (requires daily aspirin maintenance after desensitization)

Cystic Fibrosis Basics

- Pathophysiology: Autosomal-recessive defect in chloride ion channel
- Etiology: Multiple mutations in CF conductance transmembrane conductance regulator (CFTR); F508 deletion is most common
- Clinical sinonasal manifestations
  - Severe chronic inflammation and polyposis
  - Chronic and recurrent bacterial infections (*Pseudomonas aeruginosa*, *S. aureus*, *Escherichia coli*, *Burkholderia cepacia*, *Acinetobacter* species, *Stenotrophomonas maltophilia*, *H. influenzae*, Streptococci, and anaerobes)
  - CT scans reveal underdeveloped paranasal sinuses
  - Viscous mucus secretions
- Medical treatment
  - Saline irrigations
  - Topical and oral steroids
  - Oral antibiotics
  - Topical antibiotics
  - Mucolytics (dornase alfa)

- Novel therapies
  - Ivacaftor (potentiates mutant CFTR on cell surface)
  - Lumacaftor (improves delivery of CFTR to cell surface)
  - Ataluren (induces translational reading of nonsense CFTR mutations)
  - Combination therapy, for example, Trikafta (elexacaftor/ivacaftor/tezacaftor)
- Surgical treatment
  - FESS allows improved debridement and irrigations
    - Modified endoscopic medial maxillectomy to promote gravity drainage of maxillary sinuses and allow for improved irrigations and debridement
  - Endoscopic debridements (in-office or under anesthesia)

Granulomatosis With Polyangiitis (Formerly Wegener Disease) Basics

- Small, medium vessel vasculitis; etiology unknown
- C-ANCA antibodies often present
- Clinical sinonasal manifestations
  - Severe chronic inflammation
  - Presence of granulation tissue
  - Concurrent infection (*S. aureus*)
  - Chronic mucosal crusting
  - Septal perforation and erosion of sinonasal structures (turbinates)
  - Saddle nose deformity
- Treatment
  - Oral corticosteroids
  - Immunosuppressive agents (cyclophosphamide and methotrexate)
  - Sulfamethoxazole and trimethoprim (Bactrim) for disease in remission
  - Topical saline rinses and steroids for symptomatic relief
  - FESS in quiescent disease (disease in remission)

Sarcoidosis Basics

- Noncaseating granulomatous disease
- Systemic clinical manifestations
  - Bi-hilar lymphadenopathy on chest x-ray
  - Fatigue, night sweats, and weight loss
  - Erythema nodosum
  - Uveitis
  - Peripheral lymphadenopathy
  - Heerfordt syndrome (enlarged parotid glands, facial nerve palsy, uveitis, and fever)
- Clinical sinonasal manifestations
  - Severe chronic inflammation and polyps
  - Presence of mucosal nodules and/or cobblestoning of mucosa
  - Mucosal crusting
- Treatment
  - Oral corticosteroids
  - Immunosuppressive agents (cyclophosphamide and methotrexate)
  - Topical saline rinses and steroids for symptomatic relief
  - FESS in controlled inflammatory disease

Churg-Strauss Basics

- Small-to-medium vessel vasculitis, etiology unknown
- P-ANCA antibodies often present
- American College of Rheumatology criteria for diagnosis
  1. Asthma
  2. Eosinophilia of more than 10% in peripheral blood

3. Paranasal sinusitis
4. Pulmonary infiltrates
5. Histological proof of vasculitis with extravascular eosinophils
6. Mononeuritis multiplex or polyneuropathy
- Three clinical phases
7. Prodromal phase (asthma and upper-respiratory involvement)
8. Peripheral eosinophilia (pulmonary or gastrointestinal [GI] involvement)
9. Disseminated (lung, CNS, kidney, GI, and skin)
- Treatment
  - Oral corticosteroids
  - Immunosuppressive agents (cyclophosphamide and methotrexate)
  - FESS

SINONASAL NEOPLASMS

Differential Diagnosis of Benign Sinonasal Neoplasms

1. Osteoma
2. Fibrous dysplasia
3. Ossifying fibroma
4. Chordoma
5. Cementoma
6. Hemangioma
7. Inverted papilloma (Figs. 4.13–4.16)
8. JNA (Figs. 4.17–4.19)
9. Pleomorphic adenoma
10. Schwannoma
11. Neurofibroma

Differential Diagnosis of Malignant Sinonasal Neoplasms

1. Esthesioneuroblastoma
2. Lymphoma
3. Ewing sarcoma
4. Chondrosarcoma
5. Rhabdomyosarcoma
6. Nasopharyngeal carcinoma
7. Small cell carcinoma
8. Squamous cell carcinoma
9. Sinonasal undifferentiated carcinoma (SNUC)
10. Adenocarcinoma
11. Adenocystic carcinoma
12. Mucoepidermoid carcinoma
13. Hemangiopericytoma (both benign and malignant types)
14. Melanoma
15. Peripheral nerve sheath tumor

Differential Diagnosis of Congenital Sinonasal Neoplasms

1. Dermoid
2. Teratoma
3. Glioma
4. Encephalocele

Differential Diagnosis of Inflammatory Sinonasal Neoplasms

1. Nasal polyp
2. Antrochoanal polyp
3. Inverting papilloma

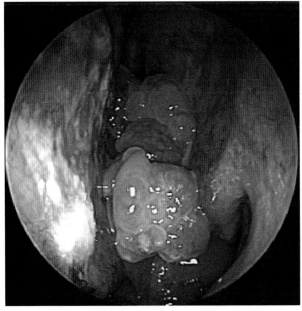

Fig. 4.13 Typical endoscopic appearance of an inverted papilloma. A polypoid lesion with a pale, papillary surface protrudes from the middle meatus and extensively fills the left nasal cavity. (From Flint PW, Haughey BH, Lund VJ, et al. *Cummings Otolaryngology—Head and Neck Surgery.* 6th ed. Philadelphia, PA: Saunders; 2015, Fig. 48.1.)

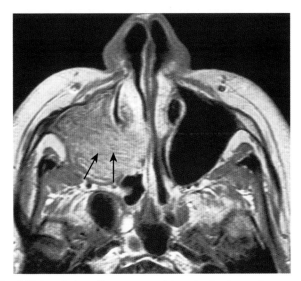

Fig. 4.14 Inverted papilloma on an axial contrast-enhanced, T1-weighted, spin-echo magnetic resonance image. The maxillary sinus is occupied by a solid mass that protrudes into the nasal fossa through an accessory ostium. The lesion exhibits a cerebriform-columnar pattern, which is typically seen in inverted papilloma (*arrows*). (From Flint PW, Haughey BH, Lund VJ, et al. *Cummings Otolaryngology—Head and Neck Surgery.* 6th ed. Philadelphia, PA: Saunders; 2015, Fig. 48.2.)

Differential Diagnosis of Vascular Sinonasal Neoplasms

1. Hemangioma
2. Lobular capillary hemangioma (pyogenic granuloma)
3. Hamartoma

Differential Diagnosis of Traumatic Sinonasal Neoplasms

1. Encephalocele
2. Septal hematoma
3. Pyogenic granuloma

Differential for Sinonasal "Blue Cell" Tumors

1. Rhabdomyosarcoma
2. Esthesioneuroblastoma
3. Lymphoma
4. Melanoma
5. Poorly differentiated carcinoma (SNUC)
6. Hemangiopericytoma

7. Immature teratoma
8. Carcinoid
9. Peripheral nerve sheath tumor

Staging Systems for Juvenile Nasopharyngeal Angiofibroma

- UPMC
  - Stage I: Nasal cavity, medial pterygoid fossa

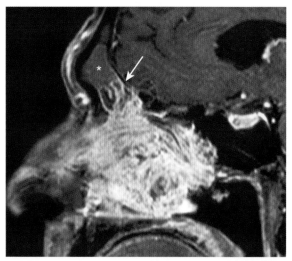

Fig. 4.16 Inverted papilloma on a sagittal contrast-enhanced magnetic resonance image. The advantage of this acquisition plane is the excellent assessment of tumor growth into the most caudal part of the frontal sinus. The upper part of the sinus is filled with inflammatory secretions (*asterisk*). The sagittal plane also permits accurate evaluation of the relationships between the tumor and the floor of the anterior cranial fossa, which is not invaded (*arrow*). (From Flint PW, Haughey BH, Lund VJ, et al. *Cummings Otolaryngology—Head and Neck Surgery.* 6th ed. Philadelphia, PA: Saunders; 2015, Fig. 48.5.)

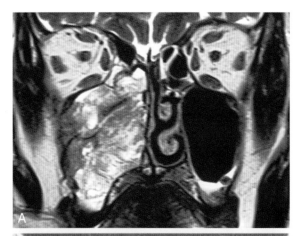

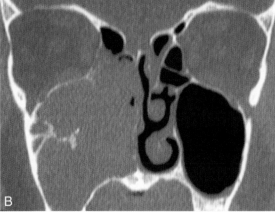

Fig. 4.15 Inverted papilloma on a magnetic resonance imaging (MRI) scan and a CT scan, both in the coronal plane. The maxillary sinus is completely occupied by an expansile lesion that destroyed the medial wall and invaded the right nasal fossa. (**A**) The T2-weighted spin-echo MRI scan demonstrates the cerebriform-columnar pattern of the lesion and permits visualization of the bony spur along the lateral maxillary sinus wall, where the lesion originates. (**B**) The CT scan does not provide a good characterization of soft tissue–density opacification but gives a superior view of the sclerotic bony spur. (From Flint PW, Haughey BH, Lund VJ, et al. *Cummings Otolaryngology—Head and Neck* Surgery. 6th ed. Philadelphia, PA: Saunders; 2015, Fig. 48.3.)

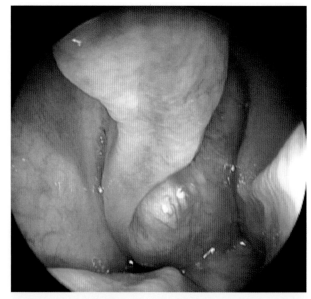

Fig. 4.17 Juvenile angiofibroma. On endoscopy, the lesion typically appears as a polypoid hypervascularized mass that bulges from the lateral wall behind the middle turbinate, which is laterally compressed. The choana is completely obstructed. (From Flint PW, Haughey BH, Lund VJ, et al. *Cummings Otolaryngology—Head and Neck Surgery.* 6th ed. Philadelphia, PA: Saunders; 2015, Fig. 48.7.)

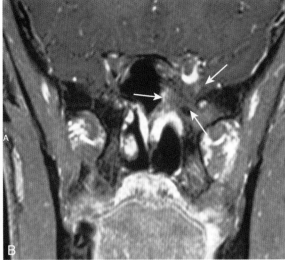

Fig. 4.18 Juvenile angiofibroma on coronal contrast-enhanced magnetic resonance images (MRIs) obtained before and after endoscopic resection. (**A**) Pretreatment image shows encroachment of both the floor and lateral wall of the left sphenoid sinus (SS) and infratemporal fossa. Intracranial extension is demonstrated in close proximity to the superior orbital fissure (*arrows*). (**B**) MRI obtained after surgical resection shows solid tissue (*arrows*) along the lateral SS wall; the lack of contrast enhancement suggests residual scar tissue. (From Flint PW, Haughey BH, Lund VJ, et al. *Cummings Otolaryngology—Head and Neck Surgery.* 6th ed. Philadelphia, PA: Saunders; 2015, Fig. 48.8.)

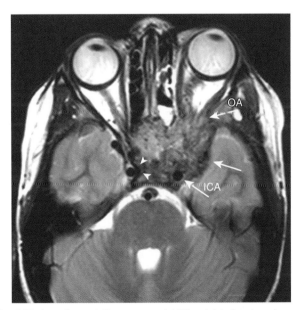

Fig. 4.19 Juvenile angiofibroma on axial T2-weighted, spin-echo magnetic resonance image. The lesion invades the left orbital apex (OA); the lateral wall of the left sphenoid sinus (*arrows*) is completely destroyed, and the internal carotid artery (ICA) is encased. On the right side, a bony barrier (*arrowheads*) still separates the lesion from the ICA. (From Flint PW, Haughey BH, Lund VJ, et al. *Cummings Otolaryngology—Head and Neck Surgery.* 6th ed. Philadelphia, PA: Saunders; 2015, Fig. 48.9.)

- Stage II: Paranasal sinuses, lateral pterygoid fossa; no residual vascularity
- Stage III: Skull base erosion, orbit, infratemporal fossa, no residual vascularity
- Stage IV: Skull base erosion, orbit, infratemporal fossa, residual vascularity
- Stage V: Intracranial extension, residual vascularity, medial extension, lateral extension
- Radkowski (most universally accepted system)

- Stage IA: Limited to nose or nasopharynx
- Stage IB: Extension into at least one paranasal sinus
- Stage IIA: Minimal extension through the sphenopalatine foramen; includes a minimal part of the medial pterygomaxillary fossa
- Stage IIB: Full occupation of pterygomaxillary fossa with Holman-Miller sign (bowing of the posterior wall of the maxillary sinus on CT); lateral or anterior displacement of maxillary artery branches; may have superior extension with orbital bone erosion
- Stage IIC: Extension through the pterygomaxillary fossa into the cheek, temporal fossa, or posterior to the pterygoids
- Stage IIIA: Skull-base erosion with minimal intracranial extension
- Stage IIIB: Skull-base erosion with extensive intracranial extension ± cavernous sinus
- Modified sessions
- Fisch

Staging Systems for Esthesioneuroblastoma

- Kadish
  - Stage A: Tumor limited to the nasal cavity
  - Stage B: Extension to the paranasal sinuses
  - Stage C: Extension beyond the nasal cavity/paranasal sinuses
  - Stage D: Metastatic disease
- Dulgerov
  - Stage T1: Tumor of the nasal cavity and/or paranasal sinuses, sparing the most superior ethmoid cells
  - Stage T2: Tumor involving the nasal cavity and/or paranasal sinuses (including sphenoid) with extension to or erosion of the cribriform plate
  - Stage T3: Tumor extending to the orbit or protruding into the anterior fossa
  - Stage T4: Tumor involving the brain
- Biller
  - Stage T1: Tumor of the nasal cavity/paranasal sinuses (excluding sphenoid) with or without erosion of the anterior fossa bone

- Stage T2: Extension into the orbit or protrusion into the anterior fossa
- Stage T3: Involvement of the brain that is resectable with margins
- Stage T4: Unresectable
- Hyams (histological grade)
  - Grade I: Prominent neurofibrillary matrix, tumor cells with uniform nuclei, some rosettes, and absence of nuclear pleomorphism, mitotic activity, or necrosis
  - Grade II: Some neurofibrillary matrix, nuclear pleomorphism, and mitotic activity; absence of mitoses and necrosis
  - Grade III: Minimal neurofibrillary matrix and rosettes; more prominent mitotic activity and nuclear pleomorphism; some necrosis may be seen
  - Grade IV: no neurofibrillary matrix or rosettes seen; marked nuclear pleomorphism and necrosis, and increased mitotic activity

Staging Systems for Inverted Papilloma

- Han
  - Group 1: Limited to nasal cavity, lateral nasal wall, medial maxillary sinus, ethmoid sinus and sphenoid sinus
  - Group II: Extension to lateral maxillary medial maxillary wall with or without group I critreria
  - Group III: Extension into frontal sinus
  - Group IV: Extension into outside sinuses
- Krouse
  - Stage T1: Limited to one area of the nasal cavity
  - Stage T2: Involvement of the medial wall of the maxillary or ethmoid sinuses and/or the osteomeatal unit
  - Stage T3: Involvement of the superior, inferior, posterior, anterior, or lateral walls of the maxillary sinus
  - Stage T4: Tumors with extrasinonasal spread or malignancy
- Cannaday
  - Group A: Confined to the nasal cavity, medial maxillary sinus, and ethmoid sinus (recurrence rate = 3%)
  - Group B: Involving the lateral maxillary sinus, sphenoid sinus, or frontal sinus (recurrence rate = 19.8%)
  - Group C: Extrasinus extension (recurrence rate = 35.5%)

Surgical Approaches

1. Open craniofacial
2. Endoscopic assisted (combined open and endoscopic)
3. Endoscopic and expanded endoscopic approaches

SURGERY OF THE PARANASAL SINUSES

Indications for Endoscopic Sinus Surgery

- Chronic sinusitis with or without polyps refractory to medical treatment: Most common indication, to relieve obstruction and allow for delivery of medication
- Recurrent sinusitis (≥4 episodes a year): Should be confirmed endoscopically or on CT scan while the patient is symptomatic to rule out disorders that mimic sinusitis, such as migraines
- Acute complications of rhinosinusitis (i.e., intracranial or orbital)
- Antrochoanal polyps
- Sinus mucoceles: Marsupialized to avoid continued expansion and risk of intracranial and orbital complications
- Excision of sinonasal tumors
- Excision of skull-base tumors
- CSF leak repair
- Orbital decompression (e.g., Graves ophthalmopathy)

- Optic nerve decompression
- Dacryocystorhinostomy (DCR)
- Choanal atresia repair
- Foreign body removal
- Intractable epistaxis control
- Noninvasive fungal sinusitis
- Invasive fungal sinusitis
- Headache and facial pain—controversial—contact points on CT and/or endoscopy with clear reduction in headache in response to intranasal decongestants after both thorough neurological and radiographical evaluation and failure of medical therapy

Indications for Surgical Intervention in Acute Bacterial Sinusitis

- Impending complications of sinusitis
- Nonresponse to medical therapy
- Immunosuppressed patient

Functional Endoscopic Sinus Surgery Principles

- Restore mucociliary function by reestablishing physiological sinus ventilation and drainage
- Remove irreversibly diseased mucosa and bone and preserve normal tissue
- Allow for delivery of topical therapies
- Ostiomeatal complex is the primary target of ESS because minimal inflammation in this area can lead to disease in the maxillary, anterior ethmoid, and frontal sinuses

External Approaches to the Paranasal Sinuses

- Maxillary sinus: Caldwell-Luc procedure and canine fossa trephination
- Ethmoid sinuses: External ethmoidectomy (results in external scar; loss of bone lateral to the frontal recess and loss of mucosa often result in scar tissue and stenosis of the frontal recess)
- Frontal sinus: Frontal sinus trephination, osteoplastic flap with or without obliteration (has significant rate of long-term failure and mucocele formation)

Major Complications of Endoscopic Sinus Surgery

- CSF leak
- Blindness
- Diplopia
- ICA injury
- Major bleeding
- Orbital hematoma

Other Complications of Endoscopic Sinus Surgery

- Nasolacrimal duct injury
- Hyposmia
- Minor epistaxis
- Adhesions
- Periorbital ecchymosis
- Facial pain

Management of Postoperative Orbital Hematoma

- Surgical emergency
- Immediate decompression of the orbit via a lateral canthotomy with inferior cantholysis and/or formal external or endoscopic orbital decompression
- Surgical hemostasis of bleeding vessels

BOX 4.3 Basic Steps in Endoscopic Sinus Surgery

1. Patient positioning
2. Diagnostic nasal endoscopy
3. Topical anesthetic injections
4. Medialization of the middle turbinate (MT) to expose the ostiomeatal complex (basal lamella–relaxing incision is optional)
5. Uncinectomy with a zero-degree endoscope
6. Maxillary antrostomy: Use a 30- or 45-degree endoscope to identify the maxillary sinus ostium and floor of the orbit and then follow it up to the medial orbital wall (lamina papyracea)
7. Removal of the ethmoid bulla; identification of the lamina papyracea in its medial wall
8. Identification of the basal lamella of the MT in the horizontal and oblique segments
9. Removal of the inferomedial part of the vertical MT basal lamella to penetrate into the posterior ethmoid sinus
10. Ethmoidectomy; stay low, between the superior turbinate medially and the lamina papyracea laterally
11. Identification of the sphenoid face
12. Identification of the posterior skull base, in either the posterior ethmoid (possible in the absence of polyps or in a single tier of cells) or following the sphenoid face up to the skull base
13. Clearance of the skull base in a posterior to anterior direction, removing the ethmoid partitions
14. Sphenoid sinusotomy (if needed) through the medial inferior triangle of the posterior ethmoid box or by identifying it in the sphenoethmoidal recess
15. Optional: Identification of the frontal recesses, frontal sinusotomy
16. Optional: Medialization of the medial MT by creating adhesion between the medial surface and septum (suture or pack)
17. Optional: Placement of a middle meatal spacer

From Flint PW, Haughey BH, Lund VJ, et al. *Cummings Otolaryngology— Head and Neck Surgery*. 6th ed. Philadelphia, PA: Saunders; 2015, Box 49.3.

- Ophthalmology consultation
- IV mannitol
- IV acetazolamide
- IV steroids

Factors Increasing Risk of Orbital or Skull-Base Injuries (Box 4.3)

- Lamina papyracea lies medial to maxillary ostium
- Dehiscence of the lamina
- Maxillary sinus hypoplasia
- Low or sloping fovea ethmoidalis
- Sphenoid sinus septations are attached to the carotid canal
- Carotid canal or optic nerve dehiscence
- Presence of sphenoethmoid (also known as Onodi) cell

Common Causes of Failure of Endoscopic Sinus Surgery

- Lateralized MT
- Missed ostium sequence and recirculation
- Maxillary ostium stenosis
- Frontal recess scarring
- Residual ethmoidal air cells
- Adhesions
- Recurrent polyposis

Indications for Use of Image Guidance

- Revision sinus surgery
- Distorted sinus anatomy of development, postoperative, or traumatic origin

- Extensive sinonasal polyposis
- Pathology involving the frontal, posterior ethmoid, and sphenoid sinuses
- Disease abutting the skull base, orbit, optic nerve, or carotid artery
- CSF rhinorrhea or conditions in which there is a skull-base defect

Revision Sinus Surgery

- Initial surgery represents the greatest chance for long-term success
- Comprehensive postsurgical care with directed debridement, sinonasal irrigations, and appropriate medical therapy is critical to achieving high success rates in primary surgery
- Causes of failure
  - Misattribution of symptoms: Initial surgery performed for misattributed symptoms (e.g., headache, facial pain, odontogenic disease, temporomandibular joint [TMJ] dysfunction, and reflux)
  - Medical factors
    - Persistent microbial disease
    - Biofilm formation
    - Persistent inflammatory disease (e.g., chronic sinusitis with nasal polyposis, presence of asthma, and AERD)
    - Systemic comorbidities (e.g., granulomatous diseases, allergy, CF, immunoglobulin deficiencies, and HIV)
  - Environmental factor: Smoking
  - Iatrogenic factors

  - Submaximal dissection of the instrumented sinuses (e.g., retained ethmoid cells and residual agger nasi remnants)
  - Incomplete uncinate dissection and posteriorly placed maxillary antrostomy not incorporating natural os, resulting in possible recirculation phenomenon
  - MT lateralization and middle meatal obstruction, common in setting of partial middle turbinectomy
  - Failure to recognize and address anatomical variants such as infraorbital ethmoid (Haller) and sphenoethmoid (Onodi) cells

Frontal Sinus Surgery

- Use an instrument in the frontal recess only with good reason. Remove all cells obstructing the frontal recess, including agger nasi, frontal, suprabullar and supraorbital cells.
- Functional drainage of the frontal sinus relies on preservation of the mucosa of the frontal recess
- If the mucosa of the frontal recess cannot be preserved, a Draf III procedure is the remaining endoscopic option
- Maintain bony support around the frontal recess whenever possible

Endoscopic Frontal Sinus Approaches

- Balloon dilation
- Draf I: Complete ethmoidectomy with removal of the bulla and suprabullar cells
- Draf IIa: Enlargement of the frontal outflow tract with removal of all occupying cells (frontal sinusotomy)
- Draf IIb (unilateral frontal sinus drill out): Removal of the floor of the frontal sinus, from the lamina papyracea to the septum, to produce the largest possible unilateral outflow tract
- Draf III (endoscopic modified Lothrop): Complete drill out of the floor of the frontal sinuses, frontal beak, and intersinus septum and an adjacent part of the nasal septum

External Frontal Sinus Approaches

- Frontal trephine
- External ethmoidectomy
- Osteoplastic flap with or without obliteration
  - If obliteration of the sinus is required, remove all mucosa and drill the cavity
  - Obliteration is associated with a high rate of long-term failure

Approaches to Benign or Malignant Nasal Masses

- Endoscopic excision
- Midface degloving
- Lateral rhinotomy ± lip-split and subciliary incisions
- Combined craniofacial (facial incisions with bicoronal incisions)
- Transpalatal
- Infratemporal fossa
- Facial translocation

Endoscopic Skull-Base Reconstruction Options

- Septal mucosal flap: Septal branch of sphenopalatine artery
- MT flap: MT branch of sphenopalatine artery
- Inferior turbinate flap: Inferior turbinate branch of sphenopalatine artery
- Tunneled pericranial flap: Supraorbital and supratrochlear arteries
- Temporoparietal fascia flap: Anterior branch of the superficial temporal artery
- Palatal flap: Descending palatine artery

ENDOSCOPIC DACRYOCYSTORHINOSTOMY

Classification of Lacrimal Obstruction

- Anatomical
  - 70% of cases have complete blockage; better outcome with DCR
    - Children with nasolacrimal duct obstruction often have imperforate Hasner valve amenable to probing
    - Young adults tend to have pathology of the canaliculi
    - Middle-aged patients tend to have dacryoliths, which are amenable to DCR
    - Elderly patients tend to have lacrimal duct obstruction, which is amenable to DCR
  - Functional failure in 30% of cases: Of proximal pump mechanism or critical narrowings

Physical Examination

- Exclude lid laxity, malposition, punctal anomalies, and blepharitis
- Palpate over lacrimal sac to search for reflux of mucopurulence
- Dye disappearance test: Drop of 2% fluorescein into both conjunctival fornices—normal test is symmetric and with complete disappearance of dye within 5 minutes
- A cotton swab is used in the inferior meatus to confirm the flow of fluorescein (positive Jones I test)
- For abnormal results, perform Jones II test.
  - Bowman lacrimal probe places an inferior or a superior canaliculus to palpate the common internal punctum.
    - Soft stop: Impeded progress of the lacrimal probe before entering the lacrimal sac requires further assessment

- Hard-stop: Probe impacts the medial bony wall of the lacrimal sac, which implies no stenosis of the canalicular system
- Finally, a 25-G blunt lacrimal needle is placed into the inferior punctum to irrigate the lacrimal system with clear (nonfluorescein dyed) saline
  - If the patient tastes saline, this rules out a complete obstruction but not a functional problem
  - If the patient does not taste saline, anatomical obstruction is likely

Interpretation of Jones II Test Results

1. Reflux of clear saline fluid from the same punctum being irrigated indicates obstruction proximal to the common canaliculus because fluorescein did not fill the lacrimal sac during Jones I and is not present in sufficient quantity to stain refluxing saline
2. Reflux of clear fluid from the opposite punctum indicates obstruction of the common canaliculus or common internal punctum
3. Reflux of fluorescein-stained fluid through the opposite punctum indicates nasolacrimal duct obstruction (fluorescein present in lacrimal sac stains refluxing saline

Radiological Evaluation

- Scintillogram: Nuclear medicine equivalent of the dye disappearance test; assesses functional and anatomical obstructions
- Dacryocystogram (DCG) requires syringing the lacrimal puncta with radiopaque dye; gives results similar to Jones II test results

Surgical Technique

- Advantages over external DCR
  - Lack of an incision
  - No disruption of the lacrimal pump mechanism
- Key elements
  - Creation of the widest possible marsupialization of the medial wall of the lacrimal sac
  - Identification of the common internal punctum (most proximal portion of the lacrimal system that can be successfully managed by DCR)
- Endoscopic anatomical landmarks
  - Axilla of the MT: Upper one-third of the sac just superior to the anterior insertion of the MT
  - Maxillary line: Corresponds intranasally to the junction of the uncinate and maxilla, extranasally to the suture line between the lacrimal bone and maxilla within the lacrimal fossa; inferior two-thirds of the sac is oriented vertically, just under the maxillary line
- Steps of surgery
  - Flap elevation or removal of mucosa around maxillary line
  - Frontal process of the maxilla covering the anterior portion of the lacrimal sac is now removed with punch or drill; frontal process of the maxilla and the lacrimal bone are the two bone segments on either side of the lacrimomaxillary suture that need to be removed
  - Superior and inferior lacrimal puncta dilated and cannulated with Bowman probes
  - Once the probe is evident in the lacrimal sac, the sac is incised from top to bottom
  - May consider stenting (e.g., with silicone Crawford tubes) for a period of several weeks to months

Outcomes of Dacryocystorhinostomy

- Anatomical obstruction >95% success rate (free flow of fluorescein; asymptomatic patient)
- Functional obstruction approximately 80% success rate
- Lacrimal sump syndrome may be cause of failure due to inadequate marsupialization of the lacrimal sac inferiorly
- 5% rate of complications, including hemorrhage, orbital fat exposure, orbital hematoma, and synechiae/granulation tissue obstruction of the ostium

FURTHER READINGS

American Academy of Otolaryngology—Head and Neck Surgery (AAO-HNS) Clinical practice guideline (update): Adult sinusitis. *Otolaryngol Head Neck Surg.* 2015;152(suppl 2):S1–S39.

Cannaday SB, Batra PS, Sautter NB, et al. New staging system for sinonasal inverted papilloma in the endoscopic era. *Laryngoscope.* 2007;117:1283–1287.

Fokkens WJ, Lund VJ, Mullol J, et al. EPOS 2012: European position paper on rhinosinusitis and nasal polyps 2012. A summary for otorhinolaryngologists. *Rhinology.* 2012;50:1–12.

Han JK, Smith TL, Loehrl T, et al. An evolution in the management of sinonasal inverting papilloma. *Laryngoscope.* 2001;111:1395–1400.

Krouse JH. Development of a staging system for inverted papilloma. *Laryngoscope.* 2000;110:965–968.

Poetker DM, Jakubowski LA, Lal D, et al. Oral corticosteroids in the management of adult chronic rhinosinusitis with and without nasal polyps: An evidence-based review with recommendations. *Int Forum Allergy Rhinol.* 2013;3:104–120.

Reh DD, Woodworth BA, Poetker D, et al. Rhinology maintenance of certification review. *Am J Rhinol Allergy.* May–Jun 2014;28(suppl 1): S18.

Rudmik L, Hoy M, Schlosser RJ, et al. Topical therapies in the management of chronic rhinosinusitis: An evidence-based review with recommendations. *Int Forum Allergy Rhinol.* 2013;3(4):281–298.

Snyderman CH, Pant H, Carrau RL, Gardner P. A new endoscopic staging system for angiofibromas. *Arch Otolaryngol Head Neck Surg.* 2010;136(6):588–594.

Soler ZM, Oyer SL, Kern RC, et al. Antimicrobials and chronic rhinosinusitis with or without polyposis in adults: An evidenced-based review with recommendations. *Int Forum Allergy Rhinol.* 2013;3:31–47.

5   Head and Neck Surgery

Kiran Kakarala, Charissa Kahue, and Allen S. Ho

PRINCIPLES OF RADIATION THERAPY

Types of Radiation

- Photon: Most common form
- Electron: Superficial penetration, ideal for skin
- Neutron: High-energy particle and highly toxic
  - Selectively used for salivary gland malignancies
- Proton: Low-energy particle with a sharp falloff of dose beyond the target (Bragg peak)
  - Increasingly used for skull base, where dose to critical adjacent structures must be minimized
- Carbon ion: High-energy particle with a sharp Bragg peak

Units of Radiation Energy

- Gray (Gy): 1 Gy equals 1 Joule (J) of energy deposited per kilogram material
- Radiation-absorbed dose (rad): 100 rad = 1 Gy

Radiation Sources

- Cobalt (Co-60), iridium (Ir-192), and cesium (Cs-137)
- Linear accelerator
- X-rays and electron energy of 4 to 25 MeV
- Accelerated electrons strike tungsten to produce x-rays

Radiation Delivery

- Conventional radiation
- Intensity-modulated radiation therapy (IMRT)
- Brachytherapy
- Stereotactic body radiation therapy (SBRT)

Conventional Radiation

- Manual blocks are cut to shape the beam
- Multileaf collimators are introduced to shape the radiation field

Intensity-Modulated Radiation Therapy

- Inverse planning
  - Ideal radiation dose distribution is based on imaging
  - Computer algorithm is applied to achieve the ideal distribution
- Precise control
  - Multiple small "beamlets" converge on targets
  - Multiple beamlet conformations contour the dose
  - Minimization of the dose to critical structures
    - Salivary glands
    - Pharyngeal constrictors
    - Temporal lobe
    - Optic nerve
    - Cochlea
    - Spinal cord

Brachytherapy

- Radioisotopes applied to tumor bed
- Permanent implants (beads) or interstitial catheters
- Rapid dose falloff of radiation
- Lip cancer
- Nasopharyngeal recurrence
- Base of tongue recurrence

Indications for Postoperative Radiotherapy

- Advanced-stage disease: pT3, pT4
- Multiple positive nodes
  - Without extracapsular extension (radiation alone)
  - With extracapsular extension (concurrent chemoradiation)
- Positive surgical margins
  - Reresection preferable if possible
  - Concurrent chemoradiation if re-resection is not possible
- Perineural invasion

Timing of Radiation Therapy

- Primary: 2 weeks after any necessary dental extractions
- Adjuvant: Within 4 to 6 weeks after surgery
  - Delays in initiation and completion of postoperative adjuvant radiation are associated with decreased locoregional control and overall survival

Pretreatment Considerations

- Dental evaluation
- Nutritional status
  - Avoid prophylactic gastrostomy tube unless patient has preexisting dysphagia, aspiration, or severe weight loss
    - Longer duration of tube use compared with as-needed tube placement or temporary nasogastric tube use
    - Higher likelihood of long-term dysphagia
- Swallowing evaluation
- Airway safety: Determination of the potential need for a tracheotomy
- Treatment planning and simulation
  - Thermoplastic mask immobilization

Fractionation Schemes (Box 5.1)

- Conventional fractionation
  - Daily treatment, 5 days/week × 7 weeks
  - Example: 2 Gy/fraction, 1 fraction/day, 5 days/week × 7 weeks (60–70 Gy total)
- Hyperfractionation
  - Decreased dose per fraction, increased number of fractions, larger total dose
  - Example: 1.15 Gy/fraction, 2 fractions/day, 5 days/wk, 7 weeks (81.5 Gy total)
  - Theoretical improvement in locoregional control

BOX 5.1 Salient Features of Altered Fractionation Schemes

Hyperfractionation
- Smaller fraction size (115–120 cGy) compared with conventional fractionation (180–200 cGy)
- BID to TID fractionation
- Larger total dosage (7440–8460 cGy) than conventional fractionation (7000 cGy)
- Similar overall treatment duration as conventional fractionation

Accelerated Fractionation
- Similar fraction size as conventional fractionation (180–200 cGy)
- BID to TID fractionation
- Similar total dosage as conventional fractionation
- Shortened overall treatment duration compared with conventional fractionation

Hypofractionation
- Larger fraction size (600–800 cGy) compared with conventional fractionation (180–200 cGy)
- Fractions delivered several days apart
- Lower total dosage (2100–3200 cGy) than conventional fractionation (7000 cGy)
- Shortened overall treatment duration compared with conventional fractionation

BID, twice a day; *TID,* three times a day.
Modified from Shah JP, Patel SG, Singh B. *Jatin Shah's Head and Neck Surgery and Oncology.* 4th ed. Philadelphia, PA: Mosby; 2012, Fig. 19.4.

- Possible therapeutic advantage over conventional radiation, but greater burden on patients leads to poorer compliance
- Accelerated fractionation
  - Conventional dose per fraction, increased number of fractions
  - Similar total dose and decreased treatment duration
  - Example: 1.6 Gy/fraction, 3 fractions/day, 5 days/wk, for 5 weeks
  - Reduce tumor repopulation as a cause of radiotherapy (RT) failure
  - Increased toxicity
- Hypofractionation
  - Larger doses per fraction, decreased number of fractions
  - Smaller total dose and decreased treatment duration
  - Decreased side effects
  - Examples: 6 Gy/fraction, 1 fraction q3day (every 3 days) for 15 days (30 Gy total)
  - Used in melanoma or in palliative regimens

Complications of Radiation Therapy

- Mucositis (World Health Organization scale)
  - Grade 1: Soreness with erythema
  - Grade 2: Erythema, ulcers, and can eat solids
  - Grade 3: Ulcers and liquid diet only
  - Grade 4: Alimentation is not possible
- Xerostomia
  - Prevention
    - IMRT to spare salivary glands
    - Submandibular gland transfer
  - Treatment
    - Saliva substitutes and mucosal lubricants
    - Stimulation of saliva
      - Sugar-free hard candy or gum
      - Pilocarpine: Nonselective parasympathomimetic agent that is often limited by side effects of bronchospasm, bradycardia, sweating, headaches, flushing, and increased bowel and bladder function

- Cevimeline: Selective (M1/M3 muscarinic receptors) parasympathomimetic agent; fewer cardiopulmonary side effects than pilocarpine, but use still limited by side effects
- Dental caries
- Osteoradionecrosis (ORN)
  - Mandible
    - Risk factors
      - Radiation dose >60 Gy
      - Poor oral hygiene or poor dentition
      - Location of primary tumor: The posterior mandible is most commonly affected
      - Extent of mandible in radiation field
      - Poor nutritional status
      - Concurrent chemoradiation
    - IMRT is less likely to cause ORN than conformal radiation fields are
    - Marx classification system
      - Staging based on response to hyperbaric oxygen (HBO)
      - Stage I: Exposed bone treated with HBO alone
      - Stage II: Diagnosed if there was no response to HBO at stage I and debridement is undertaken followed by further HBO
      - Stage III: Diagnosed if there was no response to stage II treatment and resection and reconstruction are undertaken
  - Temporal bone
  - Maxilla
- Chondroradionecrosis of the larynx
- Soft-tissue fibrosis
- Dysphagia: Potential gastrostomy tube dependence
- Hypothyroidism
- Cranial neuropathy
- Atherosclerosis and long-term risk of stroke
- Long-term risk of secondary malignancies such as sarcomas

Prevention of Radiation Complications

- Pretreatment dental examination
  - Extraction of diseased teeth (at least 2 weeks before starting radiation treatments)
  - Fabrication of custom molded fluoride trays for use during radiation
- Posttreatment dental care
  - Routine dental follow-up and daily fluoride application
  - HBO treatments before dental extractions: 20 dives at 2.4 atmospheres for 90 minutes before extraction and 10 dives after extraction

PRINCIPLES OF CHEMOTHERAPY
Role of Chemotherapy

- Sensitizes radiation
- Palliation
- Not curative as a single agent

Drugs Used

- Platinum agents
  - Cisplatin
    - Most common chemotherapy used
    - Leads to DNA cross-link formation and subsequent apoptosis
    - High-dose q3 week cisplatin protocol: Delivered every 3 weeks (100 mg/m² on days 1, 22, and 43)

- Category-1 evidence
- More toxic
- Low-dose weekly cisplatin protocol: Weekly (40 mg/m²)
  - Category-2b evidence
  - Better tolerated
- Side effects: Nephrotoxicity, ototoxicity, alopecia, nausea/vomiting, neutropenia
- Carboplatin
  - Similar mechanism of action as cisplatin
  - More myelosuppressive
  - Better tolerated than cisplatin (less ototoxic)
  - Mixed results in studies comparing its efficacy to cisplatin
- 5-Fluorouracil (5-FU)
  - Causes derangements in DNA synthesis and repair
  - Causes severe mucositis
  - Less commonly used now in favor of platinum agents
- Taxanes
  - Stabilize microtubules and arrest cells in G2/M phase
  - In induction chemotherapy regimens, addition of taxanes to cisplatin and 5-FU (TPF) leads to better outcomes compared with cisplatin and 5-FU alone
- Targeted therapy
  - Cetuximab
    - Epidermal growth factor highly overexpressed in head and neck squamous cell carcinoma (HNSCC)
    - Cetuximab is a monoclonal antibody that binds epidermal growth factor receptor (EGFR)
    - Improved survival when given concurrently with radiation compared with radiation alone
  - Vemurafenib, dabrafenib/trametinib
    - *BRAF V600E* mutation implicated in aggressiveness of melanoma and follicular-derived thyroid cancers
    - Vemurafenib and dabrafenib are *BRAF V600E* inhibitors (trametinib is an *MEK* inhibitor)
    - Approved for use in advanced/metastatic cutaneous melanoma and anaplastic thyroid cancer (*BRAF*-mutant cases only)
  - Vismodegib
    - Hedgehog pathway inhibitor
    - Approved for use in advanced/metastatic basal cell carcinoma
- Immunotherapy
  - Pembrolizumab and nivolumab
    - Programmed cell death protein 1 (PD-1) is an immune checkpoint receptor with pro-apoptotic effects
    - PD-1 is inactivated by programmed death ligand 1 (PD-L1), which can be overexpressed in some cancers
    - Pembrolizumab and nivolumab are monoclonal antibodies that bind PD-1 and prevent PD-L1 binding, allowing immune upregulation against tumor cells
    - Approved by the US Food and Drug Administration (FDA) for use in metastatic/unresectable recurrent head and neck squamous cell carcinoma and melanoma
  - Cemiplimab
    - Monoclonal antibody against PD-1
    - Approved for use in advanced/metastatic cutaneous squamous cell carcinoma
  - Ipilimumab
    - Cytotoxic T-lymphocyte-associated protein 4 (CTLA-4) raises the threshold for activation of T-cells, decreasing the immune response to cancer
    - Ipilimumab is a monoclonal antibody that binds CTLA-4 and blocks its inhibitory effects, allowing immune upregulation against tumor cells
    - First FDA-approved immunotherapy agent of any kind, approved for unresectable or metastatic melanoma

Rationale for Concurrent Chemotherapy and Radiation

- Improves the therapeutic ratio of radiation
  - Chemotherapeutic drug affects tumor and normal tissues differently
    - RTOG 95-01 Trial
    - High-risk patients (positive margins, extracapsular extension or ≥2 positive nodes) received 60 to 66 Gy plus concurrent cisplatin
    - Improved locoregional control and disease-free survival, with no significant difference in overall survival compared with RT alone
  - EORTC 22931 Trial
    - High-risk patients (positive margins, extracapsular extension, perineural invasion, vascular tumor embolism, oral cavity, or oropharynx primary with level IV or level V lymph nodes) received 66 Gy plus concurrent cisplatin
    - Improved locoregional control, disease-free survival, and overall survival compared with RT alone
  - Meta-analysis of these two trials determined that the addition of cisplatin to adjuvant radiation was helpful only in cases with extracapsular extension or positive margins
  - MACH-NC meta-analysis: Patient age—decrease in the efficacy of concurrent chemotherapy with increasing age; no benefits noted in patients over age 7

Induction Chemotherapy

- Chemotherapy given before definitive surgery or radiation
- With few exceptions, this has not resulted in better outcomes
- Induction with TPF (taxane, platinum, and fluorouracil) is superior to a two-drug induction regimen but not superior to concurrent chemoradiation
- PARADIGM and DeCIDE randomized control trials failed to show benefit with induction chemotherapy

Management of the Neck

- Management of regional lymphatics is determined by the extent of disease at initial staging
- Anatomical landmarks of neck levels (Fig. 5.1)
  - Level Ia: Bounded by the anterior bellies of the digastric muscle laterally, the mandible superiorly, the hyoid inferiorly, and the mylohyoid deeply
  - Level Ib: Bounded anteriorly by the anterior belly of the digastric, superiorly by the body of the mandible, and posteriorly by the posterior belly of the digastric
  - Level II: Upper jugular group that extends from the skull base superiorly to the hyoid bone inferiorly
    - Level IIa: Inferior to the spinal accessory nerve
    - Level IIb: Superior to the spinal accessory nerve
  - Level III: Midjugular group that extends from the carotid bifurcation (surgical landmark) or the hyoid (radiographic landmark) to the junction of the omohyoid muscle and the internal jugular vein (surgical landmark) or the inferior border of the cricoid cartilage (radiographic landmark)
  - Level IV: Lower jugular group that extends from the junction of the omohyoid with the internal jugular vein (surgical landmark) or the inferior border of the cricoid cartilage (radiographic landmark) to the clavicle
  - Level V: Posterior triangle nodes that are bordered by the trapezius muscle posteriorly and the posterior border of the sternocleidomastoid muscle anteriorly; the inferior border is the clavicle
    - Level Va: Nodes located above a horizontal plane at the inferior border of the cricoid cartilage
    - Level Vb: Nodes located below a horizontal plane at the inferior border of the cricoid cartilage

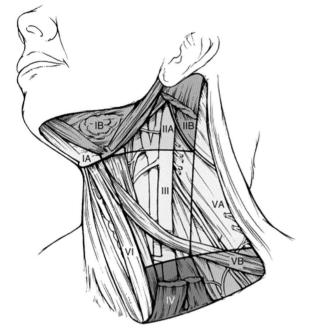

Fig. 5.1 Neck dissection levels. The six sublevels of the neck used to describe the location of lymph nodes within levels I, II, and V. Level Ia, submental group; level Ib, submandibular group; level IIa, upper jugular nodes along the carotid sheath, including the subdigastric group; level IIb, upper jugular nodes in the submuscular recess; level Va, spinal accessory nodes; and level Vb, the supraclavicular and transverse cervical nodes. (From Flint PW, Haughey BH, Lund V, et al. *Cummings Otolaryngology—Head and Neck Surgery.* 7th ed. Philadelphia, PA: Saunders; 2021, Fig. 118.2.)

- Level VI: Central compartment nodes bounded by the hyoid bone superiorly, the common carotid arteries laterally, and the innominate artery inferiorly; includes the paraesophageal, paratracheal, precricoid (Delphian), and perithyroidal nodes
- Level VII: Superior mediastinal nodes bounded by the superior border of the manubrium superiorly, the left common carotid artery and the innominate artery on the left, and the arch of the aorta inferiorly

- Types of neck dissection
  - Radical: Resection of levels I to V with sacrifice of internal jugular vein, sternocleidomastoid muscle, and spinal accessory nerve
  - Modified radical: Resection of levels I to V with sparing of at least one of the nonlymphatic structures taken in a radical neck dissection

  - Selective neck dissection
    - Supraomohyoid neck dissection: levels I to III
    - Lateral neck dissection: Levels II to IV
    - Posterolateral neck dissection: Levels II to V, suboccipital lymph nodes
      - Most often employed for cutaneous melanoma or Merkel cell carcinoma of the posterior scalp
    - Central neck dissection: Level VI nodal contents
    - Extended: Removal of an additional lymphatic group or nonlymphatic structure (e.g., retropharyngeal node dissection, supraclavicular node dissection, external carotid artery, or the vagus nerve)

NECK DISSECTION IN THE N0 NECK

- Elective neck dissection for detection of occult disease
  - Diagnostic: Additional pathological information for risk stratification and determination of adjuvant needs
  - Therapeutic: Occult N1 disease without adverse features may not require postoperative radiation
  - Treatment of the neck (surgery or radiation) indicated when the risk of nodal involvement reaches 20%
- Indications
- Oral cavity: primary with >4-mm depth of invasion and radiation is not already planned
  - Supraomohyoid neck dissection (levels I–III)
  - Consider bilateral dissection for midline lesions (floor of mouth and tongue)
- Oropharynx: T1 or T2 primary treated surgically where radiation is not already planned
  - Ipsilateral dissection for tonsil primary (at least levels II to IV)
  - Bilateral dissections for the base of the tongue
- Supraglottis: T1 or T2 primary treated surgically where radiation is not already planned (bilateral levels II–IV)
- Hypopharynx: T1 or T2 primary treated surgically where radiation is not already planned (ipsilateral vs. bilateral levels II–IV)

- T3 or T4 primary disease with N0 neck
  - Surgical management of primary should include neck dissection
  - Ipsilateral: Lateral tongue not crossing the midline, retromolar trigone, buccal mucosa, lateral alveolar ridge, and tonsil
  - Bilateral: Oral tongue crossing the midline, anterior floor of the mouth, soft palate, base of tongue, supraglottis, glottis, and hypopharynx

Neck Dissection for N+ Disease

- Neck dissection is indicated when the primary site is managed surgically
  - Modified radical neck dissection is indicated for positive disease
  - Selective neck dissections should be considered in small-volume neck disease
- Salvage neck dissection
  - Removal of metastatic disease of the neck that was previously treated
  - Common practice is to perform a positron emission tomography (PET) scan 3 months after completion of the nonsurgical treatment followed by salvage neck dissection for fluorodeoxyglucose (FDG)-avid residual disease
  - Perform surgery if needed within 3- to 6-month window after chemoradiation to avoid radiation-induced fibrosis
- Incisions for radical neck dissection (Fig. 5.2)

- Complications of neck dissection
  - Nerve injury: Marginal mandibular nerve (more common with level Ib), hypoglossal nerve (levels Ib, IIa), spinal accessory nerve (level IIb), vagus nerve, recurrent laryngeal nerve (RLN; more common with level VI), phrenic nerve, sympathetic chain, brachial plexus
  - Hematoma
  - Seroma
  - Infection
  - Chyle (left)/lymphatic leak (right)
  - Injury to great vessels

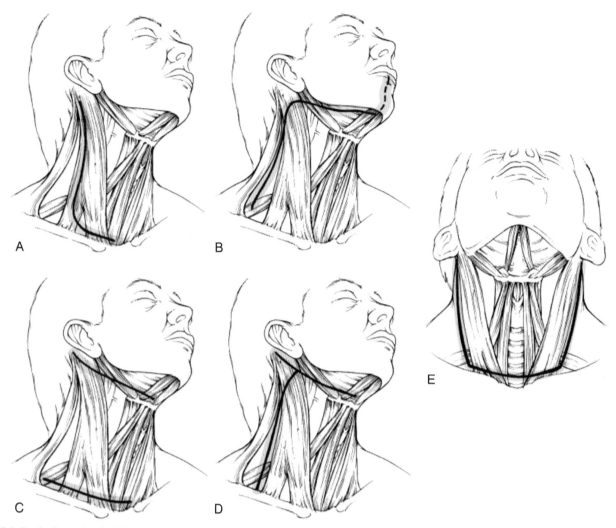

Fig. 5.2 Neck dissection incisions. Incisions for radical and modified radical neck dissections. (**A**) Hockey stick. (**B**) Boomerang. (**C**) McFee. (**D**) Modified Schobinger. (**E**) Apron or bilateral hockey stick. (From Flint PW, Haughey BH, Lund V, et al. *Cummings Otolaryngology—Head and Neck Surgery*. 7th ed. Philadelphia, PA: Saunders; 2021, Fig. 118.4.)

Lymphomas of the Head and Neck

- Second most common primary malignancy of the head and neck
- 8% of supraclavicular masses are found to be lymphoma

Presentation

- "B symptoms": temperatures >38°C, night sweats, and >10% weight loss
- Persistent cough and mediastinal adenopathy

Types

- Hodgkin lymphoma
  - Often presents with an enlarged node in the neck that may wax and wane
  - Histological feature: Reed-Sternberg cells (binucleated giant cells with eosinophilic inclusions) (Fig. 5.3)
- Non-Hodgkin lymphoma
  - Most are B-cell types
  - Oropharyngeal or nasopharyngeal mass
  - Waldeyer's ring
  - Epstein-Barr infection

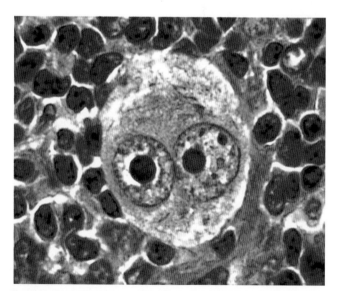

Fig. 5.3 Reed Sternberg cells. Characteristic histological finding of Hodgkin lymphoma. (From Goldblum JR, Lamps LW, McKenney JK, et al. *Rosai and Ackerman's Surgical Pathology*. 11th ed. Philadelphia, PA: Elsevier; 2018, Fig. 37.47.)

- Extranodal natural killer (NK)/T-cell lymphoma
  - Midline lethal granuloma
  - Destruction of the nose, sinuses, or the face
- Thyroid lymphoma (more common than anaplastic thyroid carcinoma)
  - Hashimoto disease is a risk factor
- Burkitt lymphoma: Endemic in Africa and may present as a jaw mass (Fig. 5.4)
- Salivary gland involvement
  - Mucosa-associated lymphoid tissue lymphoma
  - Sjögren syndrome

Diagnosis

- Requires fresh tissue (no formalin)
- Fine-needle aspiration inadequate
- Requires excisional biopsy or core needle biopsy

Lugano Staging (Updated from Prior Ann Arbor Classification) (Table 5.1)

ORAL CAVITY MALIGNANCIES

Oral Cavity Subsites

- Lips (skin-vermilion junction to the gingiva)
- Buccal mucosa
- Oral tongue
- Floor of the mouth

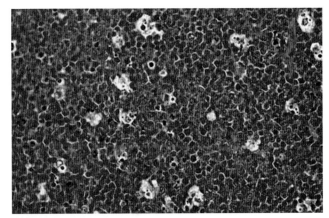

Fig. 5.4 Burkitt lymphoma. Characteristic histology "starry sky" appearance of Burkitt lymphoma. (From Goldblum JR, Lamps LW, McKenney JK, et al. *Rosai and Ackerman's Surgical Pathology.* 11th ed. Philadelphia, PA: Elsevier; 2018, Fig. 37.93.)

TABLE 5.1 Lugano Lymphoma Staging Classification

Stage I	Involvement of a single lymph node region or lymphoid structure (e.g., spleen, thymus, Waldeyer's ring)
Stage II	Involvement of 2 or more lymph node regions or lymphoid structures on the same side of the diaphragm
Stage III	Involvement of lymph node regions or lymphoid structures on both sides of the diaphragm
Stage IV	Diffuse or disseminated involvement of 1 or more extranodal organs or tissue beyond that designated "E," with or without associated lymph node involvement

Adapted from Cheson BD, Fisher RI, Barrington SF, et al. Recommendations for initial evaluation, staging, and response assessment of Hodgkin and non-Hodgkin lymphoma: the Lugano classification. *J Clin Oncol* 2014; 32:3059.

- Hard palate
- Alveolar ridge
- Retromolar trigone

Risk Factors for Oral Cavity Cancer

- Tobacco (smoking imparts greater risk than chewing tobacco)
- Alcohol (synergistic risk with tobacco)
- Betel nut (commonly used in Asia)
- Inflammatory disorders of the oral cavity
  - Submucosal fibrosis (often associated with Betel nut use)
  - Lichen planus (erosive and atrophic subtypes)
  - Poor oral hygiene
- Sun exposure (lip cancer)

Presentation

- Pain: At oral site, referred otalgia, odynophagia
- Bleeding
- Neck mass
- Weight loss

Physical Exam

- Leukoplakia: White patch that does not rub off (no histopathologic correlate)
  - May represent mild, moderate, or severe dysplasia
  - Most commonly hyperkeratosis secondary to irritant
- Erythroplakia: red, velvet-textured lesion that cannot be classified as another entity; high likelihood of dysplasia or carcinoma on biopsy

Differential Diagnosis of Oral Cavity Lesions

- Benign
  - Frictional keratosis
  - Mucocele
  - Hairy leukoplakia: Epstein-Barr mediated, more common in human immunodeficiency virus (HIV)/acquired immunodeficiency syndrome (AIDS)
  - Papilloma
  - Pyogenic granuloma
  - Fibroma (typically buccal and labial mucosa)
  - Pleomorphic adenoma (often on hard palate)
  - Granular cell tumor (dorsal surface of tongue)

- Malignant
  - Squamous cell carcinoma (90%–95%)
  - Minor salivary gland tumors (mucoepidermoid carcinoma, adenoid cystic carcinoma, adenocarcinoma)
  - Mucosal melanoma
  - Lymphoma
  - Sarcoma

Imaging of Oral Cavity Tumors

- Computed tomography (CT) scan: Good for evaluation of bone involvement; fast, inexpensive; dental artifacts can limit use for evaluation of the oral cavity
- Magnetic resonance imaging (MRI): Excellent for evaluation of soft tissues, perineural invasion, and bone involvement; limitations include motion artifact, cost, and claustrophobic conditions
- Positron emission tomography (PET)/CT scan: May improve definition of the extent of primary disease and detection of pathological nodes that do not meet size criteria on CT/MRI; limitations include cost and availability

Oral Cavity Cancer Staging (Table 5.2)

Management

- Surgery is the preferred modality
  - Less morbidity than radiation therapy with equivalent efficacy
  - No randomized trials comparing surgery to radiation for early-stage disease
- Radiation considered in patients unable to tolerate surgery

Lip

- 25% of oral cavity cancers
- Lower lip more common than upper lip because of sun exposure
- Prognosis is better for lower lip than for upper lip or oral commissure
- Optimal resection margins are not well defined
  - Final margins >5 mm are generally recommended
  - Initial operative margin may shrink by 50%; thus, at least a 1-cm operative margin is generally recommended
- Brachytherapy has a high success rate in lip cancer

- Reconstruction depends on the extent of resection
  - A <50% defect of the lip can often be closed primarily
  - Larger lesions may require local flaps (Abbe, Estlander, Karapandzik, or Gilles fan flap) or free tissue transfer (Fig. 5.5)

Floor of Mouth

- Locally invasive with a higher rate of occult metastasis; bilateral lymphatic drainage to central floor of mouth (FOM)
- Must carefully examine for tongue/mandible involvement
- Surgical considerations: Lingual nerve and Wharton's duct (must be prepared to re-route), reconstruct to prevent tongue tethering
- Defect closure/reconstruction: Primary closure for small lesions, secondary intention, skin grafts, local flaps (e.g., platysmal flap, supraclavicular flap), free tissue transfer for larger defects

Oral Tongue

- Speech and swallowing considerations affect reconstructive considerations
- Depth of invasion directs decision on management of the N0 neck
  - Depth >4 mm imparts risk of occult disease >20%
    - Supraomohyoid neck dissection
    - Consider sentinel lymph node biopsy (SLNB) at high-volume centers
- Deep margin assessment can be difficult
  - Skeletal muscle is often friable, leading to unreliable association with tumor
  - Muscle fibers contract with resection, leading to a narrower pathological margin
  - Low threshold to treat close margins (re-resection or radiation)

Retromolar Trigone

- Mucosal space between the third mandibular molar and the maxillary tuberosity
- Continuous with buccal mucosa, hard and soft palate, anterior tonsillar pillar, maxillary tuberosity, and the upper and lower alveolar ridges

TABLE 5.2 American Joint Committee on Cancer Oral Cavity TNM Staging

Primary Tumor	
TX	Unable to assess primary tumor
T0	No evidence of primary tumor
Tis	Carcinoma in situ
T1	Tumor <2 cm in greatest dimension and depth of invasion (DOI) ≤5 mm
T2	Tumor ≤2 cm and DOI >5 mm yet ≤10 mm or tumor >2 cm ≤4 cm in greatest dimension and DOI ≤10 mm
T3	Tumor >4 cm in greatest dimension or any tumor with DOI >10 mm
T4 (lip)	Primary tumor invades cortical bone, inferior alveolar nerve, floor of mouth, or skin of face (e.g., nose, chin)
T4a (oral)	Tumor invades adjacent structures (e.g., cortical bone, into deep tongue musculature, maxillary sinus) or skin of face
T4b (oral)	Tumor invades masticator space, pterygoid plates, or skull base or encases the internal carotid artery

REGIONAL LYMPHADENOPATHY	
NX	Unable to assess regional lymph nodes
N0	No evidence of regional metastasis
N1	Metastasis in a single ipsilateral lymph node, <3 cm in greatest dimension and extranodal extension-negative (ENE)
N2a	Metastasis in a single ipsilateral lymph node, <3 cm in greatest dimension and extranodal extension-positive (ENE) or metastasis to a single ipsilateral lymph node >3 cm but <6 cm and ENE-negative
N2b	Metastasis in multiple ipsilateral lymph nodes, all nodes <6 cm, and ENE-negative
N2c	Metastasis in bilateral or contralateral lymph nodes, all nodes <6 cm, and ENE negative
N3a	Metastasis in a lymph node >6 cm in greatest dimension and ENE-negative
N3b	Metastasis to a single ipsilateral lymph node >3 cm in greatest dimension and ENE-positive or metastasis to multiple ipsilateral, contralateral, or bilateral lymph nodes with any that are ENE-positive

DISTANT METASTASES	
MX	Unable to assess for distant metastases
M0	No distant metastases
M1	Distant metastases

TNM STAGING			
Stage 0	Tis	N0	M0
Stage I	T1	N0	M0
Stage II	T2	N0	M0
Stage III	T3	N0	M0
	T1–T3	N1	M0
Stage IVa	T4a	N0	M0
	T4a	N1	M0
	T1–T4a	N2	M0
Stage IVb	Any T	N3	M0
	T4b	Any N	M0
Stage IVc	Any T	Any N	M1

From Flint PW, Haughey BH, Lund VJ, et al. *Cummings Otolaryngology—Head and Neck Surgery.* 7th ed. Philadelphia, PA: Saunders; 2021, Table 91.1.

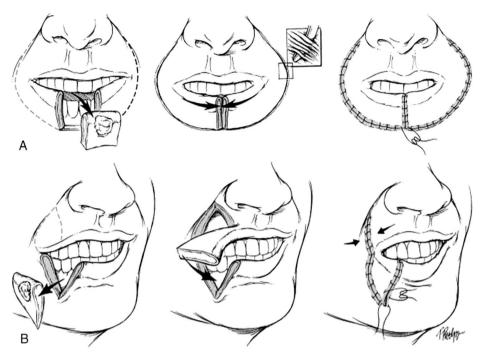

A

B

Fig. 5.5 (A) Abbe-Estlander flap for a left lower-lip resection that extended to the oral commissure. **(A1)** Wedge resection of lateral lower-lip carcinoma. **(A2)** Initial mobilization of upper-lip tissue that preserves the commissure, consistent with Abbe-Estlander flap reconstruction. **(A3)** Final inset of flap; arrows mark the site of advancement and tension with closure. **(B)** Karapandzic fan flap for midline lower-lip defect. **(B1)** Rectangular-shaped full-thickness resection of lower-lip carcinoma. **(B2)** Initial mobilization of circumoral advancement flaps; the neurovascular pedicle (inset) is preserved bilaterally. **(B3)** Final inset of reconstruction. (From Flint PW, Haughey BH, Lund V, et al. *Cummings Otolaryngology—Head and Neck Surgery*. 7th ed. Philadelphia, PA: Saunders; 2021, Figs. 91.11 and 91.12.)

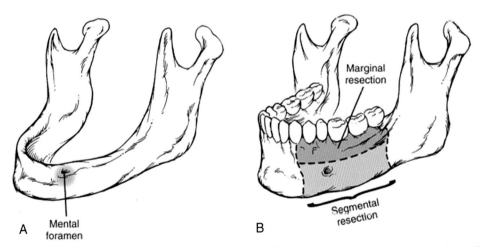

A Mental foramen   B

Fig. 5.6 Mandible variants and surgical approaches. (A) Edentulous mandible, which demonstrates why marginal mandibulectomy is difficult to perform without iatrogenic fracture in these patients. **(B)** Examples that compare marginal versus segmental mandibulectomy. (From Flint PW, Haughey BH, Lund V, et al. *Cummings Otolaryngology—Head and Neck Surgery*. 7th ed. Philadelphia, PA: Saunders; 2021, Fig. 91.13.)

- Early extension to the closely approximated mandible
- 5-Year survival of early-stage disease is 70%
- Surgery is the first-line treatment
  - Difficult exposure
  - May require a lip split for access
  - Marginal mandibulectomy is often necessary for deep margin (Fig. 5.6)
  - Edentulous patients are more likely to have mandibular invasion
    - Porous bone
    - Lower threshold for segmental resection

Hard Palate and Alveolar Ridge

- Hard palate: Reverse smoking is a risk factor

- Mucosa lies directly on the bone
  - Marginal mandibulectomy for early-stage (T1/T2) disease
  - Segmental mandibulectomy indications: Mandible enveloped by tumor, cortical bone erosion, tooth root involvement
  - Infrastructural maxillectomy reconstruction options: Regional flaps, free flaps, obturator prosthetics

Buccal Mucosa

- Often misdiagnosed as traumatic lesion
- 5-Year survival is 75% to 85% for stage I, 65% for stage II, 18% to 27% for stage III/IV
- Oral submucous fibrosis: 19-fold increased risk of buccal cancer
- Minority of oral cancers in North America, but common in India/Southeast Asia (betel nut quid use)
- Buccal space involvement common
- 40% of T2 tumors are node positive; 50% of T3 tumors are node positive
- Perifacial and submandibular nodes are typically first echelon
- Most common site of verrucous carcinoma
- Difficult exposure
- All defects must be reconstructed to prevent trismus
  - Skin graft for small tumors
  - Regional or free tissue transfer for larger tumors
- Adjuvant radiation or chemoradiation is commonly indicated

Neck Management in Early-Stage Disease

- Risk of occult metastasis is dependent on the depth of invasion
- Selective neck dissection with (clinical) thickness >2 to 4 mm
- Preoperative assessment of tumor depth is difficult
  - Imaging unreliable
  - Consider full-thickness punch biopsy
- Intermediate thickness lesions may be approached in two stages
  - Primary >2 mm thick: Perform neck dissection
  - Primary <2 mm thick: Observe the neck clinically

Consideration of Oral Cavity Sentinel Lymph Node Biopsy

- Equivalent survival versus elective neck dissection in early-stage oral cancer cases
- First-echelon nodes from floor of mouth may be unreliable due to "shine-through" signal from primary site
- Often requires radiotracer injection by surgeon instead of nuclear medicine
- If any sentinel lymph nodes positive: Perform therapeutic neck dissection

Extent of Prophylactic Neck Dissection

- Levels I to III (supraomohyoid)
- Oral tongue cancers may skip to level IV
- Level IIB lymph nodes controversial
  - May be unnecessary in absence of gross disease
  - Level IIB dissection can cause spinal accessory nerve weakness and injury
- Midline lesions may drain bilaterally and require bilateral neck dissection

Indications for Adjuvant Treatment

- Positive or close margins (if not reresected)
- Bone invasion
- Pathologically positive nodes: Controversy regarding N1 disease
- Perineural invasion

OROPHARYNGEAL MALIGNANCIES

Oropharynx Subsites

- Palatine tonsils
  - Most common site of oropharyngeal squamous cell carcinoma (OP SCC; 75%)
- Base of tongue/lingual tonsils (tissue posterior to the circumvallate papillae)
- Soft palate and uvula
- Anterior and posterior tonsillar pillars (palatoglossus and palatopharyngeus muscles)
- Posterior pharyngeal wall

Cancers of the Oropharynx

- SCC
  - Traditional: Negative for human papillomavirus (HPV; p16 negative) and mediated by alcohol and tobacco
    - Spindle cell variant (sarcomatoid): Highly aggressive
    - Verrucous: Relatively radioresistant
    - Basaloid
    - Adenosquamous
    - Often larger primary site disease and smaller nodal disease
  - HPV-mediated (p16-positive)
    - HPV is a double-stranded, nonenveloped DNA virus
    - HPV-16 is the most common virus subtype in HNSCC
    - Oncogenic HPV types: 16, 18, 31, and 33
    - Affects younger patients compared with HPV-negative HNSCC
    - Better prognosis (less so in patients with >10 pack-year smoking history)
    - Often presents with larger and more cystic/necrotic nodal disease and smaller primary site disease
    - p16
      - Tumor suppressor, overexpressed in HPV-mediated SCC
      - Used as histological biomarker for diagnosis of HPV
- Lymphoma: Two-thirds of Waldeyer's ring resides in the oropharynx
  - Palatine tonsil is the most common extranodal site of non-Hodgkin lymphoma
- Minor salivary gland neoplasms
  - Adenoid cystic carcinoma (most common minor salivary gland tumor of the oropharynx)
  - Mucoepidermoid carcinoma (second most common minor salivary gland tumor of the oropharynx)
- Sarcomas (rare)

Presentation

- Early-stage disease is often asymptomatic
- Neck mass (most common presenting symptom)
- Otalgia
- Odynophagia
- Dysphagia ± associated weight loss and malnutrition
- Globus sensation
- Voice changes
- Hemoptysis
- Difficulty breathing

Workup

- Physical exam
  - Flexible fiberoptic laryngoscopy
  - Oral exam (visual and palpation)
  - Neck exam for lymphadenopathy
  - Evaluate access to oropharynx (e.g., status of dentition, presence of trismus)
- Biopsy
  - Primary site and/or lymph node
    - Fine-needle aspiration (FNA) of lymph node
  - HPV testing (p16 testing as a surrogate for HPV)

- Imaging
  - CT scan with contrast
  - MRI with contrast
  - PET/CT scan

Oropharynx Staging (Table 5.3)

Treatment

- Early stage (stage I or II)
  - Single modality therapy

- Radiation
- Surgery
- Advanced stage (stages III and IV)
  - Concurrent chemoradiation (surgery reserved for salvage)
  - Surgery with adjuvant radiation or chemoradiation

Surgical Approaches

- Transoral approaches
  - Transoral robotic surgery (TORS; Fig. 5.7)

TABLE 5.3 American Joint Committee on Cancer Oropharynx TNM Staging

Primary Tumor (T) — Clinical and Pathologic T-Category

	Non-HPV-Associated (p16-negative)	HPV-associated (p16-positive)
Tx	Primary tumor cannot be assessed	NA
T0	NA	No primary identified
Tis	Carcinoma in situ	
T1	Tumor ≤2 cm in greatest dimension	Tumor ≤2 cm in greatest dimension
T2	Tumor >2 cm but ≤4 cm in greatest dimension	Tumor >2 cm but ≤4 cm in greatest dimension
T3	Tumor >4 cm in greatest dimension or extension to lingual surface of epiglottis	Tumor >4 cm in greatest dimension or extension to lingual surface of epiglottis
T4	Moderately or very advanced local disease	Moderately advanced local disease; tumor invades the larynx, extrinsic muscle of tongue, medial pterygoid, hard palate, or mandible or beyond (mucosal extension to lingual surface of epiglottis/vallecula does not constitute invasion of larynx)
T4a	Moderately advanced local disease; tumor invades the larynx, deep or extrinsic muscle of tongue, medial pterygoid, hard palate, or mandible (mucosal extension to lingual surface of epiglottis/vallecula does not constitute invasion of larynx)	NA
T4b	Very advanced local disease; tumor invades lateral pterygoid muscle, pterygoid plates, lateral nasopharynx, or skull base or encases carotid artery	NA

Regional Lymph Nodes (N) category

	Clinical and Pathologic N category	*Clinical N category*
Nx	Regional lymph nodes cannot be assessed	Regional lymph nodes cannot be assessed
N0	No regional lymph node metastasis	No regional lymph node metastasis
N1	Metastasis in a single ipsilateral lymph node ≤3 cm in greatest dimension and ECE-negative	One or more ipsilateral lymph nodes, none >6 cm
N2	Metastasis in a single ipsilateral lymph node >3 cm but ≤6 cm in greatest dimension and ECE-negative; or in multiple ipsilateral lymph nodes, none >6 cm in greatest dimension and ECE-negative; or in bilateral or contralateral lymph nodes, none >6 cm in greatest dimension and ECE-negative	Contralateral or bilateral lymph nodes, none >6 cm
N2a	Metastasis in a single ipsilateral lymph node >3 cm but ≤6 cm in greatest dimension and ECE-negative	NA
N2b	Metastasis in multiple ipsilateral lymph nodes, none >6 cm in greatest dimension and ECE-negative	NA
N2c	Metastasis in bilateral or contralateral lymph nodes, none >6 cm in greatest dimension and ECE-negative	NA
N3	Metastasis in a lymph node >6 cm in greatest dimension and ECE-negative; or metastasis in any lymph node(s) and clinically overt ECE-positive	Lymph node(s) >6 cm
N3a	Metastasis in a lymph node >6 cm in greatest dimension and ECE-negative	
N3b	Metastasis in any nodes (s) and clinically overt ECE-positive	
	Pathologic N category same as clinical N category for p16-negative OPSCC	*Pathologic N-category different from clinical N category for p16-positive OPSCC*
		Nx — Regional lymph nodes cannot be assessed
		N0 — No regional lymph node metastasis
		N1 — Metastasis in ≤4 lymph nodes
		N2 — Metastasis in >4 lymph nodes

Distant Metastasis (M) category

MX	Distant metastasis cannot be assessed	Distant metastasis cannot be assessed

(Continued)

TABLE 5.3 American Joint Committee on Cancer Oropharynx TNM Staging—cont'd

Primary Tumor (T) — Clinical and Pathologic T-Category			
M0	No distant metastasis	No distant metastasis	
M1	Distant metastasis	Distant metastasis	
T and N Category			
Non–human Papillomavirus-Associated (p16-Negative)	Human Papillomavirus–Associated (p16-Positive)		
TNM Stage	Clinical and Pathologic TNM Stage	Clinical TNM Stage	Pathologic TNM Stage
Stage I	T1N0	T0-T2N0-N1	T0-T2N0-N1
Stage II	T2N0	T0-T2N2 or T3N0-N2	T3-T4N0-N1 or T0-T2N2
Stage III	T3N0 or T1-3N1	T4 or N3	T3-4N2
Stage IV	NA	Any M1	Any M1
Stage IVA	T4aN0-N2c or T1-T3N2a-2c	NA	NA
Stage IVB	T4bN0-N3 or T1-T3N3	NA	NA
Stage IVC	Any M1	NA	NA

From Flint PW, Haughey BH, Lund VJ, et al. *Cummings Otolaryngology—Head and Neck Surgery.* 7th ed. Philadelphia, PA: Saunders; 2021, Tables 96.2 and 96.3.

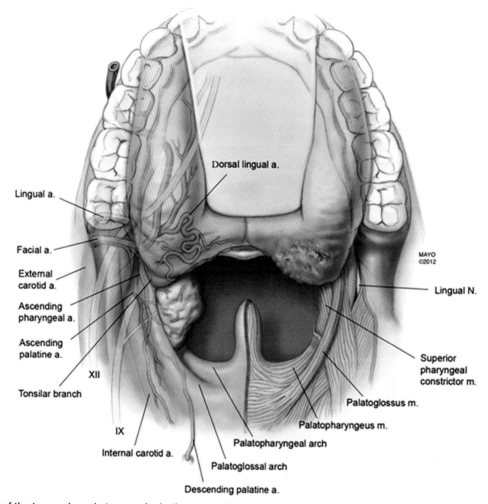

Fig. 5.7 Anatomy of the tongue base in transoral robotic surgery. Important adjacent structures include the lingual artery, facial artery, and lingual nerve. (From Van Abel KM, Moore EJ. Surgical management of the base of tongue. *Oper Tech Otolaryngol.* 2013;24:74–85, Fig. 4.)

- Intuitive da Vinci (2009) and Medrobotics Flex (2015) robotic systems: FDA approved for T1 and T2 oropharyngeal cancers
- Three-dimensional, high-definition view
- Assistant sits at the head of the bed and surgeon sits at the operating console
- Close margins are acceptable because of proximity to the carotid artery

- Bleeding risk up to 18.5% (major bleeding decreased with prophylactic ligation of external carotid branches)
- Contraindications
  - Tonsil cancer with retropharyngeal carotid
  - Tumor is in midline of the tongue/vallecula (risks injury to both lingual arteries)
  - Tumor is adjacent to carotid bulb/internal carotid (results in exposed vessel)
  - Carotid encasement by primary tumor (T4b) or node
  - Tumor requires resection of >50% of deep base of tongue musculature, posterior pharyngeal wall, up to 50% of the base of tongue and entire epiglottis
  - Posterolateral fixation of tonsil to prevertebral fascia
  - Cancer-related trismus
  - Unresectable neck disease
  - Multiple distant metastases
  - Inability to stop antiplatelet agents/anticoagulants
  - Cervical spine disease preventing suspension/positioning
- Transoral laser microsurgery (TLM)
  - Micrographic surgical technique
  - Initial cuts are made through the tumor to define the normal tissue/tumor interface
  - Careful communication with pathology and inking of margins are required
- Benefits of transoral techniques
  - No facial disassembly to access the tumor (e.g., lip split, mandibulotomy, pharyngotomy)
  - Shorter hospital stay
  - Faster resumption of oral diet
  - Tracheostomy often unnecessary
- Open Approaches
  - Transhyoid pharyngotomy (Fig. 5.8)
    - Dissection superior to the hyoid with pharyngotomy in the vallecular space
    - Pharyngotomy must be made away from the tumor: Best for lateral lesions of the base of the tongue or inferior tonsil

- Advantage: Preservation of pharyngeal plexus
- Disadvantage: Less exposure compared with other open approaches
- Lip split with mandibulotomy (Fig. 5.9)
  - Midline or parasymphyseal cut
  - Plating performed before mandibulotomy
  - Advantages: Wide exposure and preservation of alveolar nerve and pharyngeal plexus
  - Disadvantage: Facial scar and potential for mandible nonunion or malocclusion
- Visor flap (Fig. 5.10)
  - With or without lingual release/pull through
  - Cosmetically preferable
  - May require transection of bilateral mental nerves
  - By itself, it may limit posterior access

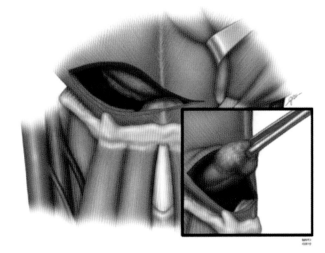

Fig. 5.8 Transhyoid pharyngotomy. A suprahyoid incision leads to the pharyngotomy, leaving a cuff of muscle along the hyoid bone for closure. The point of entry is at the hyoepiglottic ligament. (From Van Abel KM, Moore EJ. Surgical management of the base of tongue. *Oper Tech Otolaryngol.* 2013;24:74-85, Fig. 7).

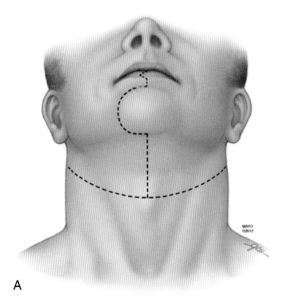

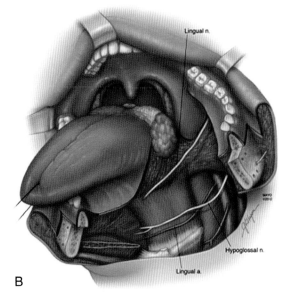

A   B

Fig. 5.9 Lip split with mandibulotomy. (A) Cervical incision for lip-split mandibulotomy approach. **(B)** Demonstration of the important neurovascular, bony, and muscular structures exposed through the mandibulotomy. The mandible bony cuts are performed in stair-step fashion. (From Van Abel KM, Moore EJ. Surgical management of the base of tongue. *Oper Tech Otolaryngol.* 2013;24:74–85, Figs. 8 and 9.)

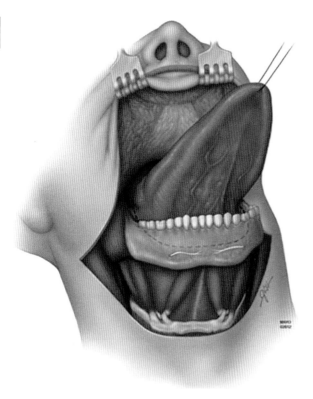

Fig. 5.10 Visor flap. The superior flap is raised in the subplatysmal plane up to the submandibular level. Intraoral mucosal cuts are then performed transorally along the lingual surface of the mandible (hatched line). (From Van Abel KM, Moore EJ. Surgical management of the base of tongue. *Oper Tech Otolaryngol.* 2013;24:74–85, Fig. 10.)

- Lingual release (Fig. 5.11)
  - Circumferential incision at the floor of the mouth: alveolar ridge junction
  - Used for total glossectomy
  - Advantage: Wide exposure of the oral tongue in conjunction with the base of the tongue
  - Disadvantage: Release of all lingual attachments to the mandible

Surveillance

- 3-Month posttreatment PET/CT
  - If negative findings, may follow clinically with no further imaging required
  - If equivocal, further imaging may be warranted
- Salvage surgery
  - Approximately 90% of recurrences occur within the first 2 years
  - Salvage surgery has been shown to improve survival if resectable
  - Confers importance of close and routine clinical follow-up

LARYNGEAL MALIGNANCIES
Sites of Larynx

- Supraglottis
- Glottis
- Subglottis

Subsites of Supraglottis

- Epiglottis
- Aryepiglottic (AE) folds

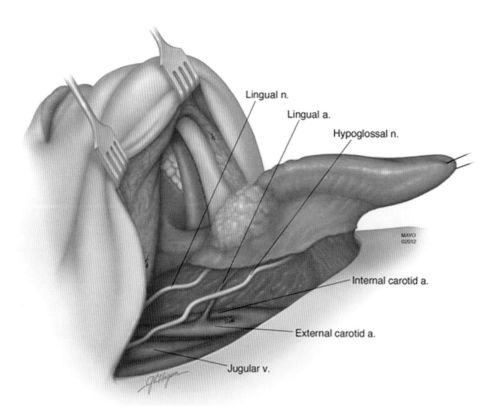

Lingual n.
Lingual a.
Hypoglossal n.
Internal carotid a.
External carotid a.
Jugular v.

Fig. 5.11 Lingual release (pull through). Extension of cuts to the retromolar trigone and into the tonsillar fossa and pharynx allows for enough mobility of the tongue so that it can be dropped beneath the mandible and visualized in the neck. (From Van Abel KM, Moore EJ. Surgical management of the base of tongue. *Oper Tech Otolaryngol.* 2013;24:74–85, Fig. 11.)

- Arytenoids
- False vocal cords

Subsites of Glottis

- True vocal cords
  - Layers (Fig. 5.12)
    - Squamous epithelium
    - Superficial lamina propria (Reinke's space)
    - Intermediate lamina propria (vocalis ligament)
    - Deep lamina propria (vocalis ligament)
    - Vocalis muscle (vocal fold body)
- Anterior commissure
- Posterior commissure
- Ventricle

Barriers to Spread of Cancer (Fig. 5.13)

1. Quadrangular membrane (above false cords) for supraglottis
2. Conus elasticus (between true cords and cricoid) for glottis and subglottis
3. Cricothyroid membrane
4. Thyrohyoid membrane
5. Thyroid cartilage inner perichondrium

Anatomic Pathways to Spread of Cancer (Fig. 5.14)

- Broyle's tendon: Vocalis tendon insertion into thyroid cartilage at anterior commissure (lacks perichondrium here)
- Preepiglottic space
- Paraglottic space

Laryngeal Lymphatic Drainage

- Prelaryngeal/pretracheal
- Paralaryngeal/paratracheal
- Upper, mid- and lower jugular
- Mediastinal (considered distant metastasis)

Laryngeal Cancer Staging (Table 5.4)

Treatment

Supraglottic Cancer

Early-Stage (T1-T2) Supraglottic Cancer
1. Primary radiation
2. Transoral endoscopic or robotic supraglottic partial laryngectomy and elective vs. therapeutic neck dissections
3. Open supraglottic partial laryngectomy and elective versus therapeutic neck dissections

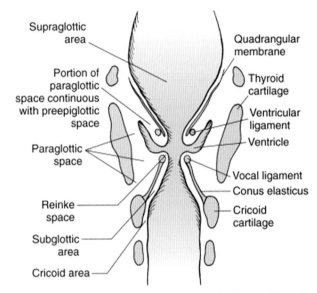

Fig. 5.13 Connective tissue barriers within the larynx. (From Flint PW, Haughey BH, Lund VJ, et al. *Cummings Otolaryngology—Head and Neck Surgery.* 7th ed. Philadelphia, PA: Saunders; 2021, Fig. 108.7.)

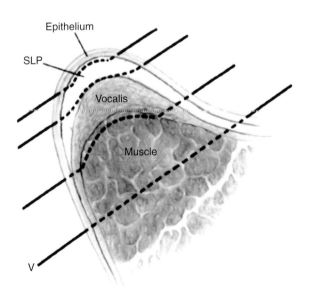

Fig. 5.12 Vocal fold layers showing potential planes of dissection: epithelium, superficial lamina propria (*SLP*), vocalis ligament, and thyroarytenoid (*vocalis*) muscle (*V*). (From Myers EN, Carrau RL. *Operative Otolaryngology: Head and Neck Surgery.* 2nd ed. Philadelphia, PA: Saunders; 2008, Fig. 46.2.)

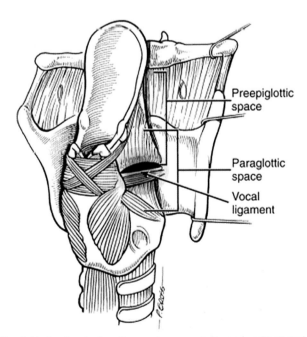

Fig. 5.14 Anatomical pathways to spread of cancer. Posterior/oblique view of larynx showing confluence of preepiglottic and paraglottic spaces. (From Flint PW, Haughey BH, Lund VJ, et al. *Cummings Otolaryngology—Head and Neck Surgery.* 7th ed. Philadelphia, PA: Saunders; 2021, Fig. 105.2.)

TABLE 5.4 American Joint Committee on Cancer Larynx TNM Staging

Primary Tumor (T)	
TX	Primary tumor cannot be assessed
T0	No evidence of primary tumor
TIS	Carcinoma in situ
SUPRAGLOTTIS	
T1	Tumor limited to one subsite of supraglottis with normal vocal cord mobility
T2	Tumor invades mucosa of more than one adjacent subsite of supraglottis or glottis or region outside the supraglottis (e.g., mucosa of base of tongue, vallecula, and medial wall of piriform sinus) without fixation of the larynx
T3	Tumor limited to larynx with vocal cord fixation and/or invades any of the following: postcricoid area, preepiglottic space, paraglottic space, and/or inner cortex of thyroid cartilage
T4a	Moderately advanced local disease
	Tumor invades through the outer cortex of the thyroid cartilage and/or invades tissues beyond the larynx (e.g., trachea, soft tissues of neck, including deep extrinsic muscle of the tongue, strap muscles, thyroid, or esophagus)
T4b	Very advanced local disease
	Tumor invades prevertebral space, encases carotid artery, or invades mediastinal structures
GLOTTIS	
T1	Tumor limited to the vocal cord(s) with normal mobility; may involve anterior or posterior commissure
T1a	Tumor limited to one vocal cord
T1b	Tumor involves both vocal cords
T2	Tumor extends to supraglottis and/or subglottis and/or with impaired vocal cord mobility
T3	Tumor limited to the larynx with vocal cord fixation and/or invasion of paraglottic space and/or inner cortex of the thyroid cartilage
T4a	Moderately advanced local disease
	Tumor invades through the outer cortex of the thyroid cartilage and/or invades tissues beyond the larynx (e.g., trachea, cricoid cartilage, soft tissues of neck including deep extrinsic muscle of the tongue, strap muscles, thyroid, or esophagus)
T4b	Very advanced local disease
	Tumor invades prevertebral space, encases carotid artery, or invades mediastinal structures
SUBGLOTTIS	
T1	Tumor limited to the subglottis
T2	Tumor extends to vocal cord(s) with normal or impaired mobility
T3	Tumor limited to larynx with vocal cord fixation and/or invasion of paraglottic space and/or inner cortex of the thyroid cartilage
T4a	Moderately advanced local disease
	Tumor invades cricoid or thyroid cartilage and/or invades tissues beyond the larynx (e.g., trachea, soft tissues of neck, including deep extrinsic muscles of the tongue, strap muscles, thyroid, or esophagus)
T4b	Very advanced local disease
	Tumor invades prevertebral space, encases carotid artery, or invades mediastinal structures
REGIONAL LYMPH NODES (N)	
cNX	Regional lymph nodes cannot be assessed
cN0	No regional lymph node metastasis
cN1	Metastasis in a single ipsilateral lymph node, ≤3 cm in greatest dimension
cN2	Metastasis in a single ipsilateral lymph node, >3 cm but not >6 cm in greatest dimension, or in multiple ipsilateral lymph nodes, none >6 cm and ENE(–); or metastasis in multiple ipsilateral lymph nodes, none >6 cm and ENE(–); or bilateral or contralateral lymph nodes, none >6 cm and ENE(–)
cN2a	Metastasis in a single ipsilateral lymph node, >3 cm but not >6 cm and ENE(–)
cN2b	Metastasis in multiple ipsilateral lymph nodes, none >6 cm and ENE(–)
cN2c	Metastasis in bilateral or contralateral lymph nodes, none >6 cm and ENE(–)
cN3	Metastasis in a lymph node >6 cm and ENE(–); or metastasis in any lymph node(s) with clinically overt ENE(+)
cN3a	Metastasis in a lymph node, >6 cm and ENE(–)
cN3b	Metastasis in any lymph node(s) with clinically overt ENE(+)
pNX	Regional lymph nodes cannot be assessed
pN0	No regional lymph node metastasis
pN1	Metastasis in a single ipsilateral lymph node, ≤3 cm and ENE(–)
pN2	Metastasis in a single ipsilateral lymph node, ≤3 cm and ENE(+); or >3 cm but not >6 cm and ENE(–); or multiple ipsilateral nodes, ≤6 cm and ENE(–); or bilateral or contralateral lymph node(s) ≤6 cm and ENE(–)
pN2a	Metastasis in a single ipsilateral lymph node, ≤3 cm and ENE(+)
pN2b	Metastasis in multiple ipsilateral lymph nodes, none >6 cm and ENE(–)
pN2c	Metastasis in bilateral or contralateral lymph nodes, none >6 cm in greatest dimension and ENE(–)

TABLE 5.4 American Joint Committee on Cancer Larynx TNM Staging—cont'd

REGIONAL LYMPH NODES (N)

pN3	Metastasis in a lymph node >6 cm in greatest dimension and ENE(−); or metastasis in a single ipsilateral node, >3 cm and ENE(+); or multiple ipsilateral, contralateral, or bilateral lymph nodes any with ENE(+); or a single contralateral node of any size and ENE(+)
pN3a	Metastasis in a lymph node, >6 cm in greatest dimension and ENE(−)
pN3b	Metastasis in a single ipsilateral node >3 cm and ENE(+); or multiple ipsilateral, contralateral or bilateral lymph nodes any with ENE(+); or a single contralateral node of any size and ENE(+)

Stage	T	N	M
0	TIS	N0	M0
I	T1	N0	M0
II	T2	N0	M0
III	T3	N0	M0
	T1	N1	M0
	T2	N1	M0
	T3	N1	M0
IVA	T4a	N0	M0
	T4a	N1	M0
	T1	N2	M0
	T2	N2	M0
	T3	N2	M0
	T4a	N2	M0
IVB	T4b	Any N	M0
	Any T	N3	M0
IVC	Any T	Any N	M1

From Flint PW, Haughey BH, Lund VJ, et al. *Cummings Otolaryngology—Head and Neck Surgery.* 7th ed. Philadelphia, PA: Saunders; 2021, Box 105.1 and Table 105.1.

Advanced Stage (T3-T4) Supraglottic Cancer

1. Primary chemoradiation
2. Open supraglottic partial laryngectomy in special cases and elective versus therapeutic neck dissections
3. Total laryngectomy and elective versus therapeutic neck dissections

Glottic Cancer

Early Stage (T1-T2) Glottic Cancer

1. Primary radiation
2. Endoscopic cordectomy for T1 tumor of middle third of true vocal fold (TVF); see Table 5.5
3. Open laryngofissure and cordectomy for T1 tumor of middle third of TVF; see Table 5.5
4. Open vertical partial laryngectomy

Advanced Stage (T3-T4) Glottic Cancer

1. Primary chemoradiation
2. Open partial supracricoid laryngectomy ± elective vs. therapeutic neck dissection(s)
3. Total laryngectomy ± elective vs. therapeutic neck dissection(s)

Advantages of Surgery for Glottic Cancer

- Equivalent voice outcomes for T1 disease
- Faster than radiation
- Better salvage options for recurrence that are less morbid
- Avoid long-term speech/swallow dysfunction from radiation

TABLE 5.5 Types of Cordectomy

Type	Description
Type I	Subepithelial
Type II	Subligamental
Type III	Transmuscular
Type IV	Total/complete
Type Va	Extended, including contralateral true vocal cord
Type Vb	Extended, including arytenoid
Type Vc	Extended, including ventricular fold
Type Vd	Extended, including subglottis

Advantages of Radiation for Glottic Cancer

- Better voice outcomes, especially in patients with T2-T4 disease
- Equivalent local control
- Avoid issues with unfavorable surgical access
- Avoid need for second-look OR procedures

Subglottic Cancer

- Subglottic cancer seldom diagnosed in early stages

Early Stage (T1-T2) Subglottic Cancer

1. Primary radiation
2. Total laryngectomy (partial laryngectomy, cricotracheal resection are not oncological options) and elective versus therapeutic neck dissections

Advanced Stage (T3-T4) Subglottic Cancer

1. Primary chemoradiation
2. Total laryngectomy and elective versus therapeutic neck dissections

Principles of Organ Preservation (Partial Laryngectomy) Surgery

- Must achieve local control
  - Organ preservation procedures should be used only when local control rates approximate that of total laryngectomy
  - Difficult to diagnose recurrences following preservation procedures
- Need for accurate assessment of the three dimensional extent of the tumor
  - Comprehensive appreciation of the extent of the tumor is necessary
  - May result in need for total laryngectomy when a different partial procedure may have been appropriate
- The cricoarytenoid unit is the basic functional unit of the larynx
  - Consists of an arytenoid, cricoid cartilage, associated musculature, superior laryngeal nerve, and RLN
  - Preservation of the cricoarytenoid unit (not vocal folds) allows for physiological speech/swallow without need for permanent tracheostomy
- Must resect normal tissue to achieve an expected functional outcome: Additional resection of normal tissue in a standard approach is necessary to achieve consistent functional outcomes

Contraindications to Partial Laryngectomy

- Older age (relative)
- Poor pulmonary function (must have good enough baseline function to be able to tolerate postoperative aspiration)
- Fixed vocal folds
- Cartilage invasion
- Subglottic extension (see specific procedures)

- Interarytenoid/posterior surface of arytenoid cartilage involvement
- Cervical metastasis (relative)

Open Partial Laryngectomy Procedures

Supraglottic Laryngectomy

- Indications: T1, T2, limited T3 (preepiglottic space) supraglottic cancers
- Contraindications: T3 (vocal cord fixation), interarytenoid involvement, posterior arytenoid mucosa involvement, thyroid cartilage invasion, extralaryngeal spread (including limited base of tongue mobility)
- Removes: Epiglottis, AE folds, false cords, preepiglottic space, portion of the hyoid, portion of the thyroid cartilage above the ventricles (Fig. 5.15)
- Spares: Arytenoids, both TVFs

Supracricoid Laryngectomy

- Indications: Select T3 glottic (paraglottic space) and supraglottic (ventricle/false cord) cancers
- Contraindications: Arytenoid fixation, cricoid cartilage contact/invasion, major preepiglottic space/hyoid involvement, posterior arytenoid mucosa involvement, thyroid cartilage outer perichondrium invasion, extralaryngeal spread
- Removes: Entire thyroid cartilage, bilateral true and false cords, one arytenoid and the paraglottic space, ± epiglottis (Fig. 5.16)
- Spares: Cricoid, hyoid, and at least one arytenoid
- Reconstruction
  - Cricohyoidoepiglottopexy if epiglottis spared (see Fig. 5.16)
  - Cricohyoidopexy if epiglottis removed (worse swallowing outcomes; Fig. 5.17)

Vertical Partial Laryngectomy

- Indications: T1 (including anterior commissure and may be bilateral if no more than anterior 1/3 of the contralateral cord is involved), T2 (transglottic) glottic cancers

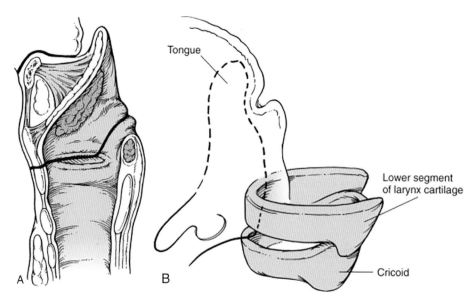

Fig. 5.15 Supraglottic laryngectomy. (**A**) Supraglottic laryngectomy superior to inferior of the false cord, to the level of the ventricle, and anterior to the arytenoids. (**B**) Laryngoplasty is performed with three closure stitches circumferentially around the inferior half of the thyroid cartilage and submucosally into the tongue base, as is done in the supracricoid partial laryngectomy. (From Flint PW, Haughey BH, Lund VJ, et al. *Cummings Otolaryngology—Head and Neck Surgery.* 7th ed. Philadelphia, PA: Saunders; 2021, Figs. 108.13 and 108.14.)

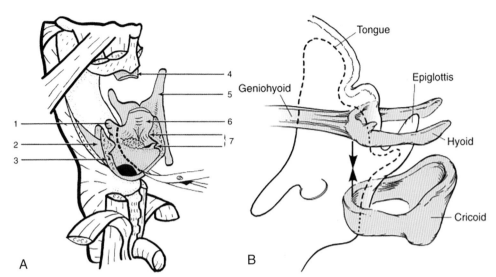

Fig. 5.16 Supracricoid laryngectomy with cricohyoidoepiglottopexy (CHEP). (A) Exposure of malignancy in a supracricoid partial laryngectomy with CHEP. 1, Arytenoid; 2, internal thyroid perichondrium; 3, vocal process; 4, inferior aspect of transected epiglottis; 5, thyroid cartilage; 6, petiole of the epiglottis; 7, false and true vocal cords. **(B)** Laryngoplasty is performed using circumferential cricoid, hyoid, epiglottic, and tongue-base sulures. (From Flint PW, Haughey BH, Lund VJ, et al. *Cummings Otolaryngology—Head and Neck Surgery.* 7th ed. Philadelphia, PA: Saunders; 2021, Figs. 108.11 and 108.12.)

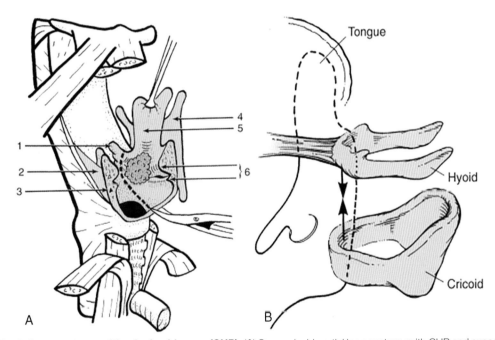

Fig. 5.17 Supraglottic laryngectomy with cricohyoidopexy (CHP). (A) Supracricoid partial laryngectomy with CHP and exposure of malignancy. 1, Arytenoid; 2, external thyroid perichondrium; 3, vocal process; 4, thyroid cartilage; 5, epiglottis; 6, false and true cords. **(B)** Supracricoid partial laryngectomy with CHP using three circumferential cricoid, hyoid, and tongue base stitches. (From Flint PW, Haughey BH, Lund VJ, et al. *Cummings Otolaryngology—Head and Neck Surgery.* 7th ed. Philadelphia, PA: Saunders; 2021, Figs. 108.16 and 108.17.)

- Contraindications: Bilateral cord involvement (see above), >10 mm anterior subglottic extension, >5 mm posterior subglottic extension, posterior commissure involvement, bulky transglottic disease, T3 disease (fixed vocal cord, paraglottic space involvement), cricoarytenoid joint involvement, posterior arytenoic mucosa involvement, AE fold involvement, thyroid cartilage invasion
- Removes: One entire true vocal cord from vocal process to anterior commissure (may also resect anterior commissure and up to anterior one-third of contralateral cord), false cord, ventricle, paraglottic space, overlying thyroid cartilage

Total Laryngectomy

- Indications
  - T3/T4 tumors with thyroid cartilage destruction
  - Posterior commissure or bilateral arytenoid involvement (seen in advanced supraglottic tumors)
  - Circumferential submucosal disease
  - Subglottic extension with cricoid cartilage involvement
  - Radiation or chemoradiation failures
  - Completion laryngectomy for failed conservation laryngeal surgery

- Hypopharyngeal tumors that spread to the postcricoid mucosa
- Thyroid tumors that invade both sides of the larynx
- Advanced tumors of unusual histology that are incurable by conservation surgery or chemoradiation (e.g., adenocarcinoma and sarcomas)
- Extensive pharyngeal or tongue-base resections in patients at high risk for aspiration
- Radiation necrosis of the larynx
- Severe irreversible aspiration

Measures to Prevent Laryngectomy Stomal Stenosis

- Bevel tracheal cuts
- Minimize tracheal tension
- Cut medial heads of sternocleidomastoid muscles
- Minimize suctioning
- Minimize laryngectomy tube use

Complications From Total Laryngectomy

- Early complications
  - Hypoglossal nerve injury
  - Hematoma
  - Infection
  - Pharyngocutaneous fistula
  - Wound dehiscence
- Late complications
  - Stomal stenosis
  - Pharyngoesophageal stenosis or stricture
  - Hypothyroidism

Considerations for Total Laryngectomy

- Neck dissection
  - Bilateral selective neck dissections recommended for supraglottic involvement
  - Unilateral neck dissection can be considered for T3 glottic carcinoma
  - Salvage neck dissection recommended for chemoradiation failures

- Concurrent thyroidectomy
  - Higher risk of thyroid involvement with subglottic tumor (paratracheal and parapharyngeal lymphatic spread)
  - Tumor can extend directly through thyroid/cricoid cartilages into thyroid gland
  - Depending on extent, ipsilateral hemithyroidectomy may be performed versus total thyroidectomy for advanced disease
- Pharyngeal closure in radiated patients
  - 30% risk of pharyngocutaneous fistula in salvage laryngectomy patients
  - Pharyngeal mucosal closure options: Primary closure, constrictor muscle overlay, pedicled flap buttress, and free-flap buttress
  - Controversial whether pedicled flap or free flap decreases fistula incidence
- Primary versus secondary tracheoesophageal puncture (TEP)
- Primary TEP
  - Performed at time of laryngectomy (fewer procedures)
  - Able to be done in salvage laryngectomies
- Secondary TEP
  - Staged procedure weeks to months after laryngectomy
  - Ideal for patients at high-risk for wound complications (high radiation doses, poor nutrition, hypothyroid), with subglottic disease with need for postoperative radiation

Vocal Rehabilitation After Total Laryngectomy (Fig. 5.18)

- Esophageal voice
- Electrolarynx
- TEP

Treatment of Pharyngocutaneous Fistula

- NPO with alternate nutrition source (nasogastric/gastrostomy tube, total parenteral nutrition)
- Local wound care and debridement
- Strict glycemic control
- Correction of hypothyroidism
- Surgery: Local closure versus regional flaps

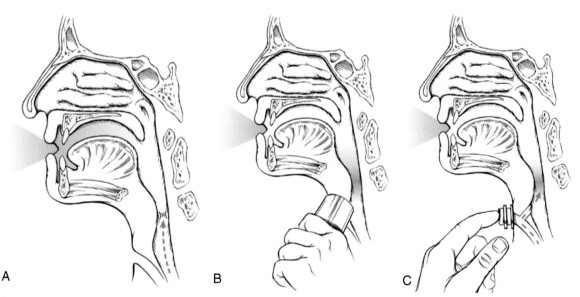

Fig. 5.18 Forms of speech after total laryngectomy. (A) Electrolarynx speech. **(B)** Esophageal speech. **(C)** Tracheoesophageal puncture speech. (From Flint PW, Haughey BH, Lund VJ, et al. *Cummings Otolaryngology—Head and Neck Surgery.* 7th ed. Philadelphia, PA: Saunders; 2021, Figs. 111.4, to 111.6.)

LANDMARK LARYNGEAL CANCER TRIALS

Department of Veterans Affairs Laryngeal Cancer Study Group (1991)

- 332 randomized stages III-IV glottic or supraglottic SCC patients
- Arms
  - Cohort 1: Total laryngectomy + postoperative radiation
  - Cohort 2: Induction chemotherapy + radiation
    - Proceed to total laryngectomy + postoperative radiation if not at least a partial response with induction chemotherapy + radiation
- No significant difference in 2-year overall survival (68% vs. 68%), but 64% of Cohort 2 had their larynx preserved
- Controversy: Whether the 64% of patients with preserved larynges were functional
- Effect: Supports that chemoradiation is as effective as laryngectomy with the potential to preserve function

Radiation Therapy Oncology Group (RTOG) 91-11 Intergroup Trial (2003, 2013)

- 547 randomized patients with stages III-IV glottic or supraglottic SCC
- Excluded T1 node-positive or large-volume T4 disease
- Arms
  - Cohort 1: Induction chemotherapy + radiation (or laryngectomy if no response)
  - Cohort 2: Concurrent chemoradiation
  - Cohort 3: Radiation alone
- Larynx preservation is superior with concurrent chemoradiation (88%) versus induction (75%, $p = 0.005$) or versus radiation alone (70%, $p < 0.001$)
- Locoregional control is superior with concurrent chemoradiation (78%) versus induction (61%) or versus radiation alone (56%)
- Decreased distant metastasis in chemotherapy groups (Cohorts 1 and 2), but 2-year and 5-year overall survival no different among the 3 cohorts
- Use of induction chemotherapy + radiation (Cohort 1) not supported
- Effect: Supports that concurrent chemoradiation protocols should become the standard of care
- 10-year follow-up: No significant difference in overall survival, with chemotherapy groups (Cohorts 1 and 2) showing improved larynx preservation over radiation alone

HYPOPHARYNGEAL MALIGNANCIES

Subsites of Hypopharynx (Fig. 5.19)

- Pyriform sinuses
  - Medial border: Aryepiglottic fold
  - Lateral border: Thyroid cartilage
  - Superior border: Glossoepiglottic fold
  - Inferior border: Cricopharyngeus
  - Posterior border: Lateral pharyngeal walls
- Postcricoid space
  - Superior border: Posterior arytenoid mucosa
  - Inferior border: Cricopharyngeus
  - Lateral border: Tracheoesophageal groove
- Posterior pharyngeal wall
  - Superior border: Level of vallecula
  - Inferior border: Cricopharyngeus
  - Lateral border: Lateral pharyngeal walls

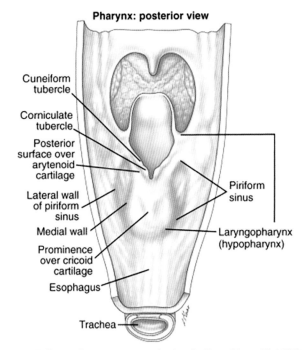

Fig. 5.19 Hypopharynx anatomical subsites. (From Flint PW, Haughey BH, Lund VJ, et al. *Cummings Otolaryngology—Head and Neck Surgery*. 7th ed. Philadelphia, PA: Saunders; 2021, Fig. 101.1.)

Innervation

- Motor
  - Superior pharyngeal nerve
  - Pharyngeal branches of the CN IX and CN X
  - External branch of the superior laryngeal nerve
- Sensory
  - Internal branch of the superior laryngeal nerve (CN X)
  - Glossopharyngeal nerve (CN IX)
  - Vagus nerve (CN X)

Lymphatic Drainage of the Hypopharynx (Fig. 5.20)

- Jugulodigastric
- Midjugular
- Spinal accessory chain
- Paratracheal (pyriform sinus apex)
- Paraesophageal
- Retropharyngeal (pyriform sinus and posterior pharyngeal wall)

Presentation

- Dysphagia
- Neck mass
- Sore throat
- Hoarseness
- Otalgia

Differential Diagnosis

- SCC (>95%)
- Lymphoma
- Adenocarcinoma
- Sarcoma

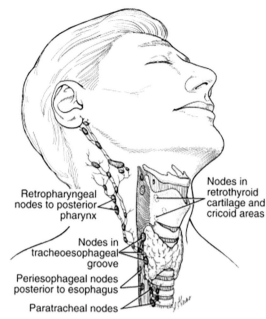

Fig. 5.20 Hypopharynx lymphatic drainage. Hypopharyngeal carcinomas metastasize primarily to the superior jugular and midjugular nodes. However, metastasis to the retropharyngeal, paratracheal, paraesophageal, and parapharyngeal space nodes may be present. (From Flint PW, Haughey BH, Lund VJ, et al. *Cummings Otolaryngology—Head and Neck Surgery.* 7th ed. Philadelphia, PA: Saunders; 2021, Fig. 101.2.)

Hypopharyngeal Squamous Cell Carcinoma

- More likely to present in advanced stages (>75% are stages III-IV at time of diagnosis)
- Frequent submucosal spread (may lead to underestimation of tumor size)
- More direct correlation with alcohol intake than other HNSCC
- Association with Plummer-Vinson syndrome
  - Specifically associated with postcricoid SCC
  - Female predominance (85%)
  - Diagnostic triad: Dysphagia, iron deficiency anemia, and hypopharyngeal/esophageal webs
  - Chronic inflammation from webs can progress to SCC
  - Syndrome etiology likely the result of nutritional deficiency

Hypopharynx and Cervical Esophagus Staging (Table 5.6)

Treatment

- Radiation alone (stages I-II)
- Chemoradiation (organ preservation; stages III-IV)
- Surgery + postoperative radiation ± chemotherapy (variable stages)
- Neck Management
  - Elective neck dissection warranted for N0 disease based on risk of occult metastasis (>20%)
  - Bilateral necks should be addressed in nearly all cases with surgery or radiation (except early T1 lesions) given rich lymphatic drainage
  - Radiation frequently used because retropharyngeal lymph node metastases are common and not typically removed with standard neck dissection
  - Neck Dissection Considerations
    - N0 disease: Bilateral levels II-IV

- Clinically node-positive disease: Bilateral levels I-V
- Pyriform sinus apex tumors: Level VI
- Posterior pharyngeal wall tumors: Retropharyngeal nodes

Surgical Management

Surgical Approaches

- Transoral laser or robotic partial pharyngectomy
  - Indications: Small tumors with adequate endoscopic exposure, best for lateral pyriform sinus base/posterior pharyngeal wall tumors
- Open partial pharyngectomy
  - Via lateral pharyngotomy
  - Indications: Pyriform sinus base/posterior pharyngeal wall tumors
- Open partial laryngopharyngectomy
  - Very limited use
- Total laryngectomy with partial pharyngectomy
  - Indications: Pyriform sinus apex and postcricoid tumors
- Total laryngopharyngectomy
  - Indications: Postcricoid mucosa tumors, extension across midline, large tumor of posterior pharyngeal wall
- Total laryngopharyngoesophagectomy
  - Indications: Same as total laryngopharyngectomy plus cervical esophagus involvement

Advantages of Transoral Excision

- Tracheostomy seldom required
- Preservation of suprahyoid musculature facilitates more normal swallowing
- No reconstruction needed
- Voice preservation
- Decreased hospital stay

Complications From Open Surgery

- Pharyngocutaneous fistula
- Stricture
- Gastrostomy tube dependency
- Tracheostomy dependency

Reconstruction Options

- Primary closure
- Recommend a minimum of 3 cm of pharynx mucosa (side to side)
- Must estimate the extent of resection before surgery (requires 1.5 cm minimum margins)
- Contraindications to primary closure
  - Cancer extension past the midline
  - Involvement of postcricoid mucosa or cervical esophagus
- Regional flap (pectoralis major, supraclavicular, platysma)
- Secondary intention (transoral approaches)
- Gastric pull-up (when resection extends below the cervicothoracic junction of the esophagus)
- Colonic interposition
- Free flaps: Radial forearm, anterolateral thigh, jejunal
  - Jejunal free flap
  - Advantages
    - Large segment that can be used for anastomosis as high as the nasopharynx
    - Intrinsic mucous production may assist in swallowing
    - Tolerates postoperative radiation
    - Lower mortality/morbidity rates compared with gastric pull-up

TABLE 5.6 American Joint Committee on Cancer Hypopharynx and Cervical Esophagus TNM Staging

Primary Tumor (T)

HYPOPHARYNX

TX	Primary tumor cannot be assessed
T0	No evidence of primary tumor
T1	Tumor limited to one subsite of hypopharynx and ≤2 cm in greatest dimension
T2	Tumor invades more than one subsite of hypopharynx or an adjacent site or measures >2 cm but not >4 cm in greatest dimension without fixation of the hemilarynx
T3	Tumor >4 cm in greatest dimension or with fixation of the hemilarynx
T4a	Tumor invades thyroid/cricoid cartilage, hyoid bone, thyroid gland, esophagus, or central compartment soft tissue (including prelaryngeal strap muscles and subcutaneous fat)
T4b	Tumor invades prevertebral fascia, encases carotid artery, or involves mediastinal structures

CERVICAL ESOPHAGUS

TX	Primary tumor cannot be assessed
T0	No evidence of primary tumor
Tis	Carcinoma in situ
T1	Tumor invades lamina propria, muscularis mucosae, or submucosa
T1a	Tumor invades lamina propria or muscularis mucosae
T1b	Tumor invades submucosa
T2	Tumor invades muscularis propria
T3	Tumor invades adventitia
T4	Tumor invades adjacent structures
T4a	Resectable tumor invades pleura, pericardium, or diaphragm
T4b	Unresectable tumor invades other adjacent structures, such as aorta, vertebral body, trachea, etc.

REGIONAL LYMPH NODES (N)

HYPOPHARYNX

NX	Regional lymph nodes cannot be assessed
N0	No regional lymph node metastasis
N1	Metastasis in a single ipsilateral lymph node ≤3 cm in greatest dimension and ENE negative
N2a	Metastasis in a single ipsilateral or contralateral lymph node ≤3 cm in greatest dimension and ENE positive; ormetastasis in a single ipsilateral lymph node >3 cm but not >6 cm in greatest dimension and ENE negative
N2b	Metastasis in multiple ipsilateral lymph nodes, none >6 cm in greatest dimension and ENE negative
N2c	Metastasis in bilateral or contralateral lymph nodes, none >6 cm in greatest dimension and ENE negative
N3a	Metastasis in a lymph node >6 cm in greatest dimension and ENE negative
N3b	Metastasis in a single ipsilateral node >3 cm in greatest dimension and ENE positive; or metastasis in multiple ipsilateral, contralateral, or bilateral lymph nodes, with any ENE positive

CERVICAL ESOPHAGUS

NX	Regional lymph nodes cannot be assessed
N0	No regional lymph node metastasis
N1	Metastasis in one to two regional lymph nodes
N2	Metastasis in three to six regional lymph nodes
N3	Metastasis in seven or more regional lymph nodes

DISTANT METASTASIS (M)

MX	Distant metastasis cannot be assessed
M0	No distant metastasis
M1	Distant metastasis present

GRADE (G)

GX	Grade cannot be assessed, stage as G1
G1	Well differentiated
G2	Moderately differentiated
G3	Poorly differentiated
G4	Undifferentiated, stage as G3

Stage	T	N	M	Grade
HYPOPHARYNX				
0	Tis	N0	M0	

(Continued)

TABLE 5.6 American Joint Committee on Cancer Hypopharynx and Cervical Esophagus TNM Staging—cont'd

Stage	T	N	M	Grade
I	T1	N0	M0	
II	T2	N0	M0	
III	T3	N0	M0	
	T1	N1	M0	
	T2	N1	M0	
	T3	N1	M0	
IVa	T4a	N0	M0	
	T4a	N1	M0	
	T1	N2	M0	
	T2	N2	M0	
	T3	N2	M0	
	T4a	N2	M0	
IVb	T4b	Any N	M0	
	Any T	N3	M0	
IVc	Any T	Any N	M1	
CERVICAL ESOPHAGUS				
0	Tis	N0	M0	1, X
Ia	T1	N0	M0	1, X
Ib	T1	N0	M0	2, 3
IIa	T2, T3	N0	M0	1, X
IIb	T1, T2	N1	M0	Any
	T2, T3	N0	M0	2, 3
IIIa	T1, T2	N2	M0	Any
	T3	N1	M0	Any
	T4a	N0	M0	Any
IIIb	T3	N2	M0	Any
IIIc	T4a	N1, N2	M0	Any
	T4b	Any	M0	Any
	Any	N3	M0	Any
IV	Any T	Any N	M1	Any

From Flint PW, Haughey BH, Lund VJ, et al. *Cummings Otolaryngology—Head and Neck Surgery.* 7th ed. Philadelphia, PA: Saunders; 2021, Tables 101.2 and 101.3.

- Disadvantages
  - Flap tolerates short ischemia time
  - Dysphagia from jejunum peristalsis
  - Poor vocal rehabilitation from TEP prosthesis (wet "gurgly" voice) compared with anterolateral thigh (ALT)
  - Morbidity from abdominal incision
  - Need for two microvascular anastomoses

NASOPHARYNGEAL MALIGNANCIES

Nasopharyngeal Carcinoma (NPC)

- Etiologies
- Genetic factors
  - Family clusters: 15% of Chinese patients have a first-degree relative with NPC
  - HLA-B, C, D haplotypes associated with increased risk
- Environmental factors
- High-nitrosamine diet
  - Type of preservative used with salted fish, eggs, and vegetables
  - Risk associated with early exposure or during weaning period
- Wood dust
- Chemical fumes
- Dermatomyositis patients have 10% risk of NPC, should be screened regularly
- Epstein-Barr virus (EBV)
  - Viral capsid antigen (VCA) and early antigen (EA)
  - Majority of general population (w/o NPC): Elevated immunoglobulin G (IgG) VCA and IgG EA
  - Majority of general population has elevated IgG VCA and IgG EA
  - NPC patients have elevated IgA VCA (highly sensitive) and IgA EA (highly specific), elevated EBV nuclear antigens and latent membrane proteins

Demographics

- Male predominance (75%)
- 20% of NPC patients will have a first-degree relative with NPC
- >50% of NPC patients are diagnosed between age 30 and 50 years
- Highest world incidence is in Guangzhou, China (Guangdong Province; <30 per 100,000) among ethnic Chinese
- Other groups with higher incidence: Eskimos, Polynesians, indigenous Mediterranean population

Presentation

- 99% of patients symptomatic at diagnosis
- Neck mass present in 60% (usually level II and high level V, although 80% will have radiographically enlarged lymph nodes present)
- Otitis media with effusion/Eustachian tube dysfunction/unilateral hearing loss/tinnitus
- Blood-tinged saliva/sputum (epistaxis is not common)
- Nasal obstruction
- Cranial nerve palsies (10%): CNs V, VI, IX, X, XII

Differential Diagnosis of Nasopharyngeal Masses

- NPC
- Juvenile nasopharyngeal angiofibroma (JNA)
- Adenoid cystic carcinoma
- Chordoma
- Craniopharyngioma
- Angiofibroma
- Lymphoma
- Thornwaldt cyst
- Adenoid hypertrophy

Nasopharyngeal Carcinoma Staging (Table 5.7)

World Health Organization Classification of Nasopharyngeal Carcinoma

- Type I: SCC (keratinizing)—5-year survival is 35%
  - Poorer response to radiation than type II
- Type IIa: Nonkeratinizing carcinoma (EBV+)
- Type IIb: Undifferentiated carcinoma (EBV+)
  - Most common type in endemic regions
  - More aggressive, distant metastases more common
  - 5-year survival: 60%

Workup

- Nasopharyngeal endoscopy (10% of NPCs may be entirely submucosal)
- MRI for evaluation of tumor extent and skull-base involvement
- PET/CT for evaluation of distant metastasis (bone most common)
- Audiogram
  - Baseline (especially if patient has conductive hearing loss from otitis media)
  - Radiation may worsen Eustachian tube dysfunction
  - Platinum-based chemotherapies may cause sensorineural hearing loss
- EBV serology: IgA VCA (highly sensitive) and IgA EA (highly specific)
- Dental evaluation
- Speech and swallow evaluation

Treatment

- Stages I-II: Radiation alone
- Stages II-IV: Chemoradiation
  - Concurrent chemoradiation for stage II disease with parapharyngeal extension due to higher risk of distant metastasis (communication of pterygoid venous plexus and prevertebral plexus)
  - Possible induction chemotherapy first for locally advanced stage IV disease)
- Persistent disease: Salvage surgery
- Recurrent disease: Reirradiation or salvage surgery

TABLE 5.7 American Joint Committee on Cancer Nasopharynx TNM Staging

Stage	Description
T Classification	
TX	Primary tumor unable to be assessed
T0	No evidence of tumor, but EBV-positive cervical node(s) involvement
T1	Confined to nasopharynx or extends to oropharynx and/or nasal cavity without parapharyngeal involvement
T2	Tumor extends to parapharyngeal space, and/or adjacent soft tissue involvement (medial pterygoid, lateral pterygoid, prevertebral muscles)
T3	Tumor involves bony structures at skull base, paranasal sinus, cervical vertebrae, and/or pterygoid structures.
T4	Intracranial extension, involvement of cranial nerves, hypopharyx, orbit, parotid and/or extensive soft tissue infiltration beyond lateral surface of the lateral pterygoid muscle
N Classification	
N0	No nodal involvement
N1	Unilateral cervical lymph nodes ≤6 cm, or unilateral or bilateral retropharyngeal nodes ≤6 cm, above caudal border of cricoid cartilage
N2	Bilateral cervical lymph nodes ≤6 cm, above caudal border of cricoid cartilage
N3	Lymph node >6 cm and/or extension below the caudal border of cricoid cartilage
M Classification	
M0	No distant metastasis
M1	Distant metastasis (includes mediastinal nodes)
Stage Classification	
I	T1N0M0
II	T1N1M0, T0N1M0, T2N0M0, T2N1M0
III	T3N0M0, T3N1M0, T0 to T3N2M0
IVa	T4, any NM0 or any T, N3M0
IVb	Any T, any N, M

From Flint PW, Haughey BH, Lund VJ, et al. *Cummings Otolaryngology—Head and Neck Surgery.* 7th ed. Philadelphia, PA: Saunders; 2021, Table 95.1.

Radiation Side Effects

- Early: Mucositis, xerostomia, sinusitis, nasal crusting, otitis media with effusion, conductive hearing loss, Eustachian tube dysfunction
- Late: sensorineural hearing loss (CN VIII damage), CN XII palsy, trismus (particularly if skull base is treated)

Locoregional Recurrence

- 5% to 10% of NPC patients develop local recurrence (50% of these eligible for salvage surgery)
- Success of salvage surgery correlates with T-stage (must follow patients closely with low threshold for biopsy to detect recurrence early)
- 10% of patients develop neck recurrence or have residual neck disease (should determine if eligible for neck dissection)
- Reirradiation carries significant risk (transverse myelitis, temporal lobe necrosis, trismus, sensorineural hearing loss, choanal stenosis, palatal dysfunction, cranial nerve palsies)

Surgical Management

- Contraindications: Internal carotid encasement/involvement, clival erosion, intracranial extension
- Surgical Approaches
  - Endoscopic
    - Best for small tumors on the central nasopharyngeal wall
    - Can be used for more lateral tumors by experienced surgeons
    - Deep margin should include prevertebral muscle
    - Nasoseptal flap improves healing
  - Lateral rhinotomy with medial maxillectomy (Fig. 5.21)
    - For tumors limited to nasopharynx ± pterygopalatine fossa extension ± orbital extension
    - Can be combined with transoral approach
    - Exposure gained by removing middle turbinate and posterior nasal septum
  - Maxillary swing (Fig. 5.22)
    - Modified Weber-Ferguson incision
    - For tumors in the pterygopalatine fossa, require control of internal carotid
    - Maximum exposure, but requires palatal split
    - Allows for free flap inset

Prognosis

- Patients with stages I-II disease treated with radiation alone have a 5-year overall survival (OS) of 80% or higher
- Patients with stages III-IV disease treated with chemoradiation have a 5-year OS of 70%
- N3 disease is associated with poorer survival and higher rates of distant metastasis
- Distant metastasis remains the main cause of death

SINONASAL MALIGNANCIES

Sinonasal Subsites

- Nasal cavity
- Paranasal sinuses
- Pterygopalatine fossa
- Infratemporal fossa
- Orbital cavity
- Anterior cranial fossa

Differential Diagnosis of Sinonasal Masses

- Papillomas: Fungiform, cylindrical, keratotic, inverted
- Osteoma/ossifying fibroma
- Fibrous dysplasia
- JNA
- Nasopharyngeal carcinoma
- SCC
- Adenocarcinoma
- Adenoid cystic carcinoma
- Sarcoma: Rhabdomyosarcoma, leiomyosarcoma, chondrosarcoma, fibrosarcoma
- Hemangiopericytoma
- Lymphoma
- Mucosal melanoma
- Esthesioneuroblastoma
- Plasmacytoma

Most Common Sites of Sinonasal Malignancies

- Maxillary sinus (50%–70%)
- Nasal cavity (15%–30%)
- Ethmoid sinus (10%–20%)

Risk Factors

- Wood-dust exposure (adenocarcinoma)
- Leather-related occupational exposure (adenocarcinoma)
- Smoking (SCC)

Presentation

- Nasal symptoms: Obstruction, discharge, epistaxis
- Localized facial pain
- Ocular symptoms (advanced disease): Epiphora, diplopia, decreased vision, proptosis
- Palatal/facial numbness (CN VII; advanced disease)
- Trismus (advanced disease)

Physical Exam

- Ophthalmological exam (proptosis, epiphora, visual acuity changes, and extraocular muscle impingement)
- Neurological exam (numbness, paresthesias)

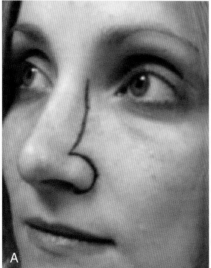 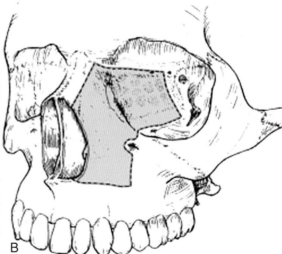

Fig. 5.21 Lateral rhinotomy and medial maxillectomy. (A) Lateral rhinotomy incision. **(B)** Medial maxillectomy cuts encompass the inferior and middle turbinates, portions of the maxillary and ethmoid sinuses, and lamina paprycea. (From Flint PW, Haughey BH, Lund VJ, et al. *Cummings Otolaryngology—Head and Neck Surgery.* 7th ed. Philadelphia, PA: Saunders; 2021, Figs. 94.7A and 94.8A.)

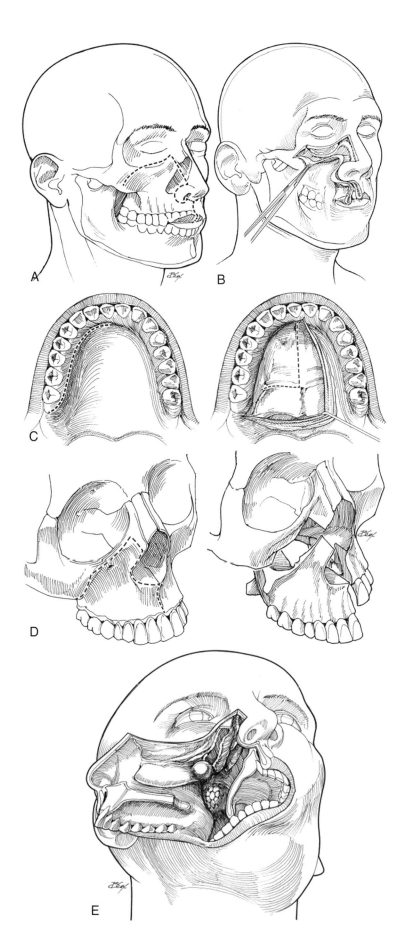

Fig. 5.22 Maxillary swing. (**A**) Modified Weber-Ferguson incision with subciliary lower lid extension. (**B**) Skin and soft tissues under the incision are not elevated more than a few millimeters laterally over the anterior surface of the maxilla, maintaining all soft tissue attachments intact on the anterior surface of the maxilla. (**C**) Incision in the mucosa of the hard palate is made from the ipsilateral incisor along the alveolus extending posteriorly onto the soft palate adjacent to the maxillary tuberosity. The flap is raised subperiosteally toward the soft palate and beyond the midline of the hard palate before the midline osteotomy. (**D**) Osteotomies are made in the anterior maxillary wall (alveolar process in midline, nasal process of maxilla, inferior orbital rim), zygomatic arch, hard palate. (**E**) Maxilla and attached soft tissue is rotated and reflected anteriorly and laterally, preserving blood supply. There is wide access to the nasopharynx, infratemporal fossa, parapharyngeal space and middle fossa. (From Shuman AG, Shah JP. Maxillary swing approach for removal of recurrent nasopharyngeal carcinoma. *Oper Tech Otolaryngol.* 2014:25:248–53, Fig. 2.6.)

- Dental exam (trismus, palatal lesions, loose dentition)
- Nasal endoscopy exam (outflow obstruction, cerebrospinal fluid leakage)

Workup

- Imaging
  - Computed Tomography (CT)
    - Faster than MRI
    - Less expensive than MRI
    - Evaluates bony expansion, remodeling, or destruction
    - Evaluates calcifications (associated with esthesioneuroblastomas, sarcomas)
    - Evaluates widening of bony fissures or foramina
  - Magnetic Resonance Imaging (MRI)
    - Helps rule out encephalocele before biopsy
    - Evaluates perineural invasion
      - Asymmetric nerve enlargement or enhancement
      - Obliteration of perineural fat planes
      - Denervation changes in end organs (muscles of facial expression or mastication)
      - Widening of nerve foramina
    - Differentiates postobstructive changes from tumor
    - Better evaluation of orbital invasion (differentiates periorbita from tumor)
    - Better evaluation of intracranial invasion (differentiates dura from tumor)
  - Positron emission tomography/computed tomography (PET/CT)
    - Evaluates for distant metastases
    - Posttreatment surveillance

Ohngren's Line (Fig. 5.23)

- Imaginary plane from the medial canthus of the eye to the angle of mandible
- Infrastructural lesions (anterior and inferior to line)
  - Earlier presentation
  - More amenable to resection
  - Patterns of spread (from the maxillary sinus): Medial into the nasal cavity, lateral into the masticator space, inferior into the oral cavity, anterior into the soft tissues of the cheek
- Suprastructural lesions (posterior and superior to line)
  - More advanced presentation
  - More likely to involve critical structures, less amenable to resection
  - Patterns of spread (from the maxillary sinus): Superior into the orbit, superior/medial into the ethmoid sinuses, posterior into the pterygopalatine fossa

STAGING SYSTEMS

Nasal Cavity and Paranasal Sinus Carcinoma Staging (Table 5.8)

Mucosal Melanoma Staging (Table 5.9)

Kadish System for Esthesioneuroblastoma (Table 5.10)

Treatment

Surgical Approaches

- Endoscopic maxillectomy
  1. Contraindications: Involvement of facial soft tissue, anterolateral frontal sinus, palate, dura beyond midpupillary line, mandible, orbit
- Open maxillectomy

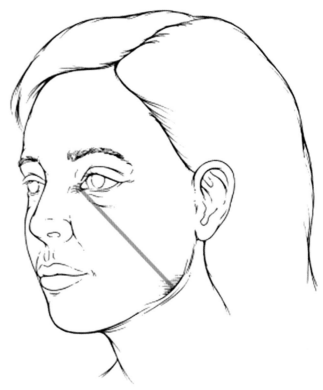

Fig. 5.23 Ohngren's Line. An imaginary line is drawn from the medial canthus to the angle of the jaw, which gives a rough estimate of the dividing line between tumors that may be resected with a good prognosis (below the line) and those with a poor prognosis (above the line). (From Flint PW, Haughey BH, Lund VJ, et al. *Cummings Otolaryngology—Head and Neck Surgery.* 7th ed. Philadelphia, PA: Saunders; 2021, Fig. 94.4.)

  1. Contraindications: Trismus (pterygoid muscle involvement), skull base invasion, significant brain parenchyma involvement, carotid encasement)
  2. Transoral
  3. Midface degloving approach (Fig. 5.24)
  4. Lateral rhinotomy approach (Fig. 5.25)
     1. Lynch incision: Extend superiorly to the medial eyebrow (access the medial canthal ligament and lacrimal duct)
     2. Subciliary incision: Extend across the lower-eyelid crease (access the orbital floor)
  5. Weber-Ferguson incision: Extend inferiorly as the upper-lip split (access to the palate) (Fig. 5.26)
  6. Craniofacial resection (Fig. 5.27)
- Robotic approach
  1. Medial maxillectomy (middle turbinate, inferior turbinate, ethmoid sinus, and maxillary sinus)
  2. Infrastructural maxillectomy (medial maxillectomy plus the maxillary alveolar ridge and adjoining hard palate)
  3. Subtotal maxillectomy (entire maxilla)
  4. Total maxillectomy (entire maxilla and orbital floor)
  5. Radical maxillectomy (total maxillectomy plus orbital exenteration)
  6. Craniofacial resection (anterior cranial-base removal, including the cribriform plate, ethmoid sinuses, and dura)

Reconstruction

- Obturator coverage with facial and dental prostheses
  - Faster with shorter hospitalization

TABLE 5.8 American Joint Committee on Cancer Nasal Cavity and Paranasal Sinus Staging

Maxillary sinus

T category	T criteria
TX	Primary tumor cannot be assessed
Tis	Carcinoma in situ
T1	Tumor limited to maxillary sinus mucosa with no erosion or destruction of bone
T2	Tumor causing bone erosion or destruction, including extension into the hard palate and/or middle nasal meatus, except extension to posterior wall of maxillary sinus and pterygoid plates
T3	Tumor invades any of the following: Bone of the posterior wall of maxillary sinus, subcutaneous tissues, floor or medial wall of orbit, pterygoid fossa, ethmoid sinuses
T4	Moderately advanced or very advanced local disease
T4a	Moderately advanced local disease
	Tumor invades anterior orbital contents, skin of cheek, pterygoid plates, infratemporal fossa, cribriform plate, sphenoid or frontal sinuses
T4b	Very advanced local disease
	Tumor invades any of the following: Orbital apex, dura, brain, middle cranial fossa, cranial nerves other than maxillary division of trigeminal nerve (V2), nasopharynx, or clivus

Nasal cavity and ethmoid sinus

T category	T criteria
TX	Primary tumor cannot be assessed
Tis	Carcinoma in situ
T1	Tumor restricted to any one subsite, with or without bony invasion
T2	Tumor invading two subsites in a single region or extending to involve an adjacent region within the nasoethmoidal complex, with or without bony invasion
T3	Tumor extends to invade the medial wall or floor of the orbit, maxillary sinus, palate, or cribriform plate
T4	Moderately advanced or very advanced local disease
T4a	Moderately advanced local disease
	Tumor invades any of the following: Anterior orbital contents, skin of nose or cheek, minimal extension to anterior cranial fossa, pterygoid plates, sphenoid or frontal sinuses.
T4b	Very advanced local disease
	Tumor invades any of the following: Orbital apex, dura, brain, middle cranial fossa, cranial nerves other than V2, nasopharynx, or clivus.

Regional lymph nodes (N)

Clinical N (cN)

N category	N criteria
NX	Regional lymph nodes cannot be assessed
N0	No regional lymph node metastasis
N1	Metastasis in a single ipsilateral lymph node, ≤3 cm in greatest dimension and ENE(−)
N2	Metastasis in a single ipsilateral node >3 cm but not >6 cm in greatest dimension and ENE(−); or
	Metastases in multiple ipsilateral lymph nodes, none >6 cm in greatest dimension and ENE(−); or
	In bilateral or contralateral lymph nodes, none >6 cm in greatest dimension and ENE(−)
N2a	Metastasis in a single ipsilateral node >3 cm but not >6 cm in greatest dimension and ENE(−)
N2b	Metastasis in multiple ipsilateral nodes, none >6 cm in greatest dimension and ENE(−)
N2c	Metastasis in bilateral or contralateral lymph nodes, none >6 cm in greatest dimension and ENE(−)
N3	Metastasis in a lymph node >6 cm in greatest dimension and ENE(−); or
	Metastasis in any node(s) with clinically overt ENE(+)
N3a	Metastasis in a lymph node >6 cm in greatest dimension and ENE(−)
N3b	Metastasis in any node(s) with clinically overt ENE (ENEc)

Pathologic N (pN)

N category	N criteria
NX	Regional lymph nodes cannot be assessed
N0	No regional lymph node metastasis
N1	Metastasis in a single ipsilateral lymph node, ≤3 cm in greatest dimension and ENE(−)
N2	Metastasis in a single ipsilateral lymph node, ≤3 cm in greatest dimension and ENE(+); or
	Larger than 3 cm but not >6 cm in greatest dimension and ENE(−); or
	Metastases in multiple ipsilateral lymph nodes, none >6 cm in greatest dimension and ENE(−); or
	In bilateral or contralateral lymph node(s), none >6 cm in greatest dimension and ENE(−)
N2a	Metastasis in a single ipsilateral lymph node, ≤3 cm in greatest dimension and ENE(+); or
	A single ipsilateral node >3 cm but not >6 cm in greatest dimension and ENE(−)

(Continued)

TABLE 5.8 American Joint Committee on Cancer Nasal Cavity and Paranasal Sinus Staging—cont'd

Maxillary sinus

N category	N criteria
N2b	Metastasis in multiple ipsilateral nodes, none >6cm in greatest dimension and ENE(−)
N2c	Metastasis in bilateral or contralateral lymph node(s), none >6cm in greatest dimension and ENE(−)
N3	Metastasis in a lymph node >6cm in greatest dimension and ENE(−); or
	In a single ipsilateral node >3cm in greatest dimension and ENE(+); or
	Multiple ipsilateral, contralateral, or bilateral nodes, any with ENE(+); or
	A single contralateral node ≤3cm and ENE(+)
N3a	Metastasis in a lymph node >6cm in greatest dimension and ENE(−)
N3b	Metastasis in a single ipsilateral node >3cm in greatest dimension and ENE(+); or
	Multiple ipsilateral, contralateral, or bilateral nodes, any with ENE(+); or
	A single contralateral node ≤3cm and ENE(+)

NOTE: A designation of "U" or "L" may be used for any N category to indicate metastasis above the lower border of the cricoid (U) or below the lower border of the cricoid (L).

Similarly, clinical and pathologic ENE should be recorded as ENE(−) or ENE(+).

Distant metastasis (M)

M category	M criteria
M0	No distant metastasis (no pathologic M0; use clinical M to complete stage group)
M1	Distant metastasis

Prognostic stage groups

When T is…	And N is…	And M is…	Then the stage group is…
Tis	N0	M0	0
T1	N0	M0	I
T2	N0	M0	II
T3	N0	M0	III
T1, T2, T3	N1	M0	III
T4a	N0, N1	M0	IVA
T1, T2, T3, T4a	N2	M0	IVA
Any T	N3	M0	IVB
T4b	Any N	M0	IVB
Any T	Any N	M1	IVC

From Flint PW, Haughey BH, Lund VJ, et al. *Cummings Otolaryngology—Head and Neck Surgery.* 7th ed. Philadelphia, PA: Saunders; 2021, Table 94.1.

TABLE 5.9 American Joint Committee on Cancer Mucosal Melanoma TNM Staging

Primary tumor (T)

T category	T criteria
T3	Tumors limited to the mucosa and immediately underlying soft tissue, regardless of thickness or greatest dimension; for example, polypoid nasal disease, pigmented or nonpigmented lesions of the oral cavity, pharynx, or larynx
T4	Moderately advanced or very advanced
T4a	Moderately advanced disease
	Tumor involving deep soft tissue, cartilage, bone, or overlying skin
T4b	Very advanced disease
	Tumor involving brain, dura, skull base, lower cranial nerves (IX, X, XI, XII), masticator space, carotid artery, prevertebral space, or mediastinal structures

Regional lymph nodes (N)

N category	N criteria
NX	Regional lymph nodes cannot be assessed
N0	No regional lymph node metastases
N1	Regional lymph node metastases present

Distant metastasis (M)

M category	M criteria
M0	No distant metastasis
M1	Distant metastasis present

From Flint PW, Haughey BH, Lund VJ, et al. *Cummings Otolaryngology—Head and Neck Surgery.* 7th ed. Philadelphia, PA: Saunders; 2021, Table 94.3.

TABLE 5.10 Kadish Classification of Esthesioneuroblastoma Staging

Kadish A	Confined to nasal cavity
Kadish B	Extends to paranasal sinuses
Kadish C	Extends beyond nasal cavity and paranasal sinuses
Kadish D	Lymph node or distant metastases

From Flint PW, Haughey BH, Lund VJ, et al. *Cummings Otolaryngology—Head and Neck Surgery.* 7th ed. Philadelphia, PA: Saunders; 2021, Table 94.2.

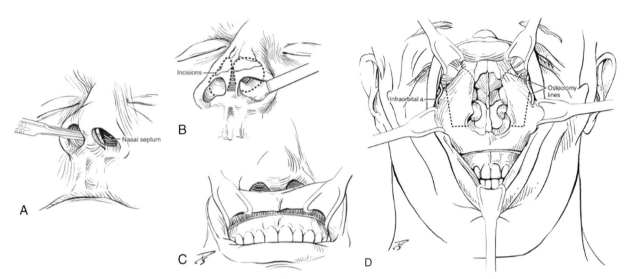

Fig. 5.24 Midface degloving. (**A**) Release of the nasal septum. (**B**) Further incisions are extended over the alar cartilages to the pyriform aperture. (**C**) Mucosal incisions are made into the soft tissues of the gingivolabial sulcus. (**D**) The upper-lip and midface tissues are retracted superiorly to expose the tumor. (From Cohen JI, Clayman GL. *Atlas of Head & Neck Surgery.* 1st ed. Philadelphia, PA: Saunders; 2011, Figs. 42.6A–42.6C and 42.7.)

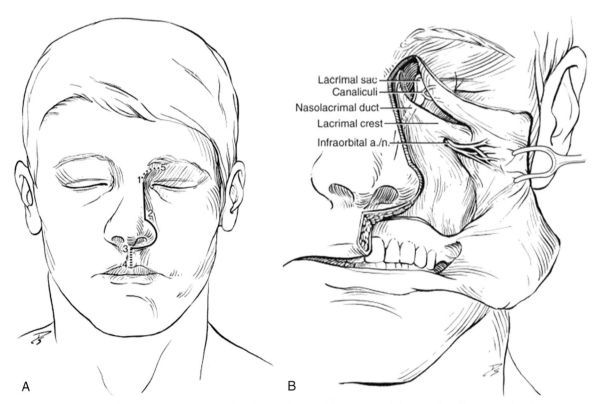

Fig. 5.25 Lateral rhinotomy. (**A**) Lateral rhinotomy incision. The basic lateral rhinotomy incision is outlined by connecting three surface points. The first (1) is marked halfway between the nasion and medial canthus. The second (2) is where the alar crease begins and the third (3) is at the base of the columella. (**B**) Soft-tissue dissection, exposing critical structures, including the lacrimal sac, nasolacrimal duct, and infraorbital nerve. (From Cohen JI, Clayman GL. *Atlas of Head & Neck Surgery.* 1st ed. Philadelphia, PA: Saunders; 2011, Fig. 42.1.)

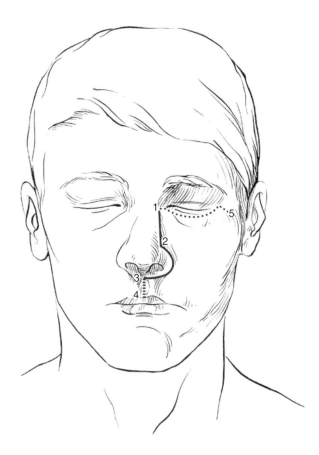

Fig. 5.26 Weber-Ferguson incision. The lateral rhinotomy incision is extended laterally along the infraorbital crease. (From Cohen JI, Clayman GL. *Atlas of Head & Neck Surgery*. 1st ed. Philadelphia, PA: Saunders; 2011, Fig. 42.2.)

- Easier to survey for recurrence
- Requires prosthodontics team with specialized expertise
- Radiation and healing cause contraction that requires numerous obturator adjustments
- Microvascular free flap reconstruction
  - May better restore facial contour and profile
  - May better support orbital floor
  - Can accept dental implants
  - May better withstand effects of postoperative radiation
  - May have better mastication and speech intelligibility and less oronasal reflux

Nonsurgical Management

- Very advanced or nonresectable cases
- Unlikely to improve survival but may slow tumor growth into critical structures
- Options
  - Induction chemotherapy followed by surgery if there is a response
  - Surgical debulking followed by topical 5-FU
  - Proton beam or carbon ion radiation

SALIVARY NEOPLASMS
Distribution of Salivary Neoplasms

- Parotid: 70% (75% benign, 25% malignant)
- Submandibular: 22% (57% benign, 43% malignant)
- Minor salivary: 8% (18% benign, 85% malignant)

Parapharyngeal Space Anatomy

- Prestyloid compartment: Deep lobe parotid tumors and minor salivary gland tumors
- Poststyloid compartment: Neurogenic and glomus tumors
  - Neurogenic tumors: Enhance with gadolinium
  - Glomus tumors: Serpiginous flow voids (salt-pepper)

Differential Diagnosis of Parotid Swelling/Masses

- Viral parotitis
- Bacterial parotitis: Often in elderly, malnourished, dehydrated, or immunocompromised patients
- Sialolithiasis
- Sjögren syndrome
- Inflammatory/reactive lymph node
- Benign neoplasm
  - Pleomorphic adenoma (45%)
  - Warthin tumor (papillary cystadenoma lymphomatosum; 6%)
  - Benign cyst (1%)
- Malignant neoplasm
  - Mucoepidermoid carcinoma (16%)
  - Adenoid cystic carcinoma (10%)
  - Adenocarcinoma (8%)
  - Malignant mixed tumor (6%)
  - Acinic cell carcinoma (3%)
  - Squamous cell carcinoma (4; not salivary in origin, most often metastasis from a cutaneous primary)

Presentation

- Concerning for malignancy
  - Pain
  - Facial nerve paresis or paralysis
  - Tongue weakness or numbness (submandibular malignancies)
  - Fixation of mass to overlying skin or underlying structures
  - Cervical lymphadenopathy
- Suggestive of parotid deep lobe/parapharyngeal space involvement
  - Decreased gag reflex (CN IX and CN X)
  - Aspiration (CN IX and CN X)
  - Asymmetric palate elevation (CN X)
  - Hoarseness (CN X)
  - Dysphagia (CN X)
  - Shoulder weakness (CN XI)
  - Tongue atrophy/paresis (CN XII)
  - Ptosis (sympathetic chain)

Workup
Fine-Needle Aspiration

- High sensitivity, specificity
- Higher diagnostic accuracy for benign salivary tumors
- Helps avoid unnecessary surgical resection for lymphomas and inflammatory masses
- Cytology difficulties with salivary neoplasms
  - Multiple cell types in pleomorphic adenoma
  - Benign versus malignant lesions with similar cytological appearance
    - Basal cell adenoma versus adenoid cystic carcinoma
    - Salivary duct obstruction versus mucoepidermoid carcinoma
    - Oncocytic lesion versus acinic cell carcinoma

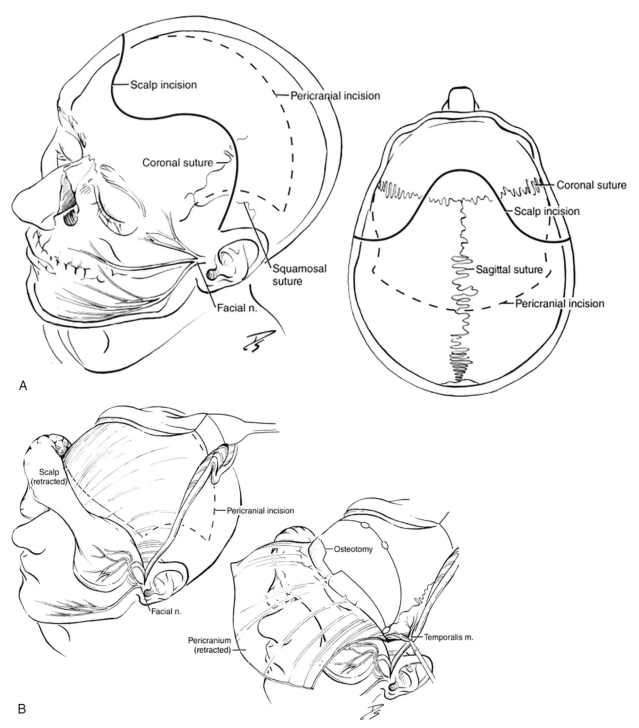

Fig. 5.27 Bifrontal Approach. (A) The incision begins in a preauricular crease anterior to the tragus, and then is elevated in a subgaleal plane superficial to the pericranium between the superior temporal lines. An incision is made through the temporalis fascia (superficial and deep layers) 1.5 cm posterior to the superior orbital rim, extending parallel to the zygomatic arch. Dissection proceeds deep to the deep layer of the temporalis fascia to preserve the frontal branch of the facial nerve, which is superficial to the fascia. **(B)** The scalp flap is elevated anteriorly to expose the superior orbital rims and supraorbital nerves. (From Cohen JI, Clayman GL. *Atlas of Head & Neck Surgery*. 1st ed. Philadelphia, PA: Saunders; 2011, Fig. 44.3.)

Imaging

- Routine use for small masses not warranted (does not change the treatment plan)
- Useful for lesions that may be malignant
  - Provides accurate delineation of location and extent of tumor
  - Provides relationship to major neurovascular structures
  - Provides information on perineural spread, skull base invasion, and intracranial extension
- MRI characteristics of salivary tumors
  - Bilateral masses with nonenhancing hyperintense T2: Most likely Warthin tumor

- Unilateral mass with enhancing hyperintense T2 signal: Most likely pleomorphic adenoma
- Mass with intermediate to low T2 signal: More likely to be malignant

Warthin Tumor (Papillary Cystadenoma Lymphomatosum)

- Benign, smoking associated
- 10% to 15% are multicentric, bilateral
- Histology: Oncocytic (eosinophilic), prominent lymphoid tissue (with germinal centers) (Fig. 5.28)

Pleomorphic Adenoma

- Most common salivary neoplasm
- Histology: Mixture of epithelial and myoepithelial cells with chondromyxoid stroma
- Recommended to resect with cuff of normal tissue to capture satellite nodules/pseudopodia (these structures increase risk of recurrence)
- Risk of malignant transformation 1.5% within the first 5 years, increases to 10% if observed for >15 years

American Joint Committee on Cancer Major Salivary Gland TNM Staging (Table 5.11)

Mucoepidermoid Carcinoma

- Most common salivary malignancy (adult and pediatric)
- Cytological diagnostic similarities: Necrotizing sialometaplasia (hard palate) and adenosquamous carcinoma
- Grading: Low, intermediate, and high grades correlate with clinical aggressiveness and adjuvant treatment

Adenoid Cystic Carcinoma (Fig. 5.29)

- Second most common salivary malignancy in the parotid gland
- Patterns: Tubular, cribriform, and solid
- Frequent perineural invasion
- Slowly progressive, infiltrative growth with distant metastases developing over years

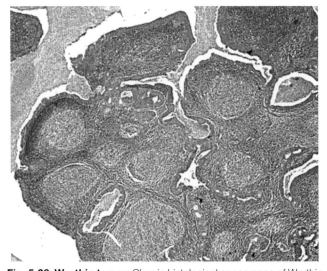

Fig. 5.28 Warthin tumor. Classic histological appearance of Warthin tumor with lymphoid germinal centers and surrounding eosinophilic oncocytic cells. (From Goldblum JR, Lamps LW, McKenney JK, et al. *Rosai and Ackerman's Surgical Pathology.* 11th ed. Philadelphia, PA: Elsevier; 2018, Fig. 6.18.)

TABLE 5.11 American Joint Committee on Cancer Major Salivary Gland TNM Staging

Primary Tumor (T)	
TX	Primary tumor cannot be assessed
T0	No evidence of primary tumor
Tis	Carcinoma in situ
T1	Tumor is ≤2 cm in greatest dimension without extraparenchymal extension [a]
T2	Tumor is >2 cm but not >4 cm in greatest dimension without extraparenchymal extension [a]
T3	Tumor is >4 cm in greatest dimension and/or having extraparenchymal extension [a]
T4a	Moderately advanced disease Tumor invades skin, mandible, ear canal, and/or facial nerve
T4b	Very advanced disease Tumor invades skull base and/or pterygoid plates and/or encases carotid artery
REGIONAL LYMPH NODES	
CLINICAL (C)	
NX	Regional lymph nodes cannot be assessed
N0	No regional lymph node metastasis
N1	Metastasis in a single ipsilateral lymph node ≤3 cm in greatest dimension and ENE(−)
N2a	Metastasis in a single ipsilateral node >3 cm, not >6 cm in greatest dimension and ENE(−)
N2b	Metastases in multiple ipsilateral lymph nodes, none >6 cm in greatest dimension and ENE(−)
N2c	Metastases in bilateral or contralateral lymph nodes, none >6 cm in greatest dimension and ENE(−)
N3a	Metastasis in a lymph node >6 cm in greatest dimension and ENE(−)
N3b	Metastasis in any node(s) with clinically overt ENE(+)
REGIONAL LYMPH NODES	
PATHOLOGIC (P)	
NX	Regional lymph nodes cannot be assessed
N0	No regional lymph node metastasis
N1	Metastasis in a single ipsilateral lymph node ≤3 cm in greatest dimension and ENE(−)
N2a	Metastasis in a single ipsilateral or contralateral lymph node ≤3 cm and ENE(+); or A single ipsilateral node >3 cm but not >6 cm in greatest dimension and ENE(−)
N2b	Metastases in multiple ipsilateral lymph nodes, none >6 cm in greatest dimension and ENE(−)
N2c	Metastases in bilateral or contralateral lymph nodes, none >6 cm in greatest dimension and ENE(−)
N3a	Metastasis in a lymph node >6 cm in greatest dimension and ENE(−)
N3b	Metastasis in a single ipsilateral node >3 cm in greatest dimension and ENE(+); or Multiple ipsilateral, contralateral, or bilateral nodes and ENE(+) in any node; or Single contralateral node of any size and ENE(+)
DISTANT METASTASIS (M)	
MX	Distant metastasis cannot be assessed
M0	No distant metastasis (no pathologic M₀; use clinical M to complete stage group for surgically resected patient staging)
M1	Distant metastasis

[a] *Extraparenchymal extension* is clinical or macroscopic evidence of invasion of soft tissues. Microscopic evidence alone does not constitute extraparenchymal extension for classification purposes.

From Flint PW, Haughey BH, Lund VJ, et al. *Cummings Otolaryngology—Head and Neck Surgery.* 7th ed. Philadelphia, PA: Saunders; 2021, Table 85.3.

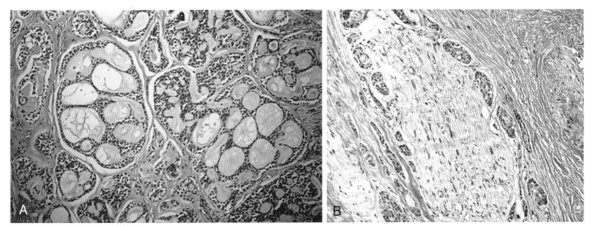

Fig. 5.29 Adenoid cystic carcinoma. (A) Classic histological appearance of adenoid cystic carcinoma. **(B)** Adenoid cystic carcinoma with perineural invasion. (From Goldblum JR, Lamps LW, McKenney JK, et al. *Rosai and Ackerman's Surgical Pathology*. 11th ed. Philadelphia, PA: Elsevier; 2018, Figs. 6.34 and 6.37.)

Polymorphous Low-Grade Adenocarcinoma

- Primarily arises mainly from minor salivary glands
- Most common location: Hard/soft palate junction
- Second most common minor salivary gland carcinoma
- Low-grade malignancy with excellent prognosis

Acinic Cell Carcinoma

- Arises mainly in the parotid gland (90% of cases)
- Second most common childhood salivary gland malignancy
- Low-grade malignancy
- 10% to 15% will develop regional or distant metastases

Malignant Mixed Tumors

- True malignant mixed tumor (carcinosarcoma)
- Carcinoma ex pleomorphic adenoma
  - Any pleomorphic adenoma with carcinoma of any kind
  - Carcinoma form most commonly poorly differentiated adenocarcinoma not otherwise specified (NOS), salivary duct carcinoma, or undifferentiated carcinoma
  - Prognosis is dependent on type of carcinoma
- Metastasizing pleomorphic adenoma

Salivary Duct Carcinoma

- Very aggressive
- Presents as rapidly growing parotid mass
- Significant minority present with facial nerve paresis
- All are high grade by definition
- 30% to 40% develop local recurrence
- 50% to 75% develop distant metastases
- Minority are positive for ERBB2 (Her2/neu) receptors

SURGERY

Parotidectomy

Landmarks to Identify the Facial Nerve During Parotidectomy

- Tragal pointer (1 cm medial and anteroinferior)
- Tympanomastoid suture line (6–8 mm medial)
- Retrograde dissection (marginal mandibular branch at the mandible superficial to facial vessels; buccal branch deep to the parotidomasseteric fascia, parallel to the parotid duct)

- Posterior belly of the digastric muscle (superior)
- Mastoid (vertical segment within mastoid bone)

Facial Nerve Management

- If the facial nerve is fully intact before surgery, attempts should be made to preserve it via an R1 resection
- If the facial nerve is paretic or paralyzed before surgery, it should be resected to negative margins
- Reconstruction options
  - Primary neurorrhaphy
    - Nerve mobilization via mastoidectomy
  - Cable/interposition graft
    - Greater auricular nerve
    - Hypoglossal descendans/ansa cervicalis
    - Sural nerve

Surgical Approaches to Parapharyngeal Space

- Transoral
- Transcervical ± mandibulotomy
- Transcervical-transparotid combined
- Transcervical-transmastoid combined
- Infratemporal fossa

Complications of Parotidectomy

- Seroma
- Hematoma
- Facial nerve paresis or paralysis
  - Immediate postoperative facial nerve dysfunction: 46%
  - Permanent facial nerve paralysis: 1% to 4%
  - Higher risk of paralysis in revision cases or for extended parotidectomy
- Sensory abnormalities (greater auricular nerve)
- Gustatory sweating (Frey syndrome)
  - Aberrant cross-innervation between postganglionic secretomotor parasympathetic fibers (parotid) to postganglionic sympathetic fibers (sweat glands of the skin)
  - Estimated incidence 35% to 60%
  - Diagnosis: Minor starch/iodine test
  - Treatment: Topical antiperspirant, glycopyrrolate lotion, tympanic neurectomy, botulinum toxin injections
- First-bite syndrome
  - Most common after deep lobe parotidectomy/parapharyngeal space exploration

- Symptoms: Severe cramping/spasm in the parotid with the first bite of a meal
- Etiology: Loss of sympathetic innervation causes denervation hypersensitivity activated by parasympathetic hyperactivation, which stimulates exaggerated parotid myoepithelial cell contraction
  - Treatment: Analgesics, acupuncture, botulinum injections
- Salivary fistula: Treatment includes aspiration, pressure dressings, botulinum toxin injections

Prognostic Variables

- Primary tumor site (submandibular and minor salivary glands more aggressive)
- Primary tumor size (T classification)
- Age (>50 years worse outcomes)
- Presenting symptoms (facial nerve paralysis, pain)
- Histological type/grade (high-grade)
- Perineural and bone invasion
- Histological stains: Her2 (ERBB2) and Ki-6: 7 overexpression, low p27 expression

Radiation

Indications for Adjuvant Radiation

- Advanced stage
- Positive resection margins
- High-grade histological types
- Local tissue invasion, perineural, or bone invasion

Neutron Beam Radiation

- Delivers more energy than conventional photon/electron radiation
- Historically considered for salivary tumors, which are thought to be radioresistant
- RTOG-MRG study on unresectable salivary cancers
  - Only prospective randomized trial of radiation for salivary tumors
  - Compared fast neutron therapy with conventional photon RT (not IMRT)
  - Neutrons demonstrated significantly improved locoregional control but not overall survival
- Benefits of neutrons compared with modern IMRT techniques are controversial
  - Neutrons may have higher toxicity
  - Neutrons are less widely available

Cutaenous Nonmelanoma Malignancies

Basal cell carcinoma (BCC)

- 80% of nonmelanoma skin cancer
- Arises from basal layer of epidermis
- 80% of BCCs occur on the head and neck, 25% on the nose
- Primary risk factor: Ultraviolet (UV) exposure
- Histology: Nests of uniform, basaloid cells with oval nuclei, small amounts of cytoplasm (Fig. 5.30; nodular BCC)
- Most common subtypes
  - Nodular: Most common; pearly dome-shaped nodule with central ulceration (Fig. 5.31)
  - Superficial: Multifocal, red-brown patches, common on trunk (Fig. 5.32)
  - Sclerosing/morpheaform: Atrophic, telangiectatic plaque; typically arises around ears/nose; more aggressive, with high recurrence rate; desmoplastic reaction in tissue makes tumor margins difficult to discern (Fig. 5.33)

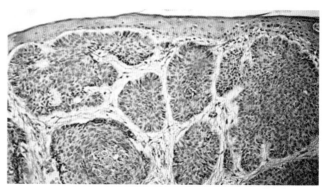

Fig. 5.30 Nodular basal cell carcinoma. Classic histological appearance of nodular basal cell carcinoma with basaloid cells organized in nests with peripheral palisading. (From Dinulos JG. *Habif's Clinical Dermatology.* 7th ed. Philadelphia, PA: Elsevier; 2021, Fig. 21.1.)

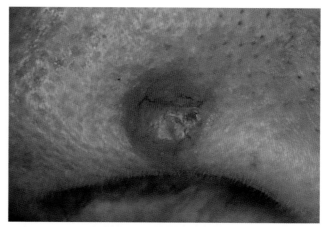

Fig. 5.31 Nodular basal cell carcinoma. (From Dinulos JG. *Habif's Clinical Dermatology.* 7th ed. Philadelphia, PA: Elsevier; 2021, Fig. 21.7.)

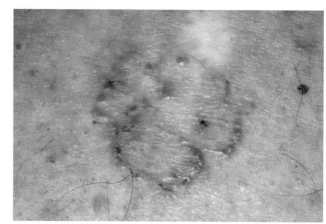

Fig. 5.32 Superficial basal cell carcinoma. The border of this flat lesion is slightly elevated and nodular, a characteristic of superficial basal cell carcinoma. (From Dinulos JG. *Habif's Clinical Dermatology.* 7th ed. Philadelphia, PA: Elsevier; 2021, Fig. 21.15.)

- Treatment
  - Surgery offers best chance of cure, but not always feasible depending on size/location of tumor (surgery can be standard excision with postoperative margin assessment or Mohs micrographic surgery)

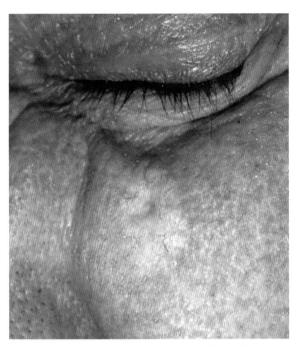

Fig. 5.33 Sclerosing/morpheaform basal cell carcinoma.
Sclerosing basal cell carcinoma. These hard, yellow masses may have
ill-defined borders. (From Dinulos JG. *Habif's Clinical Dermatology*. 7th
ed. Philadelphia, PA: Elsevier; 2021, Fig. 21.12.)

- Radiation considered for nonsurgical candidates
- Topical treatments (imiquimod, 5 fluorouracil), photodynamic and laser therapy, cryotherapy can be considered
for low-risk, superficial BCC when surgery/radiation not
feasible
- BCC rarely metastasizes (<0.55%); thus, neck dissection
indicated only for clinically node-positive cases
- Vismodegib: Hedgehog pathway targeted inhibitor
approved for metastatic and locally advanced BCC

Cutaneous Squamous Cell Carcinoma (cSCC)

- 10% to 20% of nonmelanoma skin cancer
- Also associated with UV exposure
- American Joint Committee on Cancer high-risk features:
tumor ≥4 cm, perineural invasion, invasion of tumor beyond
subcutaneous fat or >6 mm, bone invasion
- Immunosuppressed patients are at high risk for development
of cutaneous SCCs and recurrences after treatment
- Treatment
  - Similar to BCC, surgery offers best chance of cure, but
  not always feasible depending on size/location of tumor
  (surgery can be standard excision with postoperative margin assessment or Mohs micrographic surgery)
  - cSCC more likely to metastasize than BCC; should evaluate for regional metastasis
  - Metastasis to parotid nodes common; consider parotidectomy if node-positive in basin through which the parotid
  drains
  - Selective neck dissection in advanced disease cases
  - No established consensus on criteria to perform sentinel
  lymph node biopsy for cSCC
  - Systemic chemotherapy ± radiation for nonsurgical candidates or as adjuvant therapy
  - Cemiplimab: Monoclonal antibody against PD-1
  approved for metastatic and locally advanced cSCC

Genetic Syndromes Associated With Cutaneous Malignancies

- Xeroderma pigmentosum
  - Autosomal-recessive inheritance
  - Defect in DNA repair mechanism causes extreme skin
  and eye sensitivity to UV light
  - Dry skin, irregular freckling, burns within minutes of sun
  exposure
  - Increased risk of BCC, cSCC, and melanoma
- Gorlin (basal cell nevus) syndrome
  - Autosomal-dominant inheritance
  - Multiple BCCs beginning at early age
  - Other associations: Mandibular odontogenic keratocysts,
  palmar/plantar pits, calcified falx cerebri, bifid/splayed/
  fused ribs, macrocephaly/frontal bossing

Merkel Cell Carcinoma

- Rare neuroendocrine tumor
- Most commonly occurs on the face (27%)
- Rapidly growing, nontender, firm, flesh-colored or blue-red
nodule
- Risk factors: UV exposure, Merkel cell polyomavirus,
immunosuppression
- Treatment: Surgery plus sentinel lymph node biopsy in all
clinically negative necks or neck dissection in positive necks;
adjuvant radiation frequently recommended

CUTANEOUS MELANOMA

Risk Factors

- Physical characteristics: Fair complexion, inability to tan,
freckling, blue/green eyes, blond/red hair
- Ultraviolet radiation: History of blistering/peeling sunburns, teenage outdoor activity, tanning bed use
- Medical history: Immunosuppression, actinic keratosis,
atypical (dysplastic) nevus, giant congenital melanocytic
nevus, nonmelanoma skin cancer, xeroderma pigmentosa
  - Genetic factors: family history of melanoma, CDKN2A
  (p16) mutation

Melanoma subtypes

- Superficial spreading (Fig. 5.34)
  - Most common type in fair-skinned individuals
  - ~70% of melanomas
  - 50% arise from preexisting nevi
  - Begin with slow, radial growth phase, then transition to
  rapid, vertical growth phase
  - May partially regress due to immune response to tumor
- Nodular (Fig. 5.35)
  - Second most common type in fair-skinned individuals
  - ~15% to 30% of melanomas
  - More common in men
  - Blue-black or pink-red nodule ± ulceration
  - Higher stage at diagnosis, poorer prognosis
- Lentigo maligna (Fig. 5.36)
  - ~10% of melanomas
  - Develops in chronically sun-damaged skin, most commonly
  on face
  - Slow-growing pigmented macule
  - 5% progress to invasive melanoma
- Acral lentiginous (Fig. 5.37)
  - ~5% of melanomas
  - Incidence similar across all racial/ethnic groups, but makes
  up higher proportion of melanoma in blacks and Asians
  (due to lower rates of sun exposure–related melanoma)

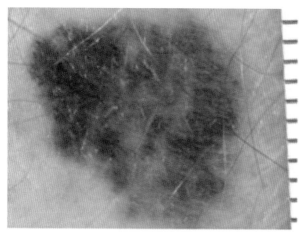

Fig. 5.34 Superficial spreading melanoma. Superficial spreading melanoma demonstrating asymmetry due to variation in color and irregularly in outline. (From Bolognia JL, Schaffer JV, Cerroni L, et al. *Dermatology.* 4th ed. Philadelphia, PA: Elsevier; 2018, Fig.113.9A.)

- Develops on palms/soles and in/under nail beds
- Higher stage at diagnosis (patient dismissal as concerning lesion, higher threshold to biopsy given location)
- Desmoplastic (Fig. 5.38)
  - <4% of melanomas
  - >50% occur in head/neck
  - Frequently hypopigmented
  - Locally aggressive/infiltrative, with up to 50% local recurrence due to neural infiltration
  - Higher stage at diagnosis
  - Pure desmoplastic subtype: Desmoplastic cells comprise >90% of lesion, 1% incidence of nodal metastasis, SLNB not recommended
  - Mixed desmoplastic subtype: 22% incidence of nodal metastasis, SLNB recommended
- Unknown primary
  - ~2% to 8% of melanomas
  - Usually presents with regional metastasis
  - Full-body skin and mucosal evaluations required

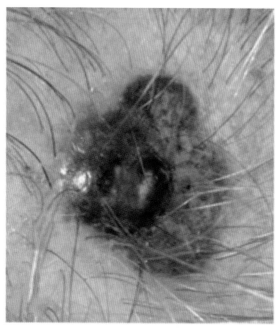

Fig. 5.35 Nodular melanoma. Darkly pigmented plaque on the scalp with eccentric nodule. (From Bolognia JL, Schaffer JV, Cerroni L, et al. *Dermatology.* 4th ed. Philadelphia, PA: Elsevier; 2018, Fig.113.13C.)

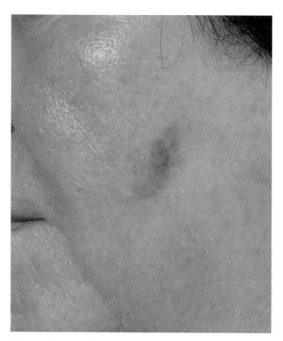

Fig. 5.36 Lentigo maligna. Early lentigo maligna presenting as a light brown patch with subtle asymmetric pigmentation. (From Bolognia JL, Schaffer JV, Cerroni L, et al. *Dermatology.* 4th ed. Philadelphia, PA: Elsevier; 2018, Fig.113.15A.)

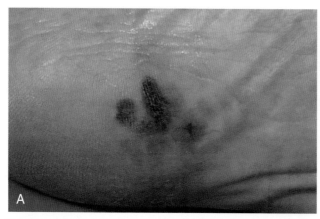
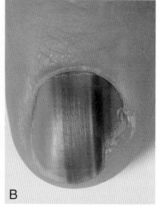

Fig. 5.37 Acral lentiginous melanoma. (A) Irregularly pigmented lesion on the plantar surface of the foot. **(B)** Melanoma of the nail matrix. (From Bolognia JL, Schaffer JV, Cerroni L, et al. *Dermatology.* 4th ed. Philadelphia, PA: Elsevier; 2018, Fig.113.16 and 113.17A.)

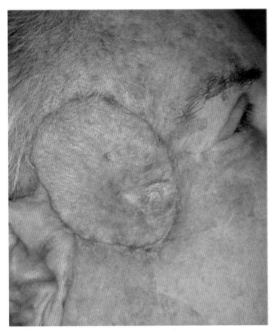

Fig. 5.38 Desmoplastic melanoma. Amelanotic nodular recurrence of a desmoplastic melanoma within a skin graft. (From Bolognia JL, Schaffer JV, Cerroni L, et al. *Dermatology.* 4th ed. Philadelphia, PA: Elsevier; 2018, Figs. 113.16 and 113.30C.)

Workup

Physical Exam

American Cancer Society ABCDE checklist for concerning signs suggestive of melanoma:
- A: Asymmetry in appearance
- B: Border irregularity
- C: Color variation
- D: Diameter >6mm
- E: Evolving changes

Differential Diagnosis

- Sebhorrheic keratosis
- Hemangioma
- Blue nevus
- Spitz nevus
- Pyogenic granuloma
- Pigmented basal cell carcinoma
- Cutaneous squamous cell carcinoma

Biopsy

Principles of Biopsy in Suspected Melanoma

- Complete excisional biopsy with narrow 1- to 3-mm margin recommended
  - Allows for evaluation of important prognostic factors (Breslow depth, ulceration, mitotic rate, angiolymphatic invasion, perineural invasion)
- If location not amenable to excisional biopsy, can perform a full-thickness punch biopsy or incisional biopsy through the thickest or darkest portion
- Shave biopsy, frozen-section biopsy, and FNA not recommended
  - Prevents evaluation of tumor thickness, which dictates treatment

- Broad shave biopsy can be used for melanoma in situ/lentigo maligna
- Excisional biopsy with wide margins (initial) not recommended (may compromise the ability to perform SLNB)
- If melanoma is diagnosed, the pathology report should include Breslow depth, ulceration status, dermal mitotic rate (#/mm²), microsatellitosis
  - Dermal mitotic rate no longer used for T1 staging in the *AJCC Cancer Staging Manual, 8th edition*, but is important for prognosis across all thicknesses
  - Microsatellitosis: Presence of tumor nests >0.05 mm in diameter in the reticular dermis, panniculus, or vessels beneath the principal invasive tumor, but separated from it by at least 0.3 mm of normal tissue on the section in which the Breslow measurement was taken
- In-transit metastasis: Metastatic tumor that is separate from the primary lesion by >2 cm and not in the lymph node basin

Histopathologic Markers for Melanoma

- S100: Most sensitive, least specific (also stains nerve sheath tumors)
- Melan-A (MART-1): More sensitive than HMB-45, more specific than S100
- HMB-45: More specific than S100

Metastatic/Genetic Workup

- Imaging recommended to evaluate specific signs/symptoms suggestive of metastasis, regardless of stage
- Stage 0, IA/B, II: No routine imaging, except may consider nodal basin ultrasound if planning SLNB; negative ultrasound is not a substitute for biopsy of clinically suspicious nodes
- Stage IIIA (positive SLNB). Baseline cross-sectional imaging for staging (CT of the neck with contrast or PET/CT)
- Stage IIIB/C/D, IV, local satellite/in-transit recurrence: Baseline cross-sectional imaging ± brain MRI with contrast for staging
- *BRAF* mutation testing when there are positive satellite/in-transit metastases or lymph nodes (clinical or pathological)

Cutaneous Melanoma Staging (Table 5.12)

Most Important Predictors of Survival

- Stages I and II (localized) disease
  - Tumor Breslow depth (most important prognostic indicator)
  - Tumor ulceration (second most important)
  - Mitotic rate for T1 lesions
- Stage III (regional) disease
  - Number of metastatic lymph nodes (most important)
  - Whether metastatic lymph nodes are clinically occult or detected (second most important)
  - Presence/absence of satellite, in-transit, microsatellite metastases
- Stage IV (distant) disease
  - Elevated lactate dehydrogenase (LDH)
    - Poor prognostic indicator regardless of site and number of metastases
    - Negative predictor of response to therapy

Treatment

- Surgery is first-line treatment when disease is resectable and surgical morbidity is reasonable
- Primary radiation almost never used

TABLE 5.12 American Joint Committee on Cancer Cutaneous Melanoma TNM Staging

Definition of Primary Tumor (T)

T Category	Thickness	Ulceration Status
TX: Primary tumor thickness cannot be assessed (e.g., diagnosis by curettage)	Not applicable	Not applicable
T0: No evidence of primary tumor (e.g., unknown primary or completely regressed melanoma)	Not applicable	Not applicable
Tis (melanoma in situ)	Not applicable	Not applicable
T1	≤1.0 mm	Unknown or unspecified
T1a	<0.8 mm	Without ulceration
T1b	<0.8 mm	With ulceration
	0.8–1.0 mm	With or without ulceration
T2	>1.0–2.0 mm	Unknown or unspecified
T2a	>1.0–2.0 mm	Without ulceration
T2b	>1.0–2.0 mm	With ulceration
T3	>2.0–4.0 mm	Unknown or unspecified
T3a	>2.0–4.0 mm	Without ulceration
T3b	>2.0–4.0 mm	With ulceration
T4	>4.0 mm	Unknown or unspecified
T4a	>4.0 mm	Without ulceration
T4b	>4.0 mm	With ulceration

Definition of Regional Lymph Node (N)

N Category	Number of Tumor-Involved Regional Lymph Nodes	Presence of in-Transit, Satellite, and/or Microsatellite Metastases
NX	Regional nodes not assessed (e.g., SLNB not performed, regional nodes previously removed for another reason)	No
	Exception: Pathologic N category is not required for T1 melanomas; use cN	
N0	No regional metastases detected	No
N1	One tumor-involved node or in-transit, satellite, and/or microsatellite metastases with no tumor-involved nodes	
N1a	One clinically occult (i.e., detected by SLNB)	No
N1b	One clinically detected	No
N1c	No regional lymph node disease	Yes
N2	Two or three tumor-involved nodes or in-transit, satellite, and/or microsatellite metastases with one tumor-involved node	
N2a	Two or three clinically occult (i.e., detected by SLNB)	No
N2b	Two or three, at least one of which was clinically detected	No
N2c	One clinically occult or clinically detected	Yes
N3	Four or more tumor-involved nodes or in-transit, satellite, and/or microsatellite metastases with two or more tumor-involved nodes, or any number of matted nodes without or with in-transit, satellite, and/or microsatellite metastases	
N3a	Four or more clinically occult (i.e., detected by SLNB)	No
N3b	Four or more, at least one of which was clinically detected, or presence of any number of matted nodes	No
N3c	Two or more clinically occult or clinically detected and/or presence of any number of matted nodes	Yes

Definition of Distant Metastasis (M)

M Category	Anatomic Site	LDH Level
M0	No evidence of distant metastasis	Not applicable
M1	Evidence of distant metastasis	See below

TABLE 5.12 American Joint Committee on Cancer Cutaneous Melanoma TNM Staging—cont'd

Definition of Distant Metastasis (M)

M Category	Anatomic Site	LDH Level
M1a	Distant metastasis to skin, soft tissue, including muscle, and/or nonregional lymph node	Not recorded or unspecified
M1a(0)		Not elevated
M1a(1)		Elevated
M1b	Distant metastasis to lung with or without M1a sites of disease	Not recorded or unspecified
M1b(0)		Not elevated
M1b(1)		Elevated
M1c	Distant metastasis to non-CNS visceral sites with or without M1a or M1b sites of disease	Not recorded or unspecified
M1c(0)		Not elevated
M1c(1)		Elevated
M1d	Distant metastasis to CNS with or without M1a, M1b, or M1c sites of disease	Not recorded or unspecified
M1d(0)		Normal
M1d(1)		Elevated

CNS, Central nervous system; LDH, lactate dehydrogenase; SLNB, sentinel lymph node biopsy.

Suffixes for M category: (0) LDH not elevated, (1) LDH elevated. No suffix is used if LDH is not recorded or is unspecified.

Clinical (c TNM)

When T Is...	And N Is...	And M Is...	Then the Clinical Stage Group Is...
Tis	N0	M0	0
T1a	N0	M0	IA
T1b	N0	M0	IB
T2a	N0	M0	IB
T2b	N0	M0	IIA
T3a	N0	M0	IIA
T3b	N0	M0	IIB
T4a	N0	M0	IIB
T4b	N0	M0	IIC
Any T, Tis	≥N1	M0	III
Any T	Any N	M1	IV

Pathologic (p TNM)

When T Is...	And N Is...	And M Is...	Then the Pathologic Stage Group Is...
Tis	N0	M0	0
T1a	N0	M0	IA
T1b	N0	M0	IA
T2a	N0	M0	IB
T2b	N0	M0	IIA
T3a	N0	M0	IIA
T3b	N0	M0	IIB
T4a	N0	M0	IIB
T4b	N0	M0	IIC
T0	N1b, N1c	M0	IIIB
T0	N2b, N2c, N3b or N3c	M0	IIIC
T1a/b–T2a	N1a or N2a	M0	IIIA
T1a/b–T2a	N1b/c or N2b	M0	IIIB
T2b/T3a	N1a–N2b	M0	IIIB
T1a–T3a	N2c or N3a/b/c	M0	IIIC
T3b/T4a	Any N ≥ N1	M0	IIIC
T4b	N1a–N2c	M0	IIIC
T4b	N3a/b/c	M0	IIID
Any T, Tis	Any N	M1	IV

From Flint PW, Haughey BH, Lund VJ, et al. *Cummings Otolaryngology—Head and Neck Surgery*. 7th ed. Philadelphia, PA: Saunders; 2021, Table 80.3.

SLNB, sentinel lymph node biopsy. Pathologic stage 0 (melanoma in situ) and T1 do not require pathologic evaluation of lymph nodes to complete pathologic staging; cN information should be used to assign their pathologic stage.

- Can be used for melanoma in situ/lentigo maligna if a poor surgical candidate for medical reasons or extent of resection would have significant surgical morbidity

Recommended Surgical Margins by Tumor Thickness (Table 5.13)

Sentinel Lymph Node Biopsy

- Nodal status is the most important prognostic factor for all melanoma patients
- 10% to 20% harbor occult microscopic nodal disease, with higher frequency correlating with higher Breslow depth
- Sentinel lymph node status is shown to represent accurately the status of the entire nodal basin
- Identifies the group that potentially warrants therapeutic neck dissection, thereby sparing the remaining 80% an unnecessary neck dissection
- Cases with known metastatic disease are not candidates for SLNB
- Cases with previous surgical disruption of lymphatics can be considered, but accuracy is decreased

National Comprehensive Cancer Network (NCCN) Indications for SLNB

- 5% to 10% probability of positive SLN for T1a–T1b disease
- >10% probability of positive SLN for T2b/clinical stage II disease
- Consider SLNB:
  - T1a with high mitotic index ($\geq 2/mm^2$) and/or lymphovascular invasion
  - T1b (Breslow depth <0.8 mm with ulceration or 0.8 to 1.0 mm without ulceration)
  - When microscopic satellitosis is present
- Offer SLNB: T2b or clinical stage II (>1 mm thick, any feature, N0)
- Non-mitogenic tumors and older patients have lower risk of positive SLN
- Acceptable to forego SLNB if patient is medically unfit or unlikely to act on information gained from SLNB

American Society of Clinical Oncology (ASCO) Clinical Practice Guidelines for SLNB

- Consider SLNB:
  - T1b (Breslow depth <0.8 mm with ulceration or 0.8 to 1.0 mm without ulceration)
  - T4 (>4.0 mm) after discussion of risks/benefits
    - Controversy: Higher risk of systemic disease; thus, SLNB may not be necessary
    - Can still be valuable for staging if no distant disease
    - Positive SLN: Consider adjuvant treatment
- Offer SLNB: T2 (1.01 to 2.0 mm) or T3 (2.01 to 4.0 mm)

TABLE 5.13 Recommended Surgical Margins for Excision of Primary Cutaneous Melanoma

Tumor Thickness (mm)	Surgical Margin (cm)
In situ	0.5–1.0 cm
≤1.0	1.0
1.01–2.0	1.0–2.0
>2.0	2.0

From Flint PW, Haughey BH, Lund VJ, et al. *Cummings Otolaryngology— Head and Neck Surgery.* 7th ed. Philadelphia, PA: Saunders; 2021, Table 80.4.

ASCO Clinical Practice Guidelines for Complete Lymph Node Dissection (CLND)

- Based on Multicenter Selective Lymphadenectomy Trial (MSLT) I/II and German Dermatologic Cooperative Oncology Group (DeCOG-SLT) Trial
- CLND versus observation acceptable for patients with low-risk micrometastatic disease
- CLND does not improve overall or disease-specific survival but does improve regional control/recurrence rates (NCCN Melanoma)
- For high-risk disease, careful observation only after thorough discussion of risk/benefit profile of CLND (high-risk defined as ENE(+), concomitant primary tumor microsatellitosis, >3 positive nodes, >2 involved nodal basins, immunosuppression)
- Therapeutic neck dissection should be performed for all clinically positive lymph nodes with adjuvant treatment if needed

Adjuvant Treatment

- Historical systemic agents
  - Interferon alpha-2b (IFN-α)
    - Immunomodulating cytokine that improves tumor immune response
    - Improvement in relapse-free survival (RFS), but not OS, poorly tolerated side effect profile
  - Interleukin-2 (IL-2)
    - Immunomodulating cytokine, drives activation-induced cell death and T-cell differentiation
    - Low but durable response rate, also has poorly tolerated side effect profile
- Non-targeted chemotherapy
  - Dacarbazine
    - DNA methylator, requires liver activation to active metabolite
    - Low response rate, short duration
    - Can be used alone or in combination with cisplatin and vinblastine
  - Temozolomide
    - Analog of dacarbazine (MTIC), does not require liver activation, alkylating agent
    - Not FDA approved
  - Platinum-based chemotherapy ± taxanes
- Targeted systemic agents
  - Ipilimumab
    - Monoclonal antibody against cytotoxic T-lymphocyte antigen 4 (CTLA-4)
    - Low but durable response
    - Moderate side effect profile
  - Nivolumab and pembrolizumab
    - Monoclonal antibodies against programmed cell death receptor 1 (PD-1)
    - Preferred adjuvant systemic treatment
    - Moderate, durable responses
    - Pembrolizumab toxicity similar to ipilimumab
  - Vemurafenib, dabrafenib/trametinib
    - *BRAF* V600E mutation inhibitors (trametinib is a MEK inhibitor)
    - Dabrafenib/trametinib combination superior to vemurafenib monotherapy with moderate, durable responses
- Adjuvant radiation
  - Primary site treatment not usually recommended except for high-risk desmoplastic melanomas (head and neck location, extensive neurotropism, pure desmoplastic subtype, close margins and unable to resect, locally recurrent)
  - Nodal basin treatment reduces regional recurrence in patient at high risk but does not improve RFS or OS (high

risk: ENE(+), ≥1 parotid or >2 cervical node involvement, ≥3 cm cervical node involvement)
  - Systemic agents and radiation may be used alone or in combination as adjuvant treatment

Treatment of Locally Advanced/Metastatic Disease

- Surgical excision to the extent possible
- Clinical satellite/in-transit metastases: Excision to the extent possible, intralesional T-VEC, adjuvant systemic agents
  - Talimogene laherparepvec (T-VEC): Genetically modified herpes oncolytic virus, stimulates tumor immune response
- Unresectable disease
  - Systemic therapy
  - Intralesional injections: T-VEC, BCG (Bacillus Calmette-Guerin), IL-2
  - Topical imiquimod for superficial dermal lesions
  - Palliative radiation

THYROID MALIGNANCIES

Epidemiology

- Increasing incidence is almost completely attributable to papillary thyroid cancer
- Increasing incidence is also due largely to improved/increased detection methods
- Palpable thyroid nodules in 4% to 7% of US population
- Subclinical thyroid nodules on ultrasonography in 19% to 67% of US population
- Only 5% of thyroid nodules are malignant
- Younger and older patients are more likely to have a malignant thyroid nodule
- Patients younger than age 20 years have 20% to 50% incidence of malignancy when presenting with a single thyroid nodule

Relevant Anatomy

Recurrent Laryngeal Nerve (RLN) (Fig. 5.39)

- Right RLN
  - Exits the vagus nerve at the base of the neck
  - Loops around the right subclavian artery (fourth arch)
  - Returns deep to the innominate artery and back to the thyroid bed diagonally
  - "Nonrecurrent" RLN may rarely occur on the right side and enter from more lateral course, associated with an aberrant retroesophageal subclavian artery (arteria lusoria)
- Left RLN
  - Exits the vagus nerve at the level of the aortic arch and ligamentum arteriosum (sixth arch), lateral to the obliterated ductus arteriosus
  - Returns to the thyroid bed along the tracheoesophageal groove via a more medial and vertical course than the right RLN
  - Crosses deep to the inferior thyroid artery 70% of the time
- Superior Laryngeal Nerve (Fig. 5.40)
  - Arises beneath the nodose ganglion of the upper vagus nerve
  - Divides into internal and external branches 2 cm above the superior pole
  - Internal branch: Travels medially, entering through the posterior thyrohyoid membrane to supply sensation to the supraglottis
  - External branch: Travels medially along, within, or deep to the inferior constrictor muscle to enter the cricothyroid muscle; travels with the superior thyroid artery, diverging 1 cm from the thyroid superior pole
- Parathyroid Glands
  - 80% of patients have four parathyroid glands, with at least 10% having greater than four glands

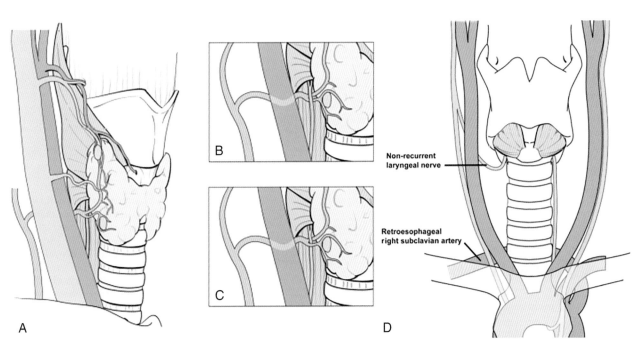

Fig. 5.39 Recurrent laryngeal nerve anatomy. Anatomical relationships of the recurrent laryngeal nerve to the inferior thyroid artery. (**A**) Posterior. (**B**) Anterior. (**C**) Between branches of the inferior thyroid artery. (**D**) Nonrecurrent right laryngeal nerve. (From Shah JP, Patel SG, Singh B. *Jatin Shah's Head and Neck Surgery and Oncology.* 5th ed. Philadelphia, PA: Mosby; 2020, Figs. 12.27 and 12.29.)

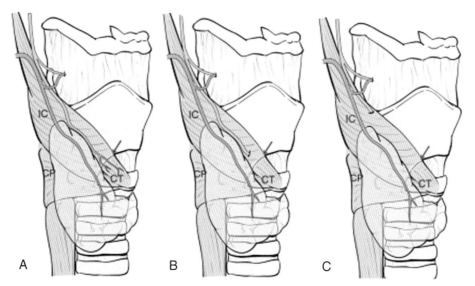

Fig. 5.40 Variant course of the external branch of the superior laryngeal nerve. (A) Type 1: The superior laryngeal nerve (SLN) runs superficial to the inferior constrictor muscle. **(B)** Type 2: The SLN dives into and runs deep to the inferior constrictor muscle. **(C)** Type 3: The SLN runs deep to the inferior constrictor muscle. (From Shah JP, Patel SG, Singh B. *Jatin Shah's Head and Neck Surgery and Oncology*. 5th ed. Philadelphia, PA: Mosby; 2020, Fig. 12.26.)

- Superior parathyroid glands: At the level of the cricoid cartilage, medial to the intersection of the RLN and inferior thyroid artery
- Inferior parathyroid glands: Lateral or posterior surface of lower thyroid pole
- Thyroid Vascular Supply
  - Inferior thyroid artery (branch of thyrocervical trunk)
  - Superior thyroid artery (branch of external carotid artery)
  - Superior, middle, and inferior thyroid veins (drain to internal jugular or innominate veins)

Risk Factors for Thyroid Cancer

- Older age
- Sex: Females 3× more likely to develop papillary thyroid carcinoma (PTC)
- Exposure to radiation: Only established environmental risk for thyroid cancer
  - Thyroid nodules with radiation history have 50% incidence of malignancy
  - Higher risk with exposure in childhood vs. adulthood
  - 1986 Chernobyl accident conferred a 60-fold increased risk in children
- Family history of thyroid cancer
  - ~6% of patients with PTC have familial disease
  - PTC
    - Increased frequency in certain families with breast, ovarian, renal, and central nervous system malignancies
    - Associated with Gardner and Cowden syndromes
  - MTC: Associated with familial MTC, MEN2A, and MEN2B syndromes

Differential Diagnosis of Thyroid Masses

- Cyst
- Goiter (diffuse, multinodular)
- Neoplasm
  - Follicular-derived neoplasms
    - Benign
      - Noninvasive follicular thyroid neoplasm with papillary-like nuclear features (NIFTP; previously considered malignancy that was called *encapsulated follicular variant of PTC*)

- Follicular adenoma
  - Hurthle cell neoplasm
- Malignant
  - Papillary thyroid carcinoma (PTC)
  - Follicular thyroid carcinoma (FTC)
  - Hurthle cell carcinoma
- Medullary thyroid carcinoma (MTC)
- Poorly differentiated thyroid carcinoma
- Anaplastic thyroid carcinoma
- Lymphoma
- Metastases to thyroid (most common: kidney, breast, lung, cutaneous SCC, and melanoma)

Thyroid Nodule Workup

- Flexible fiberoptic laryngoscopy for airway or dysphonia complaints
- Serum thyroid stimulating hormone (TSH)
  - If low (hyperthyroid), obtain thyroid radionuclide scan to evaluate for hyperfunctioning "hot" nodule
  - If normal to elevated, obtain thyroid ultrasound
- Imaging
  - Thyroid ultrasound
    - Provides key baseline information regarding nodule size and architecture
    - Noninvasive and inexpensive way to track changes in nodules
    - Obtain concurrent neck ultrasound to evaluate lateral compartments for adenopathy (operative management altered in 20% of patients)
  - Sonographic patterns and risk of malignancy
    - High suspicion (>70%–90%): Microcalcifications, hypoechoic solid nodule, irregular margins, taller than wide, extrathyroidal extension (ETE), suspicious-appearing lymph nodes (see below)
    - Intermediate suspicion (10%–20%): Hypoechoic solid nodule, regular margins
    - Low suspicion (5%–10%): Hyperechoic solid nodule, regular margins, partially cystic with eccentric solid portion
    - Very low suspicion (<3%): Spongiform, partially cystic without other suspicious features
    - Benign (<1%): Purely cystic

- Lymph nodes: Loss of fatty hilum, increased vascularity, round node configuration, microcalcifications
- CT and MRI
  - Usually unnecessary in evaluation of thyroid tumors
  - Not as effective as ultrasound in evaluation of thyroid nodules
  - Useful for characterizing substernal extension, cervical and mediastinal lymphadenopathy, and trachea invasion
  - Complements ultrasound by visualizing behind the sternum, trachea, and esophagus
  - Recommended for bulky lymph node disease to facilitate surgical planning
  - Iodinated contrast may preclude the use of postoperative radioactive iodine (RAI) for 2 to 3 months; however, this delay does not affect outcome
- PET
  - Not recommended for workup of thyroid nodules
  - Incidental FDG-avidity on PET scans obtained for other reasons
  - Diffuse uptake suggestive of Hashimoto's other diffuse thyroid conditions (2% of PETs)
  - Focal uptake in nodules carries ~35% risk of malignancy (1%–2% of PETs)
- FNA biopsy
  - High sensitivity and specificity
  - Decreases unnecessary surgery by 35% to 75%
  - 60% to 90% of FNA specimens are cytologically benign
  - 15% of FNA specimens are nondiagnostic/inadequate; repeat FNA recommended
  - Benign nodules require routine follow-up (5% false-negative rate)
  - Follicular neoplasms cannot be classified by FNA because of the need for architecture (must be able to visualize capsule and vessels to diagnose follicular carcinoma)
  - American Thyroid Association (ATA) Guidelines for Fine Needle Aspiration Biopsy of Thyroid Nodules (last updated in 2015; Table 5.14)
  - American College of Radiology (ACR) Thyroid Imaging Reporting and Data System (TI-RADS; new in 2017)
    - Scoring system based on thyroid nodule sonographic features used to recommend observation versus fine-needle aspiration biopsy
    - Reader selects one feature from composition, echogenicity, shape, margin categories, and all applicable features from echogenic foci category; total score based on features places nodule in TI-RADS categories from 1 to 5
    - System considers size in addition to sonographic features to recommend for/against FNA
    - ACR recommends biopsying no more than 2 nodules with highest scores
  - National Comprehensive Cancer Network Guidelines for Threshold for Thyroid Nodule FNA (2019)
  - Bethesda System for Reporting Thyroid Cytopathology (Table 5.15)

Staging and Risk Stratification Systems

- TNM Staging for Thyroid Cancer (Table 5.16)[96]
  - Excellent prognosis for younger PTC patients
  - PTC patients younger than 55 years old cannot be greater than stage II
- Age, Metastasis, Extent, Size (AMES) Risk Stratification System
  - Age (low risk includes men <41 years and women <51 years)
  - Metastases
  - Extent of tumor invasion
  - Size of tumor (low risk includes <5 cm)
- Metastasis, Age, Completeness, Invasion, and Size (MACIS) Score
  - Metastasis
  - Age at diagnosis
  - Completeness of surgical resection
  - Invasion (extrathyroidal)
  - Size of tumor
- American Thyroid Association (ATA) Risk Stratification for Recurrence (Box 5.2)

Papillary Thyroid Carcinoma

Histology (Fig. 5.41)

- Branching papillae with fibrovascular cores
- Enlarged nuclei with chromatin clearing ("Orphan Annie eye nuclei"), nuclear grooves
- Psamomma bodies
- Marker: Thyroglobulin

TABLE 5.14 American Thyroid Association Guidelines for Fine-Needle Aspiration Biopsy of Thyroid Nodules

Level of Suspicion	Ultrasound Features	Estimated Risk of Malignancy	Recommendation
High	Solid hypoechoic nodule or solid component of a mixed nodule with ≥1 of the following suspicious features: microcalcifications, taller and wide dimensions, irregular margin(s), extrathyroidal extension	>70%–90%	FNA if ≥1 cm
Intermediate	Solid hypoechoic nodule without above suspicious features	10%–20%	FNA if ≥1 cm
Low	Solid isoechoic or hyperechoic nodule or partially cystic nodule with eccentric solid area without above suspicious features	5%–10%	FNA if ≥1.5 cm
Very low	Spongiform or partially cystic nodules without above suspicious features	<3%	Consider FNA if ≥2 cm vs. observation
Benign	Purely cystic nodules	<1%	No FNA

FNA, Fine-needle aspiration.

TABLE 5.15 Bethesda System for Reporting Thyroid Cytopathology

FNA diagnosis	Risk of malignancy (NIFTP not considered cancer)[a]	Risk of malignancy (NIFTP considered cancer)[a]	Management
Nondiagnostic or unsatisfactory specimen	5%–10%	5%–10%	Repeat FNA under ultrasound guidance
Benign	0%–3%	0%–3%	Clinical and sonographic follow-up
Atypia of undetermined significance (AUS) or follicular lesion of undetermined significance (FLUS)	6%–18%	10%–30%	Repeat FNA vs. molecular testing[b] vs. thyroid lobectomy
Follicular neoplasm or suspicious for follicular neoplasm	10%–40%	25%–40%	Molecular testing[b] vs. thyroid lobectomy
Suspicious for malignancy	45%–60%	50%–75%	Near-total thyroidectomy vs. thyroid lobectomy
Malignant	94%–96%	97%–99%	Near-total thyroidectomy vs. thyroid lobectomy

FNA, Fine-needle aspiration; *NIFTP,* noninvasive follicular thyroid neoplasm with papillarylike nuclear features.

[a]2017 update of the Bethesda criteria includes risks of malignancy when NIFTP is (older system) and is not (newer system) considered a malignancy
[b]Molecular testing of thyroid nodules is a new addition to recommended management

Adapted with permission from Ali S, Cibas E 2018 The Bethesda System for Reporting Thyroid Cytopathology: Definitions, Criteria, and Explanatory Notes. Second edition. Springer, New York, NY.

TABLE 5.16 American Joint Committee on Cancer Thyroid TNM Staging

PRIMARY TUMOR (T)

TX	Primary tumor cannot be assessed
T0	No evidence of primary tumor
T1a	Tumor ≤1 cm in greatest dimension and limited to the thyroid
T1b	Tumor >1 cm but ≤2 cm in greatest dimension and limited to the thyroid
T2	Tumor >2 cm and ≤4 cm in greatest dimension and limited to the thyroid
T3a	Tumor >4 cm in greatest dimension and limited to the thyroid
T3b	Tumor of any size with gross extrathyroidal extension invading only strap muscles (sternohyoid, sternothyroid, thyrohyoid, omohyoid muscles)
T4a	Moderately advanced disease; tumor of any size that extends beyond the thyroid capsule to invade the subcutaneous soft tissues, larynx, trachea, esophagus, or recurrent laryngeal nerve
T4b	Very advanced disease; tumor invades prevertebral fascia or encases the carotid artery or mediastinal vessels
T4a (anaplastic)	Intrathyroidal anaplastic carcinoma,[a] surgically resectable
T4b (anaplastic)	Extrathyroidal anaplastic carcinoma,[a] surgically unresectable

REGIONAL LYMPH NODES (N)

NX	Regional lymph nodes cannot be assessed
N0	No regional lymph node metastasis
N1a	Metastasis to level VI (pretracheal, paratracheal, and prelaryngeal/Delphian) or VII (upper mediastinal) lymph nodes
N1b	Metastasis to unilateral, bilateral, or contralateral cervical (levels I through V) or retropharyngeal lymph nodes

DISTANT METASTASIS (M)

MX	Distant metastasis cannot be assessed
M0	No distant metastasis
M1	Distant metastasis
Overall	
Papillary/Follicular	

Stage	Age <55 Years	Age ≥55 Years
I	Any T, any N, M0	T1 or T2, N0 M0
II	Any T, any N, M1	T1 or T2, N1 M0 T3, any N, M0
III		T4a, any N, M0
IVA		T4b, any N, M0
IVB		Any T; any N, M1

MEDULLARY (ANY AGE)

I	T1 N0 M0
II	T2 N0 M0 T3 N0 M0

TABLE 5.16 American Joint Committee on Cancer Thyroid TNM Staging—cont'd

MEDULLARY (ANY AGE)	
III	T1 to T3, N1a M0
IVA	T4a, any N, M0
	T1 to T3, N1b M0
IVB	T4b, any N, M0
IVC	Any T, any N, M1
ANAPLASTIC (ANY AGE)	
IVA	T4a, any N, M0
IVB	T4b, any N, M0
IVC	Any T, any N, M1

[a]All anaplastic carcinomas are considered T4 tumors.

From the American Joint Committee on Cancer: AJCC cancer staging manual, ed 8, New York, 2018, Springer.

BOX 5.2 Risk Stratification for Thyroid Cancer Recurrence

Low Risk

Papillary thyroid cancer (all of the following must apply)
- No local or distant metastases
- All macroscopic tumor has been resected
- No tumor invasion of locoregional tissues or structures
- Tumor does not have aggressive histology (e.g., tall cell, insular, and columnar cell carcinoma) or vascular invasion
- If ^{131}I is given, no ^{131}I uptake occurs outside the thyroid bed on the first posttreatment whole-body radioactive isotope scan

Intermediate Risk (any of the following)
- Microscopic invasion of tumor into the perithyroid soft tissues at initial surgery
- Cervical lymph node metastases or ^{131}I uptake outside the thyroid bed on the whole-body radioactive isotope scan done after thyroid remnant ablation
- Tumor with aggressive histology or vascular invasion

High Risk (any of the following)
- Macroscopic tumor invasion
- Incomplete tumor resection
- Distant metastases
- Thyroglobulinemia out of proportion to what is seen on the post-treatment scan

From Flint PW, Haughey BH, Lund VJ, et al. *Cummings Otolaryngology—Head and Neck Surgery.* 6th ed. Philadelphia, PA: Saunders; 2015, Box 123.1.

Clinical Characteristics

- Genetic alterations: *BRAF, RET, Ras* mutations
- 75% of differentiated thyroid cancers
- Metastases occur via lymphatic spread
- Locations of recurrence: Thyroid bed (5%–6%), regional nodal basin (8%–9%), distant (4%–11%)
- Poor prognostic factors: Vascular invasion, aggressive histological subtypes (tall cell, columnar cell, hobnail variants), multifocal PTC with *BRAF V600E* mutation, ETE

Management

- Surgery generally recommended
  - ATA Guidelines
    - Thyroid lobectomy is acceptable for patients with tumors <1 to 4 cm without ETE and no clinical lymph node metastases

- Total or near-total thyroidectomy is recommended for tumors >4 cm, with gross ETE or clinically positive lymph nodes
- Total or near-total thyroidectomy is necessary if treatment plan includes postoperative radioactive iodine
  - NCCN Guidelines
    - Thyroid lobectomy acceptable if tumor ≤4 cm, patient has no prior radiation exposure, no ETE present, no cervical or distant metastases present
    - Should perform total thyroidectomy if any of these conditions are present
    - If lobectomy was performed, should perform completion thyroidectomy if any of the following are met: tumor ≥4 cm, positive margins, gross ETE, macroscopic (>1 cm) multifocal disease, macroscopic nodal metastasis, vascular invasion
- Neck management
  - Central neck dissection
    - Level VI boundaries: Carotid arteries laterally, hyoid superiorly, innominate artery inferiorly (Fig. 5.42)
    - Recommended for clinically positive central compartment nodes (known either preoperatively or discovered intraoperatively)
    - Consider ipsilateral versus bilateral central compartment dissection in cT3/T4N0
    - Compartmental dissection (not selective node plucking) is recommended
    - Higher incidence of inadvertent inferior parathyroidectomy and recurrent laryngeal nerve injury
  - Lateral neck dissection
    - Therapeutic lateral neck dissection should be performed for biopsy-proven lateral neck metastases
    - Elective lateral neck dissection not recommended
- *BRAF V600E* mutation frequently in aggressive subtypes (tall cell, columnar cell, hobnail variants, associated with higher risk of recurrence
- Recommendation for postoperative RAI depends on risk profile and risk of recurrence
- Postoperative thyroglobulin (Tg) level monitoring
- Routine neck ultrasound monitoring

Follicular Thyroid Carcinoma

Histology (Fig. 5.43)

- Resembles thyroid follicles with central colloid

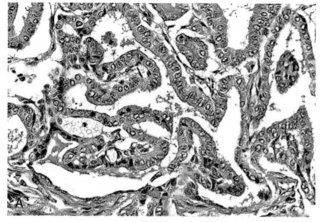
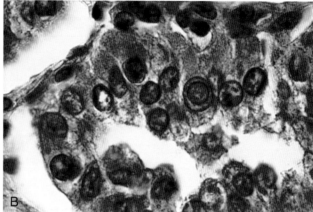

Fig. 5.41 Papillary thyroid carcinoma (PTC). Classic histological appearance of PTC. (**A**) Complex branching papillae in classic variant of PTC. (**B**) Nuclear pseudoinclusions ("Orphan Annie eye" nuclei). (From Goldblum JR, Lamps LW, McKenney JK, et al. *Rosai and Ackerman's Surgical Pathology.* 11th ed. Philadelphia, PA: Elsevier; 2018, Figs. 8.38 and 8.39B.)

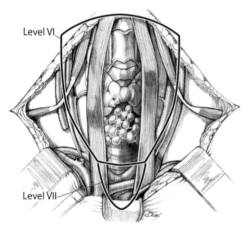

Fig. 5.42 Boundaries of the central compartment of the neck (level VI). The compartment extends from the hyoid bone to the suprasternal notch, as well as the carotid arteries laterally. (From Pai SI, Tufano RP. Central compartment lymph node dissection. *Oper Tech Otolaryngol.* 2009;20:39–43, Fig. 1.)

- Carcinoma diagnosed by vascular or capsular invasion (cannot be diagnosed by FNA or frozen specimens, requires diagnostic thyroidectomy) (Fig. 5.43)
- Considered minimally invasive if limited to capsule invasion

Clinical Characteristics

- 15% of differentiated thyroid cancers
- Genetic alterations: *Ras, PPAR-G* mutations
- Cervical lymphadenopathy less common than in PTC
- Metastases occur more commonly via hematogenous spread
- Distant metastases more common than in PTC
- Poor prognostic factors: Age >50 years, tumor >4 cm, >4 foci of vascular invasion, ETE, and distant metastasis
- Overall recurrence rate 30% (less for minimally invasive histology)
- In contrast to PTC, mortality is directly related to recurrence

Management

- Surgery
  - ATA: Indications same as with PTC (also a follicular-derived carcinoma)

- NCCN
  - Lobectomy appropriate in most cases
  - Total thyroidectomy recommended if invasive, metastatic, or based on patient preference
- Recommendation for postoperative RAI depends on risk profile and risk of recurrence

Hurthle Cell Carcinoma

Histology

- Oncocytic (eosinophilic) thyroid follicular cells with large nuclei
- Can have other features that resemble other differentiated thyroid cancers (follicular vs. papillary growth pattern, nuclear grooves, psammoma body-like calcifications)

Clinical Characteristics

- <10% of differentiated thyroid cancers
- Tend to be more aggressive than PTC or FTC with worse OS
- More likely than FTC to have cervical lymphadenopathy
- Highest incidence of distant metastasis among well-differentiated thyroid cancers

Management

- ATA: Indications same as with PTC (also a follicular-derived carcinoma)
- NCCN
  - Lobectomy appropriate in most cases
  - Total thyroidectomy recommended if invasive, metastatic, or based on patient preference
- Lower likelihood of ablation success with RAI (less likely to concentrate iodine)

Adjuvant Treatment for Follicular-Derived Thyroid Cancers

- Radioactive iodine
  - I-131 taken up by thyroid follicular cell sodium-iodide transporter

- Not useful in thyroid cancers that do not concentrate iodine (MTC, ATC, thyroid lymphoma)

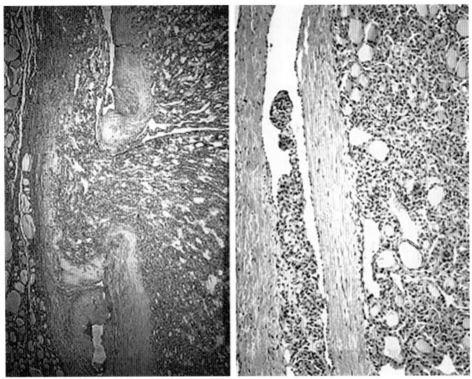

Fig. 5.43 Follicular thyroid carcinoma. Capsular (**A**) and vascular (**B**) invasion in minimally invasive FTC. (From Goldblum JR, Lamps LW, McKenney JK, et al. *Rosai and Ackerman's Surgical Pathology.* 11th ed. Philadelphia, PA: Elsevier; 2018, Fig. 8.60.)

- ATA Guidelines
  - Consider use for thyroid remnant ablation following total thyroidectomy in ATA intermediate-risk patients (Table 5.17)
  - Recommended postoperative use in ATA high-risk patients
  - Contraindications: Pregnancy and breastfeeding (risk of fetal/infantile cretinism)
- NCCN Guidelines
  - Recommendations based on presence of tumor/node features
- Improved OS following RAI in stages III and IV patients with differentiated thyroid cancer (National Thyroid Cancer Treatment Cooperative Study Group)
- Must increase TSH prior to RAI administration (uptake by thyroid tissue driven by TSH) via thyroid hormone withdrawal (3–4 weeks before RAI dose) or recombinant human TSH (injections on 2 consecutive days with RAI given on the third day)
- Iodinated contrast is typically cleared from circulation after 1 month, but RAI administration usually dosed 2 to 3 months after last contrast load
- Can be re-dosed if iodine-avid tissue is seen on follow-up uptake scans
- Complications: Sialadenitis, hypogonadism (transient), secondary malignancy
- Adjuvant systemic treatment
  - Used only if surgery not feasible
  - Lenvatinib (inhibitor of VEGF, FGF, PDGF, KIT, RET receptors)
  - Larotrectinib (NTRK fusion inhibitor; NTRK fusions more likely to be found in absence of *BRAF, Ras* mutations)

TABLE 5.17 American Thyroid Associated Risk Stratification System (2015)

Risk	Features
Low	• PTC with all of the following: No local or distant metastases, removal of all macroscopic tumor, no ETE, no aggressive histology (tall cell, columnar cell, hobnail variants), no vascular invasion, no RAI-avid foci outside the thyroid bed on first post-RAI uptake scan, clinically N0 or pathologically up to 5 micrometastases 2 mm or smaller • Intrathyroidal papillary microcarcinoma (≤1 cm) (unifocal, multifocal, *BRAF* mutated) • Intrathyroidal encapsulated follicular vartiant PTC • Intrathyroidal well-differentiated FTC with capsular invasion and <4 foci of vascular invasion
Intermediate	• Microscopic ETE • Aggressive histologic subtype • PTC with vascular invasion • Multifocal papillary microcarcinoma with ETE and *BRAF V600E* mutation • Clinically N1 or >5 lymph nodes involved (all <3 cm)
High	• Macroscopic ETE • Incomplete tumor resection • Distant metastases • Elevated postoperative thyroglobulin suggestive of distant metastases • Pathologic N1 with any metastatic node ≥3 cm • FTC with >4 foci of vascular invasion

ETE, Extrathyroidal extension; *FTC,* follicular thyroid carcinoma; *PTC,* papillary thyroid carcinoma; *RAI,* radioactive iodine.

Based on Cibas ES, Ali SZ. The 2017 Bethesda System for Reporting Thyroid Cytopathology. *Thyroid.* 2017 Nov;27(11):1341–1346. doi: 10.1089/thy.2017.0500. PMID: 29091573.

- Adjuvant external beam radiation indications
  - Consider for macroscopic residual disease that does not concentrate RAI

Medullary Thyroid Cancer (MTC)

Histology

- Neuroendocrine tumor derived from parafollicular C cells
- Markers: Calcitonin, chromogranin, carcinoembryonic antigen (CEA), amyloid

Clinical Characteristics

- <5% of all thyroid carcinomas
- Of patients with palpable MTC, 70% have cervical metastasis, 5% to 10% have distant metastasis
- 30% are familial
  - Autosomal dominant, nearly 100% penetrance
  - MEN2A syndrome: MTC, pheochromocytoma, hyperparathyroidism
  - MEN2B syndrome: MTC, pheochromocytoma, mucosal neuromas, Marfanoid body habitus
- Poor prognostic factors: Age >50 years, vascular invasion, regional/distant metastases, significantly elevated preoperative serum calcitonin level

Workup

- Serum calcitonin and CEA: Magnitude/ratio determines extent of disease
- RET oncogene mutation testing
- Determines familial versus sporadic, tumor aggressiveness (based on mutation type), and need for family screening
  - Negative RET testing precludes need to test for MEN (multiple endocrine neoplasm) syndrome (e.g., catecholamines, calcium, and abdominal MRI)
  - Negative RET testing suggests a greater likelihood that MTC is unifocal
  - Positive RET testing should prompt MEN syndrome workup
    - Serum calcium (assess for hyperparathyroidism)
    - 24-hour urine metanephrines/catecholamines (assess for pheochromocytoma)
    - Abdominal MRI (assess for pheochromocytoma)
    - Children of known patients with RET mutations should have early screening and thyroidectomy depending on mutation type (as early as in the first year of life)
- Imaging
  - Recommended thyroid and lateral neck ultrasounds if MTC diagnosis is known preoperatively
  - Low threshold to obtain axial imaging for patients with extensive neck disease or symptoms concerning for distant metastases

Management

- Surgery
  - Must address pheochromocytoma (if present) before thyroidectomy
  - Total thyroidectomy with central neck dissection recommended
  - Strongly consider lateral neck dissection if central neck nodes are involved
  - Consider elective ipsilateral lateral neck dissection when primary tumor is >1 cm

- Postoperative RAI is not effective (not a follicular-derived carcinoma)
- If MTC is diagnosed following thyroid lobectomy, completion thyroidectomy is not necessary unless the patient has a germline RET mutation, significantly elevated postoperative serum calcitonin level, or imaging suggestive of residual disease
- Adjuvant radiation
- Targeted systemic agents for recurrent metastatic disease
  - Vandetanib (inhibitor of VEGF-R, EGF-R, RET)
  - Cabozatinib (inhibitor of VEGF-R, RET)
  - Lenvatinib
- Surveillance
  - TSH suppression not necessary (not a follicular-derived carcinoma)
  - Serum calcitonin and CEA monitoring
  - Flushing and diarrhea may appear with significant disease
  - Salvage surgery preferred for recurrent or residual disease
  - External beam radiation is controversial
  - Targeted therapies are available for recurrent/metastatic disease (cabozantinib and vandetanib)

Anaplastic Thyroid Cancer Management

Histology

- May arise from prior differentiated thyroid carcinoma
- Loss of differentiation (TTF-1 and PAX-8 stains help identify thyroid origin), frequent necrosis, vascular invasion, and mitoses

Clinical Characteristics

- ~1% of thyroid cancers
- Very aggressive
- Median survival of 5 months; median 1-year OS of 20%
- Genetic alterations: *TP53*, *Ras*, *BRAF*, and *PIK3CA* mutations
- Presentation: Long-standing neck mass with subsequent rapid enlargement, pain, dysphonia, dysphagia, and dyspnea
- Most patients die of superior vena cava syndrome, asphyxiation, or exsanguination

Workup

- Core biopsy or operative biopsy is necessary given tissue heterogeneity and the possibility of lymphoma
- Airway management
- Nutritional support
- Advance care planning

Treatment

- Consider surgery if grossly negative margins (R1 resection) can be achieved
- Tumor debulking (R2 resection) does not improve locoregional control or survival
- Tracheostomy may treat acute airway distress but is not typically recommended because it may increase suffering and lead to a prolonged hospital stay
- Radiation may be used as adjuvant or palliative treatment
- Systemic treatment
  - Cytotoxic chemotherapy (doxorubicin/cisplatin combination)
  - Lenvatinib
  - Dabrefinb/trametinib (*BRAF* mutation and MEK inhibitor kinase) in ATC with *BRAF V600E* mutation

Adjuvant Treatment

- TSH suppression
  - Long-term levothyroxine administration to suppress TSH and, therefore, possible recurrence or progression of thyroid cancer
  - Goal TSH of <0.1 for intermediate- to high-risk patients
  - Goal TSH of 0.1 to 0.5 for low-risk patients
- RAI
  - For higher-risk PTC and FTC
  - Decreases risk of recurrence and disease-specific mortality
  - Indications
    - Any primary tumor >4 cm
    - ETE
    - Distant metastases
    - High-risk features (poorly differentiated subtypes, vascular invasion, and multifocal disease)
    - Not recommended for primary tumors <1 cm
- Dosage
  - Typically 100 mCi for residual thyroid bed uptake
  - Typically 100 to 200 mCi for regional or distant disease, or aggressive subtypes
  - No clear evidence on whether fixed amounts versus quantitative tumor dosimetry tailored to patient is superior
- External beam radiation, suggested indications
  - Anaplastic thyroid cancer
  - Patient older than 55 years with gross ETE and high likelihood of microscopic residual disease
  - Patient with gross residual tumor unlikely to respond to further surgery or RAI

PARATHYROID DISORDERS

Parathyroid Hormone

- Intact parathyroid hormone (PTH) (1–84) is the major circulating form of biologically active PTH
- Half-life of 3 to 5 minutes
- Cleared by liver and kidney
- Targets and functions of PTH
  - Kidney
    - Increase resorption of calcium
    - Decrease resorption of phosphorus
    - Convert 25-hydroxyvitamin (25-OH) D3 (calcifediol) to 1,25-dihydroxyvitamin (1,25-OH) D3 (calcitriol)
  - Skeletal system: Stimulate osteoclast activity via osteoblast modulation

- Intestine: Increase calcium absorption through vitamin D
- Calcitonin
  - Opposes the role of PTH by reducing serum calcium and inhibiting bone resorption
  - Much smaller role than PTH in calcium homeostasis
  - Secreted by parafollicular cells in thyroid gland

Parathyroid Glands

- Normal weight often 30 to 60 mg
- Fat content varies and hovers around 50% and increases with age
- 85% of patients have four glands, whereas 3% to 6% have three glands
- Approximately 1% of patients have a hyperfunctioning fifth parathyroid gland
- Supernumerary glands commonly are mediastinal (thymus and aortic arch)
- Rare incidence of intrathyroidal parathyroid glands (0.5% to 3%)
- Locations (Fig. 5.44)
  - Superior parathyroid glands
    - Cricothyroid junction approximately 1 cm cranial to the juxtaposition of the RLN and inferior thyroid artery
    - Paraesophageal location in 1% of cases
    - More consistent position compared with inferior parathyroid glands
    - Embryologically deep (dorsal) to the RLN
  - Inferior parathyroid glands
    - Inferior pole of the thyroid and along the thyrothymic ligament
    - Migratory pathway into the anterior-superior mediastinum
    - Up to 33% of missed parathyroid glands are found in the anterior-superior mediastinum
    - More variable position compared with superior parathyroid glands (longer migratory descent during development)
  - Ectopic parathyroid glands
  - Can be found in other locations, including mediastinum/thymus (most common), retroesophageal, in the carotid sheath, within the thyroid gland
- Arterial supply
  - Inferior thyroid artery supplies the large majority of both superior and inferior parathyroid glands (>80%)
  - However, abundant plexus of vessels may provide additional vascularization

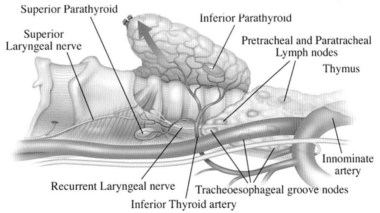

Fig. 5.44 Parathyroid location relative to adjacent thyroid neurovascular structures. The thyroid gland is mobilized medially. The inferior parathyroid must be distinguished from neighboring pretracheal and paratracheal lymph nodes as well as fat lobules and thyroid tissue. (From Friedman M, Kelley K, Maley A. Central neck dissection. *Oper Tech Otolaryngol.* 2011;22:169–172, Fig. 2.)

- Superior thyroid artery may provide dominant arterial supply for superior parathyroid glands in up to 10% to 20% of patients

Pathological Conditions

Hyperparathyroidism

Primary Hyperparathyroidism

- Can be caused by parathyroid adenoma, hyperplasia, lipoadenoma, carcinoma
- Lab findings
  - High calcium
  - Elevated PTH
  - Normal creatinine
  - Low or low-normal phosphate
  - Urinary calcium >125 mg/24 hours
  - Normal 25-OH vitamin D and 1,25-OH vitamin D
- Symptoms of hypercalcemia
  - Renal: Nephrolithiasis and urolithiasis; most stones are calcium oxalate
  - Skeletal system: Osteitis fibrosis cystica (bone pain, pathological fracture, and cystic bone change), osteoporosis; hyperparathyroidism-related bone loss occurs at cortical bone sites and spares trabecular bone
  - Neuromuscular system: Muscle weakness (40% incidence), fatigue, and aches; muscle weakness improves after parathyroidectomy in 80% to 90% of patients
  - Neurological: anxiety, psychosis, depression, deafness, dysphagia, and dysosmia; depression improves after parathyroidectomy in 50% of patients
  - Gastrointestinal: Peptic ulcer, pancreatitis, and cholelithiasis
  - Cardiovascular: Hypertension

Secondary Hyperparathyroidism

- Renal insufficiency or failure
- Insufficient calcium intake, decreased calcium absorption, and vitamin D deficiency
- Requires subtotal parathyroidectomy or total parathyroidectomy with autotransplantation (considered equivalent)

Tertiary Hyperparathyroidism

- Long-standing renal insufficiency/failure leads to autonomous parathyroid hyperfunction

Untreated Mild Hyperparathyroidism

- Most patients show no significant progression of symptoms
- Disease progression in 27% of patients, including marked hypercalcemia, hypercalciuria, and loss of bone mineral density
- Impossible to predict which patients will progress
  - 33% of patients who develop hypercalcemic crisis had initial symptoms of mild hypercalcemia
  - Younger patients appear more prone to progressive hypercalcemia
- Risk of occult symptoms and end-organ damage increases over time

Hyperparathyroidism With Normal Calcium Levels (Normocalcemic Hyperparathyroidism)

- May have physiological secondary hyperparathyroidism
- Before parathyroidectomy, must rule out:
  - Low calcium or vitamin D intake

- Calcium or vitamin D malabsorption
- Inability to convert 25-OH vitamin D to 1,25-OH vitamin D
- Hypercalciuria
- Lithium and thiazide diuretics may falsely elevate calcium and PTH (must be off for at least 1 month before reevaluation)

Multiple Gland Disease

- Double parathyroid adenoma
  - Between 1% and 2% incidence
  - Up to 10% incidence in patients older than 60 years
- Sporadic diffuse hyperplasia
  - Up to 10% to 15% incidence
  - 40% of equivocal sestamibi scans found to have diffuse multigland hyperplasia
  - 3.5-gland parathyroidectomy performed after all hypercellular glands are found
- Familial hyperparathyroidism
  - Familial types are more likely to have multiglandular disease and persistent hyperparathyroidism after surgery
  - MEN I: High and early penetrance with four gland hyperplasia
  - MEN IIA: Less frequent multigland involvement and lower incidence of persistent hyperparathyroidism after surgery compared with MEN I
  - Non-MEN familial hyperparathyroidism: more aggressive than MEN or sporadic subtypes

Medical Management of Hyperparathyroidism

- Adequate hydration
- Furosemide (loop diuretics)
- Bisphosphonates (alendronate): Decrease calcium gut absorption and 1,25-OH vitamin D
- Estrogen
- Calcitonin
- Calcimimetic (cinacalcet): Sensitizes PTH receptor to calcium

Hypercalcemia of Malignancy

- PTH-related protein secretion (lung, esophagus, head and neck, renal cell, ovary, bladder, and pancreatic)
- Ectopic PTH secretion by small cell lung cancer, small cell ovarian cancer, and squamous cell lung cancer
- Ectopic 1,25-OH D production by B-cell lymphoma and Hodgkin disease
- Lytic bone metastasis (multiple myeloma, lymphoma, breast cancer, and sarcoma)
- Tumor cytokines

Familial Hypercalcemic Hypocalciuria

- Autosomal-dominant disorder
- Inactivating mutations in the calcium-sensing receptor of the parathyroid gland
- Low 24-hour urine calcium relative to their hypercalcemia
  - 24-hour calcium-to-creatinine clearance ratio
  - Familial hypercalcemic hypocalciuria: Ratio <0.01
  - Hyperparathyroidism: Ratio >0.01

Parathyroid Carcinoma

- Presents with hypercalcemia (frequently >14 mg/dL) and high PTH (frequently 5× the upper limit of normal or higher)
- Indolent growth, frequent recurrence common
- Morbidity associated with uncontrolled PTH secretion

- May be difficult to distinguish from benign parathyroid adenoma
- Challenging histological diagnosis
- Only reliable indicators of carcinoma are invasion of surrounding structures and metastasis

Imaging Localization Studies for Hyperparathyroidism

- Ultrasound
  - Well tolerated, inexpensive
  - Poor localization of retroesophageal, retrotracheal, retrosternal, deep thoracic inlet glands
- Technetium 99 m sestamibi scintigraphy
  - Mitochondria-rich glands take up Tc-99 intensely and clear slowly compared with thyroid gland parenchyma
  - Reported 100% sensitivity and 90% specificity
  - Can identify double adenomas but is inaccurate for smaller adenoma size and four gland parathyroid hyperplasia
- Single-photon emission CT/CT (single-photon emission computed tomography [SPECT]/CT)
  - Provides greater anatomical localization
  - Helps aid in minimally invasive directed approach
  - Helps accurately locate ectopic glands (thymic, retroesophageal, mediastinal, and intrathyroid)
  - Helps in directed re-exploratory surgery
- Four-phase "4-D" CT scan
  - Precontrast, immediate, early delayed, and late-delayed phases
  - Allows visualization of early enhancement and early washout of parathyroid candidates relative to thyroid tissue and lymph nodes
- CT
  - Less effective than MRI
  - High false-positive rates
  - Subject to distortion from metal clips in reoperative cases
- MRI
  - Parathyroid adenomas have low T1-intensity and high T2-intensity
  - More effective for finding ectopic parathyroid candidates

Consensus Indications for Surgery for Asymptomatic Primary Hyperparathyroidism

- Serum calcium >1 mg/dL above the upper limit of normal
- Creatinine clearance reduced >60 mL/min
- Age <50 years old
- Bone mineral density (lumbar spine, femoral neck, hip, and distal radius) T-score ≤2.5
- Pathological bone fracture
- 24-hour urine calcium >400 mg/dL (optional)
- Nephrolithiasis or nephrocalcinosis
- Surgery requested by patient, or patient unsuitable for surveillance

Surgical Approach

- Approaches
  - Bilateral cervical exploration
  - Directed unilateral cervical exploration
  - Minimally invasive techniques
- Abnormal gland identified and sent for frozen section analysis
- Intraoperative serum PTH labs
  - Half-life of PTH is 3 to 5 minutes
  - Goal is >50% decrease in PTH and drop to normal PTH range
  - If PTH remains elevated, a bilateral four gland exploration is required

- Ectopic areas should be examined, including thymic tissue, carotid sheath, paraesophageal space, and hemithyroidectomy if necessary
- Experience of surgeon
  - Experienced surgeons (>10 parathyroidectomies per year): 90% success rate
  - Inexperienced surgeons: 70% success rate, with 15% remaining hypercalcemic and 14% becoming permanently hypocalcemic

Elevated PTH After Curative Parathyroidectomy (Normal Calcium and Intraoperative Parathyroid Hormone)

- Occurs in up to 20% of patients
- Possible explanations
  - Development of secondary hyperparathyroidism in response to rapidly changed calcium levels
  - Vitamin D deficiency
  - Changes in renal function
  - Peripheral resistance to PTH
- Surgical re-exploration
  - Additional single adenomas are frequently found in "standard" locations
  - Ectopic adenomas: Most commonly in the thymus, but should also inspect the tracheoesophageal groove, retropharyngeal/retroesophageal spaces, carotid sheath, thyroid gland
  - Risks: Higher risk of injury to RLN in revision surgery (6% vs. 1%), permanent hypocalcemia

FURTHER READINGS

Alkureishi LW, Ross GL, Shoaib T, et al. Sentinel node biopsy in head and neck squamous cell cancer: 5-year follow-up of a European multicenter trial. *Ann Surg Oncol.* 2010;17(9):2459–2464.

Aubry K, Vergez S, de Mones E, et al. Morbidity and mortality revue of the French group of transoral robotic surgery: a multicentric study. *J Robot Surg.* 2016;10(1):63–67.

Bernier J, Cooper JS, Pajak TF, et al. Defining risk levels in locally advanced head and neck cancers: a comparative analysis of concurrent postoperative radiation plus chemotherapy trials of the EORTC (#22931) and RTOG (# 9501). *Head Neck.* 2005;27(10):843–850.

Bernier J, Domenge C, Ozsahin M, et al. Postoperative irradiation with or without concomitant chemotherapy for locally advanced head and neck cancer. *N Engl J Med.* 2004;350(19):1945–1952.

Bilezikian JP, Khan AA, Potts JT Jr, et al. Guidelines for the management of asymptomatic primary hyperparathyroidism: summary statement from the Third International Workshop. *J Clin Endocrinol Metab.* 2009;94(2):335–339.

Blanchard P, Baujat B, Holostenco V, et al. Meta-analysis of chemotherapy in head and neck cancer (MACH-NC): a comprehensive analysis by tumour site. *Radiother Oncol.* 2011;100(1):33–40.

Bollig CA, Gilley DR, Ahmad J, et al. Prophylactic arterial ligation following transoral robotic surgery: A systematic review and meta-analysis. *Head Neck.* 2020;42(4):739–746.

Bolognia JL, SJ., Cerroni L. *Dermatology.* 4th ed. Philadelphia, PA: Elsevier; 2018.

Bonner JA, Harari PM, Giralt J, et al. Radiotherapy plus cetuximab for squamous-cell carcinoma of the head and neck. *N Engl J Med.* 2006;354(6):567–578.

Byers RM, El-Naggar AK, Lee YY, et al. Can we detect or predict the presence of occult nodal metastases in patients with squamous carcinoma of the oral tongue? *Head Neck.* 1998;20(2):138–144.

Carhill AA, Litofsky DR, Ross DS, et al. Long-Term Outcomes Following Therapy in Differentiated Thyroid Carcinoma: NTCTCS Registry Analysis 1987–2012. *J Clin Endocrinol Metab.* 2015;100(9):3270–3279.

Cheson BD, Fisher RI, Barrington SF, et al. Recommendations for initial evaluation, staging, and response assessment of Hodgkin and non-Hodgkin lymphoma: the Lugano classification. *J Clin Oncol.* 2014;32(27):3059–3068.

Cibas ES, Ali SZ. The 2017 Bethesda System for Reporting Thyroid Cytopathology. *Thyroid.* 2017;27(11):1341–1346.

Crocetta FM, Botti C, Pernice C, et al. Sentinel node biopsy versus elective neck dissection in early-stage oral cancer: a systematic review. *Eur Arch Otorhinolaryngol.* 2020;277(12):3247–3260.

Cohen EE, Karrison TG, Kocherginsky M, et al. Phase III randomized trial of induction chemotherapy in patients with N2 or N3 locally advanced head and neck cancer. *J Clin Oncol.* 2014;32(25):2735–2743.

Cohen JI, Clayman GL. *Atlas of Head and Neck Surgery.* 1st ed. Philadelphia, PA: Saunders; 2011.

Cooper DS, Doherty GM, Haugen BR, et al. Revised American Thyroid Association management guidelines for patients with thyroid nodules and differentiated thyroid cance. *Thyroid.* 2009;19(11):1167–1214. https://doi.org/10.1089/thy.2009.0110.

Cooper JS, Zhang Q, Pajak TF, et al. Long-term follow-up of the RTOG 9501/intergroup phase III trial: postoperative concurrent radiation therapy and chemotherapy in high-risk squamous cell carcinoma of the head and neck. *Int J Radiat Oncol Biol Phys.* 2012;84(5):1198–1205.

Department of Veterans Affairs Laryngeal Cancer Study G, et al. Induction chemotherapy plus radiation compared with surgery plus radiation in patients with advanced laryngeal cancer. *N Engl J Med.* 1991;324(24):1685–1690.

Fakhry C, Zhang Q, Nguyen-Tan PF, et al. Human papillomavirus and overall survival after progression of oropharyngeal squamous cell carcinoma. *J Clin Oncol.* 2014;32(30):3365–3373.

Faries MB, Thompson JF, Cochran AJ, et al. Completion Dissection or Observation for Sentinel-Node Metastasis in Melanoma. *N Engl J Med.* 2017;376(23):2211–2222.

Flint PW, Haughey BW, Lund V, et al.*Cummings Otolaryngology-Head and Neck Surgery.* 7th ed. Philadelphia, PA: Elsevier; 2021.

Flint PW, Haughey BH, Lund VJ, et al.*Cummings Otolaryngology—Head and Neck Surgery.* 7th ed. Philadelphia, PA: Elsevier; 2021.

Forastiere AA, Goepfert H, Maor M, et al. Concurrent chemotherapy and radiotherapy for organ preservation in advanced laryngeal cancer. *N Engl J Med.* 2003;349(22):2091–2098.

Forastiere AA, Zhang Q, Weber RS, et al. Long-term results of RTOG 91-11: a comparison of three nonsurgical treatment strategies to preserve the larynx in patients with locally advanced larynx cancer. *J Clin Oncol.* 2013;31(7):845–852.

Friedman M, Kelley K, Maley A. Central neck dissection. *Operative Techniques in Otolaryngology.* 2011;22:169–172.

Goldblum JR, Lamps LW, McKenney JK, Myers JL. 2018. 11th ed. *Rosai and Ackerman's Surgical Pathology.* Philadelphia, PA: Elsevier; 2018.

Goodwin WJ. Jr. Salvage surgery for patients with recurrent squamous cell carcinoma of the upper aerodigestive tract: when do the ends justify the means? *Laryngoscope.* 2000;110(3 Pt 2 Suppl 93):1–18.

Griffin TW, Pajak TF, Laramore GE, et al. Neutron vs photon irradiation of inoperable salivary gland tumors: results of an RTOG-MRC Cooperative Randomized Study. *Int J Radiat Oncol Biol Phys.* 1988;15(5):1085–1090. https://doi.org/10.1016/0360-3016(88)90188.

Haddad R, O'Neill A, Rabinowits G, et al. Induction chemotherapy followed by concurrent chemoradiotherapy (sequential chemoradiotherapy) versus concurrent chemoradiotherapy alone in locally advanced head and neck cancer (PARADIGM): a randomised phase 3 trial. *Lancet Oncol.* 2013;14(3):257–264.

Haugen BR, Sawka AM, Alexander EK, et al. American Thyroid Association Guidelines on the Management of Thyroid Nodules and Differentiated Thyroid Cancer Task Force Review and Recommendation on the Proposed Renaming of Encapsulated Follicular Variant Papillary Thyroid Carcinoma Without Invasion to Noninvasive Follicular Thyroid Neoplasm with Papillary-Like Nuclear Features. *Thyroid.* 2017;27(4):481–483.

Ho AS, Tsao GJ, Chen FW, et al. Impact of positron emission tomography/computed tomography surveillance at 12 and 24 months for detecting head and neck cancer recurrence. *Cancer.* 2013;119(7):1349–1356.

Huang TB, MH. Epidemiology of nasopharyngeal carcinoma. *Nasopharyngeal Carcinoma Research.* 1998:6–12.

Janot F, de Raucourt D, Benhamou E, et al. Randomized trial of postoperative reirradiation combined with chemotherapy after salvage surgery compared with salvage surgery alone in head and neck carcinoma. *J Clin Oncol.* 2008;26(34):5518–5523.

Karia PS, Morgan FC, Califano JA, et al. Comparison of Tumor Classifications for Cutaneous Squamous Cell Carcinoma of the Head

and Neck in the 7th vs 8th Edition of the AJCC Cancer Staging Manual. *JAMA Dermatol.* 2018;154(2):175–181.

Laramore GE, Krall JM, Griffin Neutron versus photon irradiation for unresectable salivary gland tumors: final report of an RTOG-MRC randomized clinical trial. Radiation Therapy Oncology Group. Medical Research Council. *Int J Radiat Oncol Biol Phys.* 1993;27(2):235–240.

Leiter U, Stadler R, Mauch C, et al. Complete lymph node dissection versus no dissection in patients with sentinel lymph node biopsy positive melanoma (DeCOG-SLT): a multicentre, randomised, phase 3 trial. *Lancet Oncol.* 2016;17(6):757–767.

Leiter U, Stadler R, Mauch C, et al. Final Analysis of DeCOG-SLT Trial: No Survival Benefit for Complete Lymph Node Dissection in Patients With Melanoma With Positive Sentinel Node. *J Clin Oncol.* 2019;37(32):3000–3008.

Marx RE. A new concept in the treatment of osteoradionecrosis. *J Oral Maxillofac Surg.* 1983;41(6):351–357.

Mercadante V, Al Hamad A, Lodi G, et al. Interventions for the management of radiotherapy-induced xerostomia and hyposalivation: A systematic review and meta-analysis. *Oral Oncol.* 2017;66:64–74.

Moley JF. Medullary thyroid carcinoma: management of lymph node metastases. *J Natl Compr Canc Netw.* 2010;8(5):549–556.

Morton DL, Cochran AJ, Thompson JF, et al. Sentinel node biopsy for early-stage melanoma: accuracy and morbidity in MSLT-I, an international multicenter trial. *Ann Surg.* 2005;242(3):302–311. discussion 311-3.

Morton DL, Thompson JF, Cochran AJ, et al. Final trial report of sentinel-node biopsy versus nodal observation in melanoma. *N Engl J Med.* 2014;370(7):599–609.

Myers EN, CR. *Operative Otolaryngology: Head and Neck Surgery.* 2nd ed. Philadelphia, PA: Saunders; 2008.

NCC Network. NCCN Clinical Practice Guidelines in Oncology: Cutaneous Melanoma (Version 1.2020). 2019; Available from: https://www.nccn.org/professionals/physician_gls/pdf/cutaneous_melanoma.pdf.

NCC Network. *NCCN Clinical Practice Guidelines in Oncology: Thyroid Carcinoma (Version 2.2020).* 2020; Available from: https://www.nccn.org/professionals/physician_gls/pdf/thyroid.pdf.

Pai SI, Tufano R. Central compartment lymph node dissection. *Operative Techniques in Otolaryngology.* 2009;20:39–43.

Palmer SR, Erickson LA, Ichetovkin I, et al. Circulating serologic and molecular biomarkers in malignant melanoma. *Mayo Clin Proc.* 2011;86(10):981–990.

Pignon JP, le Maître A, Maillard E, et al. Meta-analysis of chemotherapy in head and neck cancer (MACH-NC): an update on 93 randomised trials and 17,346 patients. *Radiother Oncol.* 2009;92(1):4–14.

Randolph G. *Surgery of the Thyroid and Parathyroid Glands.* 3rd ed. Philadelphia, PA: Saunders; 2021.

Rubin AI, Chen EH, Ratner D. Basal-cell carcinoma. *N Engl J Med.* 2005;353(21):2262–2269.

Sanguineti G, Geara FB, Garden AS, et al. Carcinoma of the nasopharynx treated by radiotherapy alone: determinants of local and regional control. *Int J Radiat Oncol Biol Phys.* 1997;37(5):985–996.

Santoro R, Franchi A, Gallo O, et al. Nodal metastases at level IIb during neck dissection for head and neck cancer: clinical and pathologic evaluation. *Head Neck.* 2008;30(11):1483–1487.

Shah JP, Patel SG, Singh B, Wong R.*Jatin Shah's Head and Neck Surgery and Oncology.* 4th ed. Philadelphia, PA: Mosby; 2012.

Shuman AG, Shah JP. Maxillary swing approach for removal of recurrent nasopharyngeal carcinoma. *Operative Techniques in Otolaryngology.* 2014;25:248–253.

Tessler FN, Middleton WD, Grant EG, et al. ACR Thyroid Imaging, Reporting and Data System (TI-RADS): White Paper of the ACR TI-RADS Committee. *J Am Coll Radiol.* 2017;14(5):587–595.

Van Abel KM, Moore EJ. Surgical management of the base of tongue. *Operative Techniques in Otolaryngology.* 2013;24:74–85.

Weinstein GS, O'Malley BW Jr, Rinaldo A, et al. Understanding contraindications for transoral robotic surgery (TORS) for oropharyngeal cancer. *Eur Arch Otorhinolaryngol.* 2015;272(7):1551–1552.

Wong SL, Faries MB, Kennedy EB, et al. Sentinel Lymph Node Biopsy and Management of Regional Lymph Nodes in Melanoma: American Society of Clinical Oncology and Society of Surgical Oncology Clinical Practice Guideline Update. *J Clin Oncol.* 2018;36(4):399–413.

6 Pediatric Otolaryngology

Shelby Leuin, Aaron Lin, Sarah N. Bowe, and Karen Hawley

OTOLOGY

Pediatric Otologic Embryology and Anatomy

- Pinna
  - Develops from six hillocks of His originating from the first and second branchial arches and grooves
  - Grows rapidly during the first 2 to 3 years, reaching 90% adult size by age 8 years
  - Normal adult ear ranges from 5.5 to 6.5 cm
  - Microtia is often associated with hypoplasia or aplasia of the middle ear
- Tympanic membrane (TM) and external auditory canal (EAC)
  - The EAC has a transient obstruction during development. Ectoderm from first branchial cleft contacts endoderm of tubotympanic recess and the TM is formed.
  - TM: Adult dimensions at birth (approximate diameter of 8–10 mm)
- Eustachian tube
  - Derived from first pharyngeal pouch
  - Patent during embryologic development (allowing amniotic fluid in middle ear space)
  - As the child ages, the angle becomes less acute and the Eustachian tube lengthens; coupled with a more developed and mature immune system, older children (>7 years of age) are less susceptible to otitis media
  - Approximately 50% of adult length at birth
  - Tensor veli palatini develops with time to act as the primary dilator
  - Other muscles contributing to dilation: Tensor tympani, levator veli palatine, salpingopharyngeus and dilator tubae
- Middle ear/ossicles
  - The ossicles are formed by the first and second pharyngeal arch (Meckel's and Reichert's, respectively). Exception: Stapes footplate is derived from the otic capsule
  - Adult sized at birth
- Inner ear/temporal bone
  - Petrous and mastoid portion of the temporal bone, including the bony labyrinth, develop from the otic capsule
  - Cortex of the mastoid is very thin, predisposing for subperiosteal spread of mastoiditis in children
  - Mastoid pneumatization continues through early childhood; infant's mastoid bone and marrow can bleed substantially during mastoidectomy, often requiring bone wax and diamond burr to stop bleeding
  - Styloid process is underdeveloped at birth, making the extratemporal portion of the facial nerve at risk from external trauma such as in forceps delivery

Congenital Malformations of the Outer and Middle Ear

- Microtia/atresia (also see Craniofacial section)
  - Microtia is a congenital malformation of the auricle
    - ~75% to 90% are unilateral
    - High prevalence in Hispanic and Native American/Alaska Native populations

- Grades I to IV
  - Grade I: All structures identifiable but auricle is small
  - Grade II: Deficiencies of the helix/missing structures
  - Grade III: No identifiable structures ("peanut ear")
  - Grade IV: Anotia
- Congenital aural atresia (CAA)/congenital external auditory canal stenosis (CEACS)
  - May occur in isolation, but most frequently in the setting of microtia
  - Cholesteatoma occurs more commonly in CEACS (1 in 5) and must be closely monitored
  - Prompt audiological assessment is key as patients may have various degrees of conductive hearing loss (CHL) and about 10% may have sensorineural hearing loss (SNHL) as well
  - Surgical candidates for CAA repair are determined primarily on the Jahrsdoerfer criteria
- Congenital cholesteatoma
  - Most commonly anterior superior and extending into posterior superior quadrant
  - Potsic stage of lesion determines surgical approach and risk for recurrence
    - I: Confined to one quadrant of the mesotympanum
    - II: Two quadrants involved but no erosion of ossicles
    - III: Confined to the mesotympanum but there is ossicular erosion
    - IV: Extension into the mastoid

Congenital Malformations of the Inner Ear

- Membranous
  - Bony labyrinth is unaffected, and computed tomography (CT) or magnetic resonance imaging (MRI) of the inner ear is normal
  - Scheibe aplasia, also known as *cochleosaccular dysplasia*, is the most common membranous malformation and most common cause of congenital deafness
    - Associations with Scheibe malformation include Usher syndrome, Down syndrome, Waardenburg syndrome, and Refsum disease
  - Complete membranous labyrinthine dysplasia (rare), associated with Jervell and Lange-Nielsen syndrome and Usher syndrome
  - Alexander dysplasia: Cochlear basal turn dysplasia; high-frequency SNHL
- Osseous and membranous
  - Can be recognized radiographically
  - Michel aplasia: Characterized by the absence of the cochlea and labyrinth; cessation of the otic capsule at the third week of development
  - Cochlear anomalies (Fig. 6.1)
    - Cochlear aplasia (arrest at fifth week): No hearing
    - Common cavity (arrest at fourth week): Severe-to-profound hearing loss
    - Cochlear hypoplasia (arrest at sixth week): 15% of cochlear anomalies, and with variable hearing
    - Incomplete partition type 2 has replaced "Mondini deformity" (arrest at seventh week of gestation)

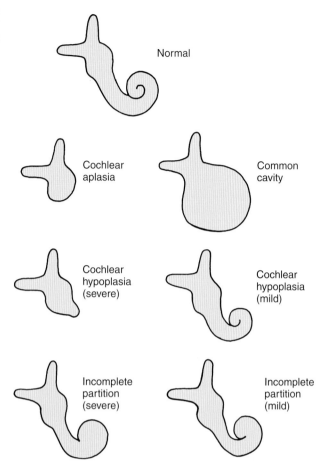

Fig. 6.1 Cochlear malformations. Drawings were made from coronal computed tomography scans. (From Jackler RK, Luxford WM, House WF. Congenital malformations of the inner ear: a classification based on embryogenesis. *Laryngoscope.* 1987;97(suppl 40):2; and Flint PW, Haughey BH, Lund VJ, et al. *Cummings Otolaryngology—Head and Neck Surgery.* 6th ed. Philadelphia, PA: Saunders; 2015.)

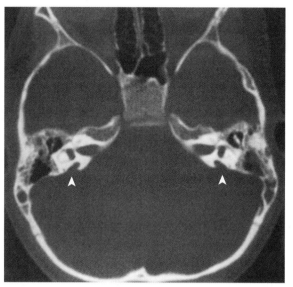

Fig. 6.2 Bilateral enlargement of the vestibular aqueducts (*arrow-heads*) as seen on an axial computed tomography scan. (From Flint PW, Haughey BH, Lund VJ, et al. *Cummings Otolaryngology—Head and Neck Surgery.* 6th ed. Philadelphia, PA: Saunders; 2015.)

- It is defined by a cochlea with 1.5 turns, with cystic middle and apical turns
- It is the most common cochlear malformation
- Associated with dilated vestibule, enlarged vestibular aqueduct (EVA); Pendred syndrome (SLC26A4); predisposition to meningitis; variable degrees of SNHL
- Labyrinthine anomalies (40% of radiologically abnormal cochlea will have a lateral semicircular canal [SCC] abnormality)
  - Cochlear abnormalities are common in patients with SCC aplasia
  - Degree of hearing loss does not necessarily correlate with severity of labyrinthine deformity
  - SCC dysplasia: 4 times as common as SCC aplasia, associated with CHL
  - SCC aplasia (horizontal canal): Found with CHARGE (**c**oloboma of the eye, **h**eart defects, **a**tresia of the nasal choanae, **r**etardation of growth and/or development, **g**enital and/or urinary abnormalities, and **e**ar abnormalities and deafness) association
- Aqueduct anomalies
  - Vestibular aqueduct: Normally 0.4 to 1.0 mm in diameter when measured halfway between the common crus and its external aperture

- EVA (Fig. 6.2) is the most common identified temporal bone abnormality in children imaged for SNHL; defined by vestibular aqueduct size of >1 mm at the midpoint and >2 mm in diameter at the operculum
  - Progressive and sudden decrements in hearing with approximately 40% eventually developing profound SNHL; the likelihood of hearing loss progression increases as the size of the vestibular aqueduct increases
  - Type of hearing loss can be SNHL, mixed, or purely conductive
- Enlarged cochlear aqueduct: Usually 3 to 4 mm in diameter and ranges from 1 to 10 mm; significance is controversial
- Internal auditory canal (IAC) abnormalities
  - Narrow IAC: <3 mm; if facial function is present, then CN VIII will most likely be absent; MRI of the temporal bone should be ordered to determine further the presence of the cochlear nerve
  - Widened IAC: >10 mm is associated with a cerebrospinal fluid (CSF) gusher in the cochlear implantation and stapedectomy

Infant and Pediatric Audiology

- Joint Committee on Infant Hearing (JCIH) Position Statement
  - Benchmarks for early hearing detection and intervention (EHDI) programs include the "1-3-6 rule"
    - Newborns are to be screened for hearing loss (and rescreened if refer on first screen) prior to discharge from the hospital or no later than 1 month of age
    - Diagnostic audiology testing (auditory brainstem response [ABR]) by 3 months of age
    - Enrollment in early intervention by 6 months of age if a hearing loss is confirmed
  - Newborns who have been in the neonatal intensive care unit (ICU) or who have been exposed to high-risk infections in utero should be screened with automated auditory brainstem response (A-ABR)
  - Newborns who pass their initial screen but have risk factors for progressive or delayed-onset hearing loss should be closely followed and reassessed with audiometric testing (Table 6.1)

TABLE 6.1 Joint Commission on Infant Hearing Recommendations for Follow-Up Regarding Infants Who Are at High Risk for Progressive or Delayed Onset Hearing Loss

Risk Factor Classification	Risk Factor	Recommended Audiology Testing/ Follow-Up
Perinatal		
	In utero infections: TORCHES, Zika (mother + infant with laboratory +/- clinical findings of Zika)	Initial screen should be with A-ABR. Follow-up within 3–9 months of age and then yearly until school aged
	Extracorporeal membrane oxygenation	3 months after occurrence and then every 12 months until school aged
	Medical/genetic conditions associated with hearing loss: • Craniofacial malformations • Microcephaly or hydrocephalus • Neurodegonerative disorders • Other physical exam findings associated with syndromic hearing loss	By 9 months and then based on hearing skills/milestones or known associated progressive hearing loss
	Hyperbilirubinemia with exchange transfusion	By 9 months and then based on hearing skills/milestones
	Neonatal intensive care stay for more than 5 days	By 9 months and then based on hearing skills/milestones
	Aminoglycosides for more than 5 days	By 9 months and then based on hearing skills/milestones
	Asphyxia or hypoxic ischemic encephalopathy	By 9 months and then based on hearing skills/milestones
	Family history of congenital/progressive hearing loss	By 9 months and then based on etiology of family hearing loss/ caregiver concern
Perinatal or Postnatal		
	Caregiver or provider concern regarding speech, language or hearing	Immediate referral
	Events associated with hearing loss: • Head trauma (especially basilar or temporal fracture) • Chemotherapy	Within 3 months of event and continue based on findings
	Meningitis/encephalitis	Within 3 months and yearly until school age

A-ABR, automated auditory brainstem response testing, *TORCHES*, neonatal infections including **to**xoplasmosis, **r**ubella, **c**ytomegalovirus, **he**rpes, **s**yphilis.

- Methods of audiological evaluation (newborn to 48 months)
  - ABR, also known as a *brainstem auditory evoked response test*
  - For hearing screens: Automated ABR (A-ABR) or screening (S-ABR) systems test for the presence or absence of wave V at soft stimulus

- Stimulus is usually click stimuli at 35 to 40 dB, with no operator interpretation
- Results are given as Pass or Refer for each ear
- It is a highly effective screening with sensitivity/specificity of 96% to 98%, but it does not rule out minimal or mild hearing loss
  - Diagnostic ABR: Used when hearing loss is suspected because of an abnormal A-ABR screening result (*or* absent otoacoustic emissions [OAEs] screening result; see OAE section)
    - Used to determine frequency-specific hearing thresholds as well as type of hearing loss (sensorineural, conductive, or mixed)
    - Child must be completely asleep throughout testing; often requires sedation after 6 months of age
    - An ABR is not a "functional" test of hearing—rather, it is an estimated hearing test in which the child does not actively participate; there is no cortical processing; results should always be confirmed or supported by behavioral testing when possible (see Behavioral auditory testing section)
  - Auditory steady-state response (ASSR) testing: A newer and less studied form of diagnostic testing for infants
    - Uses a statistical algorithm to determine responses, significantly reducing the subjective component of an ABR to interpret waves
    - Simultaneous frequencies are tested and, thus, the testing is possibly shorter in duration than ABR
    - There is still limited validation of ASSR; thus, it is not recommended as an alternative to ABR at this time
  - OAEs: Performed for hearing screens or as part of an audiological test battery (Note: Can be used as a screen only for well babies, not high-risk newborns, as mentioned earlier)
    - OAEs test cochlear outer hair cell function; if present, cochlear outer hair cell function is normal and normal-to-near-normal hearing is assumed; there are two types of OAEs:
    - Transient evoked OAE (TEOAE)
      - Click stimuli at 80 to 86 dB; typically tests only a small range of frequencies
      - May be present/pass even with mild hearing loss (about 30 dB)
    - Distortion product OAE (DPOAE)
      - More frequency-specific compared with TEOAE and can test a wider range of frequencies
      - May be present even with mild hearing loss (about 30 dB)
    - Factors that may adversely affect testing:
      - Debris or cerumen in the EAC
      - Poor probe fit because of stenotic canal
      - Middle ear effusion (MEE) or any conductive component
      - Patient compliance—patient must be relatively quiet and still throughout testing
    - OAE testing may miss auditory neuropathy spectrum disorder (ANSD): in this case, children will have present OAEs, but an abnormal ABR
- Behavioral auditory testing
  - For infants/children of 6 months and older corrected age
  - A functional test: The child participates in the task, and testing involves cortical processing of sound
  - Generally three types of test methods depending on age/developmental status:
    - Visual reinforcement audiometry (VRA)
      - Child must be at least 6 months corrected age
      - Child should have good head control and be able to make an orienting movement to sound stimuli (turn head left and right in response to sound)

- Child should be able to see visual stimuli approximately 3 feet away
  - The child is presented with a sound and when the child turns the head toward that sound, the child is rewarded with a visual stimulus (such as a toy lighting up or an animation on a screen)
- Conditioned play audiometry
  - For children usually 2 to 2.5 years (corrected age) and older
  - Child responds to an auditory stimulus with a conditioned play paradigm (drop a block in a bucket when you hear the sound)
  - Play activity can vary from child to child, but the child must be able to self-regulate, which requires a longer attention span
- Standard audiometry
  - For children 4 to 5 years and older into adulthood
  - Standard "raise your hand when you hear the beep" task
- Behavioral testing should minimally include tonal *and* speech stimuli; a full audiological evaluation should also include immittance testing (tympanometry and acoustic reflex thresholds) and OAEs

NOTE: If there are parental or primary care provider concerns at any point during child development, results of screening should be corroborated with behavioral testing. Likewise, if screening, diagnostic, or behavioral testing was normal in the past but new concerns have arisen or there is regression in speech, language, or auditory skills, refer the patient to an audiologist.

Work up and Evaluation of Pediatric Hearing Loss

- A thorough history should be obtained to identify any risk factors associated with hearing loss; see Table 6.1
- Complete head and neck exam should be performed and attention should be paid to any additional physical exam findings associated with hearing loss. Examples include a cleft palate, white forelock or heterochromia iridis (associated with Waardenburg syndrome) or anterior cervical pits/draining fistulas (associated with branchio-oto-renal [BOR] syndrome)
- Genetic testing and evaluation of congenital cytomegalovirus (cCMV) should be considered in the primary evaluation of a child with SNHL
  - cCMV must be diagnosed within the first 3 weeks of life with urine or saliva testing
  - Newborn bloodspots may be retroactively obtained and tested, but the sensitivity is significantly lower than the specificity (34%–100% and 9%–100%, respectively); therefore, a positive test is helpful but a negative test does not rule it out
- Pediatric ophthalmology consultation is recommended due to the 2- to 3-fold increased risk in ocular disease for children with hearing loss
- Electrocardiogram (EKG) is recommended for children with bilateral severe to profound SNHL or a personal/family history of syncope, cardiac arrhythmias, or childhood sudden death
- Temporal bone imaging should be considered in certain conditions but can be avoided when another diagnosis has been clearly made
  - Concordance between CT and MRI is ~70% to 80%
  - Consider imaging in the following scenarios:
    - Asymmetric, unilateral, mixed, or progressive hearing loss

- Temporal bone fracture and hearing loss with head trauma
- Planning and evaluation for cochlear implantation; cochlear nerve aplasia can present similarly to other causes of auditory neuropathy; MRI can distinguish cochlear nerve presence, which has prognostic value in cochlear implantation
- Meningitis
- Suspected auditory neuropathy
- CHL without clear evidence of the cause on exam; consider CT
- Auditory neuropathy
  - Presence of OAEs and/or cochlear microphonics and absent ABRs
  - Undergo trial of binaural amplification; if no progress with speech and language development, then consider cochlear implantation
  - Intact outer hair cell function, but absent or severely abnormal ABR
  - Lesion may be located at or between inner hair cells and the auditory nerve
  - 20% to 30% of patients ultimately develop loss of outer hair cell function and SNHL
  - Several etiologies, including genetic, anatomical, and environmental causes
  - Patients should consider using American Sign Language or another form of manual communication in addition to spoken language

Etiology of Pediatric Hearing Loss

- Acquired hearing loss
  - cCMV: cCMV causes hearing loss in about 20% of infected infants but up to 75% of infants with "symptomatic" cCMV (thrombocytopenia, petechiae, hepatosplenomegaly, intrauterine growth restriction, hepatitis, chorioretinitis, central nervous system [CNS] involvement)
  - Other causes of acquired hearing loss: ANSD in the setting of severe jaundice, ototoxicity from chemotherapy, or SNHL following meningitis
- Congenital hearing loss
  - Inner ear abnormalities: Imaging may reveal abnormalities in 27% to 39% of cases of congenital hearing loss; some, however, are in the setting of genetic/syndromic hearing loss
    - EVA: Most common radiographic finding
      - Bilateral EVA is associated with Pendred syndrome
    - Hypoplastic cochlear nerve: Most common finding in unilateral SNHL
  - Genetic cause is the most common etiology; at least 50% of congenital hearing loss is genetic (Table 6.2)
    - Autosomal recessive (AR) accounts for 75% to 80%; autosomal dominant (AD) approximately 20%; sex-linked approximately 2% to 5%; and mitochondrial <1%
      - 70% of AR causes are nonsyndromic
        - Connexin 26: Most common cause of AR nonsyndromic SNHL
    - Product of the *GJB2* gene
    - Nonfunctional gap junction protein
    - Mutations in the *GJB2* gene account for 30% to 50% of recessive deafness
    - Found in 50% of nonsyndromic severe-to-profound SNHL
  - AD syndromes associated with SNHL
    - BOR syndrome
      - Branchial cleft anomalies: Cervical fistulas, sinuses, and cysts

TABLE 6.2 Genetic Syndromes Associated With Hearing Loss

Genetic Classification	Diagnosis/Syndrome	Overall Phenotype	Hearing Phenotype	Gene Locus/Loci
Autosomal Dominant				
	Branchio-oto-renal	Branchial cleft anomalies; external, middle, or inner ear abnormalities; renal dysplasia	Mixed (90%), CHL/SNHL	EYA1, SIX-1
	Neurofibromatosis 2	Bilateral acoustic neuromas/vestibular schwannomas (often <20 years), other CNS benign tumors	SNHL; progressive	Tumor suppressor on chromosome 22
	Crouzon	Craniosynostosis, maxillary hypoplasia, proptosis, brachydactyly	CHL>SNHL	FGFR2
	Stickler	Myopia, PRS, joint hypermobility	SNHL (increases with age), CHL, mixed	COL2A1, COL11A1/2
	Waardenburg	White forelock, heterochromia iridis, dystopia canthorum, ± limb abnormalities or Hirschsprung	SNHL; profound	PAX-3 mostly associated, but there are multiple
	Treacher Collins	Craniofacial anomalies of mid- and lower face, outer and middle ear anomalies, ocular colobomas	CHL>SNHL	TCOF1
Autosomal Recessive				
	Pendred	Bilateral EVA and euthyroid goiter	SNHL; severe to profound, progressive	SLC264A
	Jervell and Lange-Nielsen	Prolonged QT, syncope	SNHL; severe to profound	KVLQT1, KCNE1
	Usher	Retinitis pigmentosa, vestibular dysfunction	SNHL; varies	MYO7A most common, but there are multiple
X-Linked				
	Alport	Hematuric nephritis, ocular disease	SNHL; progressive high frequency	COL4A5
	Mohr-Tranebjaerg	Visual and intellectual disability, dystonia and fractures	SNHL, postlingual	TIMM8A
	Norrie	Progressive ocular disease; pseudoglioma	SNHL; later onset and progressive	NDP
	Oto-palato-digital	Hypertelorism, midface hypoplasia/cleft palate, broad digits, short stature	CHL; ossicular malformation	FLNA
	Wildervanck (cervico-oculo-acoustic)	Klippel-Feil (fused cervical spine), cranial nerve VI abnormality	CHL, SNHL or mixed	Polygenic
	X-linked gusher	Bulbous fundus IAC, widened/absent bony modiolus	CHL/SNHL progressive	DFNX2

CHL, Conductive hearing loss; *EVA,* enlarged vestibular aqueduct; *IAC,* internal auditory canal; *PRS,* Pierre-Robin sequence; *SNHL,* sensorineural hearing loss.

- Otologic malformations: Conductive, sensorineural, or mixed hearing loss (nearly 90%); preauricular pits or tags (82%); auricular malformations (32%); middle and inner ear anomalies
- 2% of children with severe/profound SNHL are affected with BOR
- Individuals with ear pits and branchial defects warrant renal ultrasound
- Central neurofibromatosis (neurofibromatosis type 2 [NF 2])
  - Bilateral acoustic neuromas (vestibular schwannomas) often before age 20 years; may be unilateral
  - NF 2 is linked to mutation of a tumor suppressor gene on chromosome 22
  - Café-au-lait spots and cutaneous neurofibromas are fewer in number than in NF type 1
  - NF 2 results in other cranial, spinal, and peripheral nerve schwannomas, intracranial meningiomas, and optic gliomas
  - Radiosurgery can retard the growth of a tumor, but resection after radiation is more difficult
  - Auditory brainstem implants have been used with some hearing and spatial attention, but with limited language and speech skills
- Stickler syndrome
  - Severe myopia, which may lead to retinal detachment or cataracts
  - Joint hypermobility and enlargement with early-onset arthritis
  - Pierre Robin sequence: micrognathia is common and may result in a cleft palate
- Waardenburg syndrome
  - Four different types of Waardenburg syndrome have been classified based on phenotype and genetic mutation (*MITF* gene/*PAX3* gene)
  - Type 1: Unilateral or bilateral SNHL, white forelock, iris pigment anomalies (heterochromia iridis), dystopia canthorum, and broad nasal root
  - Type 2 is identical to type 1, but without dystopia canthorum: SNHL is more common in type 2 than in type 1
  - Type 3: Features of type 1 with upper limb abnormalities
  - Type 4: Type 1 features and Hirschsprung disease

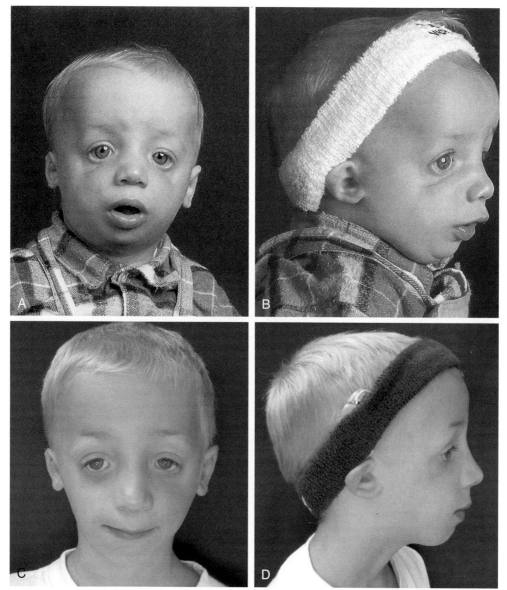

Fig. 6.3 (**A**) Characteristic facial appearance of a 10-month-old child with mandibulofacial dysostosis (Treacher Collins syndrome). (**B**) Oblique view of the same patient. Note the absent external ear canal, which is bilateral, and the headband, which holds bone conduction hearing aids. (**C**) Frontal view of the same patient at age 6 years. (**D**) Oblique view of the same patient at age 6 years. (From Flint PW, Haughey BH, Lund VJ, et al. *Cummings Otolaryngology—Head and Neck Surgery.* 6th ed. Philadelphia, PA: Saunders; 2015.)

- Treacher Collins syndrome (mandibulofacial dysostosis; Fig. 6.3)
  - CHL is secondary to ossicular abnormalities but can be accompanied by SNHL, aural atresia, and ear canal stenosis
  - Hypoplastic mandible and cleft palate
  - Downward slanting palpebral fissures and coloboma of the lower eyelids
  - Bilateral symmetric facies and eyelid coloboma distinguish Treacher Collins from similar but unilateral findings of Goldenhar
- AR syndromes associated with SNHL
  - Pendred syndrome
    - Most common syndromic form of SNHL
    - Associated with an organification defect in the thyroid
    - Bilateral EVA and bilateral incomplete partition type 2 cochlear defect visible on temporal bone imaging, resulting in mild to profound SNHL and usually progressive hearing loss
  - Can develop euthyroid goiter in childhood or as young adult; thyroid dysfunction, thus, endocrine testing is important
  - Abnormal *pendrin*, a chloride/bicarbonate exchange protein; abnormal ion exchange causes abnormal cochlear potential
  - Pendrin genetic testing is the preferred diagnostic tool
    - Alternatively, perchlorate discharge test can demonstrate an abnormal organification of nonorganic iodine; however, because of radioactive exposure, it is used infrequently
- Jervell and Lange-Nielsen syndrome
  - Heart disease: Prolonged QT interval, ventricular arrhythmias, syncopal episodes, and death

- High rate of cardiac and fatal events despite β-blockers, which do lower mortality
- Prevalence is low in children with congenital SNHL
- EKG is important in young infants with severe-to-profound hearing loss to rule out cardiac conductive anomalies
- Usher syndrome
  - 50% of concomitant deafness and blindness
  - Three clinically distinct subtypes, which differ with severity of each component
    - Type I: Congenital bilateral profound hearing loss, clinically apparent retinitis pigmentosa (RP) in first 10 years of life, significantly impaired vestibular dysfunction (may present as delayed crawling or walking)
    - Type II: Moderate, often progressive, down-sloping SNHL, normal vestibular function, and onset of RP in the first/second decade
    - Type III: Progressive Hodgkin lymphoma (HL), variable vestibular dysfunction, and variable onset of RP
    - RP: diagnosed with electroretinography; requires ophthalmology consultation
- X-linked syndromes associated with SNHL (can be X-linked recessive or dominant)
  - Mohr-Tranebjaerg syndrome
  - X-linked deafness associated with perilymphatic gusher
  - Alport syndrome (80% X-linked but can be AR or AD)
    - Results from abnormal basement membrane structure with basilar membrane, stria vascularis, and renal glomerulus
    - "Red diaper" → hematuric nephritis, family history of hematuria, and chronic renal failure
    - Eye lesions (anterior lenticonus with bulging lens) and retinopathy
  - Norrie syndrome
    - Congenital/rapidly progressive blindness because of pseudoglioma development and cataracts
    - SNHL and congenital or progressive blindness
  - Oto palato-digital syndrome
    - Hypertelorism, flat midface, small nose, cleft palate, short stature, broad fingers, toes of variable length, and wide space between the first and second toe
    - CHL: Potentially amenable to surgical correction of CHL for ossicular malformation
  - Wildervanck syndrome
    - Encompasses Klippel-Feil malformation; cervical spinal fusions
    - SNHL or mixed hearing loss because of bony inner ear malformation
    - CN VI paralysis with eye retraction on lateral gaze (i.e., Duane syndrome)

Hearing Implants in Children

- Bone-conducting hearing aids: Nonsurgical or surgical via direct (transcutaneous post) or indirect (magnet) osseointegration. Indications include:
  - Atresia and/or microtia (inability to use traditional hearing aids)
  - CHL with an air–bone gap of >30 dB
  - Mixed hearing loss with an air–bone gap of >30 to 35 dB, but with mild-to-moderate SNHL
    - Baha sound processor can compensate for SNHL of up to 65 dB
  - Single-sided deafness with normal hearing in the good ear
    - Improved speech understanding by overcoming head shadow effect and giving 360-degree sound awareness

- Inability to fit a traditional hearing aid or contralateral routing of signals because of skin allergy with ear mold or chronic draining ears
- Cochlear implants
  - Indications have been expanding
    - Bilateral severe-to-profound SNHL
      - 9 months of age and older
      - Limited benefit (speech progression) with appropriate amplification trial
      - Special consideration: Meningitis (risk of cochlear ossification), asymmetric hearing loss with known risk of progression, such as EVA or cCMV
      - <20% to 30% on Multisyllabic Lexical Neighborhood Test (MLNT) or Lexical Neighborhood Test (LNT)
    - ANSD with limited benefit from traditional hearing aids
    - Single-sided deafness: Children aged 6 years and older
  - Contraindications include cochlear aplasia (Michel deformity), cochlear nerve aplasia (most severe form of ANSD)
  - Complications
    - Acute/subacute: Bleeding, wound infection, otitis media, incomplete electrode insertion, perilymph gusher, facial paralysis, dysgeusia
    - Chronic/delayed: Hard or soft failure of the device requiring explantation, meningitis (predominantly *Streptococcus pneumoniae*), otitis media

Inflammatory and Infectious Middle Ear Disease in Children

- Risk factors for pediatric acute otitis media
  - Early onset of infections: Younger than 8 months of age
  - Daycare attendance: Grouping of six or more infants or children
  - Family history of severe or recurrent infections in siblings
  - Craniofacial abnormalities (Down syndrome, cleft palate, and Crouzon syndrome)
  - Breastfeeding <3 months' duration
  - Tobacco exposure: Smoking in the household of parents, grandparents, or other caregivers
  - Immunodeficiency: Human immunodeficiency virus (HIV) and low immunoglobulin G (IgG), IgA
  - Male gender
  - Allergies: Dietary, medications, lotions, and creams (suspected)
- Most common etiological agents in pediatric acute otitis media
  - *S. pneumoniae*
  - *Haemophilus influenzae*
  - *Moraxella catarrhalis*
  - Group A *Streptococcus*
- Complications and sequelae of acute or chronic otitis media
  - Intratemporal
    - CHL; generally transient
    - Tympanic membrane perforation
    - Speech and language delay
    - Chronic suppurative otitis media
    - Atelectasis of the middle ear/adhesive otitis media with potential for ossicular fibrosis, discontinuity, and/or fixation
    - Tympanosclerosis
    - Cholesteatoma
    - Vestibular and balance problems
    - Mastoiditis and petrositis
    - Subperiosteal abscess
    - Facial paralysis

- Intracranial
  - Meningitis
  - Intracranial abscess; cerebral, subdural or epidural
  - Sigmoid/lateral sinus thrombus
  - Otic hydrocephalus
- Indications for tympanostomy tube placement
  - Patulous eustachian tube
  - Hyperbaric oxygen therapy
  - Infectious complication of otitis media
  - Chronic otitis media with effusion (OME) for >3 months bilaterally or >6 months unilaterally
  - Recurrent acute otitis media with evidence of disease at the time of otolaryngology evaluation
  - May proceed earlier if:
    - Persistent, severe acute otitis media
    - Suspected antimicrobial resistance
    - Significant hearing loss
    - Speech/language delay
    - Developmental delay
    - Severe TM retraction
    - Disequilibrium/vertigo/tinnitus
- Complications of tympanostomy tubes
  - Otorrhea
  - Granuloma formation at the tube site
  - Persistent TM perforation
  - Early extrusion (<6 months)
  - Obstructed (nonfunctioning) tympanostomy tube
  - Cholesteatoma
  - Tympanosclerosis
  - Migration of the tube into the middle ear
- Bacteriology of acute mastoiditis (without cholesteatoma)
  - *S. pneumoniae*
  - *H. influenzae*
  - *Streptococcus pyogenes*
  - *Staphylococcus aureus*
- Differential diagnosis of aural polyp in a child
  - Foreign body (prior tympanostomy tube history)
  - Otitis externa
  - Cholesteatoma
  - Histiocytosis X (eosinophilic granuloma)
  - Malignant lesion (e.g., rhabdomyosarcoma)

HEAD AND NECK

History and Exam Findings for a Child With a New-Onset Neck Mass (Fig. 6.4)

- History
  - Time of onset and duration
  - Change in size (enlargement, fluctuation)
  - Fevers
  - Recent infection, for example, upper respiratory infection (URI)
  - Drainage
  - Skin changes (erythema, violaceous, ecchymosis)
  - Airway distress and/or signs of obstruction (stertor, stridor, snoring)
  - Dysphagia or drooling
  - Previous neck surgery
  - Recent trauma
  - Sick contacts, flu, or tuberculosis (TB) exposure
  - Exposure to cats, ticks, mosquitos, and/or insects
  - Travel history: Regional or international
  - Immunization history: Absence of routine vaccinations
  - History of radiation exposure
  - Weight loss and night sweats (B symptoms)

- Physical exam
  - Location
  - Size
  - Head tilt or torticollis
  - Skin changes and overlying skin color
  - Tenderness to palpation
  - Fluctuance
  - Mobility in relation to skin (dermal) or subcutaneous tissue (muscle/fascia)
  - Movement with swallowing (midline neck mass)
  - Range of neck motion
  - Inability to handle secretions, stridor, or other signs of respiratory distress
  - Presence of fistula or sinus

Differential Diagnosis of a Child With a New-Onset Neck Mass, by Location

- Midline neck mass
  - Thyroglossal duct cyst (TGDC)
  - Dermoid cyst
  - Lymphadenopathy/lymphadenitis
  - Sialocele of the floor of the mouth, "plunging ranula"
  - Thyroid mass
- Lateral neck mass
  - Lymphadenopathy/lymphadenitis
  - Branchial cleft cyst, sinus, and fistula
  - Lymphatic or vascular malformation
  - Mycobacterial infection
  - Hemangioma
  - Fibromatosis coli (sternocleidomastoid [SCM] tumor of infancy)
  - Neoplastic
- Base of the tongue mass
  - TGDC
  - Lingual thyroid gland
  - Vallecular cyst
  - Dermoid cyst
  - Teratoma
  - Malignant neoplasm

Differential Diagnosis of a Child With a New-Onset Neck Mass by Etiology

- Congenital
  - Branchial cleft cyst
  - TGDC
  - Dermoid cyst
  - Bronchogenic cyst
  - Thymic cyst
  - Epidermal inclusion cyst
  - Pilomatrixoma
  - Fibromatosis coli (SCM tumor of infancy; Fig. 6.5)
  - Ectopic thymus
  - Ectopic thyroid
  - Foregut duplication cyst
- Infectious/inflammatory
  - Lymphadenopathy, lymphadenitis, phlegmon, and abscess (bacterial, viral)
  - Mycobacterial infection, including atypical
  - Fungal
  - Cat scratch/*Bartonella henselae*
  - Protozoal—toxoplasmosis
- Vascular anomalies
  - Lymphatic malformation
  - Hemangioma
  - Venous
  - Arteriovenous malformation (AVM)

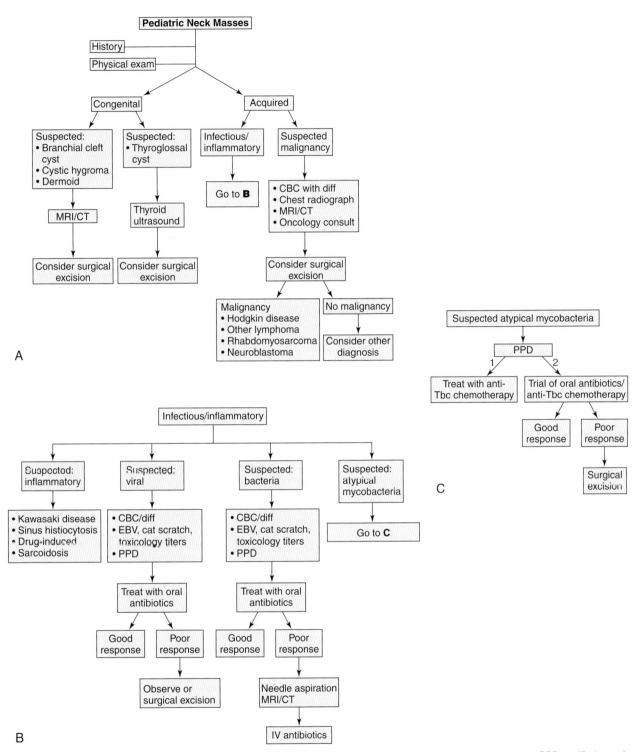

Fig. 6.4 Algorithms for the differential diagnosis of neck masses. *anti-Tbc*, Antituberculous; *CBC*, complete blood count; *PPD*, purified protein derivative. (From Flint PW, Haughey BH, Lund VJ, et al. *Cummings Otolaryngology—Head and Neck Surgery*. 6th ed. Philadelphia, PA: Saunders; 2015.)

- Autoimmune/inflammatory
  - Kawasaki disease
    - Fever >5 days
    - Conjunctivitis
    - Oral ulcers and strawberry tongue
    - Erythematous rash
    - Edema, erythema, and peeling of the hands and feet
  - Nonpurulent cervical lymphadenopathy
  - Need EKG to assess for coronary artery aneurysms
  - Treatment with immunoglobulins and aspirin
  - Rosai-Dorfman disease
  - Castleman disease
- Acquired anomalies
  - Laryngocele

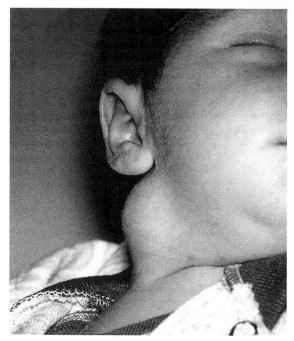

Fig. 6.5 Infant with congenital torticollis. Note the firm mass in the midportion of the sternocleidomastoid muscle. (From Flint PW, Haughey BH, Lund VJ, et al. *Cummings Otolaryngology—Head and Neck Surgery*. 6th ed. Philadelphia, PA: Saunders; 2015.)

- Ranula
- Thyroid nodule/cyst
- Lymphoproliferative disorder
- Neoplastic (benign and malignant)
  - Lymphoma
  - Rhabdomyosarcoma
  - Neuroblastoma
  - Salivary gland tumor
  - Thyroid mass/carcinoma (CA)
  - Nasopharyngeal (NP) CA

Congenital Neck Masses

- Branchial cleft anomalies
  - Incomplete closure of the branchial arch apparatus between the cleft and pouch
  - Lined with stratified squamous epithelium
    - Contains other dermal structures, such as hair follicles, sebaceous glands, and sweat glands
  - Five mesodermal arches (first to fourth and sixth) contain their own arterial and nerve supply
  - Cyst—No communication to body surface
  - Sinus—Communicates with single body surface, either skin or pharynx
  - Fistula—Communicates with two body surfaces
  - Branchial cleft anomaly classification
    - First branchial anomaly, Work Type 1: Cyst near ear canal, may course medially or laterally to the facial nerve
      - Ectodermal in origin and duplications of membranous EAC
      - Located in the periparotid and preauricular area, parallel to the EAC
      - Expression of material from the ear canal helps confirm the embryological origin of the lesion
      - Tract may open into the medial canal or middle ear space
      - Extremely rare

- First branchial anomaly, Work Type 2: Cyst near tail of parotid, may be intimately involved with the facial nerve (medial or lateral)
  - Composed of both ectoderm and mesoderm
  - Considered duplication of membranous and cartilaginous EAC
  - Otoscopy should be performed to determine whether fistula/sinus tract may end near the EAC close to the bony/cartilage junction
  - Expression of material from the ear canal helps confirm the embryologic origin of the lesion
  - More common than Type 1
- Second branchial anomaly
  - Most common overall branchial anomaly (cysts, sinuses, and fistulas)
  - Cyst and/or sinuses may be found along the anterior border of the SCM in the lower one-third of the neck
  - Tract passes superiorly and laterally to the common carotid artery, superficially to CN IX and CN XII
  - Tract splits the internal/external carotid artery
  - May enter the pharynx close to the middle constrictor or open into the tonsillar fossa
  - At the time of neck surgery may need tonsillectomy if the fistula tract opens into the tonsillar fossa region
- Third branchial anomaly
  - Very rare
  - Along the anterior border of the SCM in the lower neck, the tract goes laterally and superiorly (superficial) to the common carotid, superficially to CN XII, but deeply to the CN IX and internal carotid artery
  - Passes through the thyrohyoid membrane
  - Opens into the upper piriform sinus
  - Direct laryngoscopy with cauterization of the piriform sinus is an option for initial treatment; if this fails, then comprehensive surgical resection is required
- Fourth branchial anomaly
  - Very rare and usually on the left
  - On the left side, it starts along the anterior border of the SCM, tracks inferiorly deep to the common carotid, and loops around the aortic arch
  - On the right side, the tract loops around the right subclavian artery before ascending in the neck
  - Opens into the apex of the piriform sinus of the hypopharynx
  - Commonly presents as an abscess/cyst within or adjacent to the thyroid gland
- Nerve, muscle, cartilage, and artery derivatives of the branchial arches
  - First arch (first mandibular) structures
    - Nerve: Trigeminal (V)
    - Artery: Internal maxillary
    - Cartilage (Meckel): Malleus (except manubrium), incus (except long process), sphenomandibular ligament, anterior malleolar ligament, mandible, premaxilla, maxilla, zygoma, and part of the temporal bone
    - Muscle: Muscles of mastication, tensor tympani, tensor veli palatini, anterior belly of the digastric muscle; mylohyoid
  - Second arch structures
    - Nerve: Facial (VII)
    - Artery: Stapedial
    - Cartilage (Reichert): Manubrium of the malleus, long process of the incus, stapes (except foot plate),

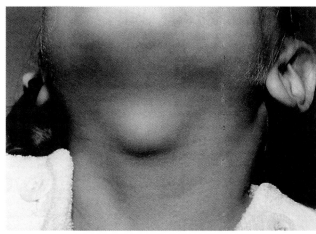

Fig. 6.6 Thyroglossal duct cysts are often found in the midline of the neck at or near the hyoid bone. (From Flint PW, Haughey BH, Lund VJ, et al. *Cummings Otolaryngology—Head and Neck Surgery.* 6th ed. Philadelphia, PA: Saunders.)

lesser cornu and upper body of the hyoid, and stylohyoid ligament
- Muscle: Muscles of facial expression, auricularis, stapedius, posterior belly digastric, and stylohyoid
- Third arch structures
  - Nerve: Glossopharyngeal (IX)
  - Artery: Common and internal carotid
  - Cartilage: Greater cornu and lower body of the hyoid
  - Muscle: Stylopharyngeus
- Fourth arch structures
  - Nerve: Superior laryngeal nerve (X)
  - Artery: Subclavian on the right and arch of the aorta on the left
  - Cartilage: Thyroid and cuneiform cartilages
  - Muscle: Pharyngeal and laryngeal muscles
- Sixth arch structures
  - Nerve: Recurrent laryngeal nerve (X)
  - Artery: Pulmonary artery on the right and ductus arteriosus on the left
  - Cartilage: Cricoid, arytenoid, and corniculate cartilages
  - Muscle: Pharyngeal and laryngeal muscles
- Thyroglossal duct cysts (TGDCs; Fig. 6.6)
  - The majority present at or below the hyoid bone in the midline, less commonly can occur superiorly
  - The tract leads into the base of the tongue, and infections are polymicrobial, consistent with oral pathogenic flora
  - Ultrasound is the preferred diagnostic modality to confirm the diagnosis and verify presence of normal thyroid gland
  - Although rare, papillary adenocarcinoma has been found in the cyst
  - Tests to consider in base of tongue mass
    - CT scan or MRI: Define depth and extent of the mass
    - Thyroid ultrasound: Assess for the presence of a normal thyroid; thyroid can be within TGDC or at the tongue base (lingual thyroid)
    - Thyroid technetium scan if there is a possible lingual thyroid
  - Sistrunk procedure for TGDC
    - Excision of the cyst, the central portion of the hyoid bone ± surrounding cuff of muscle
    - Excision of the central hyoid bone reduces the recurrence rate from 46% to 5.8%

- Acute infection should be treated initially with antibiotics, incision, and drainage if an abscess with the cyst has developed; definitive surgery with Sistrunk procedure should be undertaken after resolution of acute infection
- Dermoid cysts
  - Epithelial-lined cysts that gradually expand due to keratin deposition
  - Arise along embryonic fusion plates, can occur in submentum and anterior neck
  - Ultrasound can help to distinguish from TGDCs
  - Treatment is surgical excision of the cyst

Vascular Anomalies

- Hemangioma of infancy, also known as *infantile hemangioma* (Fig. 6.7)
  - Absent at birth and appears during infancy
  - Proliferates for 6 to 9 months and then involutes (partially or completely) over 3 to 5 years
  - Glucose transporter 1 (GLUT-1) staining positive
  - Separate from congenital hemangioma
  - Lesions described as focal versus segmental; superficial versus deep versus mixed
  - MRI: Enhancement and flow voids are present on T1 and T2
  - Complications: Airway compromise, cutaneous ulceration, visual obstruction, high-output cardiac failure, and psychosocial consequences
  - PHACE syndrome: Association with large infantile hemangioma on a child's face in conjunction with defects in the brain, blood vessels, eyes, heart, and chest (posterior fossa brain malformations [Dandy-Walker cysts], hemangioma, arterial lesions, cardiac abnormalities, eye/endocrine abnormalities)
- Congenital hemangioma
  - Present at birth (unlike hemangioma of infancy)
  - GLUT-1 staining negative
  - Two types
    - Rapidly involuting congenital hemangioma
    - Noninvoluting congenital hemangioma
- Management of hemangiomas
  - Observation, *except* for those compromising the airway, impairing vision, or causing skin ulceration or bleeding
  - Propranolol is the mainstay of treatment
  - Other treatment options:
    - Oral or intralesional steroids
    - Surgical excision: Cold knife or laser; ideally best to wait until after the proliferation stage
    - Interferon-α2a: Rarely used because of the risk of spastic diplegia
    - Pulsed-dye laser: Ideal for superficial hemangioma; can be combined with surgical excision
- Subglottic hemangioma
  - Usually present with biphasic stridor, diagnosed by laryngoscopy and bronchoscopy (lesion is most often on the left posterolateral subglottis)
  - 50% will have a cutaneous hemangioma
  - Propranolol is the first-line therapy, possibly combined with systemic steroids
  - If airway compromise despite first-line therapy: Intralesional steroids, interferon-α2a, and surgery (open excision vs. tracheotomy)
- Kasabach-Merritt syndrome
  - Platelet-trapping coagulopathy resulting in an enlarging hemangioma-like tumor
  - May be associated with tufted angioma or kaposiform hemangioendothelioma
  - Not associated with hemangioma of infancy

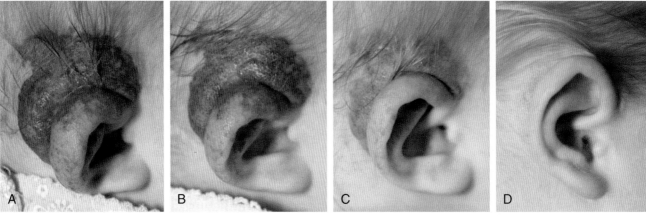

Fig. 6.7 Superficial segmental hemangioma treated with propranolol. (**A**) Pretreatment with postauricular ulceration. (**B**) After 1 month of corticosteroid treatment. (**C**) After 1 month of propranolol treatment. (**D**) After 4 months of propranolol treatment. (From Flint PW, Haughey BH, Lund VJ, et al. *Cummings Otolaryngology—Head and Neck Surgery.* 6th ed. Philadelphia, PA: Saunders; 2015.)

- Thrombocytopenia resulting in bleeding, with scattered petechiae when platelet levels fall below 10,000 mm³
- Chemotherapy (interferon-2α) is reserved for patients with life-threatening coagulopathy
- Vascular malformations
  - Present at birth, though some appear later in childhood in response to infection
  - Sudden enlargement can be seen with infection, trauma, or adolescence
  - Divided into high-flow (arteriovenous malformation) and low-flow (lymphatic, venous, and capillary) lesions
  - MRI or CT diagnostic
  - Lymphatic malformation is the most common vascular malformation of the head and neck in children
  - Lymphatic malformation can distort the facial skeleton such as the mandible; arteriovenous malformation can cause bony destruction
- Management of vascular malformations
  - Lymphatic malformations (Fig. 6.8)
    - Classified as macrocystic versus microcystic, infrahyoid versus suprahyoid and unilateral versus bilateral
    - Large suprahyoid microcystic malformations are more problematic
    - MRI or CT for diagnosis and characterization of lesions
    - Sclerotherapy (doxycycline, alcohol, and OK-432) is useful for macrocystic lesions
    - Surgical excision is most effective for localized macrocystic lesions
    - Cranial nerve or great vessel injury is possible with excision of extensive microcystic lesions
    - Laser (carbon dioxide [CO₂], Nd:YAG [neodymium-doped yttrium aluminum garnet]) or radiofrequency ablation for oral cavity and tongue
  - Venous malformations
    - May be present in muscle tissue under skin or mucosa; will enlarge with Valsalva maneuver and have a bluish hue
    - CT scan may show phleboliths
    - May have associated coagulopathy
    - Treatment with sclerotherapy and/or surgery
  - Capillary malformations
    - Persistently dilated skin capillaries
    - Serial pulse-dye laser therapy
    - If involving the upper face and eyelid, need brain MRI and ophthalmology evaluation to assess for Sturge-Weber syndrome

- Arteriovenous malformations
  - High-flow vascular malformations
  - Pulsatile mass or diffuse area of increased blood flow
  - Diagnosed with MRI or CT angiography
  - Four clinical stages: Dormancy, expansion, destruction, and heart failure
  - Treatment: Observation versus surgical excision with preoperative embolization
- Sturge-Weber syndrome
  - Capillary malformation that involves the eye and skin (CN V1) as well as the leptomeninges
  - Presents as port wine stain of the upper face and eyelid
  - Requires brain MRI and ophthalmology evaluation
  - Associated with seizures, developmental delay, and focal neurological deficits

Infectious Neck Masses

- Atypical mycobacterial infection (Fig. 6.9)
  - Also known as *nontuberculous mycobacterial infection*; must be distinguished from mycobacterium tuberculosis
  - Node enlarging slowly over weeks to months in the jugulodigastric or submandibular area, possibly with fluctuance; less often involves the periparotid or submandibular regions
  - Classically involves the skin with violaceous hue and may spontaneously drain; therefore, diagnosis can be made on clinical grounds
  - Fever is rare, and there are few systemic effects with no pulmonary involvement; however, chest x-ray (CXR) should be obtained
  - Purified protein derivative may be negative or with an intermediate reaction (5–15 mm induration) in atypical infection; cultures may take several weeks to grow and may also be negative in culture-positive specimens
  - Infectious disease consultation
    - Antimycobacterial drug therapy may be offered
    - Clarithromycin/azithromycin may also be effective
  - Natural history is of resolution in the immunocompetent patient
  - May lead to chronic draining fistula for 3 to 6 months
  - Curettage treatment may be safely offered
  - Superficial parotidectomy/submandibular gland excision for refractory infections
- Pediatric acute sialadenitis
  - Reduced salivary flow is a common initiator
  - Ductal metaplasia can occur

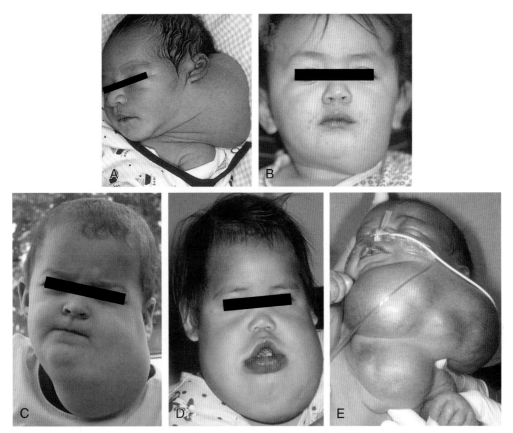

Fig. 6.8 Head and neck lymphatic malformation stages. (**A**) Stage 1, unilateral infrahyoid. (**B**) Stage 2, unilateral suprahyoid. (**C**) Stage 3, unilateral suprahyoid and infrahyoid. (**D**) Stage 4, bilateral suprahyoid. (**E**) Stage 5, bilateral suprahyoid and infrahyoid. (From Flint PW, Haughey BH, Lund VJ, et al. *Cummings Otolaryngology—Head and Neck Surgery.* 6th ed. Philadelphia, PA: Saunders; 2015.)

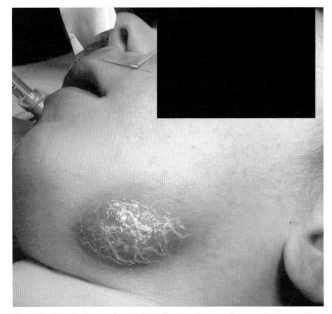

Fig. 6.9 Atypical mycobacterial infection in an advanced stage with skin erosion. (From Flint PW, Haughey BH, Lund VJ, et al. *Cummings Otolaryngology—Head and Neck Surgery.* 6th ed. Philadelphia, PA: Saunders; 2015.)

- Rule out autoimmune disease
  - Sjögren syndrome
  - Sarcoidosis

- Rule out obstruction
  - Stricture
  - Stone
- Rule out functional disease
  - Medication
  - Metabolic (diabetes)
- Rule out infectious etiology
  - Microbiology
    - *S. aureus*
    - *Streptococcus viridans*
    - *S. pneumoniae*
    - *Escherichia coli*
- First initiate conservative therapy with hydration, sialogogues, and glandular massage
- If this fails or bacterial infection is suspected, then add antibiotics
- If stone identified, consider sialendoscopy

Neoplastic Neck Masses

- Most common head and neck malignancies in children under 1 year old
  1. Retinoblastoma
  2. Neuroblastoma
  3. Germ cell neoplasms
  4. Rhabdomyosarcoma
- Most common head and neck malignancies in children 1 to 5 years old
  1. Retinoblastoma
  2. Rhabdomyosarcoma
  3. Non-Hodgkin lymphoma (NHL)
  4. Hodgkin lymphoma (HL)

- Most common head and neck malignancies in children 6 to 10 years old
  1. HL
  2. Rhabdomyosarcoma
  3. NHL
  4. Thyroid cancer
- Most common head and neck malignancies in children 11 to 18 years old
  1. Thyroid cancer
  2. HL
  3. NHL
  4. Melanoma
- Red flags for children with neck mass
  - Age <12 months
  - Lymph node is nontender and hard
  - Diameter >3 cm
  - Supraclavicular location
  - Persistent generalized lymphadenopathy
  - Mediastinal or abdominal mass
  - Persistent unexplained: Pruritis, fever, weight loss, pallor, fatigue, petechiae, hemorrhagic lesions, or hepatosplenomegaly
- Pediatric thyroid cancer
  - Associated with radiation exposure
  - 90% papillary thyroid CA; others are follicular and medullary (multiple endocrine neoplasia [MEN] syndromes)
  - Thyroid nodules more likely to be malignant in children (25%) than adults (<10%)
  - Management with fine needle aspiration (FNA), total thyroidectomy for papillary thyroid CA, neck dissection for nodal involvement, ± radioactive iodine
  - 5-year survival >95%
- Pediatric salivary gland cancer
  - Most commonly mucoepidermoid CA, and usually low grade
  - Acinic cell CA second most common in children
  - Treatment is surgical with possible adjuvant therapy
- Considerations for pediatric parotid masses
  - Pleomorphic adenoma is the most common benign epithelial tumor
  - Hemangioma is the most common mesenchymal benign mass
  - Mucoepidermoid CA (low grade and well differentiated) is the most common malignant tumor
- Nasopharyngeal carcinoma
  - Rare
  - Associated with Epstein-Barr virus (EBV) infection
  - Often presents as painless neck mass; may also have nasal obstruction, otological complaints
    - May have unilateral otitis media and/or rhinorrhea
  - Increased incidence in African and Asian teenagers
  - Treatment with chemotherapy and radiation
- Differential diagnosis of small blue cell malignancies of childhood
  - Neuroblastoma
  - Lymphoma
  - Rhabdomyosarcoma
  - Peripheral primitive neuroectodermal tumors
- Presentation and assessment for lymphoma
  - Third most common childhood cancer
  - Most common pediatric malignancy of the head and neck
  - History
    - Painless neck swelling
    - Rapid enlargement may cause tenderness
    - Stage B symptoms, which confer worse prognosis
      - Fever above 38.0°C for three consecutive days
      - Unexplained weight loss of 10% or more in 6 months
      - Drenching night sweats

- Physical exam
  - Painless supraclavicular or cervical mass
  - Lymphadenopathy firm on palpation, "rubbery"
  - Explore other lymph node basins
  - Spleen is the most common extranodal site
- Lab work
  - Complete blood count
  - Erythrocyte sedimentation rate
  - C-reactive protein
  - Liver function tests
- Imaging
  - CXR
  - CT neck and chest
  - CT or MRI of abdomen and pelvis
  - Positron emission tomography (PET) has been found to be more accurate than CT for staging: used to track disease response to therapy
- Surgery
  - Mainly for biopsy for diagnosis
  - Specimen should be sent fresh to the pathologist to facilitate flow cytometry, immunohistochemical staining, molecular genetic testing, and electron microscopy
  - Resection is rarely indicated
- Bone marrow biopsy
- Lumbar puncture
- World Health Organization classification of Hodgkin lymphoma
  - HL most commonly found in teenage children
  - Association between HL and EBV infection, may have evidence of prior exposure and in situ hybridization showing EBV genomes and pathognomonic Reed–Sternberg cells
- Classic HL
  - 90% of HL, composed of lymphocyte-depleted, nodular sclerosing, mixed cellularity, and lymphocyte-rich subtypes
  - Mixed cellularity: Pleomorphic lymphocytes, more numerous Reed–Sternberg (RS) cells
  - Nodular sclerosis: Most common classic variant, fibrosis comprising neoplastic and inflammatory cells resulting in nodules
  - Lymphocyte-depleted: Few lymphocytes with many RS cells, associated with HIV, rare in children; when disease is localized and nonbulky, is usually treated by limited cycles of chemotherapy and minimal radiation
  - Lymphocyte predominant: Many small B lymphocytes; can be treated with radiation alone or sometimes surgical excision and observation
- Ann Arbor staging of Hodgkin lymphoma
  - HL treatment is dependent on staging via Ann Arbor
    - Stage 1: Involvement of a single lymph node region (stage I) or single extralymphatic site (stage IE)
    - Stage 2: Involvement of two or more lymph node regions (stage II) or extralymphatic sites (stage IIE) on the same side of the diaphragm
    - Stage 3: Involvement of two or more lymph node regions (stage III) or extralymphatic sites (stage IIIE) on both sides of the diaphragm, the spleen (stage IIIS), or both (stage IIISE)
    - Stage 4: Diffuse or disseminated involvement of one or more extralymphatic organs and tissues with or without associated lymph node involvement (stage IV)
      - A: No systemic symptoms
      - B: Weight loss, fever, or night sweats
- Treatment of Hodgkin lymphoma
  - Combined chemotherapy and radiation therapy is favored approach
    - Reduces side effects compared with radiation therapy or chemotherapy alone

- Long-term disease survival of 85% to 100% in early-stage disease
- Disease survival of 60% in advanced-stage disease
- Non-Hodgkin lymphoma
  - Critical distinction is that almost all pediatric NHLs are high grade
  - Most important prognostic factors are the amount of tumor burden, the stage, and the serum lactate dehydrogenase level
    - Low grade
      - Small lymphocyte
      - Follicular, small cleaved
      - Follicular, small cleaved and large cell mixed
    - Intermediate grade (diffuse)
      - Small cleaved cell
      - Mixed small and large cell
      - Large cell
    - High grade
      - Large cell
      - Lymphoblastic
      - Small cell non-cleaved, Burkitt lymphoma
- St. Jude staging of non-Hodgkin lymphoma
  - Stage I: Single tumor (extranodal) or single anatomical area (nodal) with exclusion of the mediastinum and abdomen
  - Stage II: Single tumor (extranodal) with regional node involvement
    - Two or more nodal areas on the same side of the diaphragm
    - Two single (extranodal) tumors with or without regional node involvement on the same side of the diaphragm
    - Primary gastrointestinal tumor with or without involvement of associated mesenteric nodes only
  - Stage III: Two single tumors (extranodal) on opposite sides of the diaphragm
    - Two or more nodal areas above and below the diaphragm
    - All primary intrathoracic tumors
    - All extensive primary intraabdominal disease
    - All paraspinal or epidural tumors regardless of other tumor sites
  - Stage IV: Any of the abovementioned criteria with initial CNS and/or bone marrow involvement
- Burkitt lymphoma
  - Most common pediatric NHL
  - Cytogenetic evidence of the C-myc rearrangement is the gold standard for diagnosis of Burkitt lymphoma
  - B-cell lineage, classic "starry sky" pattern of ingested apoptotic cells on histology
  - Endemic and sporadic variants: EBV positivity 90% to 95% in endemic cases and 15% to 20% in sporadic cases
- Rhabdomyosarcoma of the head and neck (Table 6.3)
  - 4.5% of all pediatric malignancies and the most common sarcoma of childhood
  - 35% of all cases occur in the head and neck
  - Primary site in the head and neck is the orbit (most common, 25%–35% of cases)
  - Parameningeal tumor sites include the nasopharynx and nasal cavities, paranasal sinuses, infratemporal and pterygopalatine fossae, as well as the middle ear; increased likelihood of cranial nerve palsy and intracranial extension
  - Nonparameningeal sites include all other sites within the head and neck, such as the parotid and submandibular area, and represent more favorable prognostic sites
  - PET CT is the imaging modality of choice
  - Metastatic sites
    - Lungs
    - Bone
    - Bone marrow
- Rhabdomyosarcoma histopathology

- Embryonal: Most common in infants and children; spindle-shaped cells with interspersed large rhabdomyoblasts
  - Botryoidal and pleomorphic variants
  - Higher incidence in Beckwith-Wiedemann syndrome
- Alveolar: Poorer prognosis; worse with PAX3/FOX01 translocation gene; most common in adolescents; small round cells in a dense configuration resembling pulmonary alveoli
- Treatment is multimodal (surgery/chemo/external beam radiation therapy)
  - Primary treatment is combination chemotherapy
  - Surgery not recommended unless able to achieve clear margins; debulking does not improve outcomes
  - Distant metastases may still be surgical candidates
- Neuroblastomas of the head and neck
  - Most common extracerebral solid tumors of infancy and childhood
  - Embryonal tumors of the sympathetic nervous system, along the sympathetic chain from the neck to the pelvis
  - 40% of diagnoses occur before patients are 1 year old, 80% before 5 years old
  - Primary sites in the head and neck (2%–5% of neuroblastomas)
  - Can present with impingement of head and neck structure, such as jugular foramen cranial nerves or upper aerodigestive structures
  - Neck (sympathetic chain): May result in ipsilateral ptosis (Horner syndrome)
  - Orbit: May result in proptosis and periorbital ecchymoses ("panda eyes")
  - Spontaneous regression can occur in infants with small primary tumor
  - Metastatic lesions can occur in the head and neck
  - Check urine or serum catecholamines and metabolites (homovanillic acid, vanillylmandelic acid, and dopamine)
  - Imaging with CT and/or MRI of the neck, chest, abdomen, pelvis
  - Staging system reflects tumor burden, surgical resectability, and pattern of metastases
  - Management consists of surgical removal and chemotherapy

TABLE 6.3 Tumor-Node-Metastasis Pretreatment Staging Classification

Stage	Site	T	Size	Node	Metastases
1	Nonparameningeal	T1 or T2	a or b	N0 or N1 or Nx	M0
2	Parameningeal	T1 or T2	a	N0 or Nx	M0
3	Parameningeal	T1 or T2	a	N1	M0
			b	N0 or N1 or Nx	M0
4	Any	T1 or T2	a or b	N0 or N1 or Nx	M1

T: *T1*, Confined to anatomical site of origin; *T2*, extension and/or fixative to surrounding tissue. Size: *a* ≥5 cm in diameter; *b* >5 cm in diameter. Nodes: *N0*, regional nodes not involved; *N1*, regional nodes involved; *Nx*, regional status unknown. Metastases: *M0*, no distant metastases; *M1*, metastases present (includes positive cytology in cerebrospinal fluid).

Data adapted from Lawrence W Jr., Anderson JR, Gehan EA, Maurer H. Pretreatment TNM staging of childhood rhabdomysarcoma: a report of the Intergroup Rhabdomyosarcoma Study Group. Children's Cancer Study Group. Pediatric Oncology Group. *Cancer.* 1997;80:1165–1170.

- Excisional biopsy with removal of adjacent enlarged nodes is typically performed for head and neck neuroblastoma
- Salvage therapy can be performed after chemotherapy
- Radiation therapy used, but is not curative

NOSE AND PARANASAL SINUS DISEASE

Differential for a Child With Midline Nasal Mass

- Dermoid cyst: Most common. CT scan or MRI of midline nasal masses advised
- Glioma
- Encephalocele
- Hemangioma: Often at nasal tip, but can be intranasal

Furstenberg Sign

- Enlargement of a nasal mass with crying, straining, and compression of the jugular veins; positive sign consistent with encephalocele that communicates with CSF (not glioma or dermoid)

Three Types of Nasal Masses From Developmental Errors of the Anterior Neuropore (Fig. 6.10)

- Glioma
  - Heterotopic glial tissue without patent CSF communication, but may have fibrous stalk

- 60% extranasal (commonly at glabella), 30% intranasal, and 10% combined
- Furstenberg sign: Negative
- Not associated with meningitis
- Management is surgical excisional biopsy
- Extranasal approaches: Lateral rhinotomy, external rhinoplasty, transglabellar subcranial, bicoronal, and midline nasal
- Intranasal approaches: Endoscopic excision
- Encephalocele: Extracranial herniation of cranial contents through a defect in the skull (classification in next section)
  - Pulsatile, bluish compressible lesions that transilluminate
  - Furstenberg sign: Positive
  - Meningocele: Meninges only
  - Meningoencephalocele: Meninges plus brain tissue
  - Management is surgical excision
  - Small cranial bone defect and smaller lesions may be treated endoscopically
  - Larger lesions often require a combined craniotomy
- Dermoid: Frontal nasal inclusion cyst arising from tract related to an embryological defect of the anterior neuropore
  - Midline nasal pit or mass that may occur from the nasal tip to the cranial space
  - Protruding hair from the sinus opening is pathognomonic
  - Firm, lobulated, and noncompressible mass
  - Intracranial extension in 4% to 45% of cases
  - Recurrent meningitis suggests intracranial tract

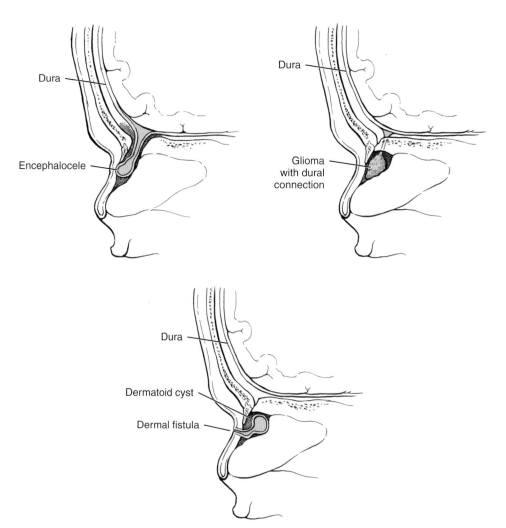

Fig. 6.10 Schematic view of the common midline nasal masses. (From Flint PW, Haughey BH, Lund VJ, et al. *Cummings Otolaryngology—Head and Neck Surgery*. 6th ed. Philadelphia, PA: Saunders; 2015.)

- Management is surgical: External rhinoplasty, lateral rhinotomy, transglabellar, subcranial, paracanthal, and bicoronal
- Intracranial extension: Craniotomy

Classification of Congenital Nasal Encephaloceles

- Sincipital: 25% of all encephaloceles, usually causes some degree of visible deformity around the nose
  - Nasofrontal: Glabellar mass causing telecanthus and inferior displacement of nasal bones
  - Nasoethmoidal: Dorsal nasal mass causing superior displacement of nasal bones and inferior displacement of alar cartilages
  - Naso-orbital: Orbital mass causing proptosis and visual disturbance
- Basal: Less common, present as intranasal masses, often not discovered until later in childhood
  - Transethmoidal (most common subtype): Passed through cribriform plate, unilateral nasal mass, may result in hypertelorism
  - Spheno-ethmoidal: Passes through defect between posterior ethmoid and sphenoid, unilateral nasal mass, may also result in hypertelorism
  - Trans-sphenoidal: Nasopharyngeal mass passing through defect to cranium, associated with cleft palate
  - Spheno-orbital: Passes through superior and inferior orbital fissures into sphenopalatine fossa, unilateral exophthalmos or diplopia

Embryologic Structures and Spaces Related to Nasal Gliomas, Encephaloceles, and Dermoids

- Anterior neuropore: Most distal end of the ectoderm-derived neural tube
- Prenasal space: Behind the nasal bones but in front of the nasal and septal cartilages
- Foramen cecum: Defect in the anterior skull base at the apex of the prenasal space that normally closes after a dural diverticulum retracts from the prenasal space into the cranium
  - May not close (encephalocele) or may close prematurely (glioma)
- Fonticulus nasofrontalis: Fontanelle between inferior frontal bones and nasal bones

Causes of Congenital Nasal Obstruction

- Choanal atresia
- Pyriform aperture stenosis
- Nasolacrimal duct cysts
- Hemangioma: Can be infantile (develops shortly after birth) or congenital (present at birth)
- Nasopharyngeal teratoma: Germ cell tumor containing tissue foreign to anatomical site; management is surgical excision

Choanal Atresia/Stenosis

- Unilateral more common than bilateral
- Commonly associated with other congenital abnormalities (e.g., CHARGE syndrome [*c*oloboma, *h*eart disease, *a*tresia of the choanae, *r*etarded growth and mental development, *g*enital anomalies, and *e*ar abnormalities])
- Mixed bony-membranous atresia more common than pure bony atresia (pure membranous atresia not seen)
- Diagnosis confirmed with endoscopy and CT imaging (Fig. 6.11)
- Bilateral choanal atresia presents with respiratory distress at birth
- Unilateral choanal atresia repair can be delayed to allow growth and ease of repair
- Transnasal repair now preferred over transpalatal

Piriform Aperture Stenosis

- May be misdiagnosed as choanal atresia
- Diagnosis confirmed by CT imaging: Reduction in width of piriform aperture (Fig. 6.12)

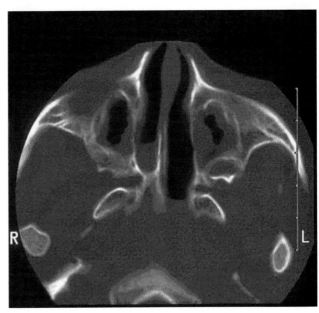

Fig. 6.11 Axial computed tomography scan of unilateral choanal atresia with a complete bony atretic plate and associated soft tissue. (From Flint PW, Francis HW, Haughey BH, et al. *Cummings Otolaryngology—Head and Neck Surgery*. 7th ed. Philadelphia, PA: Saunders; 2020, Fig. 190.18.)

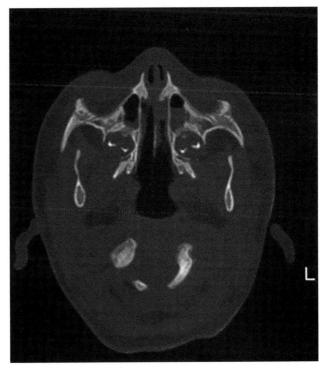

Fig. 6.12 Axial computed tomography scan showing stenosis of the piriform aperture secondary to overgrowth of the nasal process of the maxilla, causing a reduction in the width of the piriform aperture (anterior width of the floor of the nose). A pyriform aperture width of less than 6 mm in neonates is thought to be clinically significant and will likely need surgical correction. (From Flint PW, Francis HW, Haughey BH, et al. *Cummings Otolaryngology—Head and Neck Surgery*. 7th ed. Philadelphia, PA: Saunders; 2020, Fig. 190.14.)

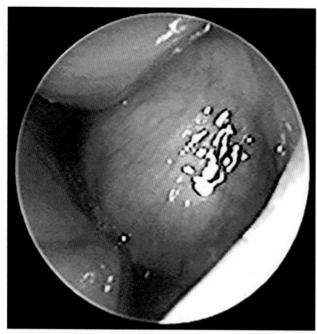

Fig. 6.13 Left nasolacrimal duct cyst in the inferior meatus as seen on anterior rhinoscopy. (From Flint PW, Francis HW, Haughey BH, et al. *Cummings Otolaryngology—Head and Neck Surgery.* 7th ed. Philadelphia, PA: Saunders; 2020, Fig. 190.16.)

- Can occur in isolation
- Commonly associated with holoproscencephaly: Failure of forebrain to cleave in hemispheres, central mega-incisor frequently present
- Medical management is possible: Steroid or decongestant drops can be used
- Surgical repair with sublabial approach with drill to enlarge lateral and inferior bony margins of aperture with subsequent stenting

Nasolacrimal Duct Cysts (Dacrocystoceles)

- Found in inferior meatus on anterior rhinoscopy or endoscopy (Fig. 6.13)
- May cause nasal obstruction and possibly respiratory distress
- CT to confirm diagnosis
- Surgical management with endoscopic marsupialization, possibly coordination with ophthalmology for nasolacrimal duct probing and stenting

Juvenile Nasopharyngeal Angiofibroma

- Benign but locally aggressive tumor that can extend to and beyond skull base
- Most commonly in adolescent males
- Unilateral epistaxis with nasal obstruction
- Imaging: CT and MRI with contrast
- Surgical management
  - Preoperative angiography and embolization
  - Endoscopic with image guidance
  - Open: Numerous approaches, such as lateral rhinotomy and midface degloving

Common Symptoms of Chronic Pediatric Sinusitis

- Cough
- Rhinorrhea
- Nasal congestion or obstruction
- Postnasal drip
- Facial pain or pressure

Diagnoses With Similar Presentations as Chronic Pediatric Sinusitis

- Adenoid hypertrophy or adenoiditis (much more common that true pediatric sinusitis)
- Allergic rhinitis
- Viral URI

Diagnosis of Chronic Pediatric Sinusitis

- Two or more symptoms
  - Nasal blockage or obstruction
  - Nasal congestion and discharge (anterior and posterior)
  - Cough
  - Facial pain or pressure
- May be difficult to differentiate from adenoid hypertrophy
- Anterior rhinoscopy and nasal endoscopy if possible
- Imaging
  - Plain film to assess adenoid size
  - CT sinus: Maxillary sinus most commonly involved on imaging

Lund-Mackay System for CT Sinus Findings

- Each sinus (anterior ethmoid, posterior ethmoid, maxillary, frontal, and sphenoid) is scored: 0 (no opacification), 1 (partial opacification), and 2 (total opacification)
- Osteomeatal complex is scored: 0 (not occluded) and 2 (total occluded)
- Right and left sinuses are scored separately and added together
- Lund score ranges from 0 to 24 in total
- Score of 5 or more predictive of chronic sinusitis

Diagnoses to Consider When Nasal Polyps Seen

- Cystic fibrosis
- Allergic fungal sinusitis: Expansile polyps
- Antrochoanal polyp (unilateral)

Conditions Associated With Chronic Pediatric Sinusitis

- Allergic rhinitis
- Asthma
- Gastroesophageal reflex disease (GERD)
- Immunodeficiency and immunoglobulin deficiency
- Primary ciliary dyskinesia: Diagnosed by mucosal biopsy (nasal or preferably tracheal) or nasal brush biopsy with electron microscopic examination of cilia
- Cystic fibrosis
  - Increased viscosity of secretions
  - Nasal polyposis (one of the few causes of polyposis in children)
  - Diagnosis with sweat chloride or genetic testing

Medical Therapy for Chronic Pediatric Sinusitis

- Nasal saline
- Nasal decongestant: Beware of overuse
- Intranasal steroids
- Consider oral steroids

- Antihistamine if there is documented allergic rhinitis
- Antibiotics
  - Frequently given despite lack of evidence
  - Amoxicillin, amoxicillin with clavulanate, cephalosporins, macrolides, and clindamycin most commonly prescribed
  - Duration: 3 to 6 weeks

Surgical Treatment for Failed Maximum Medical Therapy

- Adenoidectomy
- Sinus irrigation: May be performed with adenoidectomy
- Balloon dilation: Sinus irrigation usually performed through dilated ostia
- Functional endoscopic sinus surgery

Factors that Predispose to Functional Endoscopic Sinus Surgery Failure in Children

- Adhesions
- Maxillary sinus stenosis or missed accessory ostium
- Sinonasal polyposis
- History of allergic rhinitis
- Male gender

Bacteria Most Commonly Associated With Chronic Pediatric Sinusitis

- Aerobes: α-Hemolytic streptococci, *S. aureus*, *S. pneumoniae*, *H. influenzae*, and *M. catarrhalis*
- Anaerobes: Infrequently identified

Viruses Most Commonly Associated With Acute Sinusitis

- Rhinovirus
- Coronavirus
- Influenza
- Respiratory syncytial virus (RSV)
- Parainfluenza

Bacteria Most Commonly Associated With Acute Pediatric Sinusitis

- *S. pneumoniae*
- *H. influenzae*
- *M. catarrhalis*
- *S. aureus*
- α-Hemolytic strep

Indications for Computed Tomography Scanning for Pediatric Acute Sinusitis

- Concern for the presence of a complication (often orbital or intracranial) related to sinusitis
- Severe illness or toxic condition that does not improve with medical therapy after 48 to 72 hours
- Immunocompromise

Chandler Classification for Orbital Complications of Sinusitis

- I: Preseptal
- II: Orbital cellulitis
- III: Subperiosteal abscess
- IV: Orbital abscess
- V: Cavernous sinus thrombosis

PHARYNX, LARYNX, TRACHEA, AND ESOPHAGUS

Assessment of an Infant or Child With "Noisy Breathing"

- History
  - Onset of stridor (What is the age of onset? Sudden or gradual?)
  - Character of stridor (inspiratory, biphasic, or expiratory)
  - Strength of cry and characteristic of vocalization (e.g., strong or weak)
  - Frequency (Constant or episodic? Hourly or daily?) and progression (Better or worse?)
  - Triggers (What events make the stridor better or worse?)
  - Exacerbating and relieving factors (Medications, temperature, humidification, exercise, or position?)
  - Ability to feed (Presence of coughing, choking, or cyanosis? Volume and length of bottle/breastfeeds?)
  - Activity level (Strength to feed, play, exercise, and climb stairs?)
  - Presence of GERD symptoms (Postprandial vomiting, restless sleep, or opisthotonos?)
  - History of perinatal or neonatal events (Neonatal ICU stay? Less than 36 weeks? Prior endotracheal intubation, including length? Patent ductus arteriosus [PDA] ligation?)
- Physical examination
  - General appearance, color (e.g., cyanosis) of lips or fingers, increased work of breathing (respiratory rate: infants >40/min; toddlers >30/min)
  - Signs of distress and impending respiratory failure (Slow prolonged inspirations?)
  - Inspection of neck and thorax for retractions or accessory muscle use
  - Listening for the character of stridor (inspiratory, biphasic, or expiratory)
  - Pulse oximetry (below 90% on room air or need for supplemental oxygen)
  - Nasal patency in infants (Can a 5 Fr feeding tube pass bilaterally?)
  - Auscultation of mouth, neck, and chest (Location and intensity of stridor, wheezes, airflow, rales?)
  - Location of stridor by its auditory pattern
    - Inspiratory: Supraglottis and glottis
    - Biphasic: Glottis, subglottis, and upper trachea
    - Expiratory: Mid to lower trachea
  - Craniofacial anomalies (e.g., midface hypoplasia; retrognathic mandible; macroglossia, skeletal dysplasia; short or fused cervical spine)
- Evaluation (the "workup")
  - What should be done depends on clinical stability of child's airway (Which setting is appropriate [outpatient, emergency department, ICU]? Does the patient require intubation?)
  - Medical imaging may be of limited utility if the acuity of the child is worrisome or perilous (will often need personnel for clinical monitoring)
    - CXR anteroposterior (AP)/lateral film (pulmonary aeration/atelectasis, tracheal air column, cardiac location and size)
    - AP/lateral neck film (Are soft-tissue masses present? What is the position of tongue and patency of the nasopharynx? Any narrowing in the subglottis, i.e., steeple sign?)
    - CT scan of head, neck, and thorax (teratoma, vascular malformation, tracheal/bronchial anomalies)
    - MRI of head, neck, thorax, and abdomen (lymphatic malformation)

- Observation versus airway endoscopy is the gold standard
  - Observation for critically ill or unstable patients may be prudent depending on the clinical findings and imaging
  - Airway endoscopy requires skilled pediatric anesthesiologists, otolaryngologists, and intensivists
- Flexible fiberoptic laryngoscopy (FFL) when practical considering equipment and clinical setting and status
  - Assess nasal cavities, nasopharynx, oropharynx, hypopharynx, tongue base, and supraglottic larynx
  - Assess vocal fold appearance and mobility
- Direct laryngoscopy and bronchoscopy
  - Allows for airway visualization as well as ability to secure the airway (if not intubated already)
  - Identification and removal of supraglottic, glottic, subglottic, or tracheal lesions (e.g., cysts, papilloma, and lymphatic malformations)
  - Ability to assess for tracheal developmental anomalies (e.g., stenosis, complete rings, and mediastinal compression)
  - Indications for laryngoscopy and bronchoscopy
    - Severe stridor with impending respiratory failure (may require initial intubation)
    - Progressive and worsening stridor
    - Any event of stridor associated with cyanosis, apneic episodes, dysphagia, severe choking, progressive failure to thrive (FTT), or radiologic abnormality identifying or suggesting airway lesion
    - Stridor not explained by outpatient FFL examination
    - History or clinical findings suggestive of ingested or aspirated foreign body

One-Month-Old Infant With Inspiratory Stridor Since Birth, Worse With Crying and When Supine: What Are the Most Likely Diagnoses?

- Laryngomalacia (most likely)
- Vocal fold paralysis
- Congenital subglottic stenosis

Pediatric Airway Abnormalities That Are Worse When Supine

- Laryngomalacia
- Tongue-base lesions or collapse (e.g., vallecular cysts, micrognathia, or Pierre Robin sequence)
- Vascular compression
- Mediastinal mass

Laryngomalacia

- Clinical characteristics
  - Inspiratory stridor: Noticed shortly after birth, worse with crying, feeding, or in supine position
  - May exhibit reflux symptoms: Arching of back and frequent spit-ups
  - Most cases will improve with time as long as the child feeds well and gains weight
  - Severe cases may result in FTT, apneic events, and cyanotic episodes
  - Symptoms may be worse in the patient with neuromuscular disorders
- Anatomical characteristics (Fig. 6.14)
  - Floppy or flaccid laryngeal tissues: Mucosa of the arytenoids and aryepiglottic folds and cartilage of the epiglottis
  - Narrowed or "omega-shaped" epiglottis

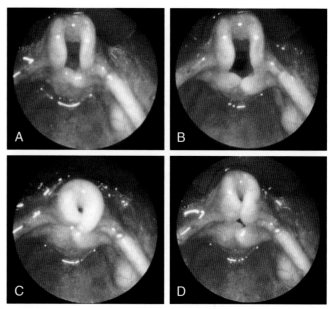

Fig. 6.14 Laryngomalacia. Progressive airway obstruction on inspiration. Note from frames A to D the progressive curling of the omega-shaped epiglottis and prolapse of the arytenoids on inspiration. (From Benjamin B. The pediatric airway. In: Slide Lecture Series, American Academy of Otolaryngology—Head and Neck Surgery. 1992; and Flint PW, Haughey BH, Lund VJ, et al. *Cummings Otolaryngology—Head and Neck Surgery.* 6th ed. Philadelphia, PA: Saunders; 2015.)

- Shortened aryepiglottic folds
- Poor visualization of vocal folds because of supraglottic collapse
- Indications for intervention in severe laryngomalacia
  - Indications
    - FTT from poor feeding
    - Airway obstruction resulting in apnea and/or cyanosis
    - Pulmonary hypertension and cor pulmonale
    - Severe chest deformity
  - Interventions
    - Medical treatment of reflux (H2 blockers; proton pump inhibitors)
    - Direct suspension laryngoscopy with bronchoscopy with supraglottoplasty: Division of aryepiglottic fold and removal of redundant arytenoid mucosa along with evaluation for secondary lesions
    - Partial epiglottectomy or epiglottopexy
    - Tracheostomy: When severe and unresponsive to prior interventions

Vocal Fold Paralysis

- Unilateral
  - Iatrogenic (most common)
    - Thoracic surgery (e.g., prior aortic arch surgery or PDA ligation)
    - Tracheoesophageal fistula (TEF) repair
  - Birth trauma
    - Cervical traction-type injury (e.g., forceps delivery)
  - Idiopathic
- Bilateral
  - Idiopathic (most common with neurological close second)
  - Neurological disease
    - Arnold-Chiari malformation
    - Meningomyelocele
    - Hydrocephalus
    - Neonatal subdural hemorrhage or hematoma

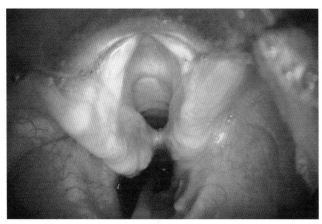

Fig. 6.15 Laryngotracheal cleft: Benjamin-Inglis Type III. (From Benjamin B. The pediatric airway. In: Slide Lecture Series, American Academy of Otolaryngology—Head and Neck Surgery. 1992; and Flint PW, Haughey BH, Lund VJ, et al. *Cummings Otolaryngology—Head and Neck Surgery.* 6th ed. Philadelphia, PA: Saunders; 2015.)

- Malignant disease (intracranial, cervical, or thoracic)
- Genetic syndrome (Mobius)

Arnold-Chiari Malformation

- Herniation of the cerebellum through the foramen magnum of the skull
- Pressure injury on the vagus nerves may result in bilateral vocal cord paralysis
- Diagnosed by MRI of the brain
- Early evaluation and neurosurgical decompression are most often recommended

Laryngeal and Laryngotracheoesophageal Clefts

- Failure of fusion of the posterior cricoid lamina
- Benjamin-Inglis Classification is most commonly used
  - Type I: Interarytenoid cleft (just above or at the level of the vocal folds)
    - Medical management (thickening liquid feeds, upright positioning for drinking, and control of reflux) may be adequate
  - Type II: Partial or complete cricoid cleft, extends below the level of the vocal cords and partially into the cricoid lamina
  - Type III: Total cricoid cleft with extension into the cervical trachea (Fig. 6.15)
  - Type IV: Laryngotracheoesophageal cleft into the intrathoracic trachea/carina

Factors That Support Surgical Repair of Laryngeal Cleft

- Recurrent aspiration and "wet" tracheal cough
- Recurrent pneumonias and hospitalizations
- Intermittent airway obstruction
- Extent of cleft (Type I, injection augmentation vs. endoscopic repair; Type II and proximal Type III, endoscopic repair vs. open repair; Types III and IV, open repair)

Recurrent Respiratory Papillomatosis

- Etiology and prevention
  - Human papillomavirus (HPV) infection (common types 6 and 11) resulting in proliferation of benign squamous papillomas within the respiratory tract

- Vertical transmission from cervical HPV in the young mother during delivery
- 9 valent HPV vaccine approved by the Centers for Disease Control and Prevention, recommended starting at ages 11 to 12 years and including all individuals up to age 26 years (and some through age 45 years)
- Types
  - Juvenile onset: More aggressive disease, typically diagnosed before the age of 5 years
    - Aggressive disease associated with more surgical procedures per year/more involved anatomical sites
  - Adult onset: Less aggressive, slower progression, with higher likelihood of becoming disease free
- Symptoms
  - Hoarseness: Principal presenting symptom (also second most frequent cause of hoarseness in pediatric patients)
  - Stridor: Second presenting symptom
  - Acute respiratory distress
  - Extralaryngeal spread
    - Oral cavity
    - Trachea
    - Bronchi
    - Lungs: May cause destruction of parenchyma (blebs, cysts, and cavitating lesions)
  - Higher risk of malignant carcinomatous transformation

Treatment Modalities for Recurrent Respiratory Papillomatosis

- Surgical debulking with preservation of normal structures
  - Microlaryngoscopy with forceps or powered microdebrider (currently the favored technique of pediatric otolaryngologists)
  - Laser
    - Direct line of sight required for CO_2 laser using micromanipulator
    - Controlled destruction with excellent hemostasis
    - Possible increased scar formation
    - Laser smoke may contain active viral DNA (requires smoke evacuation system and appropriate personal protective equipment, including N95 mask or greater)
    - Growing use of potassium-titanyl-phosphate (KTP) laser using handpiece
  - Tracheostomy for severe airway obstruction (generally try to avoid unless absolutely necessary due to concerns with distal airway spread)
- Adjuvant medical therapy: 20% of patients will require some medical treatments
  - General criteria for use:
    - More than four surgeries per year
    - Rapid regrowth of papilloma with airway compromise
    - Distal multisite spread of disease
  - Interferon therapy: Initial and most common adjuvant therapy but use has decreased because of side effects and the emergence of other therapies
  - Cidofovir
    - Broad-spectrum antiviral agent
    - Currently the most frequently used adjuvant therapy
    - Guideline indications
      - More than six surgeries per year
      - Decreasing interval between surgeries
      - Extralaryngeal spread
  - Avastin (bevacizumab)
    - Recombinant monoclonal antibody that inhibits vascular endothelial growth factors (VEGFs)
    - Most commonly used as intralesional injection in combination with surgical and laser treatment

- Photodynamic therapy
- Indole-3-carbimol: Nutritional supplement found in cruciferous vegetables
- Mumps vaccine
- HPV therapeutic vaccines

Subglottic Hemangioma (Fig. 6.16)

- Twice as common in females than in males; 50% of infants with airway hemangiomas will have cutaneous hemangiomas
- Typically present in the first 6 months of life with inspiratory or biphasic stridor: Barking cough that responds temporarily to oral steroids ("recurrent croup")
- Grows rapidly in first 6 months, stabilizes for ~1 year, and then slowly involutes
- Diagnosis by direct laryngoscopy and bronchoscopy

Treatment Options for Airway Hemangioma

- Observation with close monitoring
- Propranolol is currently first-line therapy; pretreatment cardiac evaluation is recommended
  - Children with PHACE (*p*osterior fossa abnormalities, *h*emangioma, *a*rterial abnormalities in the brain, *c*ardiac anomalies, and *e*ye abnormalities) have higher risk of stroke with propranolol use
- Systemic or intralesional steroids
- Laser excision
- Laryngotracheoplasty (may be useful for circumferential or bilateral hemangiomas)
- Tracheotomy

Subglottic Stenosis

- Etiology
  - Congenital (term newborn cricoid diameter <4mm)
    - Membranous: Fibrous connective tissue or hyperplastic dilated mucous glands, usually circumferential
    - Cartilaginous (more common than membranous and more variable): Most common is thickening or deformity of cricoid cartilage, causing a shelf-like plate
- "Elliptical cricoid ring" seen in Down syndrome
  - Acquired (more common than congenital)
    - Intubation
    - Laryngeal trauma: Prior airway surgery, inhalational injury, or external trauma
    - Chronic inflammatory, infectious, or autoimmune processes: Granulomatosis with polyangiitis (Wegener), tuberculosis, systemic lupus erythematosus, relapsing polychondritis, and sarcoidosis
    - Neoplasm: Chondroma, hemangioma, and carcinoma
- Classification System of Laryngeal and Subglottic Stenosis
  - Laryngeal
    - Grade I: <70%
    - Grade II: 70% to 90%
    - Grade III: >90%, identifiable lumen
    - Grade IV: No lumen
  - Subglottic stenosis (Myer-Cotton)
    - Grade I: <50%
    - Grade II: 51% to 70%
    - Grade III: 71% to 99%
    - Grade IV: Complete stenosis

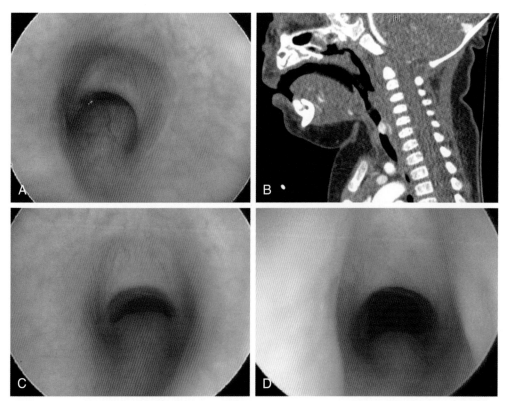

Fig. 6.16 Endoscopic and computed tomography (CT) appearance of focal tracheal hemangioma. (**A**) Before propranolol therapy. (**B**) CT angiogram of tracheal hemangioma. (**C**) After 1 month of propranolol therapy. (**D**) After 4 months of propranolol therapy. (From Flint PW, Haughey BH, Lund VJ, et al. *Cummings Otolaryngology—Head and Neck Surgery.* 6th ed. Philadelphia, PA: Saunders; 2015.)

- Reduction in the area of a subglottic airway when the radius of a full-term infant is reduced by 1 mm
  - Cross-sectional area of subglottis reduced by approximately 50% to 60%
- Approach to repair of subglottic stenosis
  - Technique depends on the patient's age and overall health (e.g., comorbidities) as well as characteristics of stenosis (e.g., location, severity, length, shape [concentric, elliptical], and maturity)
  - Tracheotomy may have already been placed depending on the severity
  - Grade I/II → observation, steroids, and nebulizers for acute exacerbations
  - Grade II/III → endoscopic or open repair
  - Grade III/IV → open repair
- Contraindications to open airway repair
  - Significant and poorly controlled reflux
  - Ventilation requirements (i.e., may benefit from continued intubation or tracheostomy)
- Surgical treatment of subglottic stenosis
  - Endoscopic: Option for symptomatic Grade II/III lesions
    - Laser (CO_2) with radial cuts
    - Microlaryngeal suspension and cup forceps or microdebrider as "cold" techniques with radial cuts
    - Balloon dilation
    - Consider adjuvant treatments (e.g., steroids and mitomycin C)
  - Open: Indicated for Grade III/IV lesions
    - Tracheostomy
    - Anterior cricoid split: Typically used in neonates with good pulmonary function; can augment with cartilage graft (e.g., auricular and thyroid ala)
    - Laryngotracheal reconstruction
      - Anterior ± posterior cricoid split and augmentation with cartilage (e.g., rib, thyroid ala, and hyoid bone)
        - Stage 1: Tracheostomy is removed or avoided and patient is kept intubated for several days to a week for stenting (Fig. 6.17)
        - Stage 2: Tracheostomy is kept and stent is placed above the trach
    - Cricotracheal resection: Severe Grade III or IV subglottic/tracheal stenosis starting at least 1 cm distal to the vocal cords
- Indications for anterior cricoid split for neonates

- Two or more failed extubations secondary to small cricoid ring or extensive submucosal fibrosis with a healthy cricoid
- Weight >1500 g
- No assisted ventilation for 10 days
- Minimal or no supplemental oxygen requirement (fraction of inspired oxygen [FiO_2] <30%)
- No congestive heart failure for 1 month
- No acute URI
- No antihypertensive medications for 10 days
- Indications for laryngotracheal reconstruction with cartilage grafts
  - Glottic or subglottic stenosis (Grade II or III)
  - No significant tracheomalacia or tracheal obstruction
- Indications for long-term stenting in airway reconstruction
  - Extensive circumferential scarring
  - Prior failed airway reconstruction
  - Lack of airway rigidity
  - Craniofacial or vertebral anomalies (avoid potentially difficult reintubation)
- Various stents used in pediatric airway reconstruction
  - Endotracheal tube
  - Montgomery T-tube
  - Aboulker fluoroplastic stent
  - Cotton-Lorenz fluoroplastic stent

Tracheostomy Recommendations

- Lower FiO_2 before entry into trachea
- Vertical tracheal incision
- Stay sutures in tracheal rings labeled "left" and "right" taped to chest until first trach change
- "Maturing" sutures connecting trachea to superior/inferior skin incision
- Flex neck and snuggly place Velcro or twill tape tracheotomy ties (able to admit fingertip only)
- Postoperative observation in pediatric ICU
- Smaller-size tracheostomy tube at the bedside
- No tracheostomy change or manipulation of sutures or ties until stoma matures (postoperative days [PODs] 3–7)
- Daily change of dressing under the tracheotomy ties to avoid moisture and skin breakdown
- Monitor neck skin twice a day at minimum
- Consult "wound care" nurse early if any concern for ulceration
- Monitor nutritional status/body weight of neonates

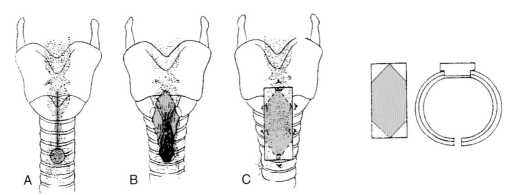

Fig. 6.17 Anterior cartilage graft. (**A**) Vertical incision is made into the thyroid cartilage from a point immediately below the anterior commissure through the upper tracheal rings, with care taken to remain in the midline. (**B**) Intraluminal scar and lining mucosa are incised along the length of the stenotic segment. (**C**) Costal cartilage is shaped into a modified boat (*inset*) and placed in position with the lining of the perichondrium facing internally. (From Flint PW, Haughey BH, Lund VJ, et al. *Cummings Otolaryngology—Head and Neck Surgery.* 6th ed. Philadelphia, PA: Saunders; 2015.)

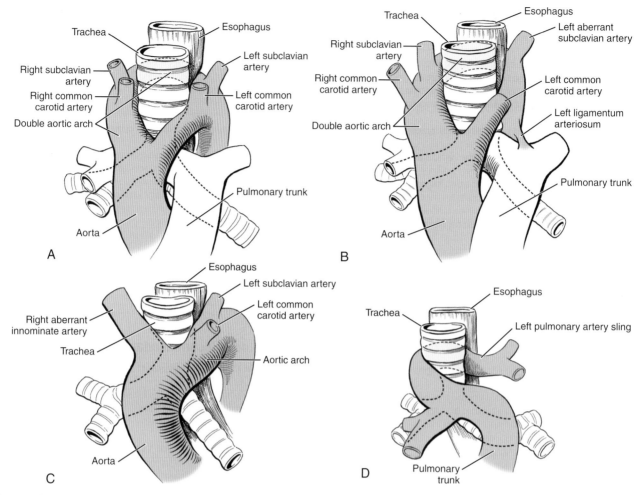

Fig. 6.18 (**A**) Double aortic arch. (**B**) Right aortic arch with aberrant left subclavian artery and left ligamentum arteriosum. (**C**) Aberrant innominate artery. (**D**) Left pulmonary artery sling. (From Flint PW, Haughey BH, Lund VJ, et al. *Cummings Otolaryngology—Head and Neck Surgery*. 6th ed. Philadelphia, PA: Saunders; 2015.)

Tracheal Anomalies

- Etiology
  - Tracheomalacia
  - Vascular compression (complete and incomplete vascular rings)
  - Segmental stenosis
  - Complete tracheal rings
  - TEF
  - Hemangioma
  - Tracheal cyst
- Most common congenital vascular anomalies that can cause tracheomalacia (Fig. 6.18)
  - Double aortic arch (most common complete vascular ring)
  - Right aortic arch with aberrant left subclavian artery and left ligamentum arteriosum (second most common complete vascular ring)
  - Innominate artery compression (most common form of incomplete vascular ring)
    - Abnormally distal takeoff from aortic arch causing anterior compression of the trachea 1 to 2 cm above the carina
  - Left pulmonary artery sling
    - Left pulmonary artery arises from the right pulmonary artery and passes between the esophagus and trachea, compressing the right main-stem bronchus and distal trachea
    - Associated with complete tracheal rings and long-segment stenosis in 50% of patients
- Tracheoesophageal fistula (TEF)
  - Symptoms and workup
    - Respiratory distress
    - Cyanosis during nursing
    - Excessive drooling
    - Inability to pass a feeding tube
    - CXR may show gastric bubble
    - Contrast radiographical studies may present a risk of significant pulmonary aspiration
    - Endoscopy is the mainstay for diagnosis
  - Types
    - Esophageal atresia (EA) and distal TEF (85%)
    - Isolated EA (8%)
    - H-type TEF (4%)
    - EA with proximal TEF (3%)
    - EA with proximal and distal TEF (<1%)
  - Management
    - Immediate gastrostomy tube placement
    - Surgical correction at 3 months of age
    - May require dilation of esophageal strictures
    - Risk of recurrent laryngeal nerve injury

- VATER association
  - V: Vertebral/vascular anomalies
  - A: Anal atresia
  - T: Tracheal anomalies (e.g., TEF)
  - E: Esophageal anomalies (e.g., distal stenosis or agenesis)
  - R: Renal/radial bone anomalies
  - VACTERL association
    - C: Cardiac anomalies (e.g., PDA and valve abnormalities)
    - L: Limb anomalies (e.g., extra digits and shortened limbs)
- Surgical management of tracheal stenosis
  - Endoscopic approach
    - Cold knife lysis
    - Laser ablation
    - Dilation (balloon dilation is the most common)
    - Stents
  - Open approaches
    - Patch tracheoplasty: Rib cartilage and pericardium
    - Segmental resection with primary anastomosis
    - Anterior wedge resection: Localized stenosis (e.g., tracheotomy site stenosis)
    - Tracheal autograft
    - Slide tracheoplasty
    - Transplant (autograft or allograft)
  - Complications
    - Granulation tissue
    - Restenosis
    - Injury to the recurrent laryngeal nerve
    - Dehiscence of repair
    - Tracheobronchomalacia
    - TEF
    - Aspiration

Aerodigestive Foreign Bodies (Table 6.4)

- Occur most commonly in boys under 3 years
- Reliable history and witnessed aspiration or ingestion are most important for diagnosis
- AP/PA (posteroanterior) and lateral x-rays are useful initial studies: Inspiratory and expiratory films or lateral decubitus films may be useful for possible airway foreign body
- Reasonable suspicion of airway foreign body mandates bronchoscopy
- Suspicion of aerodigestive battery foreign body mandates emergent removal
- Mid to distal esophageal foreign bodies in asymptomatic older children may be observed for 8 to 16 hours to see whether the object will pass

Anatomical Areas Where Esophageal Foreign Bodies Routinely Become Lodged

- Upper esophageal sphincter (i.e., cricopharyngeus)
- Aortic arch
- Left main-stem bronchus
- Lower esophageal sphincter

Caustic Ingestions

- Concentration and duration of contact affect the extent of injury
- Acid (pH <7) causes coagulation necrosis: A more superficial injury
- Alkalis (pH >7) produce liquefaction necrosis: A deeper injury
- Bleaches (pH ~7) usually a mild irritant: Does not cause substantial tissue injury

TABLE 6.4 Overview of the Management of Aerodigestive Foreign Bodies

	Airway Foreign Body	Esophageal Foreign Body
History	Witnessed aspiration Cough, dyspnea, wheezing, and stridor Refractory asthma	Witnessed ingestion Vomiting, drooling, dysphagia, odynophagia, emesis, food refusal, and chest pain
Physical examination	Decreased lung sounds, wheezing, and crackles Tachypnea and hypoxemia	Drooling, poor feeding, and choking
Imaging	PA and lateral radiographs (radiopaque foreign body, unilateral emphysema or hyperinflation, and localized atelectasis or infiltrate)	PA and lateral radiographs (radiopaque foreign body, widened prevertebral shadow, loss of lordosis)
Treatment	If adequate suspicion, proceed immediately to rigid bronchoscopy for removal	*Young symptomatic children:* FB present >24 hours or sharp metallic or caustic objects should undergo endoscopic removal *Asymptomatic children:* Recent ingestion (<24 hours), and no esophageal disorders can be observed for 8–16 hours

FB, Foreign body; *PA*, posteroanterior.
From Flint PW, Haughey BH, Lund VJ, et al. *Cummings Otolaryngology—Head and Neck Surgery.* 6th ed. Philadelphia, PA: Saunders; 2015, Table 207-1.

- General pediatric and gastrointestinal consultation
- Complications: Tongue scarring with fixation; soft palate scarring with NP reflux; hypopharyngeal, laryngeal, or esophageal strictures

Initial Management Strategy for Caustic Ingestions (Fig. 6.19)

- Presence of oral injury cannot accurately predict presence or absence of more distal involvement
- Vomiting should not be induced
- Oral dilution with water or milk (limit to 15 mL/kg)
- Intravenous (IV) fluids and nothing by mouth (NPO)
- "Blind" nasogastric tube (NGT) placement is contraindicated
- Chest and abdominal x-ray to assess for free air in the mediastinum or abdomen
- The combination of steroid, antireflux medication, and antibiotic use is controversial
- Esophagoscopy timing is controversial (<12 hours an evolving lesion may be missed; >48 hours may risk perforation)
  - Grade 0: No injury
  - Grade I: Mucosal edema and hyperemia
  - Grade IIa: Superficial, non-circumferential, whitish membranes, shallow ulcers, hemorrhage, and friable exudates
  - Grade IIb: Deep, circumferential lesions with stricture formation
  - Grade IIIa: Small, scattered areas of necrosis
  - Grade IIIb: Extensive necrosis
  - Grade IV: Perforation

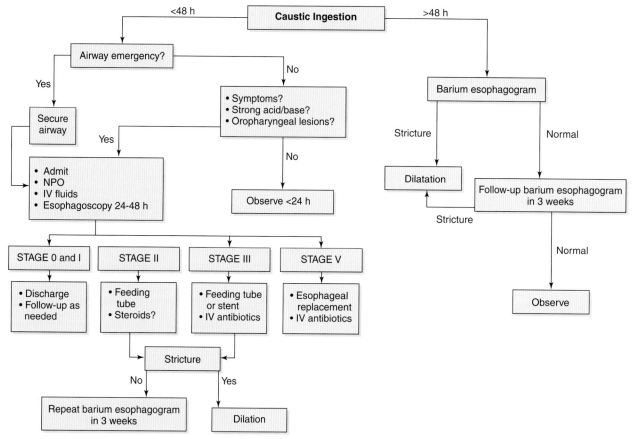

Fig. 6.19 Caustic ingestion algorithm. (From Flint PW, Haughey BH, Lund VJ, et al. *Cummings Otolaryngology—Head and Neck Surgery*. 6th ed. Philadelphia, PA: Saunders; 2015.)

- If evaluation starts >48 hours after ingestion, an esophagogram may be obtained as an initial assessment instead of esophagoscopy
- Treatment
  - Observation for Grades I and II lesions (consider steroids for Grade II)
  - Stenting with NGT if there is a risk of stricture (consider for Grades II and III)
  - If stricture is found or risk of stricture is high, repeat assessment with dilation in 3 weeks (may require long-term serial dilations)
  - For high stage, consider gastrostomy tube (G-tube) and peroral string placement for subsequent retrograde bougie esophageal dilation
  - Esophagectomy with intestinal interposition graft for severe stricture and perforation
    - Mortality rates are high

Airway Disorders in Which Gastroesophageal Reflux Disease (GERD) Should Be Considered

- Apnea or apparent life-threatening events (ALTEs) or brief resolved unexplained events (BRUEs)
- Croup
- Persistent cough
- Hoarseness or dysphonia
- Aspiration
- Laryngomalacia
- Subglottic edema

Upper Airway Infections (Table 6.5)

- Laryngotracheitis (croup)
  - Caused by parainfluenza (also influenza, RSV, measles, adenovirus, varicella, and HSV I)
  - Affects patients aged 6 months to 3 years, URI prodrome, slow onset, variable/minimal fever, hoarse with "barking" cough, and can develop respiratory difficulty with inspiratory stridor
  - Diagnosis: Clinical; radiographic "steeple sign" on AP views
  - Treatment: expectant (humidification, racemic epinephrine, steroids)
  - Direct laryngoscopy, bronchoscopy, and possible intubation if medical therapy fails: Use a tube 0.5 mm smaller than estimated, and extubate when air leak detected
- Supraglottitis (epiglottitis)
  - Caused by *H. influenzae* type B, also Group A β-hemolytic *Streptococcus*, *Staphylococcus*, pneumococcus, *Klebsiella*, and *H. parainfluenzae*
  - Affects children 1 to 8 years old, mild URI prodrome, rapid onset of high fever, toxic symptoms, drooling, dysphagia
  - Diagnosis: History, clinical presentation, do not agitate the child; radiography only if diagnosis is in question
  - Management: Intubation in the operating room, rigid/flexible bronchoscopy; IV antibiotics (ceftriaxone, cefotaxime, and ampicillin/sulbactam); extubation usually within 48 hours once swelling is down and air leak is present
- Bacterial tracheitis

TABLE 6.5 Differential Diagnosis of Upper-Airway Infections in Children

	Laryngotracheitis (Viral Croup)	Supraglottis (Epiglottitis)	Bacterial Tracheitis	Retropharyngeal Abscess
Age	6 months to 3 years	1–8 years	6 months to 8 years	1–5 years
Onset	Slow	Rapid	Rapid	Slow
Prodrome	URI symptoms	None or mild URI	URI symptoms	URI symptoms
Fever	Variable or none	High	High	Usually high
Hoarseness and barky cough	Yes	No	Yes	No
Dysphagia	No	Yes	Yes	Yes
Toxic appearance	No	Yes	Yes	Variable
Radiographs	Subglottic narrowing	Rounded, enlarged epiglottis	Subglottic narrowing, diffuse haziness, tracheal wall irregularities	Widened prevertebral space

URI, Upper respiratory infection.
From Flint PW, Haughey BH, Lund VJ, et al. *Cummings Otolaryngology—Head and Neck Surgery.* 6th ed. Philadelphia, PA: Saunders; 2015, Table 197-1.

- Caused by *S. aureus*, also *S. pyogenes*, *H. influenzae*, *M. catarrhalis*
- Affects children 6 months to 8 years old, URI prodrome, rapid onset, high fever, hoarseness with cough, dysphagia, and toxic symptoms
- Management: OR intubation, bronchoscopic suction and cultures of airway exudates; extubation when normothermic, decreased secretions, and air leak present
- Retropharyngeal abscess
  - Caused by mixed bacteria: Streptococci, *S. aureus*, *H. influenzae*, Bacteroides, peptostreptococci, and fusobacteria
  - Affects children usually <6 years old: URI prodrome, fever, sore throat, progressive dysphagia, and drooling
  - Diagnosed on the lateral soft-tissue x-ray or CT scan: Subcutaneous gas and widening of prevertebral tissues (>2× diameter of C2 body 90% sensitive)
  - Management: Secure airway, IV antibiotics, and possible OR drainage (transoral vs. transcervical)

CRANIOFACIAL

Cleft Lip/Palate: Classification and Etiology

- Unilateral or bilateral, complete or incomplete (Fig. 6.20)
  - Complete cleft lip: Involves entire lip/alveolus
  - Incomplete cleft lip: Remaining small bridge of tissue is the Simonart band
  - Complete cleft palate: Primary and secondary palate, extends anterior to incisive foramen; includes premaxilla/alveolus, often associated with cleft lip
  - Incomplete cleft palate: Posterior to incisive foramen, typically isolated cleft palate
  - Etiology
    - Multifactorial: Combination of genetics, environmental influences, and other
    - Genetics
      - 30% cleft lip and palate is associated with syndrome, and 50% cleft palate is associated with syndrome
    - Incidence of cleft lip varies by ethnic group: Highest in Native Americans (3.6 in 1000 births), Asian Americans (2.1 in 1000), and non-Hispanic Whites (1 in 1000)
    - Incidence of cleft palate does not vary by ethnicity; 0.5 in 1000 births
    - Teratogens: Alcohol, tobacco smoke, phenytoin, and retinoic acid
    - Prenatal multivitamins and folic acid may decrease risk

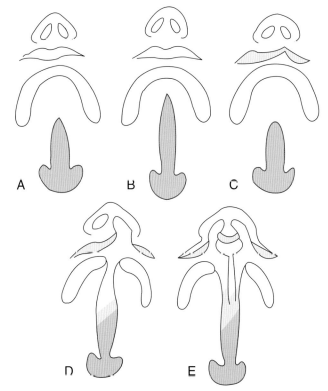

Fig. 6.20 Classification of cleft palate. The division between primary palate (prolabium, premaxilla, and anterior septum) and secondary palate is the incisive foramen. (**A**) Incomplete cleft of the secondary palate. (**B**) Complete cleft of the secondary palate (extending as far as the incisive foramen). (**C**) Incomplete cleft of the primary and secondary palates. (**D**) Unilateral complete cleft of the primary and secondary palates. (**E**) Bilateral complete cleft of the primary and secondary palates. (From McCarthy JG, Cutting CB, Hogan VM. Introduction to facial clefts. In: Mathes SJ, ed. *Plastic Surgery.* Philadelphia, PA: Saunders; 1990:2243; and Flint PW, Haughey BH, Lund VJ, et al. *Cummings Otolaryngology—Head and Neck Surgery.* 6th ed. Philadelphia, PA: Saunders; 2015.)

Anatomical Anomalies in Cleft Lip Defect (Fig. 6.21)

- Orbicularis oris muscle with abnormal orientation and insertion
- Prolabial skin deficient
- Shortened columella, which deviates to the non-cleft side in unilateral cleft
- Floor of the nose may be absent
- Central portion of the alveolar arch may be deficient
- Widened nasal tip is deflected to the non-cleft side
- Septum and anterior nasal spine are displaced to the non-cleft side

Anatomical Anomalies in Cleft Palate

- Muscles of soft palate are hypoplastic and misdirected with abnormal insertions into the posterior hard palate, primarily levator veli palatini and tensor veli palatini
- May include bony deficiency of hard palate

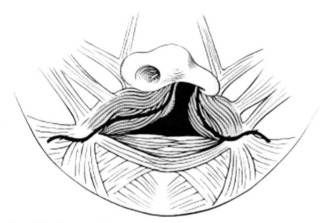

Fig. 6.21 Abnormal direction and insertion of muscle fibers of medial and lateral segments of the cleft into the cleft margin, the area of the ala nasi (laterally), and the base of the columella (medially). The black line indicates arterial supply. (From Flint PW, Francis HW, Haughey BH, et al. *Cummings Otolaryngology—Head and Neck Surgery.* 7th ed. Philadelphia, PA: Saunders; 2020, Fig. 188.16.)

Milestones for Cleft Lip/Palate Repair: Management by Multidisciplinary Cleft Team

- Lip adhesion: 2 to 4 weeks with second stage at 3 months (not as commonly done currently)
- Lip repair: 2 to 3 months
- Monitor ears/hearing/speech: Consider ear tubes
- Palate repair: 8 to 12 months
- Correction of velopharyngeal insufficiency (VPI): 4 years
- Lip revision: >4 years
- Orthodontics: >6 years
- Nasal reconstruction
  - Primary: Closure of nasal floor, repositioning of lower lateral cartilages, and repositioning of alar base, done at time of lip repair
  - Definitive (secondary) rhinoplasty: 15 to 18 years

Surgical Repair of Cleft Lip and Palate

- Lip adhesion or nasoalveolar molding (NAM): if done, performed at 2 to 4 weeks of age, with additional surgery at 3 months of age (if needed)
- Cleft lip repair: If no contraindications and no previous lip adhesion, repair is performed at 2 to 3 months
  - Millard rotation advancement technique
  - Tennison-Randall (single) triangular flap interdigitation
  - Bardach (double) triangular flap interdigitation
  - Bilateral cleft repair (Millard)
  - Straight-line closure (rarely used currently)
- Cleft palate repair: Performed 8 to 12 months up to 18 months of age if child is growing and gaining weight; restoration of the soft palate sling incorporating the tensor and levator palatini
  - Von Langenbeck
  - V-Y pushback
  - Bardach two-flap palatoplasty
  - Schweckendiek: Closure of soft palate only
  - Furlow double Z-plasty for soft palate repair

Special Considerations in Patients with Cleft Palate

- Pierre Robin Sequence (Fig. 6.22)
  - Triad of:
    - Micrognathia

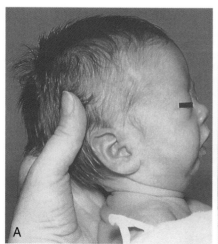
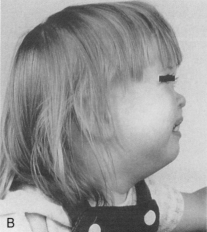
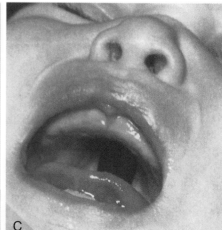

Fig. 6.22 **(A)** A newborn with Pierre Robin sequence. **(B)** The same child at age 2 years. Note the partial mandibular catch-up growth. **(C)** U-shaped cleft palate in a patient with Pierre Robin sequence. (From Flint PW, Haughey BH, Lund VJ, et al. *Cummings Otolaryngology—Head and Neck Surgery.* 6th ed. Philadelphia, PA: Saunders; 2015.)

- Glossoptosis
- Cleft palate
- Pathology: Occurs as a sequence—micrognathia (small body and short ramus) retrodisplaces the tongue, preventing secondary palate fusion
- May be syndromic or nonsyndromic
- Most common associated syndrome: Stickler
- Airway interventions
  - Prone positioning
  - Nasopharyngeal airway
  - Tongue–lip adhesion
  - Endotracheal intubation
  - Neonatal mandibular distraction osteogenesis
  - Tracheostomy
- 2.22q11 Deletion Syndrome/Velocardiofacial Syndrome/DiGeorge Syndrome
  - AD, but most patients present de novo
  - Deletion of 22q11
  - Characterized by abnormal facies, VPI, cleft palate, and cardiac anomalies
  - Long face, malar flatness, mandibular micrognathia, and microcephaly
  - Palatal clefting ranges from bifid uvula to submucosal cleft palate to true cleft palate: VPI and middle ear disease are common
  - Most common syndrome associated with isolated cleft palate
  - Cardiac anomalies are common
  - Medialized internal carotid arteries may be present: Requires contrast imaging before pharyngeal surgery such as tonsillectomy

Three Characteristics of Submucous Cleft Palate

- Bifid uvula
- Zona pellucida (translucent zone in the midline of the soft palate)
- Notched posterior hard palate

Patterns of Velopharyngeal Closure

- Coronal (55%, most common)
- Sagittal (10%–15%, least common)
- Circular (10%–20%)
- Circular with Passavant ridge (15%–20%)
- Pattern assists in surgical planning in cases of VPI
- Speech endoscopy is the standard assessment tool and is performed by the otolaryngologist and speech-language pathologist

Management of Velopharyngeal Insufficiency

- Medical
  - Speech therapy
  - Prosthetics: palatal lift, obturator
- Surgical: Preferred for long-term management of VPI not responsive to speech therapy
  - Sphincter pharyngoplasty is preferred for coronal or circular closure patterns when good palate motion
  - Superiorly based pharyngeal flap is preferred for sagittal or circular closure patterns with good lateral wall motion
  - Furlow palatoplasty (double Z-plasty) increases the thickness and length of the palate
  - Posterior pharyngeal wall augmentation can be used for a small midline gap; limited long-term success

Choanal Atresia

- Incidence 1:5000–8000 births
- Two-thirds are unilateral, usually on the right
- 50% of unilateral and 75% of bilateral are associated with other anomalies
- Four parts to the anatomical deformity
  - Narrow nasal cavity
  - Lateral bony obstruction from the pterygoid plate
  - Medial bony obstruction from the vomer
  - Membranous obstruction
- 29% bony atresia; 71% mixed bony-membranous
- Failure to pass a 6 Fr catheter to nasopharynx
- Endoscopy and CT confirm the diagnosis
- Severity of presentation depends on unilateral or bilateral atresia
  - Bilateral: Increased respiratory effort, retractions, and cyanosis
  - Unilateral: May present later in life with unilateral thick rhinorrhea
- General management approach
  - Unilateral atresia: Nonurgent repair, can wait until ~1 year of age
  - Bilateral atresia: Establish airway and gastric feeding, allow for adequate facial growth (2–4 months)
  - Oral airway
  - May require intubation
  - May require tracheotomy if multiple levels of airway obstruction or respiratory failure
- Surgical repair approaches
  - Transnasal (preferred with improved endoscopic techniques)
  - Transpalatal
  - Stenting and use of mitomycin C remain controversial
  - Transseptal
  - Recurrence and need for revision surgery is common

Syndromes Associated With Choanal Atresia

- 50% of unilateral cases and 75% of bilateral cases are associated with a syndrome
  - CHARGE syndrome
  - Crouzon
  - Apert
  - Treacher Collins
  - Velocardiofacial

Classification of Microtia (Fig. 6.23)

- Grade I: All structures are identifiable, but ear is smaller than normal
- Grade II: Deficiencies of the helix
- Grade III: Severe deformity, "peanut ear," no recognizable structures, lobule present
- Grade IV: Anotia; no auricle or lobule

General Management Approach for Microtia

- Observation
- Prosthetic
- Reconstruction
  - Autologous: Rib cartilage (age 8+ years old)
  - Alloplastic: Medpor (age 3+ years old)

Syndromes Associated With Microtia/Aural Atresia

- Goldenhar/hemifacial macrosomia/oculo-auricular-vertebral spectrum disorder

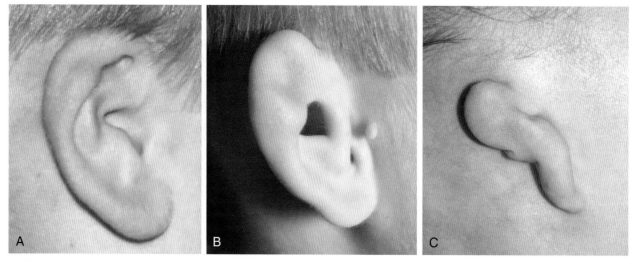

Fig. 6.23 (**A**) Type I microtia with constricted ear and minimal tissue deficiency. (**B**) Type II microtia with absence of major portions of the ear. (**C**) Type III microtia with markedly deformed and small cartilaginous remnant. (From Flint PW, Haughey BH, Lund VJ, et al. *Cummings Otolaryngology—Head and Neck Surgery.* 6th ed. Philadelphia, PA: Saunders; 2015.)

- Mandibulofacial dysostoses (Treacher Collins, Nager syndrome)
- BOR syndrome
- Crouzon

General Management Approach for Congenital Aural Atresia

- ABR within first 2 to 3 months of life
- Unilateral conductive or sensorineural hearing loss is adequate for speech and language development, but increasing evidence shows association with decreased academic performance (difficulty with sound localization in noisy classroom environment)
- Bone conduction hearing aid in children can be used starting at age 6 to 12 months
- Surgical options: BAHA Attract versus Connect versus atresiaplasty
- BAHA is Food and Drug Administration approved for children aged 5 years and older; in Europe, it is approved for children aged 3 years and older
  - Excellent closure of the air–bone gap
  - Does not interfere with associated microtia repair, although plastics repair of the outer ear is typically done first
- Atresiaplasty: Age and timing of repair is controversial, but no earlier than age 4 years

Grading Congenital Aural Atresia (Jahrsdoerfer System)

- 10-point system based on high-resolution CT findings
- 6 points or greater indicates favorable candidate for atresiaplasty
- Higher points have better hearing outcomes
  - Stapes favorable (2 points)/anomalous but present stapes (1 point)
  - Oval window open
  - Middle ear well pneumatized
  - Facial nerve favorable
  - Malleus-incus favorable

- Incus-stapes connected
- Mastoid well pneumatized
- Round window open
- Auricle normal

Complications in Aural Atresia Repair

- Facial nerve injury
- SNHL
- External auditory meatal stenosis, most common
- Lateralization of TM/delayed CHL

Facial Nerve Findings in Middle Ear Atresia

- May cover the oval window and stapes
- More acute angle is taken at the second genu, crossing more anterolateral to the middle ear instead of inferiorly
- Dehiscence of facial nerve bony canal

Considerations for Otoplasty: Indication is Prominauris

- Normal auriculocephalic angle is 25 to 35 degrees; >40 degrees is considered abnormal
- Normal distance of auricle to scalp: 10 to 12 mm superior helix, 16 to 18 mm mid-helix, and 20 to 22 mm caudal helix
- Cartilaginous growth almost complete at age 5 years
- Most common abnormalities treated with otoplasty
  - Insufficient furl at the antihelix
  - Misshapen conchal bowl
- Surgical taping and molding in neonatal period can be effective and can avoid need for reconstruction later
- Reconstruct at age 5 or 6 years (before the child starts school)
- Cartilage-sparing technique: Mustarde permanent sutures to recreate the antihelical fold
- Cartilage sculpting technique: Reshaping/scoring/splitting cartilage to weaken and recreate the antihelical fold
- Furnas sutures: Horizontal mattress sutures to anchor conchal bowl to mastoid periosteum and decrease the concho-mastoid angle

SYNDROMES AND ASSOCIATIONS WITH HEAD AND NECK MANIFESTATIONS (NOT PREVIOUSLY DESCRIBED IN DETAIL)

Achondroplasia

- Most common skeletal dysplasia
- AD, and most cases are spontaneous
- Associated with a narrow foramen magnum with the potential for brainstem compression, apnea, otitis media, and hearing loss
- Over 50% have persistent OME and require insertion of middle ear tubes
- Disorder of endochondral bone formation: Abnormal bones formed from cartilage
- Shortened limbs, frontal bossing, sunken bridge of the nose, midface hypoplasia, maxillary hypoplasia, nasal bone and septal hypoplasia, class 3 malocclusion, and cell-mediated immunodeficiencies
- High incidence of obstructive sleep apnea (OSA); central component may be secondary to narrowing of foramen magnum
- Normal cognitive function

Down Syndrome

- Extra chromosome on number 21 (aneuploidy) or partial 22 (mosaic trisomy 22)
- Brachycephaly, flat occiput, macroglossia/fissured tongue, up-slanting palpebral fissures with prominent epicanthal folds, midface hypoplasia and small nose, large fissured lips
- Dental abnormalities: Hypodontia/anodontia
- Narrow ear canals, Grade 1 microtia/small ears, mixed hearing loss
- Increased incidence of subglottic stenosis
- Short neck
- Atlantoaxial subluxation and instability
- High incidence of OSA
  - Further management required in up to 80% of cases after tonsillectomy and adenoidectomy (T&A)
  - Continuous positive airway pressure (CPAP), uvulopalatopharyngoplasty (UPPP), tongue base management, tracheostomy
  - Emerging research supporting hypoglossal nerve stimulation
- Increased association with leukemia
- High incidence of hypothyroidism
- Hypotonia

Beckwith-Wiedemann Syndrome

- Macroglossia, omphalocele, visceromegaly, and cytomegaly of the adrenal cortex
- Result of genomic imprinting
- "Overall growth syndrome," with sporadic occurrence
- Macroglossia may cause airway obstruction or chronic alveolar hypoventilation
- Tongue reduction is effective for those unable to keep the tongue in the mouth
- Associated with malignancies, including rhabdomyosarcoma, neuroblastoma, Wilms tumor and hepatoblastoma

Prader-Willi Syndrome

- Deletion of 15q11-13
- High incidence of OSA
  - Early in life: Infantile hypotonia, poor oral intake, and FTT
- Develop obesity/hyperphagia
- T&A effective in mild-to-moderate OSA but ~80% need further management for severe OSA
- VPI
- Developmental delay
- Hypogonadism and growth hormone deficiency
- Growth hormone treatment can help with weight management; assess for OSA

Goldenhar Syndrome (Part of the Oculoauriculovertebral/Hemifacial Microsomia Spectrum)

- Most cases occur sporadically and are autosomal recessive or dominant
- Characterized by hemifacial microsomia
- Unilateral microtia/atresia with conductive loss
- Facial asymmetry
- Retrognathia/micrognathia
- Asymmetric temporal, zygomatic, maxillary and mandibular hypoplasia
- Microstomia
- May have a cleft lip/palate
- Hypoplastic facial nerve and/or musculature: Range in mild-to-complete facial paralysis
- Microtia/atresia
- Also with vertebral anomalies and epibulbar dermoids

CHARGE Syndrome (or Association)

- Coloboma (75%–90%)
- Heart defects (50%–85%)
- Atresia of the choanae (35%–65%)
- Retardation of growth and/or development
- Genital hypoplasia/genitourinary defects (50%–70%)
- Ear anomalies and/or deafness (over 90%)
  - Abnormal or absent horizontal SCC is common finding on CT temporal bone

Moebius Syndrome

- Unclear pathogenesis; 98% sporadic
- Nonprogressive unilateral or bilateral facial (CN VII) and abducens (CN VI) palsy
- May affect nearly all other cranial nerves
- Monitor for feeding difficulties, hearing loss, speech/language delay
- Global delay: Motor, emotional, and speech early in childhood but generally "catch up"—10% with cognitive deficits
- Consider facial reanimation and monitor for ocular health
- Association with Pierre Robin sequence and Klippel-Feil anomaly as well as hand anomalies such as syndactyly

Mucopolysaccharidoses

- Deficiency of lysosomal enzymes that degrade mucopolysaccharides—results in large cells with vacuolated cytoplasm
- Hurler syndrome
  - AR, as is the case with most mucopolysaccharidoses
  - Leads to visceromegaly
  - Mucopolysaccharidosis type I: Deficiency of α-L-iduronidase
  - Facies: Coarse facial features and forehead prominence
  - Dwarfism
  - Mixed hearing loss
  - Macroglossia
  - Short neck

- Intellectual disability
- Skeletal disorders with joint stiffness
- May develop severe OSA
- Progressive neurological dysfunction
- Hunter syndrome
  - X-linked disorder
  - Incurable syndrome with multiple organ system mucopolysaccharidosis infiltration, usually death in teenage years from cardiomyopathy
  - Mucopolysaccharidosis type II: Iduronate sulfatase deficiency
  - Facies: Prominent supraorbital ridges, large flattened nose, low-set ears, and large jowls
  - Short stature
  - May develop severe OSA
  - Potential difficult airway
  - Short neck
  - Tracheal deposits of glycosaminoglycan, leading to airway obstruction

Craniosynostosis Syndromes

- Apert (acrocephalosyndactyly), Crouzon (craniofacial dysostosis), and Pfeiffer syndromes
  - AD, and most cases of Apert are spontaneous
  - Craniosynostosis
  - Hypertelorism/exophthalmos
  - Midface hypoplasia
  - Mandibular prognathism
  - High-arched palate
  - "Parrot-beaked nose"
  - Apert associated with symmetric syndactyly of hands and feet + other axial skeletal abnormalities
  - Pfeiffer is associated with enlarged thumbs and first toe
  - High incidence of OSA
  - Cognitive function ranges from normal to severe intellectual disability

ADENOTONSILLAR PATHOLOGY

Tonsillitis and Pharyngitis

- Viral (rhinovirus, influenza, parainfluenza, and adenovirus)
- EBV (infectious mononucleosis)
  - Diagnosis with monospot (heterophile agglutination test)
  - Can develop hepatosplenomegaly; thus, contact sports must be avoided
  - May develop a rash with amoxicillin
  - Nonsteroidal antiinflammatory drugs (NSAIDs) for pain
  - Consider steroids for obstructive tonsillar hypertrophy
- Group A β-hemolytic *Streptococcus* (GABHS)
  - 15% to 30% of children who present with tonsillitis
  - Streptococcal carrier may convert to active infection or spread the infection to another person
  - Diagnosis with rapid antigen detection test and/or throat culture
  - If rapid detection test is negative, proceed with throat culture
  - Antibiotics for a 10-day course (penicillin or amoxicillin first line; first-generation cephalosporin, clindamycin, clarithromycin, azithromycin for penicillin allergic)
  - Consider tonsillectomy for repeat infections (sore throat with fever; cervical lymphadenopathy, tonsillar exudate, or GABHS-positive testing)
  - Nonsuppurative complications

- Scarlet fever: Generalized, nonpruritic, erythematous macular skin rash lasting 3 to 7 days, with strawberry tongue, fevers, and arthralgias
- Rheumatic fever: Rare today; bacterial vegetation grows on mitral and tricuspid valves, resulting in heart murmur, relapsing fevers, and valve regurgitation or stenosis
- Acute poststreptococcal glomerulonephritis: Acute nephritic syndrome (generalized edema, hypertension, and hematuria/proteinuria) 1 to 2 weeks after infection
- Pediatric autoimmune neuropsychiatric disorders associated with streptococcal infections (PANDAS): Obsessive-compulsive disorder and/or tic disorder, episodic course, well-documented temporal relationship with GABHS, abnormal neurological exam
- Periodic fever with aphthous ulcers, pharyngitis, and adenopathy (PFAPA) syndrome
  - Constellation of symptoms, fevers lasting several days, constitutional symptoms
  - Critical to exclude autoimmune disorders and immunodeficiency (HIV) before arriving at PFAPA diagnosis
  - High fevers every 3 to 8 weeks
  - Associated with pharyngitis, aphthous stomatitis, and cervical adenitis
  - Treat with NSAIDs and consider steroids and tonsillectomy
  - Adenotonsillectomy is highly effective at resolving this condition

Peritonsillar Abscess (PTA)

- Symptoms: Severe unilateral sore throat, odynophagia, severe pain when ipsilateral soft palate is probed with a tonsil blade, trismus, and referred otalgia
- Exam: Uvular deviation, drooling, and muffled voice
- Management
  - Hydration
  - Pain control
  - Antibiotics
  - Steroids to improve trismus
  - Needle aspiration or incision and drainage
  - Quinsy tonsillectomy
- Subsequent management for recurrence
  - CT scan
  - Repeat incision and drainage
  - Quinsy tonsillectomy
- Complications
  - Dehydration
  - Airway obstruction
  - Sepsis
  - Spread to other neck spaces
  - Great vessel injury (external and internal carotid artery)

Indications for Tonsillectomy for Infections

- Recurrent acute infections: 7 in 1 year, 5 per year for 2 years, and 3 per year for 3 or more years (Paradise criteria)
- Recurrent acute infections with complications (cardiac valve disease and febrile seizures)
- Streptococcus carrier
- Recurrent PTA
- Mononucleosis with obstructing tonsils unresponsive to therapy
- Chronic tonsillitis associated with halitosis, tonsilliths, persistent sore throat, and cervical adenitis (controversial)

Obstructive Sleep Apnea (OSA)

- General criteria for abnormal pediatric polysomnogram (PSG)
  - Apnea hypopnea index (AHI) >1
    - Mild: 1 to 5
    - Moderate: 5 to 10
    - Severe: >10
  - Oxygen desaturation to below 92%
  - Peak end tidal CO_2 >53 mm Hg
  - Elevated end tidal CO_2 >50 mm Hg >10% of total sleep time
- Risk factors for OSA
  - Hypertrophied adenotonsillar tissue
  - Obesity (body mass index > 30)
  - Craniofacial abnormalities, particularly involving the mandible or maxilla (e.g., achondroplasia, Pierre Robin sequence, and hemifacial microsomia)
  - Neuromuscular disease (e.g., cerebral palsy)
  - Down syndrome
  - Mucopolysaccharidoses, such as Hunter or Hurler syndromes
- Differences between adult and pediatric OSA
  - FTT and enuresis seen in pediatrics
  - Academic, social, emotional, and behavioral changes (e.g., poor school performance, hyperactivity, attention deficit, and aggression) seen in pediatrics

Indications for Tonsillectomy for Obstruction

- Sleep disordered breathing
- OSA
- Cor pulmonale
- FTT and dysphagia
- Craniofacial growth abnormalities
- Speech/occlusion abnormalities (controversial)
- Suspicion of malignancy (such as unilateral tonsillar hypertrophy)

Causes of Subacute or Chronic Unilateral Tonsillar Hypertrophy

- Idiopathic
- Neoplastic: lymphoma
- Infectious
  - *Mycobacterium tuberculosis*
  - Atypical mycobacteria
  - Actinomycosis
  - Fungal

Criteria for Overnight Stay After Tonsillectomy Due to Increased Risk of Airway Obstruction

- Severe OSA
- Neuromuscular disease (e.g., cerebral palsy)
- Age under 3 years
- Weight under 15 kg
- Craniofacial abnormalities
- Medical comorbidities (e.g., diabetes, seizures, Down syndrome, asthma, cardiac disease)
- Emesis or hemorrhage during or after surgery
- Long distance (over 1 hour) between home and the nearest hospital

Postobstructive Pulmonary Edema

- Clinical symptoms and signs
  - Hypoxemia
  - Increased work of breathing
  - Pink, frothy oral or tracheal secretions
  - Bilateral end expiratory wheezing and rales
  - CXR findings showing increased pulmonary markings and fluid overload
- Treatment
  - Oxygen therapy
  - CPAP and possible intubation
  - IV fluid restriction
  - Diuretics
  - Consider steroids

Indications for Follow-Up PSG After Surgery

- Persistent sleep-disordered breathing symptoms
- Severe OSA, particularly with preoperative complication (e.g., pulmonary hypertension)
- Age <1 year

Adenoid Hypertrophy

- Most common cause of nasal-airway obstruction in children, but not the most common etiology in the neonate
  - Daycare, chronic allergies, and secondary-smoke exposure cause chronic inflammation
  - Best to assess the degree of obstruction with nasopharyngoscopy; lateral neck film is acceptable but is not as comprehensive and has the risk of radiation exposure
- Innervation: CN IX and CN X; very little pain should be expected after adenoidectomy
- Typical child with adenoid hypertrophy has six to eight viral URIs per year
- Techniques for removal: Suction cautery, coblation, or microdebrider

Indications for Adenoidectomy

- Infection
  - Recurrent/chronic adenoiditis or sinusitis (with or without hypertrophy)
  - Tympanostomy tube placement (with infectious or obstructive symptoms if less than 4 years old); alone or in combination with tympanostomy tube placement (without infectious or obstructive symptoms if more than 4 years old)
- Obstruction
  - Chronic nasal obstruction or obligate mouth breathing
  - OSA or sleep-disordered breathing
  - Craniofacial growth abnormalities
  - "Slack jaw" or "adenoid" faces
  - Dental occlusion abnormalities
  - Hyponasal speech
  - Before VPI surgery (prior to pharyngeal flap or to alleviate secondary nasal obstruction)
- Suspected neoplasm

Complications of Adenotonsillectomy

- Blood supply to the tonsil
  - Facial artery (tonsillar branch, ascending palatine branch)
  - Dorsal lingual branch of the lingual artery
  - Internal maxillary artery (descending palatine and greater palatine artery)
  - Ascending pharyngeal artery
- Blood supply to the adenoid
  - Pharyngeal branch of the internal maxillary (major supply)
  - Major bleeding after adenoidectomy is rare and can be indicative of an underlying bleeding disorder

- Hemorrhage
  - Primary postoperative hemorrhage within 24 hours
  - Secondary postoperative hemorrhage between POD 1 and 14
  - Bleeding history is most important in determination of preoperative risk; coagulation testing before surgery is not cost-effective
- Dehydration
- Tylenol with codeine hypermetabolizer leading to metabolically induced narcotic overdose (black box warning for use after adenotonsillectomy)
- Postoperative pulmonary edema
- Mandibular dislocation
- VPI (may occur after adenoidectomy)
- NP stenosis (rare)
- Nontraumatic atlantoaxial subluxation (Grisel syndrome)
  - Results from C1–C2 subluxation with prevertebral inflammation
  - Complication following adenoidectomy, oftentimes inflammation and infection related to electrocautery
  - Prolonged neck pain and stiffness for 2 weeks or more; head rotated away from the side where the atlas has shifted
  - Diagnosis confirmed with CT scan of the cervical spine
  - Treat with antiinflammatory medication and soft diet
  - May need neck immobilization (cervical collar)

Risk Factors for VPI After Adenoidectomy

- Symptoms that fail to resolve in 8 weeks (temporary VPI occurs and typically improves)
- History of nasopharyngeal regurgitation before surgery
- Occult submucous cleft
- Neuromuscular disorders

Nonobstructive Sleep Disorders

- Dyssomnia: Abnormality in the amount, quality, or timing of sleep that results in difficulty initiating or maintaining sleep (e.g., insufficient sleep syndrome, narcolepsy, sleep-related movement disorders, circadian sleep–wake disorders, idiopathic hypersomnia, Kleine-Levin syndrome, and chronic insomnia disorder)
- Parasomnia: Undesirable events that occur during entry into sleep, within sleep, or during arousal from sleep occurring during rapid eye movement (REM) sleep (e.g., nightmare disorder, recurrent isolated sleep paralysis, and REM sleep behavior disorder) or non-REM sleep (e.g., sleep terrors, sleepwalking, confusional arousals)

FURTHER READINGS

Isaacson G. Endoscopic anatomy of the pediatric middle ear. *Otolaryngol Head Neck Surg.* 2015;150(1):6–15.

Cotton RT, Gluckman JL, Seiden AM, Tami TA, Pensak ML. *Otolaryngology: The Essentials.* 1st ed. New York, NY: Thieme; 2001.

Jones SM, Jones TA. *Genetics, Embryology, and Development of Auditory and Vestibular Systems.* Plural Publishing Inc; 2011.

Park JH, Ahn J, Moon IJ. Transcanal endoscopic ear surgery for congenital cholesteatoma. *Clin Exper Otorhinolaryngol.* 2018;11(4):233–241.

Niparko JK. *Cochlear Implants: Principles and Practices.* Philadelphia, PA: Lippincott Williams & Wilkins; 2000.

Cureoglu S, Schachern PA, Paperella MM. Scheibe dysplasia. *Otol Neurotol.* 2003;24(1):125–126.

Gross M, Eliashar R, Eiidan J. Michel's aplasia. *Otol Neurotol.* 2005;26(3):547.

Yu KK, Mukherji S, Carrasco V, et al. Molecular genetic advances in semicircular canal abnormalities and sensorineural hearing loss: a report of 16 cases. *Otolaryngol Head Neck Surg.* 2003;129(6):637–646.

Zhou G, Gopen Q, Kenna MA. Delineating the hearing loss in children with enlarged vestibular aqueduct. *Laryngoscope.* 2008;118(11):2062–2066.

Joint Committee on Infant Hearing Year 2019 Position Statement: Principles and Guidelines for Early Hearing Detection and Intervention Programs. *J Early Interv.* 2019;4(2):1–42.

Liming BJ, Carter J, Cheng A, et al. International Pediatric Otolaryngology Group (IPOG) Consensus Recommendations: hearing loss in the pediatric patient. *Int J Pediatr Otorhinolaryngol.* 2016;90:251–258. https://doi.org/10.1016/j.ijporl.2016.09.016.

Wetmore RF, Muntz HR, McGill TJI. *Pediatric Otolaryngology: Principles and Practice Pathways.* New York, NY: Thieme; 2012:292–293.

Graham JM, Scadding GK, Bull PD. *Pediatric ENT. Berlin and New York.* NY: Springer; 2003.

Colletti L. Beneficial auditory and cognitive effects of auditory brainstem implantation in children. *Acta Otolaryngol.* 2007;127(9):943–946.

Lee KJ. *Essential Otolaryngology: Head and Neck Surgery.* 8th ed. New York, NY: McGraw-Hill; 2003.

Goldenberg I, Moss AJ, Zareba W, et al. Clinical course and risk stratification of patients with Jervell and Lange-Nielsen syndrome. *J Cardiovasc Electrophysiol.* 2006;17(11):1161–1168.

Kaplan J, Gerber S, Bonneau D, et al. A gene for Usher syndrome type 1 (USH1A) maps to chromosome 14q. *Genomics.* 1992;14(4):979–987.

Kimberling WJ, Weston MD, Moller C, et al. Localization of Usher syndrome type 2 to chromosome 1q. *Genomics.* 1990;7(2):245–249.

Mathur P, Yang J. Usher syndrome: hearing loss, retinal degeneration and associated abnormalities. *Biochim Biophys Acta.* 2015;1852(3):406–420.

Savige J, Colville D. Opinion: ocular features aid the diagnosis of Alport syndrome. *Nat Rev Nephrol.* 2009;5(6):356–360.

El-Dessouky M, Azmy AF, Raine PA, Young DG. Kasabach-Merritt syndrome. *J Pediatr Surg.* 1998;23(2):109–111.

Weiner MA, Leventhal BG, Marcus R, et al. Intensive chemotherapy and low-dose radiotherapy for the treatment of advanced-stage Hodgkin's disease in pediatric patients: a Pediatric Oncology Group Study. *J Clin Oncol.* 1991;9(9):1591–1598.

Smith RS, Chen Q, Hudson MM, et al. Prognostic factors for children with Hodgkin's disease treated with combined-modality therapy. *J Clin Oncol.* 2003;21(10):2026–2033.

Sandlund JT, Downing JR, Crist WM. Non-Hodgkin's lymphoma in childhood. *N Engl J Med.* 1996;334(19):1238–1248.

Reilly BK, Kim A, Pena MT, et al. Rhabdomyosarcoma of the head and neck in children: review and update. *Int J Pediatr Otolaryngol.* 2015;79(9):1477–1483. https://www.cdc.gov/hpv/parents/vaccine.html.

Derkay CS, Wiatrak B. Recurrent respiratory papillomatosis: a review. *Laryngoscope.* 2008;118(7):1236–1247. https://doi.org/10.1097/MLG.0b013e31816a7135.

Cassidy S, Schwartz S, Miller JL, et al. Prader-Willi syndrome. *Genet Med.* 2012;14:10–26.

Picciolini O, Porro M, Catteneo E, et al. Moebius syndrome: clinical features, diagnosis, management and early intervention. *Ital J Pediatr.* 2016;42(1):56.

Chetham MM, Roberts KB. Infectious mononucleosis in adolescents. *Pediatr Ann.* 1991;20(4):206–213.

Licameli G, Jeffrey J, Luz J, et al. Effect of adenotonsillectomy in PFAPA syndrome. *Arch Otolaryngol Head Neck Surg.* 2008;134(2):136–140.

Wald ER, Guerra N, Byers C. Upper respiratory tract infections in young children: duration of and frequency of complications. *Pediatrics.* 1991;87(2):129–133.

Cooper JD, Smith KJ, Ritchey AK. A cost-effective analysis of the coagulation testing prior to tonsillectomy and adenoidectomy in children. *Pediatr Blood Cancer.* 2010;55(6):1153–1159.

Tschopp K. Monopolar electrocautery in adenoidectomy as a possible risk factor for Grisel's syndrome. *Laryngoscope.* 2002;112:1445–1449.

7 Laryngology

Daniel Fink and Jayme Rose Dowdall

LARYNGEAL AND PHARYNGEAL FUNCTION

Three functions of the larynx
1. Voice
2. Respiration
3. Deglutition

The only laryngeal abductor (Fig. 7.1) is the posterior crico-arytenoid (PCA).
- Attaches the cricoid to the muscular process of the arytenoid
- Pulls the muscular process posteriorly and caudally, rotating the vocal process laterally and upward

The only internal muscle of the larynx not supplied by the recurrent laryngeal nerve (RLN) is the cricothyroid (supplied by the external branch of the superior laryngeal nerve [SLN]).

Primary function of the internal branch of the SLN
- Sensation to the supraglottis

What is the myoelastic-aerodynamic theory?
- Interaction of aerodynamic forces and the mechanical properties of the laryngeal tissues are responsible for inducing vocal fold vibration and generating vocal sound

What are the three components of sound creation?
1. Power source: The lungs
2. Vibrator/vibratory source: The larynx
3. Resonator: *Supraglottal vocal tract*, including the supraglottic larynx, pharynx, oral cavity, and, potentially, the nasal cavity

What is the best method for assessing vocal fold vibration?
- Laryngeal stroboscopy at multiple frequencies and intensities

What are the functions of the extrinsic muscles of the larynx in voice production?
1. Alter the position of the larynx, which, in turn, can affect the length of the vocal tract resonator
2. Stabilize the larynx within the neck when singing

What are the functions of the intrinsic muscles of the larynx in voice production?
1. Adduction and abduction
2. Fine changes in tension of the vocal folds

What are the three histological layers of the vocal fold?
1. Cover
2. Transition zone or vocal ligament
3. Body

What are the components of the vocal fold cover?
1. Squamous epithelium
2. Superficial layer of the lamina propria (Reinke space)
   - Composed of fibroblasts that produce proteins and glycoproteins
   - Forms an extracellular matrix of loose connective tissue

What are the components of the vocal fold transition zone or vocal ligament?
1. Intermediate layer of the lamina propria (composed of elastin)
2. Deep layers of the lamina propria

What are the components of the vocal fold body?
- Thyroarytenoid muscle (Fig. 7.2)

Vocal fold layers from medial to lateral
- Squamous epithelium
- Superficial layer of the lamina propria

- Vocal ligament
- Thyroarytenoid muscle
- Perichondrium and thyroid cartilage provide the lateral boundary of the vocal fold (Fig. 7.3)

VISUALIZATION OF THE LARYNX

Indirect Methods of Visualizing the Larynx

1. Mirror laryngoscopy
2. Rigid indirect laryngoscopy
3. Flexible indirect laryngoscopy

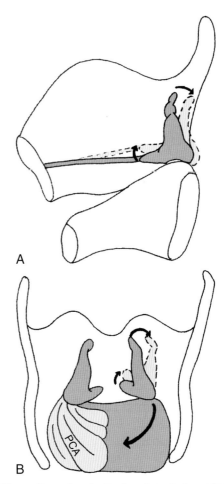

Fig. 7.1 Three-dimensional effects of posterior cricoarytenoid muscle contraction. (A) Sagittal view. **(B)** Posterior view. (From Flint PW, Haughey BH, Lund VJ, et al. *Cummings Otolaryngology—Head and Neck Surgery.* 6th ed. Philadelphia, PA: Saunders; 2015, Fig. 54.3.)

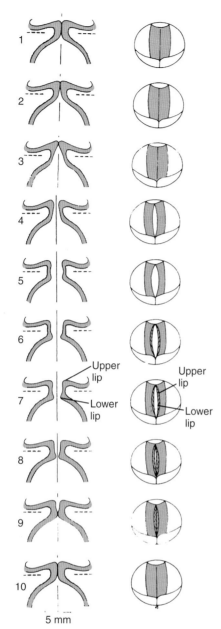

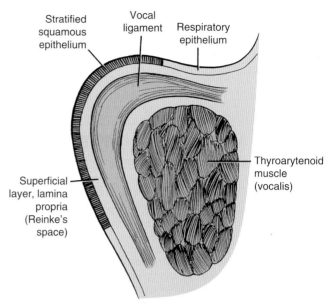

Fig. 7.3 Cross section of the vocal fold. (From Flint PW, Haughey BH, Lund VJ, et al. *Cummings Otolaryngology—Head and Neck Surgery.* 6th ed. Philadelphia, PA: Saunders; 2015, Fig. 61.1.)

Fig. 7.2 Movements of different portions of vocal folds during one cycle of vibration shown schematically in the coronal plane (*left*) and from above (*right*). Mucosal upheaval begins caudally (*1*) and then moves rostrally. The lower portion is closing as the upper margin is opening (*5*). (From Hirano M. *Clinical Examination of Voice.* New York, NY: Springer-Verlag; 1981; and Flint PW, Haughey BH, Lund VJ, et al. *Cummings Otolaryngology—Head and Neck Surgery.* 6th ed. Philadelphia, PA: Saunders; 2015, Fig. 54.11.)

Benefits of Rigid Indirect Laryngoscopy

1. Higher resolution
2. Brighter, clearer picture
3. Image is more accurately magnified
4. Generally does not require topical anesthesia

Drawbacks of Rigid Indirect Laryngoscopy

1. Cannot visualize the larynx while patient performs complex speaking tasks

2. May be difficult to visualize arytenoid abduction/adduction in certain patients

Benefits of Flexible Indirect Laryngoscopy

1. Can visualize the larynx during speaking/singing tasks
2. The larynx is in a more natural configuration for neurological evaluation

Drawbacks of Flexible Indirect Laryngoscopy

1. Generally requires topical anesthesia
2. Distortion at the periphery of the image
3. Inferior light transport/magnification versus rigid

Key Structures and Findings to Be Evaluated With Laryngopharyngeal Endoscopy

1. Overall structure of vocal folds
   • Bowed (atrophy)
   • Scar/sulcus deformity
2. Masses or lesions
3. Abduction and adduction of true vocal folds
   • Vocal fold paresis/paralysis
   • Cricoarytenoid joint fixation
   • Posterior glottic stenosis
4. Supraglottic configuration
   • Relaxed: Can see the whole vocal fold
   • Asymmetric: May imply paresis or be seen with paralysis
   • Symmetric: May be a normal variant or muscle tension dysphonia (MTD)
5. Pooling of secretions
   • Vallecula: Consider tongue-base weakness
   • Piriform sinuses/postcricoid region
     • Pharyngeal weakness
     • Lack of sensation/neurological deficit
     • Esophageal obstruction: See the dysphagia/esophageal section

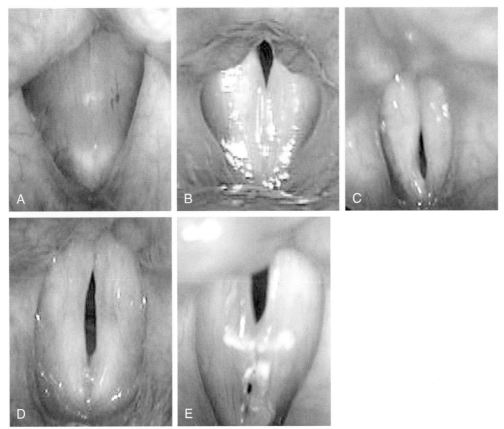

Fig. 7.4 Glottal closure and gap patterns. (**A**) Complete closure. (**B**) Posterior glottal gap. (**C**) Anterior glottal gap. (**D**) Spindle-shaped gap. (**E**) Hourglass-shaped gap. (From Flint PW, Haughey BH, Lund VJ, et al. *Cummings Otolaryngology—Head and Neck Surgery.* 6th ed. Philadelphia, PA: Saunders; 2015, Fig. 55.3.)

Videostroboscopy Basics

- Used to assess vocal fold vibration
- Microphone uses pitch to calculate frequency of vocal fold vibration
- Strobe light set just off frequency to catch the vocal fold at various phases of vibration
- "Flip book" effect
- Requires a long enough phonatory segment with regular/periodic vibration to trigger the strobe light
- Cannot provide information about the phonation onset and offset, which are very short and irregular

Components of Stroboscopy Grading

1. Mucosal wave
   - Vertical upheaval of the vocal fold cover over the vocal fold body
   - Should cover approximately ½ of the superior surface of the true vocal fold at modal pitch
2. Amplitude of vibration
   - Lateral excursion of the vocal fold
   - Should be approximately ⅓ the width of the true vocal fold at modal pitch
3. Vertical phase
   - Timing difference between the superior and inferior portions of the vocal fold
   - Inferior portion of the fold leads the superior portion in its movement away from and back to the midline
4. Phase symmetry
   - Symmetry of the motion of one vocal fold compared with the other vocal fold

5. Regularity/periodicity
   - Does one wave look the same as the next?
6. Adynamic segments
   - From scarring, sulcus, or cyst
   - May be seen better with high-speed digital imaging
7. Closure

Vocal Fold Closure Patterns (Fig. 7.4)

1. Complete
2. Anterior/posterior gap
   - May be a normal variant (females may have a posterior gap)
   - Postsurgical defect
   - Scar/sulcus
3. Spindle shaped
   - Bowed vocal folds from atrophy or presbylarynges
4. Hourglass
   - Seen with vocal fold nodules, prenodular edema, or a polyp/cyst with a reactive lesion

Voice Evaluation

History Evaluation for the Patient With Hoarseness

1. Onset and duration of symptoms (e.g., upper-respiratory infection [URI] or screaming)
2. Perceived cause
3. Relapse/remit or constant
4. What makes it better and what makes it worse?
5. Does the patient have difficulty with swallowing, breathing, coughing, or throat clearing?

6. Pain
7. Occupation
8. Reflux
9. Talkativeness profile (intrinsic, personality-based tendency to use voice)
10. Vocal commitments or activities (extrinsic requirement, invitation, or opportunity to use voice), including voice type and training if the patient is a performer
11. Vocal abuse
12. Smoker/drinker
13. Hydration status
14. History of intubation
15. Psychological stressors
16. Neurological history
17. Pulmonary history

Past Medical History Evaluation of a Patient With Hoarseness

1. Neurological disorders
2. Head and neck/esophageal cancer history and risk factors
3. Reflux/treatment of such
4. Surgical history, especially spine surgery/head and neck surgery
5. Use of medications, including immunosuppressants

Voice Patient Physical Examination

1. Complete head and neck exam with special attention to cranial nerves and nasal exam
2. Palpate laryngeal framework: Assess for tension (Fig. 7.5)
   a. There should be palpable space between the thyroid cartilage and hyoid bone
   b. There should be good lateral laryngeal mobility
3. Assess voice quality with a perceptual assessment of vocal capabilities and limitations, particularly through elicitation of vocal tasks designed to detect mucosal disturbances
4. Laryngopharyngeal endoscopy
5. Stroboscopy

Objective Tools for Voice Assessment

1. Aerodynamic measurements
2. Acoustic measurements
3. Auditory perceptual assessment

Aerodynamic Measurements

1. Subglottal air pressure
   - Pressure required to sustain vocal fold vibration
   - Usually measured indirectly, transorally to avoid tracheal puncture

2. Phonation threshold pressure
   - Pressure required to initiate vocal fold vibration
   - Often corresponds to patient's sensation of vocal effort
   - Changes with viscoelastic changes in the vocal fold
3. Airflow
   - Mean flow of air (milliliter/second) during phonation
   - May increase with vocal fold paralysis
   - May decrease with maximum phonation time (MPT)
4. Laryngeal airway resistance
   - Ratio of translaryngeal air pressure to laryngeal airflow
5. MPT
   - Maximum time the patient can sustain phonation
   - Normal MPT: Female 15 to 25 seconds and male 25 to 35 seconds

Acoustic Measurements

1. Fundamental frequency (F0)
   - Number of repeating cycles per second in the acoustic waveform
   - Pitch is a correlate of this
   - Voice disorders may manifest as altered or restricted pitch
2. Intensity
   - Loudness, measured in dB sound pressure level (SPL)
   - Conversational voice is generally approximately 70 dB SPL
3. Jitter
   - Cycle-to-cycle variation in *pitch/frequency*
   - Has not been shown to correspond to voice disorders
4. Shimmer
   - Cycle-to-cycle variation in *amplitude/loudness*
   - Has not been shown to correspond to voice disorders

Vocal Tasks to Be Performed for Assessment

- Average or anchor speech frequency
- Maximum frequency range
- Projected voice and yell
- Very-high-frequency, very-low-intensity tasks that detect mucosal disturbances
- Register use and phenomena
- MPT
- Instability and tremors
- Inconsistencies between spoken and sung capabilities

Auditory Perceptual Assessment

- Grading of voice by the trained listener
- Grade, Roughness, Breathiness, Asthenia, Strain (GRBAS) scale
- Consensus auditory-perceptual-evaluation-voice (CAPE-V)

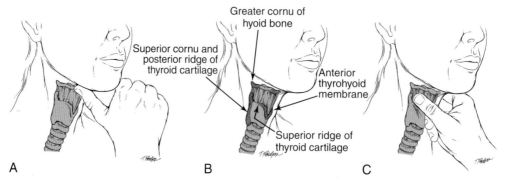

Fig. 7.5 Manual musculoskeletal tension evaluation. (A) Palpation of suprahyoid musculature. **(B)** Palpation of greater cornu of the hyoid bone, superior cornu of the thyroid cartilage, and lateral aspects of the thyroid cartilage. **(C)** Palpation of the thyrohyoid space. (From Flint PW, Haughey BH, Lund VJ, et al. *Cummings Otolaryngology—Head and Neck Surgery.* 6th ed. Philadelphia, PA: Saunders; 2015, Fig. 56.4.)

GRBAS Scale, Graded From 0 to 3

1. Grade: Overall severity
2. Roughness
3. Breathiness
4. Asthenia
5. Strain

CAPE-V, Rated by Marking Severity Along a 100-mm Line

1. Overall severity
2. Roughness
3. Breathiness
4. Strain
5. Pitch
6. Loudness

NEUROLOGICAL EVALUATION OF THE LARYNX

History Assessment for the Patient With New-Onset Dysarthria

- History of neurological defects (e.g., cerebrovascular accident [CVA])
- History of neuromuscular disease (e.g., amyotrophic lateral sclerosis [ALS]/Parkinson disease [PD])
- Presence of other areas of weakness
- Gait instability
- Dysphagia for solids and/or liquids

Physical Examination for the Patient With New-Onset Dysarthria

1. Gross-motion clues of the oral cavity and oropharynx
   - Involuntary, slow, athetoid movements: Tardive dyskinesia
   - Tongue with "bag of worms" appearance: ALS
   - Spasmodic motion of the tongue and jaw: Oromandibular dystonia
   - Regular, repetitive jerking motions of the palate and/or pharynx: Myoclonus
   - Soft voice that responds well to cuing: PD
2. Test lip motion: Repeat "Pa"
3. Test tongue motion: Repeat "Ta"
4. Test posterior tongue motion: Repeat "Ga"
   - Decreased strength of action: Lower motor neuron
   - Reduced rate with rhythm preserved: Upper motor neuron
   - Erratic rhythm: Cerebellar lesion
   - Fatigue: Myasthenia gravis
5. Flexible laryngoscopy indications of poor swallow
   - Impaired pharyngeal squeeze
   - Pooling of secretions in the hypopharynx

Laryngeal Electromyography Basics

- Assess integrity of RLN (paralysis vs. cricoarytenoid dislocation)
- May offer prognostic information in early paralysis
- Laryngeal electromyography (LEMG) will more often accurately predict poor prognosis in the setting of poor LEMG findings compared with predicting a good prognosis in the setting of positive LEMG findings

Common Laryngeal Electromyography Findings

- Intact cricothyroid signal but absent thyroarytenoid signal: RLN injury but intact vagus nerve and SLN

- Fibrillation potentials with decreased activity: Denervation
- Polyphasic action potentials: Reinnervation
- Fatiguing: Myasthenia gravis
- Decreased frequency: Neuropathy
- Decreased amplitude: Myopathy

NEUROLOGICAL DISORDERS OF THE LARYNX

Differential Diagnosis for Vocal Instability With Normal Vocal Structure and Full Abduction and Adduction of the True Vocal Folds

1. Spasmodic dysphonia (SD)
2. Vocal tremor (benign essential tremor)
3. MTD
4. Underlying neurological disease

Spasmodic Dysphonia Diagnostic Features

- Unstable voice that improves with whispering, singing, or alcohol consumption
- May worsen with stress
- If voice is unstable through multiple sounds, with whisper and with singing, consider vocal tremor versus MTD
- 16% of SD patients will have another dystonia; 10% of SD cases are familial
- Consider Meige syndrome: Dystonia of the eyelid, tongue, floor of mouth, and masseter, with 25% laryngeal involvement

Adductor Spasmodic Dysphonia

- 87% of SD cases
- Choked, strangled-strained voice with abrupt initiation/termination from thyroarytenoids (TAs)/lateral cricoarytenoids (LCAs) dysfunction
- More with voiced vowels: "We eat eggs every Easter."
- Treatment: Botulinum toxin to one or both TA muscles under electromyography (EMG) guidance
  - Demonstrated to improve speaking to mean 90% of normal function, with duration of effect between 3 and 4 months

Abductor Spasmodic Dysphonia

- 12% of SD cases
- Breathy, effortful voice with breaks; whispered segments of speech from PCA dysfunction
- Seen more in phrases with voiceless consonants: "Harry's happy hat"
- Treatment: Botulinum toxin to one or both PCA muscles
- Return to mean maximal functional performance of 70% of normal

Botulinum Toxin Basics

- Works by blocking presynaptic release of acetylcholine
- Recovery because of new nerve-terminal sprouting and increase in postjunctional receptors
- Potentiated by aminoglycosides
- Contraindicated in myasthenia gravis, Eaton-Lambert syndrome, and pregnancy

Vocal Tremor (Benign Essential Tremor)

- Tremoring persists with whisper, not sound specific, with vowel phonation
- Rhythmic at 6 to 8 Hz

- May have tremor elsewhere (e.g., hands and head)
- 10% to 20% of patients with essential tremor will have vocal involvement
- Treatment: β-Blocker, primidone is considered first-line therapy
- Botulinum toxin injections to thyroarytenoid have also been shown to be effective

Oculopalatopharyngeal Myoclonus

- Rhythmic contractions of the palate, larynx, and pharynx at a rate of approximately 1 to 2 per second
- Can involve the tensor veli palatine, causing repeating clicking noise
- Treated with botulinum toxin

Parkinson Disease

- Systemic: Resting tremor, rigidity, bradykinesia, and loss of postural reflexes
- Voice: Soft, breathy, stimulable to loud voice
- May have bowed or adynamic vocal folds
- "Parkinson plus" (multisystem atrophy/progressive supranuclear palsy), may have unilateral vocal fold immobility

Muscle Tension Dysphonia

- Strained, strangled voice with all sounds
- May cause a breathiness or a choppiness imitating a tremor or SD
- Treatment: Voice therapy

History Evaluation for the Vocal Fold–Motion-Impairment Patient

1. Recent surgery, specifically thyroid, cardiothoracic, or cervical spine surgery
2. Breathing or swallowing complaints or other signs and symptoms of lung, thyroid, or esophageal malignancy
3. History of intubations
4. History of rheumatoid disease

Possible Laryngeal Pathologies Caused by Intubation

1. Cricoarytenoid fixation
2. Posterior glottic stenosis
3. Vocal cord paralysis

Vocal Fold–Motion-Impairment Patient Voice Characteristics

1. Breathy quality
2. Phonatory dyspnea: Patient runs out of air while talking
3. Decreased MPT (normal range: 20–25 seconds)

Vocal Fold–Motion-Impairment Patient Workup

1. Direct laryngoscopy and bronchoscopy in the operating room (OR) to assess for cricoarytenoid joint dislocation/fixation
2. Imaging: Computed tomography with contrast of full course of RLNs, from the skull base to the aortic arch if no other temporal cause
3. Laboratory tests

Professional Voice

Constituents in Professional Voice User Evaluation and Treatment Team

- Laryngologist
- Speech language pathologist
- Vocal pedagogue

Ways to Increase Subglottic Pressure and Sound Intensity

1. Increase airflow: More efficient
2. Increase force of vocal fold adduction: Less efficient

Key Past Medical History Evaluation for a Professional Voice User

- Pulmonary status: Pulmonary disease and medications, especially inhalers
- Hydration: Diuretics and oral hydration
  - Singer should be drinking at least 8 glasses (64 oz) of water per day
- Posture: Musculoskeletal issues that may affect the vocal tract
- Personal habits
  - Caffeine and alcohol intake (diuretics)
  - High-fat, dairy diets will thicken mucus
- Thyroid function: May alter Reinke space

Key Physical Examination Components for a Professional Voice User

- Complete head and neck examination
- Nasal examination: Obstruction may lead to mouth breathing and dry-air exposure to the larynx
- Anterior neck/strap muscle palpation: Examine for excess tension
- Laryngeal endoscopy or stroboscopy

Vocal Misuse Basics

- Inefficient and/or excessive voice production when voice is produced with excess laryngeal tension or insufficient respiratory support
- Maladaptive patterns may begin with acute change, such as a URI

Treatment for the Singer With Laryngitis

- Voice rest: Cancel performance if laryngitis is severe
- Hydration
- Antitussives for a prominent cough
- If patient chooses to perform, inform of the increased risk of hemorrhage and potential for permanent damage to the vocal folds

Indications to Cancel Singing Performance

1. Submucosal vocal fold hemorrhage
2. Enlarging varix
3. Vocal fold mucosal break
4. Severe laryngitis

Medications to Be Avoided by a Professional Singer

- Inhaled steroids
- Antihistamines
- Aspirin
- Decongestants
- Topical analgesics
- Mentholated products

Indications for Systemic Steroids for a Professional Singer

- Edema from episodic overuse
- Mild-to-moderate laryngitis
- Vocal fold hemorrhage

Laser Surgery: Basic Principles and Safety Considerations

Three Properties of LASER Light (Fig. 7.6)

1. Monochromatic: Single color, same wavelength
2. Collimated: Emits organized light in the same direction
3. Coherent: In space and time

LASER Basics

- Light amplification by stimulated emission of radiation (LASER) has an optical resonating chamber that contains medium (e.g., argon or carbon dioxide [CO_2]) between two mirrors
- Medium is excited by a current
- Lens-focused beam to a small spot size
- Helium-neon visible aiming beam allows for visualization of wavelength in the nonvisible range

Three Variables in the Surgeon's Control

1. Power (watts)
2. Spot size (square millimeters or centimeters)
3. Exposure time (seconds)

Key LASER Formulas

- Irradiance (W/cm^2) − power/focal spot area
- Fluence (J/cm^2) = energy/target tissue = power density × time

LASER: Tissue Interactions

1. Reflection
2. Absorption (surgical interaction)
3. Transmission
4. Scattering

Argon Laser

- Blue-green light: 488 and 514 nm (tunable argon to 630 nm)
- Transmitted through clear aqueous tissues (e.g., cornea, lens, and vitreous humor)
- Absorbed and reflected to varying degrees by tissues that are white (e.g., skin, fat, and bone)
- Absorbed by hemoglobin and pigmented tissues
- Clinical use examples: Stapedotomy, port wine stains, hemangiomas, telangiectasias, and photodynamic therapy
- Drawbacks: Heat produced destroys the epidermis and upper dermis

Neodymium:Yttrium-Aluminum-Garnet LASER

- Near infrared: 1064 nm
- Transmitted through clear liquids
- Increased absorption in darkly pigmented tissues and charred debris
- Strong scattering leads to a zone of thermal coagulation and necrosis of approximately 4 mm
- Clinical use examples: Ablation of tracheobronchial and esophageal lesions and photocoagulation of vascular and lymphatic malformations
- Benefit: Control of hemorrhage is more secure because of the LASER beam's deep penetration in tissue
- Drawback: Lacks precision

Carbon Dioxide

- 10,600 nm infrared, HeNe aiming beam
- Absorbed by water
- 60°C and 65°C (140°F–149°F), protein denaturation occurs
  - Tissue effect: Blanching
- >100°C (212°F), vaporization of intracellular water occurs, craters, and tissue shrinkage occurs
  - Tissue effect: Carbonization, smoke, and gas generation
- Impact:
  - Zone of thermal necrosis about 100-µm wide
  - Adjacent zone of thermal conductivity and repair, which is usually 300 to 500 µm wide
  - Less postoperative edema, likely because heat seals vessels
- Minimize thermal damage by using a shorter pulse
- Can be used with micromanipulator, with pattern generator, or with flexible waveguide
- Clinical use examples: Stapedotomy, cosmetic skin treatment, laryngology, and bronchoesophagology (cordotomy, medial arytenoidectomy, or total arytenoidectomy)
- Very precise, with increased hemostasis and decreased intraoperative edema

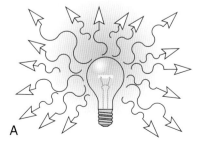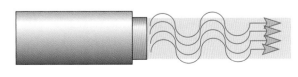

Fig. 7.6 (**A**) Light emitted from a conventional lamp. The light travels in all directions, is composed of many wavelengths, and is not coherent. (**B**) Light emitted from a laser travels in the same direction and is a single wavelength, and all of the waves are in phase; the light is coherent. (From Flint PW, Haughey BH, Lund VJ, et al. *Cummings Otolaryngology—Head and Neck Surgery*. 6th ed. Philadelphia, PA: Saunders; 2015, Fig. 60.3.)

Potassium-Titanyl-Phosphate Laser

- 532 nm
- Absorbed by hemoglobin, specifically oxyhemoglobin
- Clinical use: Otological, rhinological, and laryngological surgery; tonsillectomy, pigmented dermal lesions, and stapes surgery
- Pulsed mode to decrease thermal damage
- Fiber based

Pulsed Dye Laser

- 585 nm
- Chromophore for the pulsed dye laser (PDL) is oxyhemoglobin (577 nm)
- Selectively absorbed by intraluminal blood of vascular lesions such as papillomas, vascular polyps, vocal fold ectasias, hemangiomas, and port wine stains
- Hemoglobin absorption is maximal, with minimal scattering and absorption by melanin and other pigments

Laser Eye and Skin Safety Considerations

- Protect the eyes of the patient, surgeon, and other OR personnel
- Visible and near-infrared lasers can cause corneal or retinal burns
- CO_2 laser surgery: Place double layer of saline-moistened eye pads over the eyes of the patient
- The patient's exposed skin and mucous membranes outside the surgical field should be protected by a double layer of saline-saturated surgical towels, surgical sponges, or lap pads

Laser Smoke Safety and Evacuation Considerations

- Have two separate suction setups
  - Smoke and steam evacuation
  - Blood and mucus from the operative wound
- Papillomavirus has been detected in the laser plume, but no cases of clinical transmission of diseases have been documented

Anesthetic Considerations for Laser Surgery

- Nonflammable general anesthetic should be used (e.g., halothane and enflurane)
- Mixtures of helium, nitrogen, or air plus oxygen are commonly used
- Maintain the forced inspiratory oxygen <40%
- Nitrous oxide should not be used
- Protection should also be provided for the cuff of the endotracheal (ET) tube; saline-saturated cottonoids are placed above the cuff
- Methylene blue–colored saline may be used to inflate the cuff
- In the event of tube ignition, the tube should be withdrawn simultaneously as saline is flushed down the ET tube and ventilation is stopped
- The airway must be reestablished immediately, and bronchoscopy should be performed to assess the degree of injury
- Intravenous steroids may be delivered, and the patient should remain intubated; repeat bronchoscopy should be performed daily until it is established that the airway is stable

BENIGN VOCAL FOLD MUCOSAL DISORDERS

Risk Factors for Vocal Injury

- High intrinsic tendency to use the voice (talkativeness and extroversion)
- High extrinsic opportunity or necessity to use the voice, driven by occupation, family needs, social activities, and avocations
- Visible vocal fold lesions may not cause an audible change in the speaking voice
- Visible vocal fold lesions that cause phonatory mismatch at the free margin or mucosal stiffness that are always detectable audibly in the singing voice provided that the examiner knows how to elicit upper-range vocal tasks

Singing-Voice Symptoms of Mucosal Injury

- Loss of the ability to sing softly at high pitches
- Increased day-to-day variability of singing-voice capabilities
- Phonatory onset delays
- Reduced vocal endurance
- Sense of increased effort

Sinonasal Symptom Management in the Voice

- Sinonasal conditions should be managed locally (topically) when possible
- Systemic drugs (e.g., oral decongestants or antihistamine–decongestant combinations) dry not only nasal secretions but also secretions in the larynx, thus, should be avoided
- Profuse rhinorrhea that accompanies the common cold can also be managed with ipratropium bromide inhalations

Common Symptoms Suggesting Reflux Laryngitis

- Exaggerated "morning mouth"
- Excessive phlegm
- Scratchy or dry throat irritation that is usually worse in the morning
- Habitual throat clearing
- Huskiness or lowered pitch of the voice in the morning

Treatment of Reflux Laryngitis

- Avoid caffeine, alcohol, and spicy foods
- Eat nothing 3 hours before bed
- Elevate the head of the bed
- Take antacid at bedtime, or H2 blocker 2 to 3 hours before bed
- Proton pump inhibitor (PPI) 30 to 60 minutes before dinner

Treatment of Acute Mucosal Swelling of Overuse

- Relative vocal rest in context
- Pre-performance warm-up and solid vocal technique
- May consider short-term, high-dose tapering regimen of corticosteroids

Systemic Medications that May Affect the Larynx

- Decongestants
- Antidepressants
- Antihypertensives
- Diuretics

Voice Therapy Basics

- Success can be defined as a more consistent voice, without the exacerbations of hoarseness even if that now-more-reliable voice remains somewhat husky
- Success may require resolution of all upper-voice limitations in performers
- Some lesions are known at diagnosis to be irreversible except via surgery; aside from these exceptions, vocal fold microsurgery should follow an appropriate trial of voice therapy
- Nodules are expected to resolve, regress, or at least stabilize

SPECIFIC BENIGN VOCAL FOLD MUCOSAL DISORDERS

Vocal Fold Nodule Basics

- Vocal nodules occur most commonly in boys and in women
- Almost always vocal "over-doers"
- Formation starts with localized vascular congestion with edema at the midportion of the membranous vocal folds, where shearing and collisional forces are greatest
- Maturation occurs with hyalinization of Reinke space and, in a subset of patients, to some thickening of the overlying epithelium
- Nodules do not occur unilaterally, although one may be larger than the other
- The larynx should be examined at high frequency to visualize subtle to small swellings, which can be poorly appreciated at lower frequencies
- Initial onset may be associated with a URI or acute laryngitis, after which the hoarseness never clears completely

Common Vocal Nodule Symptoms

- Loss of the ability to sing high notes softly
- Delayed phonatory onset, particularly with high, soft singing
- Increased breathiness (air escape), roughness, and harshness
- Reduced vocal endurance ("my voice gets husky easily")
- A sensation of increased effort for singing
- A need for longer warm-ups
- Day-to-day variability of vocal capabilities that is greater than expected for the singer's level of vocal training

Vocal Nodule Treatment Options

- Voice therapy plays a primary role
- Good laryngeal lubrication should be ensured through general hydration
- Allergy and reflux, when present, should also be treated
- Surgical removal becomes an option when nodules of any size persist and when the voice remains unacceptably impaired after voice therapy for >3 months (Fig. 7.7)

Capillary Ectasia Basics

- Capillary ectasia seems to happen most often in vocal over-doers
- Repeated vibratory microtrauma can lead to capillary angiogenesis
- Hoarse after relatively short periods of singing
- Additional symptoms reminiscent of nodules
- Treatment: Voice therapy, consider stopping nonsteroidal anti-inflammatory drugs/anticoagulants if medically appropriate

Indications for Surgical Ablation of Capillary Ectasias

1. Persistent decreased vocal endurance
2. Intermittent bruising
3. Hemorrhagic polyp

Vocal Fold Hemorrhagic Polyp Basics

- Capillary rupture causes accumulation of blood; similar to a blister
- May thicken overlying epithelium and stiffen vocal fold
- More common in men
- Intermittent severe voice abuse; working in noisy environments
- Abrupt onset of hoarseness during extreme vocal effort, such as at a party or sporting event

Vocal Fold Hemorrhagic Polyp Appearance on Examination (Fig. 7.8)

- Unilateral lesion in the "node position" with a possible small contralateral lesion
- May or may not have hemorrhagic or bruised appearance

Treatment Options for Hemorrhagic Polyps and Vocal Fold Hemorrhage

- Voice therapy
- For recent large hemorrhage, evacuation of blood may be appropriate

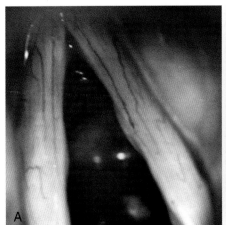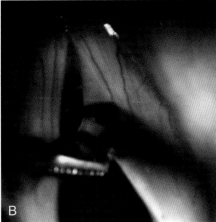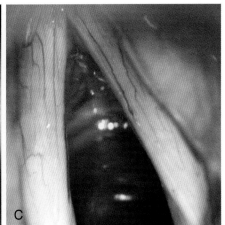

Fig. 7.7 The operative sequence in a professional musical theater actor who had been experiencing vocal symptoms and limitations compatible with fusiform vocal nodules for more than 2 years. (**A**) The operative view after many months of conservative management. Not all fusiform swellings are reversible with conservative measures alone. (**B**) A polypoid nodule is grasped superficially and tented medially with Bouchayer forceps. Scissors that curve away from the vocal fold are used for removal. The nodule is thus removed in a very superficial plane, which minimizes the risk of scar between the remaining and regenerated mucosa and the underlying vocal ligament. (**C**) Vocal fold appearance after excision. The patient experienced dramatic normalization of vocal capabilities, and no evidence of scarring was found on postoperative stroboscopic examination. The dilated capillaries may predispose to recurrent nodule formation and can be spot coagulated with a microspot laser. (From Flint PW, Haughey BH, Lund VJ, et al. *Cummings Otolaryngology—Head and Neck Surgery.* 6th ed. Philadelphia, PA: Saunders; 2015, Fig. 61.8.)

- A long-standing polyp, whether hemorrhagic or end stage and pale, should be excised at the time the spot coagulations take place
- Prognosis for full return of vocal functioning after precision surgery is excellent

Intracordal Cyst Basics

- Two types
  1. Mucus retention
  2. Epidermal inclusion
- Patients often demonstrate diplophonia in the upper vocal range
- May manifest an abrupt and irreducible transition to severe impairment at a relatively specific frequency
- Depth of lesion in superficial layer of the lamina propria (SLP) changes the vibration of the affected vocal fold

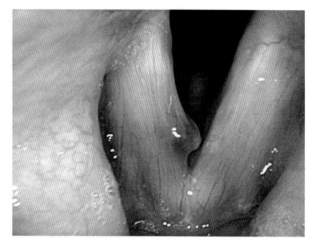

Fig. 7.8 Hemorrhagic polyp, right fold. Note the blood-blister appearance. Recent further bleeding is evident from the yellowish discoloration of the upper surface of the fold because of breakdown products of a bruise, estimated to have occurred 2 weeks earlier. Hemorrhagic polyps sometimes rebruise intermittently. (From Flint PW, Haughey BH, Lund VJ, et al. *Cummings Otolaryngology—Head and Neck Surgery.* 6th ed. Philadelphia, PA: Saunders; 2015, Fig. 61.11.)

Intracordal Cyst Findings on Examination

- Often originate just below the free margin of the fold with significant medial projection from the fold
- Reduction in mucosal wave over the lesion
- Open cyst: The sphere may be less discrete and may have a more mottled appearance on the superior surface of the vocal fold
- Opposite fold should be examined carefully because of the possibility of a more subtle cyst or sulcus

Treatment Options for Intracordal Cyst

- Voice therapy is considered
- Surgical excision should be performed with maximal mucosal preservation (Fig. 7.9)
- Surgical results are not as uniformly good as they are for nodules and polyps

Glottic Sulcus Basics

- Epidermal cyst that has spontaneously emptied, leaving the collapsed pocket behind to form a sulcus
- Can be congenital and be seen in vocal over-doers
- Similar effect as scarring: Stiffening of the mucosa inhibits oscillation and leads to dysphonia
- Not always visible during the office or voice laboratory examination: Microlaryngoscopy is often required for definitive diagnosis

Glottic Sulcus Treatment

- Trial of voice therapy
- Surgical excision: Sulcus removal is technically demanding
  - Technique: Hydrodissection via injection, circumcision of the lips of the sulcus and by dissection of the invaginated mucosal pocket from the underlying fold without injuring the vocal ligament (Fig. 7.10)
- Voice outcomes less optimal than with polyp excision

Bilateral Diffuse Polyposis Basics

- Middle-aged talkative women who have been long-term smokers
- Lower pitch than would be expected: A female being called "sir" on the telephone
- Exam: Pale, watery bags of fluid attached to the superior surface and margins of the fold

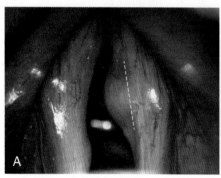
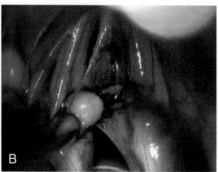
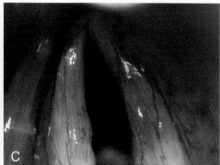

Fig. 7.9 (**A**) Mucous retention cyst of right vocal fold. Yellowish spherical mass shines through overlying mucosa and was causing the patient severe hoarseness. Incision to enter the fold is made on the dotted line. (**B**) Near completion of dissection of the cyst from its final attachments using curved scissors. (**C**) After cyst removal. The patient's voice sounded virtually normal in the recovery room, although the upper voice was still abnormal. (From Flint PW, Haughey BH, Lund VJ, et al. *Cummings Otolaryngology—Head and Neck Surgery.* 6th ed. Philadelphia, PA: Saunders; 2015, Fig. 61.17.)

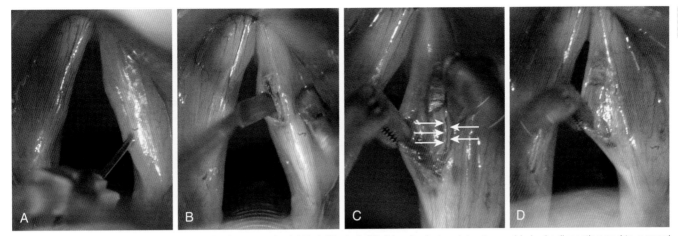

Fig. 7.10 Glottic sulcus. (A) At the beginning of surgery, the fold is infiltrated with lidocaine/epinephrine to provide hydrodissection and to expand the mucosa. The line of sulcus is seen proceeding anteriorly from the point of needle entry. **(B)** An elliptic incision has been made around the lips of the sulcus. **(C)** Right-curved alligator clip tents the medial mucosal flap. Arrows indicate the fine line that represents the opening into the sulcus. Curved scissors dissect the anterior aspect of the sulcus pocket from underlying vocal ligament. **(D)** After the sulcus pocket is removed, the gossamer mucosa is tented medially to show remaining flexibility. The voice is expected to improve, but normal upper-voice capabilities are only achieved sometimes. (From Flint PW, Haughey BH, Lund VJ, et al. *Cummings Otolaryngology—Head and Neck Surgery.* 6th ed. Philadelphia, PA: Saunders; 2015, Fig. 61.19.)

Treatment Options for Bilateral Diffuse Polyposis

- Smoking cessation
- Consider thyroid function tests
- Polyp reduction with mucosal sparing
- May consider in-office laser ablation

Contact Ulcer or Granuloma Basics

- Contact granuloma or ulceration is seen primarily in men
- Chronic coughing or throat clearing traumatizes the posterior larynx
- Reflux of acid from the stomach into the posterior larynx during sleep
- Result: Thin mucosa and perichondrium overlying the cartilaginous glottis become inflamed

Presentation of Contact Ulcer or Granuloma

- Unilateral discomfort over the midthyroid cartilage, occasionally with referred pain to the ipsilateral ear
- Hoarseness may develop when contact granulation tissue becomes large
- Exam: May appear as a depressed, ulcerated area with a whitish exudate clinging to it, or a bilobed, heaped-up lesion on the vocal process may be noted

Treatment Options for Contact Ulcer or Granuloma

- Antireflux regimen should be initiated
- Voice therapy
  - Abolish throat clearing
  - Raise average pitch for speech
- Injection of a depot corticosteroid directly into the lesion can be considered
- Botulinum injection into the thyroarytenoid muscle can be considered
- Due to high recurrence rate, removal should be limited, leaving the base or pedicle undisturbed

Intubation Granuloma Basics

- Patients who underwent acute or chronic intubation, rigid bronchoscopy, or other direct laryngeal manipulations
- Treatment: Voice therapy, reflux regimen, and time

Laryngocele and Saccular Cyst Basics (Fig. 7.11)

- Air filled: Laryngocele with patent saccular orifice
- Mucus filled: Saccular cyst with blocked orifice
- Purulence filled: Laryngopyocele with blocked orifice
- In infants, saccular disorders appear to be congenital
- Can be caused by transglottic pressure, such as that seen in trumpet players, glass blowers, and people using the voice in unusually forceful ways
- An uncommon cause of saccular cysts is laryngeal carcinoma, which causes obstruction of the saccular orifice

Laryngocele and Saccular Cyst Variants

- Anterior saccular cyst: Tends to protrude from the anterior ventricle toward the laryngeal vestibule; when large, it may "push down" on the vocal fold and cause dysphonia
- Lateral saccular cyst or laryngocele, internal only: Tends to dissect more superiorly and laterally up into the false and aryepiglottic folds, sometimes bulging not only those structures (medially) but also the medial wall of the piriform sinus (laterally), or even to fill the vallecula
- Lateral saccular cyst or laryngocele, internal/external: Tends to dissect as described for the lateral cyst but also tends to penetrate through the thyrohyoid membrane and appear as a palpable swelling in the neck

Treatment Considerations for Laryngocele and Saccular Cysts

- Researchers affirm complete endoscopic excision, instead of endoscopic marsupialization or transcervical removal, even for large recurrent lateral saccular cysts

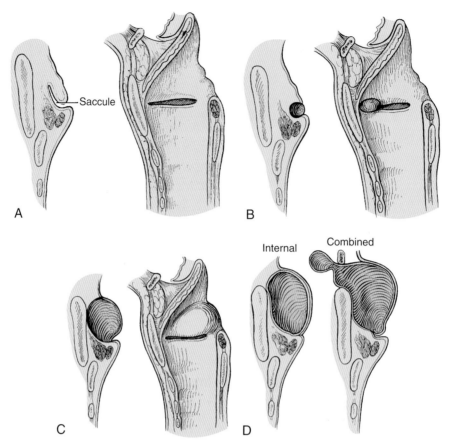

Fig. 7.11 The classification scheme for a laryngocele or saccular cyst. (**A**) Normal anatomy. (**B**) Anterior saccular cyst. (**C**) Lateral saccular cyst. (**D**) Laryngocele types. (From Flint PW, Haughey BH, Lund VJ, et al. *Cummings Otolaryngology—Head and Neck Surgery*. 6th ed. Philadelphia, PA: Saunders; 2015, Fig. 61.29.)

- During endoscopic approach should note that even a large lateral cyst that bulges dramatically during awake endoscopy can virtually disappear under conditions of direct laryngoscopy with general anesthesia
- Can begin excising the false fold, during which the wall of the cyst is invariably encountered

Recurrent Respiratory Papillomatosis Basics

- Squamous papillomata caused by the human papillomavirus (HPV)
- Most common benign neoplasms seen by laryngologists
- Majority of infections are the result of subtypes 6 and 11; type 11 appears to predispose to more aggressive disease
- Juvenile form (HPV type 6 or 11) usually manifests in infancy or childhood as hoarseness and stridor and is usually aggressive and rapidly recurrent
- Adult-onset papillomata are occasionally solitary and more localized than juvenile-onset lesions are and are more likely to be of the so-called carpet variant (Fig. 7.12)

Treatment Considerations for Recurrent Respiratory Papillomatosis

- Cold dissection, potassium-titanyl-phosphate, and 585-PDL, CO_2, and thulium lasers
  - CO_2 is the most widely accepted management for papilloma for depth control and hemostasis
  - Goal is to remove disease with preservation of vocal fold structures
  - Deep excision does not prevent recurrence

- Adjuvants
  - Intralesional cidofovir
  - Some consider bevacizumab
  - Investigational use of interferon and indole-3-carbinol

Polypoid Granulation Tissue Basics

- Most common vascular tumor in the larynx
- Can be caused by laryngeal biopsy, intubation, direct external trauma to the larynx, and external penetrating wounds
- Treatment: Conservative measures that include removal of the source of any ongoing irritation and intralesional corticosteroids
- For nonresponse and continuing symptoms, careful endoscopic removal may be considered

Laryngeal Rhabdomyoma Basics

- Most extracardiac rhabdomyomas are found in the head and neck region, in the pharynx and larynx
- Will not recur after local excision: Approach should be conservative

Other Benign Neoplasms of the Larynx

- Benign mixed neoplasm (pleomorphic adenomas)
  - Extremely rare
  - Most commonly presents as a smooth, ovoid submucosal mass in the subglottis
  - Treatment is surgical excision with type of excision to be determined by location and size of the tumor

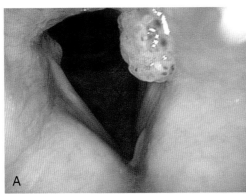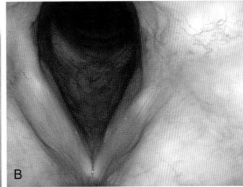

Fig. 7.12 (**A**) Papillomata at posterior vocal folds; the left side is much larger than the right. (**B**) 2 weeks after microsurgical removal, cidofovir injection, and return of normal voice. (From Flint PW, Haughey BH, Lund VJ, et al. *Cummings Otolaryngology—Head and Neck Surgery*. 6th ed. Philadelphia, PA: Saunders; 2015, Fig. 61.34.)

- Oncocytic tumor
  - Not a true neoplasm
  - Oncocytic metaplasia and hyperplasia of the ductal cell portion of glandular tissue
  - Treated with simple excision
- Chondroma
  - Clinical behavior of chondromas and low-grade chondrosarcomas are so similar that histological distinction has little practical significance
  - Slow growing and does not metastasize
  - Smooth, rounded mass in the subglottis: Posterior aspect of the cricoid
  - Treatment with excision, most commonly with laryngofissure
- Granular cell neoplasm
  - The middle to posterior part of the true vocal fold is the most common site
  - Insufficiently deep biopsy of this lesion can lead to an incorrect diagnosis of squamous cell carcinoma from overlying pseudoepitheliomatous hyperplasia of the mucosa
  - Treatment: Conservative but complete local excision
- Neurofibroma
  - Most commonly presents as lobulated nodules on the arytenoid or aryepiglottic fold
  - Recommend conservative, complete excision
- Neurilemmoma
  - Most commonly found on the aryepiglottic fold or false vocal fold
  - Treatment: Conservative but complete local excision

Postoperative Dysphonia

- Vocal fold surgery performed without extreme precision can lead to permanent dysphonia secondary to:
  - Scarring of the vocal fold cover with loss of pliability
  - Mismatch between the two vocal folds
- History must include voice-use patterns, which may explain previous lesion formation, as well as poor outcome from initial surgery
- Treatment: Voice therapy with a voice-building strategy—gradual increase in voice use, which seems to soften the vocal scar and allow greater range
- >9 to 12 months should pass before reoperation is entertained
  - If glottic insufficiency is the main issue
    - May consider injection: Collagen or fat
    - Thyroplasty
  - If scarring is the main issue, may consider incision and elevation of mucosa with early postoperative phonation to prevent reformation of scar
  - There is limited evidence to support any of these measures; proper preoperative patient education and careful surgical technique to prevent postoperative dysphonia are most important

ACUTE AND CHRONIC LARYNGITIS

Acute Laryngitis

Phonotrauma

- Vocal abuse, misuse, and overuse can contribute to phonotrauma
- Treatment: Voice rest, steroids

Viral Laryngitis

- Most common types
  - Herpes zoster
  - Coronavirus
- Treatment options
  - Supportive care, rehydration, and vocal rest
  - In severe cases that result in airway embarrassment:
    - Steroids
    - Antibiotics for secondary infections
    - PPIs
    - Humidification

Acute Bacterial Laryngitis

- Presentation: Drooling, febrile patient in respiratory distress
- Treatment options
  - Intubation in a controlled setting or awake tracheotomy may be appropriate
  - Most can be managed supportively with humidification, intravenous antibiotics, and close observation

Acute Fungal Laryngitis

- Typical history: Patient on steroids (systemic or inhaled) or antibiotics
- Most common pathogen: *Candida*

- Presentation:
  - Hoarseness with or without accompanying throat discomfort
  - Diffuse, whitish speckling of the vocal folds or supraglottis
- Differential diagnosis
  - Hyperkeratosis
  - Thick, dried mucus
  - Malignancy

Klebsiella Rhinoscleromatis

- Parts of the body are generally involved
  - Nose
  - Larynx
  - Trachea
- Pathology findings
  - Gram-negative coccobacillus, within macrophages (Mikulicz cells)
- Treatment
  - Fluoroquinolones
  - Tetracycline
  - Airway management

Chronic Laryngitis

Fungal Laryngitis

Blastomycosis

- Geographic region: Southern United States
- Pathology findings
  - Broad-based budding yeast
  - Possible *pseudoepitheliomatous hyperplasia*, which may be mistaken for the advancing front of an epithelial malignancy
- Treatment: Amphotericin B, ketoconazole, or itraconazole

Paracoccidioidomycosis

- Epidemiology: South American male farm workers
- Examination findings: Ulcerative and exophytic lesions, which can resemble carcinoma
- Treatment: Systemic antifungal therapy

Coccidioidomycosis

- Geographic region: "Valley fever" (San Joaquin Valley, California) is a disease of the southwestern United States and northern Mexico
- Can present with airway obstruction
- Treatment: Systemic antifungal therapy

Histoplasmosis

- Geographic region: Ohio and Mississippi River valleys
- Typical patient population: Immunocompromised secondary to HIV infection, posttransplant, or diabetes mellitus
- Presentation: Localized pulmonary infection or systemic dissemination
- Treatment: Amphotericin and fluconazole

Mycobacterial Laryngitis

- Geographic region: South America, Africa, and the Asian subcontinent
- Organisms: *Mycobacterium tuberculosis*, atypical mycobacteria
- Presentation: Odynophagia and dysphonia
- Pathology findings: Acid-fast bacilli and caseating granulomas
- True and false vocal folds were the most commonly affected sites
- Laryngeal manifestations of the disease are possible without systemic disease: Generally, patients had either active pulmonary disease (47%) or inactive pulmonary tuberculosis (TB; 33%), whereas 15% had isolated laryngeal TB

Noninfectious Laryngitis

Reflux Laryngitis

- Reflux irritation induces changes in the epithelium and stroma of laryngeal tissue that lead to organ dysfunction
- Bile has been implicated as a possible source of laryngeal injury
- Pepsin is active principally at acidic pH; however, pepsin was found to maintain its proteolytic activity at pH above 4 and was able to be "reactivated" after some time in a pH-neutral environment

Laryngitis Associated With Autoimmune Diseases

Pemphigoid and Pemphigus

- Presentation: 80% of the patients with pemphigus had otolaryngological signs and symptoms, of which 40% were laryngeal in nature
- Pathology: Intraepithelial (pemphigus vulgaris) or subepithelial (pemphigoid) autoantibodies
- Treatment: High-dose corticosteroids combined with immunosuppressant therapy

Granulomatosis With Polyangiitis (Wegener Granulomatosis)

- Presentation: ~20% of all patients with granulomatosis with polyangiitis (GPA) will develop subglottic stenosis
- Pathology: Small- and medium-vessel vasculitis with *necrotizing granulomas*
- Laboratory studies
  - Autoantibodies against proteinase 3 (c-ANCA) and myeloperoxidase (p-ANCA)
  - Systemic disease, 95% are ANCA positive
  - Head and neck, 75% are ANCA positive
- Treatment: Immunosuppressant therapy and surgical intervention to maintain airway

Relapsing Polychondritis

- Presentation
  - 25% to 50% demonstrate symptoms of laryngeal dysfunction
  - Most often affecting the cricoarytenoid joint, potentially causing immobility
  - Hoarseness, pain, cough, and airway obstruction
  - Most commonly manifests in the ears, nose, tracheobronchial cartilage, and joints
- Pathology
  - Inflammation in cartilages high in the glycosaminoglycans
  - Autoantibodies directed against type II collagen
- Diagnosis made clinically; no laboratory or pathology analysis
- Treatment: Local or systemic steroids and immunomodulators

Sarcoidosis

- Presentation
  - Laryngeal manifestations occur in <1% of patients
  - Pulmonary, hepatic, cutaneous, cardiac, and lymphatic system involvement is common
  - Supraglottic and glottic larynx are most often involved in the form of diffuse edema
- Pathology
  - Noncaseating granulomas
  - Possible elevated serum calcium and angiotensin-converting enzyme levels

- Treatment
  - Work with a rheumatologist to treat the underlying condition
  - First-line treatment: Systemic steroids
  - May require endoscopic resection if the mass is large enough to cause symptoms
  - Local steroid injection may also be of benefit

Amyloidosis

- Presentation
  - <1% of all benign laryngeal lesions
  - Nonulcerated, submucosal laryngeal mass or nodule often with a yellow or orange hue
  - Focal deposits can be secondary to extramedullary plasmacytomas and can occur in the mucosal-associated lymphoid tissue of the larynx
- Pathology
  - Extracellular deposition of abnormal proteinaceous debris
  - Can be associated with systemic lymphoproliferative or chronic inflammatory disorders such as multiple myeloma or rheumatoid arthritis
- Treatment
  - Consultation with pulmonary or rheumatology to assess for and treat systemic disease or underlying disorders causing the amyloidosis

Laryngeal Rhinoscleroma

- Organism: *Klebsiella rhinoscleromatis*
- Generally involves the nose and larynx and may involve the trachea
- Treatment: Fluoroquinolones, tetracycline, and supportive airway management

Vocal Fold Paralysis

Laryngeal Electromyography and Palpation

- EMG provides data regarding prognosis, which may inform the timing of intervention and choice of surgical procedures for the paralyzed larynx
- Other causes of immobility, such as joint ankylosis or cicatricle web formation, can be discerned only by palpation of the vocal process, which must be done under general anesthesia

Vocal Cord Paralysis Prognostic Factors

- Favorable prognosis: Blunt trauma, ET intubation, idiopathic vocal fold paralysis, and paralysis associated with viral pathogens (e.g., Ramsay Hunt syndrome)
- Poor prognosis: Injury after complete nerve section during surgical resection of tumor, cranial nerve involvement by tumor, paralysis associated with thoracic aneurysm, and paralysis from progressive neurological disorders

High Vagal Injury Consequences

- Loss of abductor/adductor function
- Loss of cricothyroid muscle function and deafferentation of sensory fibers
- Greater difficulty with dysphonia, dysphagia, and aspiration

Vocal Fold Medialization by Injection

Indications for Vocal Fold Injection Medialization

- Early vocal fold paralysis (<12 months from insult)
- Patients who are not candidates for thyroplasty
- Patients with limited expected survival duration (e.g., metastatic lung cancer) with severe dysphonia or aspiration symptoms

Materials Used for Vocal Fold–Injection Medialization

- Carboxymethylcellulose (Prolaryn Gel): Lasts 3 to 6 months and with no foreign body reaction
- Autologous fat: Requires overinjection; variable absorption; 62% overall success rate at 12 months
- Micronized Alloderm (Cymetra): Generally lasts 6 to 12 months and requires some overinjection and reconstitution because it comes in powdered form
- Calcium hydroxyapatite (Prolaryn Plus): Lasts 6 to 24 months and has a small potential for foreign body granulomatous reaction

Benefits and Drawbacks of In-Office Injection (Fig. 7.13)

- Safe and repeatable
- Lower cost
- Spares patient from general anesthesia

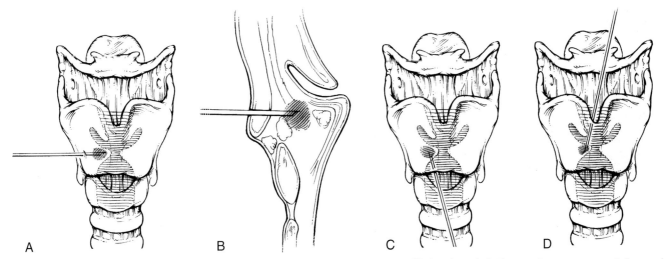

Fig. 7.13 (A) Lateral percutaneous approach for vocal fold injection. **(B)** Site of injection. **(C)** Anterior subglottic percutaneous approach for vocal fold medialization. **(D)** Superior transthyrohyoid space approach.

- Higher need for reinjection
- Higher rate of complication

In-Office Vocal Fold–Injection Medialization Approaches

1. Transoral injection
   - Requires topical laryngeal and pharyngeal anesthesia
   - Easier to assess depth
2. Transcricothyroid
   - May be performed submucosally topical anesthesia is unnecessary
   - Must be careful to assess depth
3. Transthyrohyoid
   - Requires topical laryngeal and pharyngeal anesthesia
   - Easier to assess depth
4. Transthyroid cartilage
   - Performed submucosally; thus, topical anesthesia is unnecessary
   - Must be careful to assess depth
   - Cartilage can jam the needle

Vocal Fold–Injection Medialization Under General Anesthesia

- Good for patients who do not tolerate awake injection
- Needle is placed laterally in the vocal fold just anterior to the vocal process, approximately at the depth of the lower margin of the true fold (Fig. 7.14)
- Advantages: Lower need for reinjection and lower complication rate
- Disadvantages: Cost, time, and cannot obtain vocal feedback from the patient during injection

Complications of Vocal Fold–Injection Medialization

- Underinjection
- Overinjection resulting in strained voice or potential airway compromise
- Improper placement with subglottal extension

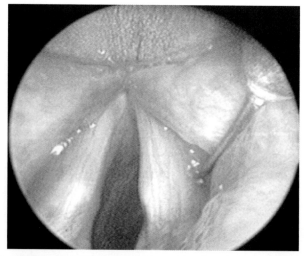

Fig. 7.14 Vocal fold injection performed by direct laryngoscopy with a Bruning syringe. The injection needle is placed lateral to the vocal process and vocal ligament to prevent infiltration into the Reinke space. (From Flint PW, Haughey BH, Lund VJ, et al. *Cummings Otolaryngology—Head and Neck Surgery*. 6th ed. Philadelphia, PA: Saunders; 2015, Fig. 63.3.)

- Laryngeal stenosis
- Migration into the superficial aspect of the vocal fold, which impairs vibratory capability
- Granuloma formation

Medialization Thyroplasty

Four Types of Laryngeal Framework Surgeries as Described by Isshiki

1. Type 1: Medial displacement—corrects glottic insufficiency
2. Type 2: Lateral displacement—used for SD
3. Type 3: Shortening or relaxation—rarely used
4. Type 4: Elongation—rarely used

Workup Before Considering Type I Thyroplasty

- Perceptual assessment: MPT and acoustic parameters
- Videostroboscopy: Provides visual assessment of glottal closure and status of the mucosal wave

Advantages of Medialization Thyroplasty

- Performed with local anesthesia with minimal or no discomfort to the patient
- Long lasting
- Reversible

Disadvantages of Medialization Thyroplasty

- Open procedure
- Technically more difficult
- Closure of the posterior glottis may be limited

Indications for Medialization Thyroplasty

1. Permanent vocal fold paralysis (>12 months from insult, nerve sacrifice, and EMG findings)
2. Vocal fold bowing because of aging or cricothyroid joint fixation
3. Sulcus vocalis
4. Soft-tissue defects from excision of pathological tissue

Medialization Thyroplasty Implants

- Factors that affect outcome include size, shape, and position of the implant
- Silastic implants can be carved to any shape but take more time during surgery to produce
- Prefabricated implants with matched sizing templates may reduce operative time
- Gore-Tex strips have increased adaptability in some situations: Better than prefabricated systems

Steps in Medialization Thyroplasty

1. Paramedian horizontal incision is outlined over the middle aspect of the thyroid lamina
2. Local anesthesia is administered subcutaneously and in four quadrants over the ipsilateral lamina
3. A 5-cm incision is made through the platysma
4. Elevate flaps
5. Strap muscles are split in the midline and are retracted laterally off the thyroid lamina, leaving the outer perichondrium intact
6. Single, large skin hook rotates the larynx
7. Cartilage window is outlined

8. Anterior aspect of the window is positioned 5 to 8 mm posterior to the ventral midline in women and 8 to 10 mm in men
9. Superior aspect of the window should be placed at the level of the true fold
10. A point half of the distance between the anterior-inferior border of the thyroid cartilage and the notch defines the level of the true fold
11. Outer perichondrium is incised and elevated
12. Window in cartilage is created
13. Size implant with flexible laryngoscopy guidance
14. Patient is asked to phonate while the template is moved through all four quadrants of the window
15. Place appropriate implant
16. Small suction drain is placed deeply to the strap muscles; the strap muscles and platysma are approximated with 4-0 absorbable suture, and the skin is closed with a running 5-0 subcuticular suture
17. Dexamethasone is given before surgery to minimize edema, and administration of prophylactic antibiotics is continued for 5 days
18. As a rule, regardless of the implant type used, it is preferable to use the largest prosthesis possible that maintains quality of voice (Fig. 7.15)

Limitations of Type I Thyroplasty

- Static change to the laryngeal framework but has no influence on dynamic function
- Average phonation time is increased from 4.6 to 15 seconds

Complications Associated With Type I Thyroplasty

- Penetration of the endolaryngeal mucosa
- Wound infection
- Chondritis
- Implant migration or extrusion
- Incomplete glottal closure: 10% to 15% of patients
- Airway obstruction
  - Potential for airway compromise requires overnight, inpatient observation
  - Combining medialization thyroplasty and arytenoid adduction increases risk of airway compromise

Arytenoid Abduction and Adduction Basics

- Variation in the position of the vocal fold and symptoms in vocal fold paralysis correlate with level of residual/regeneration of innervated vocal fold muscles

- More functional muscles: Better function, smaller gap, and less likely to need arytenoid work
- Arytenoid abduction mimics the action of the PCA muscle: Externally rotates the arytenoid to pull the vocal process superiorly and laterally
- Arytenoid adduction mimics the action of the LCA: Pulls the vocal process medially and caudally
- Can also perform cricopharyngeal myotomy to reduce dysphagia

Indications for Arytenoid Adduction

1. Large glottic gap/posterior gap
2. Insufficient voice improvement with thyroplasty alone
3. Vocal fold level (vertical height) mismatch

Steps for Arytenoid Adduction (Mimics Lateral Cricoarytenoid)

1. Create a thyroplasty window
2. Cricoid hook should then be placed on the superior cornu of the thyroid cartilage to rotate the larynx away from the field
3. Inferior constrictor muscle is transected
4. Cricopharyngeal muscle can then be resected after identification by blunt dissection, just behind its attachment to the cricoid, and then a 1- to 2-cm segment of muscle is excised
5. Identification and displacement of the piriform sinus mucosa to expose the arytenoid cartilage and avoid entry into the hypopharynx
6. Piriform sinus is separated from the medial surface of the thyroid ala by blunt dissection
7. Sac is then reflected superiorly and anteriorly to expose the PCA
8. PCA fibers are followed to their convergence and insertion on the muscular process of the arytenoid
9. Muscular process of the arytenoid cartilage appears as a white prominence between the attachments of the anterior and posterior bellies of the PCA
10. Muscle tendon is grasped near its insertion, and the needle is passed from back to front through the cartilage process; care should be taken not to injure the piriform mucosa
11. Place suture in the muscular process of the arytenoid (origin of the LCA)
12. Pass the stitch anteriorly through the paraglottic space
13. Secure to the inferior thyroid ala

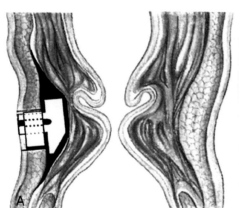
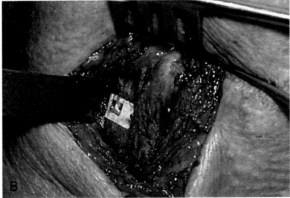

Fig. 7.15 **(A)** Schematic rendition of an implant positioned within the fenestra and secured with a shim. **(B)** Intraoperative view of hydroxyapatite implant secured with a shim.

Indication for Arytenoid Abduction

- Improve glottic airway in bilateral laryngeal paralysis, in unilateral paralysis with arytenoid prolapse into the airway; can also be used in lieu of tracheostomy in selected patients

Steps in Arytenoid Abduction (Mimics Posterior Cricoarytenoid)

1. Same approach to arytenoid as arytenoid adduction
2. Place suture in the muscular process of the arytenoid
3. Pull posteriorly and inferiorly

Laryngeal Reinnervation

Three Goals of Laryngeal Reinnervation

1. Restoration of vocal fold movement (nonselective laryngeal reinnervation does not result in *coordinated* movement)
2. Restoration of vocal fold position
3. Restoration of vocal fold bulk (tone)

Reinnervation Options for Unilateral Laryngeal Paralysis

1. Anastomosis of divided RLN
2. The neuromuscular pedicle (NMP) procedure
3. Nerve transfer to distal RLN, using the ansa cervicalis or hypoglossal
4. Direct implantation of a nerve (ansa hypoglossi) into the denervated muscle

Only Internal Laryngeal Muscle With Bilateral Innervation

- Interarytenoid muscle

Actions Involving Cricothyroid Muscle Activation

1. Deep inspiration
2. Expiration
3. Phonation

Requirements for Restoration of Function in Laryngeal Reinnervation

1. A neuron that responds to the injury with the metabolic changes necessary to support axon regrowth
2. An environment around the injured axon that permits axon growth
3. Guidance clues for restoration of function

Reinnervation of the Posterior Cricoarytenoid Using the Phrenic Nerve

- Ideal in the setting of bilateral vocal fold paralysis given goal to widen airway lumen
- Activates with inspiration
  Activity of the PCA muscle is synchronous with inspiration and precedes activation of the diaphragm by 40 to 100 μsec

Ansa Cervicalis for Laryngeal Reinnervation

- Most commonly used donor nerve
- Ansa provides motor supply to the infrahyoid muscles
- Reinnervation becomes less effective the longer a muscle is denervated
- Cricothyroid is innervated by the SLN; thus, muscle is not addressed by ansa-to-RLN reinnervation

Neuromuscular Pedicle Technique

- Transfer a nerve with a portion of its motor units intact to a denervated muscle
- Despite successful use in a few authors' experiences, widespread use of NMP has not materialized

Indications for Neuromuscular Pedicle in Bilateral Vocal Fold Paralysis

- Bilateral vocal fold paralysis that has persisted for 6 months to 1 year
- Ansa cervicalis nerve and its insertion into the appropriate strap muscle must be available and intact

Contraindications for Neuromuscular Pedicle in Bilateral Vocal Fold Paralysis

- Fixation or limitation of the cricoarytenoid joint; before planning reinnervation, must palpate the cricoarytenoid joints
- Central nervous system disease that results in bilateral vocal cord paralysis (relative contraindication)
- Only about 50% of patients are suitable candidates

Indications for Neuromuscular Pedicle in Unilateral Vocal Fold Paralysis

- Ansa cervicalis nerve intact
- Selected adductor muscle in suitable condition for reinnervation
- Mobile arytenoid on the paralyzed side
- Appropriate amount of time has passed that recovery of motion is unlikely (about 12 months)

Neuromuscular Pedicle Technique

1. NMP harvested from the omohyoid muscle
2. Branch of the ansa cervicalis nerve to the omohyoid is removed with a 2- to 3-mm attached block of muscle
3. Unilateral paralysis: NMP placed into the LCA via a window in the thyroid ala
4. Bilateral paralysis: NMP placed into the PCA after rotating the larynx and separating the fibers of the inferior constrictor

Ansa Cervicalis–to–Recurrent Laryngeal Nerve Transfer

- Procedure provides tone, position, and bulk to the denervated muscles
- Does not provide recovery of vocal fold function

Indications for Ansa Cervicalis–to–Recurrent Laryngeal Nerve Transfer

- Unilateral vocal fold paralysis without expected recovery (wait >12 months)
- Distal stump of RLN present
- Patient can tolerate general anesthesia and long delay prior to improvement from reinnervation

Contraindications for Ansa Cervicalis–to–Recurrent Laryngeal Nerve Transfer

1. Glottic airway compromise
2. Bilateral vocal fold paralysis
3. Absence of the distal RLN
4. Absence of the ansa cervicalis bilaterally
5. Poor general health

Ansa Cervicalis–to–Recurrent Laryngeal Nerve Transfer Technique

1. RLN is identified in the tracheoesophageal groove to its entrance into the larynx
2. Ansa cervicalis can be identified along the lateral border of the sternothyroid muscle at the level of the omohyoid muscle or along the internal jugular vein
3. Ansa and RLN are transected; each nerve should be divided far enough inferiorly to permit a tension-free anastomosis
4. Anastomosis is completed
5. Absorbable material can be injected at the time of surgery

CHRONIC ASPIRATION

Common Causes of Chronic Aspiration in Adults

- Lower cranial nerve deficits secondary to CVA (most common)
- Degenerative neurological disorders (e.g., PD)
- Neuromuscular and muscular disorders (e.g., myasthenia gravis, muscular dystrophy)
- Peripheral nerve disorders (Guillain-Barré, neoplasm)
- Pharyngeal disorders (postirradiation)
- Esophageal disorders (reflux)

Common Causes of Chronic Aspiration in the Pediatric Population

- Cerebral palsy
- Anoxic encephalopathy
- Sequelae of neurological trauma or surgery
- Tracheoesophageal fistula
- Other severe congenital or acquired neurological disorders

Dysphagia History Questions

1. Onset
2. Pain: Consider tumor, infection, and esophagitis
3. Solids (mass, lesion, immobility, and pouch) versus liquids (neurogenic)
4. Regurgitation
5. Weight loss
6. Aspiration/pneumonia (PNA), fever
7. Coughing while eating or drinking

Dysphagia Past Medical History Evaluation

1. Neurological disorders
2. Head and neck or esophageal cancer risk factors
3. Reflux
4. Previous spine or head and neck surgery
5. Immunosuppressant medications

Dysphagia Physical Exam

- Complete head and neck exam with special attention to cranial nerves and tongue strength
- Assess extremity motion and coordination: Rule out underlying neurological condition (e.g., PD and ALS)
- Laryngoscopy (flexible scope vs. mirror) and assess for:
  - Pooling in the vallecula, piriform sinuses, and postcricoid region
  - Masses or lesions
  - Abduction and adduction of true vocal folds
  - Tongue–base retraction
  - Pharyngeal motion

- Modified barium swallow study (MBSS)
  - Can show past the postcricoid region and upper esophageal sphincter (UES)
  - Requires transport to radiology and results in exposure to radiation
- Flexible endoscopic evaluation of swallowing
  - Allows indirect visualization of laryngeal and hypopharyngeal structures
  - Can perform at bedside without radiation
  - Can perform concurrent transnasal esophagoscopy
  - Similar sensitivity/specificity for aspiration to MBSS

Nonsurgical Management
- Swallowing therapy
- Feeding tube (nasogastric (NG), gastrostomy, jejunostomy)
  - NG tube decreases but does not eliminate aspiration

Surgical Management
- Tracheostomy for pulmonary toilet; does not prevent aspiration

LARYNGEAL AND ESOPHAGEAL TRAUMA

Laryngeal Trauma

- Often associated with intracranial and cervical injuries
- The most common injury to the hyoid bone is by strangulation
- Laryngeal injury is impacted by the degree of calcification
- The most common presenting symptom is hoarseness, followed by dysphagia and pain

Examination and Initial Management

- First priority in managing a laryngeal trauma patient: Establish a definitive, safe airway with cervical spine protection (consider awake tracheostomy)

Laryngeal Trauma Physical Examination

- Palpate the neck for:
  - Neck crepitus
  - Step-offs, deformities, and change in framework
  - Laryngeal tenderness
  - Flexible laryngoscopy—if patient is stable
    - Vocal fold mobility
      - RLN trauma
      - Structural injury
    - Particular attention at vibratory edge of the vocal fold and anterior commissure

Definitive Treatment Time frame for the Laryngeal Fracture Patient

- 24 hours (Fig. 7.16)

Schaefer Classification of Laryngeal Trauma

1. Level I: Minor hematoma/lacerations and no fractures
2. Level II: Moderate edema, lacerations, mucosal disruptions without exposed cartilage, and nondisplaced fractures
3. Level III: Massive edema, displaced fractures, and cord immobility
4. Level IV: Massive edema, >2 displaced fractures, cord immobility, instability, and anterior commissure involvement

Postoperative Care

- Voice rest 48 to 72 hours
- NG tube placement
- Humidified oxygen

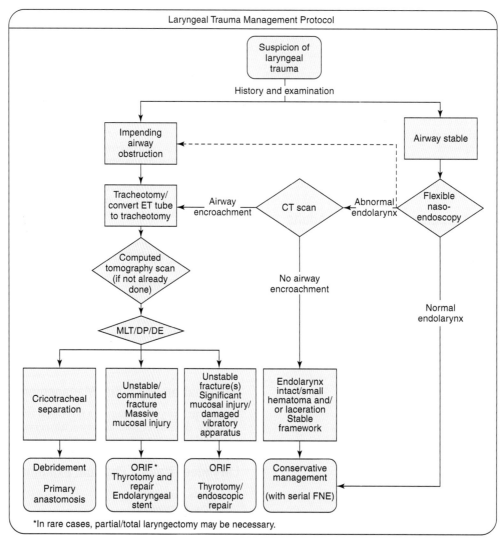

Fig. 7.16 A proposed protocol for managing laryngeal trauma. *CT*, Computed tomography; *DE*, direct esophagoscopy; *DP*, direct pharyngoscopy; *ET*, endotracheal; *FNE*, flexible nasoendoscopy; *MLT*, microlaryngoscopy; *ORIF*, open reduction with internal fixation. (From Flint PW, Haughey BH, Lund VJ, et al. *Cummings Otolaryngology—Head and Neck Surgery.* 6th ed. Philadelphia, PA: Saunders; 2015, Fig. 63.8.)

- Serial examination to assess and treat granulation tissue
- Prophylactic antibiotics and PPI if mucosal tears present
- Head of the bed elevation

Postoperative Care for Laryngeal Trauma Patients

- NG tube until safe swallow is confirmed
- Antibiotics, especially if a stent was placed
- Antacid therapies, especially if there is a denuded epithelium
- Stent should be removed in 10 to 14 days
- Postoperative serial endoscopy

Factors Influencing Laryngeal Trauma Outcomes

- Severity of initial injury
- Timing of surgery (early is better: should be <24 hours, Box 7.1)

Caustic/Thermal Airway Injury Basics

- Inhalation burns occur in 30% of all burn patients
- 20% of patients with inhalation injury have extensive laryngeal injury

- Alkali versus acid ingestion
  - Alkali injection is worse, resulting in liquefaction necrosis of muscle, collagen, and lipid, with injury worsening over time
  - Acid injection results in coagulative necrosis, which is generally superficial
- Tracheostomy versus ET intubation
  - In the setting of caustic injury, tracheostomy is favored over ET tube because of the high rate of laryngeal stenosis

Management of Caustic Laryngeal Injury

- Establish safe airway
- Cardiovascular resuscitation per standard burn-care protocol
- If laryngeal and esophageal endoscopy is to be performed, should be within the first 24 hours to avoid more severe edema and ulceration later

ESOPHAGEAL TRAUMA

Grading of Esophageal Injuries

- First degree: Mucosal erythema
- Second degree: Erythema with noncircumferential exudation

BOX 7.1 Factors that Determine the Need for and the Nature of Surgical Intervention

LARYNGEAL FRAMEWORK

Stable
  No fractures
A single undisplaced fracture

Unstable
  A single displaced fracture
  More than one fracture line
  Cricoid fracture

Potentially Nonviable
  Framework comminution with devitalized cartilage fragments

LARYNGEAL MUCOSA

Intact/Minimally Injured
  No mucosal injuries
  Small submucosal hematoma
  Linear laceration with no exposed cartilage

Injured
  Jagged/multiple linear lacerations
  Large hematoma(s)

EXPOSED CARTILAGE

Massively Injured
  Significant loss of mucosa
  Devitalized mucosal tissue

VIBRATORY APPARATUS

Intact
Injured
  Anterior commissure
  Vibrating edge of the vocal cord(s)
  Arytenoid dislocation

LARYNGOTRACHEAL JUNCTION

Intact
Any degree of laryngotracheal separation

From Flint PW, Haughey BH, Lund VJ, et al. *Cummings Otolaryngology Head and Neck Surgery*. 6th ed. Philadelphia, PA: Saunders; 2015, Table 70.4.

- Third degree: Circumferential exudation
- Fourth degree: Circumferential exudation with esophageal wall perforation

Caustic Esophageal Injury Basics

- 30% of patients with caustic esophageal injuries do not have evidence of oropharyngeal damage
- Adult injuries are generally more severe than pediatric because these are generally attempted suicide with ingestion of large volumes

Management of Caustic Esophageal Injury

- Insert large-bore NG tube to maintain patency
- Broad-spectrum antibiotics
- Antacid therapy

- Steroids
- 10% to 35% of patients will develop esophageal strictures
- One in seven patients who develop strictures will develop esophageal cancer; therefore long-term follow-up is required

SURGICAL MANAGEMENT OF UPPER-AIRWAY STENOSIS

Differential Diagnosis for Adult Laryngeal and Upper Tracheal Stenosis (Box 7.2)

BOX 7.2 Causes of Adult Laryngeal and Upper Tracheal Stenosis

TRAUMA

Internal Laryngotracheal Injury
  Prolonged ET intubation
  Tracheotomy
  Surgical procedure

External Laryngotracheal Injury
  Blunt neck trauma
  Penetrating injury of the larynx
  Radiation therapy
  ET burn
    Thermal
    Chemical

IDIOPATHIC

Chronic Inflammatory Disease
  Autoimmune
    GPA
    Sarcoidosis
    Relapsing polychondritis
  Granulomatous infection
    TB

NEOPLASMS

Benign
  Papillomas
  Chondromas
  Minor salivary gland neoplasms
  Neural neoplasms
Malignant
  Squamous cell carcinoma
  Minor salivary gland neoplasms
  Sarcomas
  Lymphoma

ET, Endotracheal; *GPA*, granulomatosis with polyangiitis; *TB*, tuberculosis. From Flint PW, Haughey BH, Lund VJ, et al. *Cummings Otolaryngology— Head and Neck Surgery*. 6th ed. Philadelphia, PA: Saunders; 2015, Box 68.1. Data from Herrington HC, Weber SM, Andersen PE. Modern management of laryngotracheal stenosis. *Laryngoscope*. 2006;116(9):1553–1557; Wester JL, Clayburgh DR, Stott WJ, et al. Airway reconstruction in Wegener's granulomatosis–associated laryngotracheal stenosis. *Laryngoscope*. 2011;121(12):2566–2571; and Parker NP, Bandyopadhyay D, Misono S, et al. Endoscopic cold incision, balloon dilation, mitomycin C application, and steroid injection for adult laryngotracheal stenosis. *Laryngoscope*. 2013;123(1):220–225.

Describe the Difference in Flow-Volume Loops Between a Patient With a Normal Airway, a Fixed Obstruction, and a Variable Extrathoracic Obstruction (Bilateral Vocal Fold Paralysis; Fig. 7.17)

Describe a Normal Flow Volume Loop

Normal result shows expiratory flow, indicated by positive deflection, and inspiratory flow, indicated by negative deflection Fig. 7.17 (A).

Extrathoracic Obstruction

Fig. 7.17 (B) Loop from a patient with bilateral vocal fold motion impairment shows variable extrathoracic obstruction with normal expiratory limb and limited mid-vital capacity inspiratory flow rate (Vi50) of <1.5 L/sec.

Fixed Obstruction

Fig. 7.17 (C) Loop from a patient with a fixed obstruction with flattening of the inspiratory and expiratory limb.

Surgical Principles

- Balance phonation, airway protection, and sustained glottic closure

  Consider

- Location
- Dimension
- Quality—soft, fibrous
- Vocal fold motion impairment
- Functional impairment

SURGICAL MANAGEMENT OF CHRONIC STENOSIS

- Supraglottic stenosis
  - Endoscopic for minimal scar

- Transhyoid pharyngotomy with tracheostomy for significant scar
- Anterior glottic stenosis
  - If web does not extend beyond inferior vocal fold and posterior commissure is normal, endoscopic repair is possible
  - Otherwise, laryngofissure approach
- Posterior glottic stenosis
  - Options based on type of stenosis, including:
    - Lysis of scar band with steroid injection
    - Arytenoidectomy, suture lateralization
    - Posterior cricoid split
- Complete glottis stenosis
  - Concomitant subglottic injury is common
  - Open laryngofissue with resection of scar with flaps and stents
- Subglottic stenosis
  - External approach when endoscopic fails or when extent is severe or factors are unfavorable for endoscopic approach
- Cicatricial membranous stenosis
  - Endoscopic in stages
  - Open approach via vertical midline so as not to disrupt blood supply laterally
- Anterior wall collapse
  - Stenting versus wedge resection
- Complete tracheal stenosis
  - Segmental resection and primary anastomosis
  - Laryngeal release procedures may be necessary

DISEASES OF THE ESOPHAGUS

Indications for Esophagoscopy

- Weight loss
- Upper gastrointestinal bleeding
- Dysphagia
- Odynophagia
- Chest pain
- Poor response to therapy
- Evaluation for Barrett esophagus

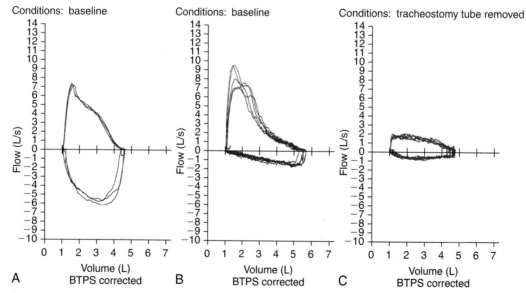

Fig. 7.17 Flow-volume loop for assessing adequacy of the upper airway. (A) Normal result shows expiratory flow, indicated by positive deflection, and inspiratory flow, indicated by negative deflection. **(B)** Loop from a patient with bilateral vocal fold motion impairment shows variable extrathoracic obstruction with a mid-vital capacity inspiratory flow rate (Vi50) of <1.5 L/sec. **(C)** Loop from a patient with an infiltrative tumor and a fixed obstruction. *BTPS,* Body temperature and pressure saturation. (From Flint PW, Haughey BH, Lund VJ, et al. *Cummings Otolaryngology—Head and Neck Surgery.* 6th ed. Philadelphia, PA: Saunders; 2015, Fig. 68.1.)

Indications for 24-Hour pH Monitoring

1. Document excessive acid reflux in patients with suspected gastroesophageal reflux disease (GERD) without endoscopic findings
2. Assess the efficacy of medical or surgical therapy

Indications for Monitoring in Lieu of Empiric Trial of Reflux Therapy With Medication and Lifestyle Changes

- Dysphagia
- Odynophagia
- Weight loss
- Chest pain
- Choking/aspiration symptoms

Most Common Symptom of Infectious Esophagitis

- Odynophagia (Fig. 7.18)

Globus Sensation

- Lump sensation in the throat that does not impede swallow
- May in fact be relieved with swallow

Manometry Basics (Table 7.1)

- Gold standard for diagnosis of motor disorders of the esophageal body and lower esophageal sphincter (LES)
- Upper sphincter pressures are highly variable, so manometry is less useful in UES assessment

Ambulatory 24-Hour pH Probe Basics

- Abnormal pH level: <4.0
- pH level at which pepsin is activated: <4.0
- Percent of time with pH <4.0 that is considered abnormal: ≥4.25%

Multichannel Intraluminal Impedance Probe Basics

- Measures both acid and nonacid refluxate
- Measures total resistance to current flow between adjacent electrodes

Esophageal Achalasia Basics

- Failure of LES to relax
- "Bird's beak" or "megaesophagus" on esophagogram
- Treatment: Esophagoscopy with Botox or myotomy; referral to gastroenterology

Esophageal Dysmotility Basics

- Normal contour on esophagogram
- Abnormal manometry
- Consider referral to gastroenterology

Scleroderma Basics

- CREST Syndrome
  - **C**alcinosis
  - **R**aynaud phenomenon
  - **E**sophageal dysmotility
  - **S**clerodactyly
  - **T**elangiectasia
- Esophagogram: Dilated *distal* esophagus
- Manometry: Normal UES and LES

Polymyositis and Dermatomyositis Basics

- Striated muscle myopathy
  - Pharyngeal weakness with upper esophageal weakness
  - Skin rash
  - Proximal muscle weakness
- Esophagogram: May see dilated *upper* esophagus

Diffuse Esophageal Spasm Basics

- High-pressure nonperistaltic contractions
- Esophagogram: "Corkscrew" esophagus

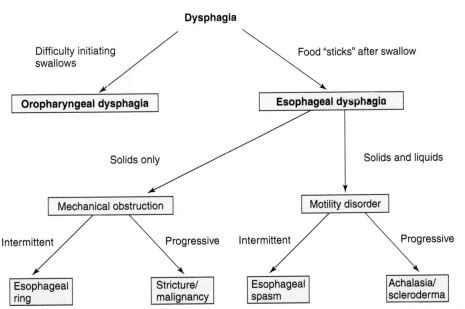

Fig. 7.18 Algorithm for the evaluation of dysphagia. (From Flint PW, Haughey BH, Lund VJ, et al. *Cummings Otolaryngology—Head and Neck Surgery.* 6th ed. Philadelphia, PA: Saunders; 2015, Fig. 69.1.)

TABLE 7.1 Esophageal Manometric Findings in Normal Patients and in Those With Motility Disorders

Finding	Normal	Achalasia	Diffuse Esophageal Spasm	Nutcracker Esophagus	Ineffective Esophageal Motility
Basal LES pressure	10–45 mm Hg	Normal or high	Normal	Normal	Low or normal
LES relaxation with swallow	Complete	Incomplete	Normal	Normal	Normal
Wave progression	Peristalsis	Aperistalsis	Peristalsis with at least 20% simultaneous contractions	Normal	30% or more failed nontransmitted contractions
Distal wave amplitude	30–180 mm Hg	Usually low (may be normal or high)	Normal	High	30% or more <30 mm Hg

LES, Lower esophageal sphincter.
From Flint PW, Haughey BH, Lund VJ, et al. *Cummings Otolaryngology—Head and Neck Surgery.* 6th ed. Philadelphia, PA: Saunders; 2015, Table 69.1.

- Manometry: Disorganized high-pressure contractions
- Treatment: Nitrates and calcium channel blockers

Transnasal Esophagoscopy

- Lower cost
- No need for sedation
- High completion rate (83%–99%); most common reason for failure is the inability to pass through the nasal vault
- High degree of correlation between the endoscopic findings (sensitivity, 89%; specificity, 97%) of transnasal esophagoscopy and conventional esophagoscopy
- No significant difference in the rate of definitive histological diagnosis
- In evaluating Barrett metaplasia, there is a 97% correlation between biopsy specimens obtained with transnasal esophagoscopy and conventional esophagoscopy

Esophageal Indications for Transnasal Esophagoscopy

- Dysphagia
- Esophageal symptoms that persist despite antireflux therapy
- Screening for Barrett esophageal metaplasia
- Visualization and biopsy of esophageal radiological abnormalities
- Long-standing (≥5 years) GERD

Extra-esophageal Indications for Transnasal Esophagoscopy

- Chronic cough
- Panendoscopy and biopsy for head and neck cancer
- Moderate to severe laryngopharyngeal reflux
- Globus pharyngeus

External Compressions of the Esophagus in Descending Order

1. Aortic compression: Pulsating anterolateral prominence
2. Left mainstem bronchus: Anterior compression 2 cm distal to aorta
3. Diaphragm: Circumferential

Transnasal Esophagoscopy–Complication Rate

- Epistaxis: Most common, 0.5% to 2%
- Vasovagal: 0.01% to 0.3%
- Minor nasal discomfort: 1.3%

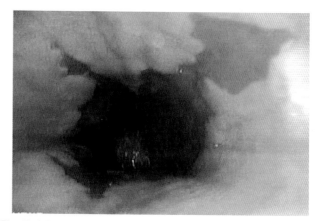

Fig. 7.19 Evidence of possible Barrett metaplasia. Salmon-colored gastric mucosa extends into the distal esophagus. This area should be biopsied to evaluate for histological changes consistent with Barrett metaplasia to make the diagnosis. (From Flint PW, Haughey BH, Lund VJ, et al. *Cummings Otolaryngology—Head and Neck Surgery.* 6th ed. Philadelphia, PA: Saunders; 2015, Fig. 70.3.)

Classic Esophagoscopy Findings

- Salmon-colored mucosa proximal to gastric rugae: Barrett esophagitis (Fig. 7.19)
- Proximal extension of gastric rugae >2 cm from the diaphragm: Hiatal hernia

Esophageal Diverticulum (Fig. 7.20)

Most Common Hypopharyngeal Diverticulum

- Zenker diverticulum

Areas of Hypopharyngeal Weakness

1. Killian's triangle (site of Zenker diverticulum)
   - Area of weakness between the inferior constrictor and the cricopharyngeus
2. Killian-Jameson dehiscence
   - Area of weakness between the oblique and transverse cricopharyngeus fibers
3. Laimer triangle
   - Area of weakness between the cricopharyngeus and the superior esophageal wall circular muscles

Traction and Pulsion Diverticula

- Pulsion: Result from pressure from within the esophagus causing the esophageal mucosa and submucosa to be herniated through an area of weakness
- Traction: Result of pulling forces external to the esophagus; for example, inflammatory, neoplastic, or following cervical spine surgery

Common Symptoms of Zenker Diverticulum

- Progressive dysphagia
- Regurgitation of food, even hours after a meal
- Unprovoked aspiration
- Noisy deglutition (borborygmi)
- Belching
- Halitosis
- Choking/coughing
- Globus pharyngeus

- Weight loss
- Recurrent respiratory infections

Van Overbeek and Groote Staging System for Zenker Diverticulum

1. Stage I: Size of one vertebral body
2. Stage II: 1 to 3 vertebral bodies
3. Stage III: >3 vertebral bodies

Treatment Options for Zenker Diverticulum

1. Diet modification
2. Gastrostomy tube
3. Endoscopic diverticulotomy with cricopharyngeal myotomy
   - Endoscopic stapler (Fig. 7.21)
   - CO_2 laser
   - Harmonic scalpel
4. Open cricopharyngeal myotomy with or without diverticulectomy, diverticulopexy, or diverticular inversion

Advantages of Endoscopic Approach to Zenker Diverticulum

1. Shorter operative time
2. Short hospital stay
3. Lower morbidity (2.6%) and mortality (0.3%)
4. Minimal risk of RLN injury
5. Shorter convalescence

Disadvantages of Endoscopic Approach to Zenker Diverticulum

1. Potential for persistent/recurrent symptoms
2. Risk of recurrent symptoms
3. May not be possible if cannot expose pouch
4. Bad option for larger pouches

Advantages of Open Approach to Zenker Diverticulum

1. Definitive procedure
2. No recurrence
3. May be the only possibility if the pouch cannot be exposed or if the pouch is >6 cm

Disadvantages of Open Approach to Zenker Diverticulum

1. Longer operative time
2. Increased morbidity (mediastinitis) and hospital stay
3. Complication rate 11.8%
4. Mortality rate 1.6%

Tracheobronchial Endoscopy

Define Lobar and Segmental Bronchi

- Lobar bronchus: Defines division of lung lobes
- Segmental bronchus: Defines division of pulmonary lobules

Number of Lobes and Lobules of Each Lung

- Right lung: 3 lobes and 10 lobules
- Left lung: 2 lobes and 9 lobules

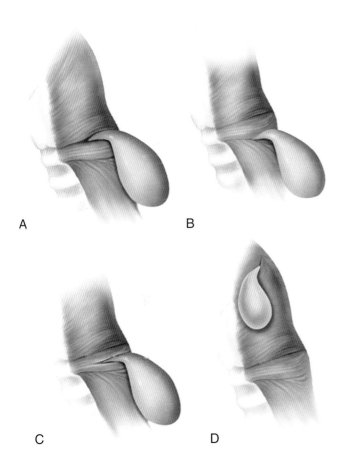

Fig. 7.20 Types of esophageal diverticulae. (**A**) Killian triangle: Region between the cricopharyngeal and inferior constrictor muscle. (**B**) Laimer triangle: Region between the cricopharyngeal and most superior esophageal circular muscle. (**C**) Killian-Jamieson triangle: Region between the oblique and transverse fibers of the cricopharyngeal muscle. (**D**) Lateral pharyngocele: Variable location above and lateral to the cricopharyngeus. (From Flint PW, Haughey BH, Lund VJ, et al. *Cummings Otolaryngology—Head and Neck Surgery*. 6th ed. Philadelphia, PA: Saunders; 2015, Fig. 71.1.)

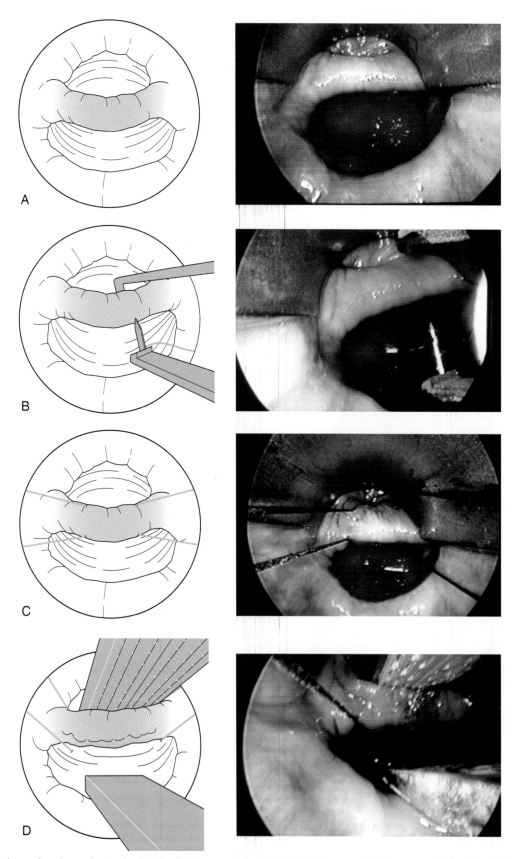

Fig. 7.21 Technique of endoscopic staple diverticulostomy as seen with a rigid telescope. (A) Common wall visualized with a Weerda laryngoscope. (**B** and **C**) With an Endo Stitch suturing device (Covidien Autosuture), retraction sutures are placed on the lateral aspects of the common wall. (**D**) The common wall is positioned between the blades of the stapler.

continued

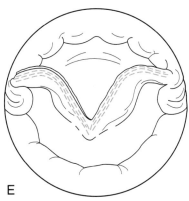 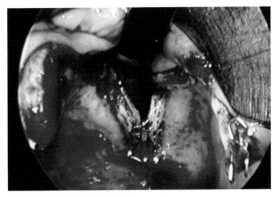

Fig. 7.21, cont'd (E) The common wall is divided after the stapler is activated. The retraction sutures are cut and removed. (From Flint PW, Haughey BH, Lund VJ, et al. *Cummings Otolaryngology—Head and Neck Surgery.* 6th ed. Philadelphia, PA: Saunders; 2015, Fig. 71.11.)

Services to Be Consulted Before Bronchoscopy for Massive Hemoptysis

- Thoracic surgery
- Interventional radiology

Topical Anesthesia

- Milligrams of lidocaine
  - 1 mL of 1% lidocaine has 10 mg lidocaine
  - 1 mL of 4% lidocaine has 40 mg lidocaine
- Maximum amount of lidocaine that can be administered at one time: 3 to 4 mg/kg

Advantages of Rigid Bronchoscopy

- Larger lumen for instrumentation/stenting
- Can ventilate through a side port using the Venturi jet ventilation system
- Can use the scope itself to tamponade bleeding or to core out the tumor

Disadvantages of Rigid Bronchoscopy

- Oral/dental trauma
- Laryngeal edema before surgery, especially with larger bronchoscope

What Is the Main Complication of Endobronchial Biopsy and How Is it Treated?

- Complication: Bleeding
- Treatment: Dispense small aliquots of oxymetazoline 0.05% or lidocaine with 1:100,000 epinephrine over the bleeding site (oxymetazoline is preferred because it causes less tachycardia (Table 71.1)

FURTHER READINGS

Adler CH, Bansberg SF, Hentz JG. Botulinum toxin type A for treating voice tremor. *Arch Neurol.* 2004;61(9):1416–1420.

Ai ZL, Lan CH, Fan LL, et al. Unsedated transnasal upper gastrointestinal endoscopy has favorable diagnostic effectiveness, cardiopulmonary safety, and patient satisfaction compared with conventional or sedated endoscopy. *Surg Endosc.* 2012;26(12):3565–3572.

Alessi DM, Berci G. Aspiration and nasogastric intubation. *Otolaryngol Head Neck Surg.* 1986;94:486.

Amin MR, Postma GN, Setzen M, et al. Transnasal esophagoscopy: a position statement from the American Bronchoesophagological Association (ABEA). *Otolaryngol Head Neck Surg.* 2008;138(4): 411–414.

Arevalo-Silva C, Eliashar R, Wohlgelernter J, et al. Ingestion of caustic substances: a 15-year experience. *Laryngoscope.* 2006;116:1422–1426.

Aronson AE, Bless DM. *Clinical Voice Disorders.* 4th ed. New York, NY: Thieme Medical Publishers; 2009.

Bastian RW. Videoendoscopic evaluation of patients with dysphagia: an adjunct to the modified barium swallow. *Otolaryngol Head Neck Surg.* 1991;104(3):339–350.

Black JD, Dolly JO. Interaction of 125I-labeled botulinum neurotoxins with nerve terminals I: ultrastructural autoradiographic localization and quantitation of distinct membrane acceptors for types A and B on motor nerves. *J Cell Biol.* 1986;103:521.

Blitzer A, Brin MF, Stewart CF. Botulinum toxin management of spasmodic dysphonia: a 12-year experience in more than 900 patients. *Laryngoscope.* 1998;108:1435.

Bogdasarian RS, Olson NR. Posterior glottic laryngeal stenosis. *Otolaryngol Head Neck Surg.* 1980;88;765.

Chang C, Payyapilli R, Scher RL. Endoscopic staple diverticulostomy for Zenker's diverticulum: review of literature and experience in 159 consecutive patients. *Laryngoscope.* 2003;113:957–965.

Childs LF, Rickert S, Wengerman OC, et al. Laryngeal manifestations of relapsing polychondritis and a novel treatment option. *J Voice.* 2012;26:587–589.

Cho S, Arya N, Swan K, et al. Unsedated transnasal endoscopy: a Canadian experience in daily practice. *Canadian J Gastroenterol.* 2008;22(3):243–246.

Donner MW, Silbiger ML. Cinefluorographic analysis of pharyngeal swallowing in neuromuscular disorders. *Am J Med Sci.* 1966;251:600.

Dean R, Dua K, Massey B, et al. A comparative study of unsedated transnasal esophagogastroduodenoscopy and conventional EGD. *Gastrointest Endosc.* 1996;44(4):422–424.

Dumortier J, Napoleon B, Hedelius F, et al. Unsedated transnasal EGD in daily practice: results with 1100 consecutive patients. *Gastrointest Endosc.* 2003;57(2):198–204.

Hale EK, Bystryn JC. Laryngeal and nasal involvement in pemphigus vulgaris. *J Am Acad Dermatol.* 2001;44:609–611.

Herrington HC, Weber SM, Andersen PE. Modern management of laryngotracheal stenosis. *Laryngoscope.* 2006;116(9):1553–1557.

Hirano M, Nozoe I, Shin T, et al. Electromyography for laryngeal paralysis. In: Hirano M, Kirchner J, Bless D, eds. *Neurolaryngology: Recent Advances.* Boston, MA: College-Hill; 1987:232–248.

Hirano M. Morphological structure of the vocal cord as a vibrator and its variations. *Folia Phoniatr (Basel).* 1974;26:89.

Hirano M, Bless DM. *Videostroboscopic Examination of the Larynx.* San Diego, CA: Singular Publishing Group; 1993.

Horner J, Massey EW, Riski JE, et al. Aspiration following stroke: clinical correlates and outcome. *Neurology.* 1988;38:1359.

Ingle JW, Young VN, Smith LJ, Munin MC, Rosen CA. Prospective evaluation of the clinical utility of laryngeal electromyography. *Laryngoscope.* 2014;124:2745–2749.

Isaak BL, Liesegang TJ, Michet CJ Jr. Ocular and systemic findings in relapsing polychondritis. *Ophthalmology.* 1986;93:681–689.

Jewett BS, Shockley WW, Rutledge R. External laryngeal trauma analysis of 392 patients. *Arch Otolaryngol Head Neck Surg.* 1999;125:877–880.

Johns MM, Garrett CG, Hwang J, Ossoff RH, Courey MS. Quality of life outcomes following laryngeal endoscopic surgery for non-neoplastic vocal fold lesions. *Ann Otol Rhinol Laryngol.* 2004;113(8):597–601.

Johnson LF, Demeester TR. Twenty-four-hour pH monitoring of the distal esophagus. A quantitative measure of gastroesophageal reflux. *Am J Gastroenterol.* 1974;62(4):325–332.

Johnson LF. 24-hour pH monitoring in the study of gastroesophageal reflux. *J Clin Gastroenterol.* 1980;2(4):387–399.

Juutilainen M, Vintturi J, Robinson S, Bäck L, Lehtonen H, Mäkitie AA. Laryngeal fractures: clinical findings and considerations on suboptimal outcome. *Acta Otolaryngol.* 2008;128(2):213–218.

Kempster GB, Gerratt BR, Verdolini Abbott K, et al. Consensus auditory-perceptual evaluation of voice: development of a standardized clinical protocol. *Am J Speech Lang Pathol.* 2009;18:124.

Koszewski IJ, Hoffman MR, Young WG, Lai Y-T, Dailey SH. Office-based photoangiolytic laser treatment of Reinke's edema: safety and voice outcomes. *Otolaryngol Head Neck Surg.* 2015;152(6):1075–1081.

Laccourreye O, Papon JF, Kania R, et al. Intracordal injection of autologous fat in patients with unilateral laryngeal nerve paralysis: long-term results from the patient's perspective. *Laryngoscope.* 2003;113:541.

Lawless ST, Cook S, Luft J, et al. The use of a laryngotracheal separation procedure in pediatric patients. *Laryngoscope.* 1995;105:198.

Lebrun Y, Devreux F, Rousseau JJ, et al. Tremulous speech: a case report. *Folia Phoniatr.* 1982;34:134.

Lebovics RS, Hoffman GS, Leavitt RY, et al. The management of subglottic stenosis in patients with Wegener's granulomatosis. *Laryngoscope.* 1992;102:1341–1345.

Lee SW, Hong HJ, Choi SH, et al. Comparison of treatment modalities for contact granuloma: a nation-wide multicenter study. *Laryngoscope.* 2013;124(5):1187–1191.

Lim JY, Kim KM, Choi EC, et al. Current clinical propensity of laryngeal tuberculosis: review of 60 cases. *Eur Arch Otorhinolaryngol.* 2006;263:838–842.

McCaffrey TV. Classification of laryngotracheal stenosis. *Laryngoscope.* 1992;102(12):1335–1340.

Meyer TK, Wolf J. Lysis of interarytenoid synechia (Type I posterior glottic stenosis): vocal fold mobility and airway results. *Laryngoscope.* 2011;121(10):2165–2171.

Mathison CC, Villari CR, Klein AM, Johns MM III. Comparison of outcomes and complications between awake and asleep injection laryngoplasty: a case control study. *Laryngoscope.* 2009;119(7):1417–1423.

Milstein CF, Akst LM, Hicks MD, et al. Long-term effects of micronized alloderm injection for unilateral vocal fold paralysis. *Laryngoscope.* 2005;115:1691–1696.

Montgomery WM, Hilman RE, Varvares MA. Combined thyroplasty type I and inferior constrictor myotomy. *Ann Otol Rhinol Laryngol.* 1995;103:858–862.

Montgomery WW. Posterior and complete glottic stenosis. *Arch Otolaryngol Head Neck Surg.* 1973;98:170.

Nordin U, Lindholm CE, Wolgast M. Blood flow in rabbit tracheal mucosa and the influence of tracheal intubation. *Acta Anesthesiol Scand.* 1977;21:84.

Nottet JB, Duruisseau O, Herve S, et al. Inhalation burns: apropos of 198 cases. *Incidence of laryngotracheal involvement. Ann Otolaryngol Chir Cervicofac.* 1997;114:220–225.

Paniello RC, Edgar JD, Kallogjeri D, Piccirillo JF. Medialization versus reinnervation for unilateral vocal fold paralysis: a multicenter randomized clinical trial. *Laryngoscope.* 2011;121:2172–2179.

Postma GN, Cohen JT, Belafsky PC, et al. Transnasal esophagoscopy: revisited (over 700 consecutive cases). *Laryngoscope.* 2005;115(2):321–323.

Ramasamy K, Gumaste VV. Corrosive ingestion in adults. *J Clin Gastroenterol.* 2003;37:119–124.

Rickert SM, Childs LF, Carey BT, et al. Laryngeal electromyography for prognosis of vocal fold paralysis: a meta-analysis. *Laryngoscope.* 2012;122(1):158–161.

Saeian K, Staff DM, Vasilopoulos S, et al. Unsedated transnasal endoscopy accurately detects Barrett's metaplasia and dysplasia. *Gastrointest Endosc.* 2002;56(4):472–478.

Scher RL, Richtsmeier WJ. Endoscopic staple-assisted esophagodiverticulostomy for Zenker's diverticulum. *Laryngoscope.* 1996;106:951–956.

Statham MM, Rosen C, Nandedkar S, et al. Quantitative laryngeal electromyography: turns and amplitude analysis. *Laryngoscope.* 2010;120:2036–2041.

Smith ME, Yanagisawa E. Physical examination of the larynx and videolaryngoscopy. In: Blitzer A, Brin M, Ramig L, eds. *Neurologic Disorders of the Larynx.* New York, NY: Thieme; 2009:54–58.

Splaingard ML, Hutchins B, Sulton LD, et al. Aspiration in rehabilitation patients: videofluoroscopy vs. bedside clinical assessment. *Arch Phys Med Rehabil.* 1988;69:637.

Sundberg J, Nordstrom PE. Raised and lowered larynx: the effect on vowel format frequencies. *J Res Sing.* 1983;6:7.

Taylor SC, Clayburgh DR, Rosenbaum JT, et al. Progression and management of Wegener's granulomatosis in the head and neck. *Laryngoscope.* 2012;122:1695–1700.

Thota PN. Zuccaro Jr G, Vargo 2nd JJ, et al. A randomized prospective trial comparing unsedated esophagoscopy via transnasal and transoral routes using a 4-mm video endoscope with conventional endoscopy with sedation. *Endoscopy.* 2005;37(6):559–565.

Tucker HM. Nerve-muscle pedicle reinnervation of the larynx: avoiding pitfalls and complications. *Ann Otol Rhinol Laryngol.* 1982;91:440–444.

van den Berg J. Myoelastic-aerodynamic theory of voice production. *J Speech Hear Res.* 1958;1:227.

Woodson GE, Zwirner P, Murry T, et al. Use of flexible laryngoscopy to classify patients with spasmodic dysphonia. *J Voice.* 1991;5:85.

Woodson GE. Configuration of the glottis in laryngeal paralysis II: animal experiments. *Laryngoscope.* 1993;103:1235–1241.

Woodson GE. Cricopharyngeal myotomy and arytenoid adduction in the management of combined laryngeal and pharyngeal paralysis. *Otolaryngol Head Neck Surg.* 1997;117:339–343.

Wu CH, Hsiao TY, Chen JC, et al. Evaluation of swallowing safety with fiberoptic endoscope: comparison with videofluoroscopic technique. *Laryngoscope.* 1997;107(3):396.

Walter T, Chesnay AL, Dumortier J, et al. Biopsy specimens obtained with small-caliber endoscopes have comparable diagnostic performances than those obtained with conventional endoscopes: a prospective study on 1335 specimens. *J Clin Gastroenterol.* 2010;44(1):12–17.

8 Otolaryngic Allergy

Lauren Miller, M. Jennifer Derebery and Elliot D Kozin

INNATE AND ADAPTIVE IMMUNE SYSTEM
Basic Types of Immunity

- Innate immune system
  - Barrier mechanisms (epithelium, mucosal, mucociliary transport)
  - Soluble bioactive molecules (complement proteins, defensins, cytokines, etc.)
  - Pattern recognition receptors
- Adaptive immune system (specific antigen recognition)
  - Humoral
  - Cellular

Cell Layers of Innate Immune System

- Epithelial cell layers
- Mucosal cell layers

Mucosal Immune System

- Organized mucosal associated lymphoid tissue (MALT)
  - Tonsils and adenoids (Waldeyer's ring)
  - Peyer's patches (small intestine)
  - Isolated lymphoid follicles throughout gut
- Diffuse mucosal immune system
  - Intraepithelial lymphocytes
  - Lamina propria

Cells of Innate Immune System

- Phagocytes: Neutrophils, macrophages, mast cells
- Monocytes
- Natural killer cells
- Mast cells
- Eosinophils
- Basophils
- Dendritic cells

Antimicrobial Peptides of Innate Immune System

- Essential to mammalian immune system as first line of defense
- Act to disrupt integrity of bacterial cell membrane
  - Cathelicidins
  - Defensins

Receptors of Innate Immune System

- Expressed on cells of innate immune system that broadly distinguish pathogen from host
  - Pattern recognition receptors: Recognize pathogen-associated molecular patterns (PAMPs)
  - Toll-like receptors: Expressed in all lymphoid tissue but most highly expressed in peripheral blood leukocytes
- Binding releases cytokines

Mechanisms of Innate Immune System

- Opsonize bacteria
- Activate coagulation
- Complement cascades (see below)

Mediators of Adaptive Immune System (Fig. 8.1)

- T lymphocytes
- B lymphocytes
- Antibodies

T Cells

- TH2: Specialize in facilitating B-cell antibody response
  - Main cytokines: IL4, IL5, IL13
    - Enable IgE production; important for clearance of helminthic and allergic response
- TH1: Evoke cell-mediated immunity, specialize in macrophage activation
  - Main cytokine: IFN-γ
    - Leads to intracellular pathogen clearance and delayed type hypersensitivity
- TH17: Involved in autoimmunity
- Regulatory T cells: Iinvolved in autoimmunity

B Cells

- Plasma: Secrete specific antibody type
- Memory: Generate robust antibody-mediated reaction in re-infection

Immunoglobulins (Fig. 8.2)

- Fc: Heavy chain, where immunoglobulin (Ig) class is determined
- Fab: Light chain, antigen-presenting cell (APC) binding site
- IgG (75%, monomer): Recall/secondary immune responses, can cross placenta
  - Four subtypes: IgG1, IgG2, IgG3, IgG4
    - IgG1 is majority
    - IgG2 deficiency is most common in children, leads to recurrent infections to polysaccharide encapsulated bacteria
    - IgG3 is most common hypogammaglobulin deficiency in adults
- IgM (10%, pentamer): Antigen receptor of B cells; first antibody to respond to infection
- IgA (15%, dimer): Found in external secretions and is primary defense against local mucosal infections, neutralizes foreign substances; found in placenta
- IgE (<0.01%, monomer): Binds to basophils and mast cells to release histamine and serotonin; involved in allergic and parasitic infections
- IgD (0.2%, monomer): Antigen receptor on B cells

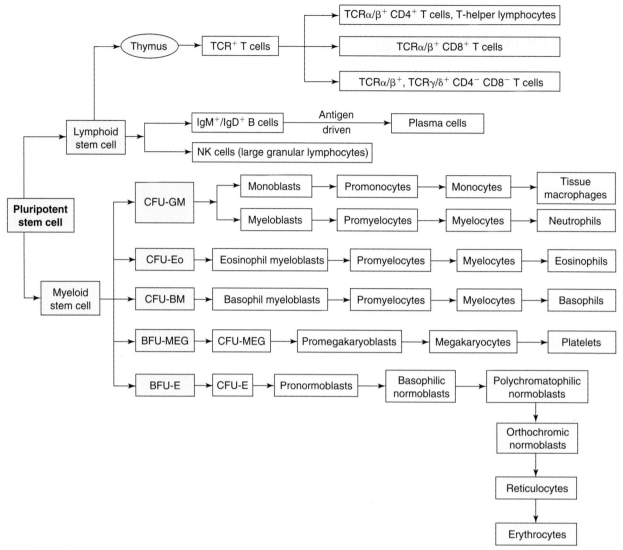

Fig. 8.1 The development of the immune cells. *BFU,* Burst-forming unit; *BM,* basophil mast cell; *CFU,* colony-forming unit; *E,* erythroid; *Eo,* eosinophil; *GM,* granulocyte-monophage; *Ig,* immunoglobulin; *MEG,* megakaryocyte; *NK,* natural killer; *TCR,* T-cell receptor. (From Flint PW, Haughey BH, Lund V, et al. *Cummings Otolaryngology—Head and Neck Surgery.* 7th ed. Philadelphia, PA: Elsevier, 2021, Fig. 35.2.)

Lymphoid Tissue of Adaptive Immune System

- Thymus: Site of T-lymphocyte maturation
- Bone marrow: Site of B-lymphocyte maturation
- Lymph nodes
- Spleen
- Epithelial immune system
- Mucosal immune system
  - Tonsils
  - Peyer's patches and lymphoid follicles
  - Lymphoid follicles
  - Intraepithelial lymphocytes and lamina propria

Human Leukocyte Antigen (HLA; Fig. 8.3)

- Major histocompatibility complex (MHC) Class I: All nucleated somatic cells
  - Antigens of endogenous origin, presented to CD8+ T cells
    - HLA-A
    - HLA-B
    - HLA-C
- MHC Class II: APCs (macrophages, dendritic cells, Langerhans cells, B cells)

- Antigens from extracellular proteins, presented to CD4+ T cells
  - HLA-DR
  - HLA-DQ
  - HLA-DP

Complement System (Fig. 8.4)

All routes lead to cleavage of C3, which results in mast cell degranulation and recruitment of phagocytic cells
- Classic pathway: Activated by C1 complex
- Lectin pathway: Activated by mannose-binding lectin
- Alternative pathway: Activated by spontaneous C3 hydrolysis

Complement System Steps

- Opsonization: Foreign particles are marked for phagocytosis
- Chemotaxis: Attraction of macrophages to a chemical signal
- Cell lysis: Destruction of the cell membrane
- Agglutination: Uses antibodies to cluster and bind pathogens together

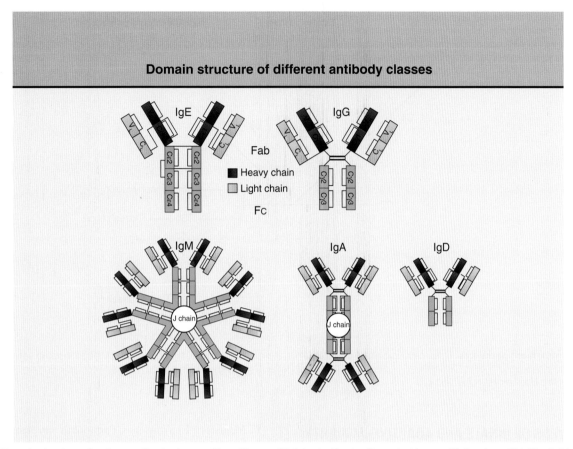

Fig. 8.2 Domain structure of various antibody classes. (From Krouse JH. Introduction to allergy. In: Krouse JH, Derebery MJ, Chadwick SJ, eds. *Managing the Allergic Patient*. 1st ed. Philadelphia, PA: Saunders Elsevier; 2008. Originally reproduced from Holgate ST. *Allergy*. 2nd ed. London: Mosby/Elsevier; 2001:245, Fig. 16.4.)

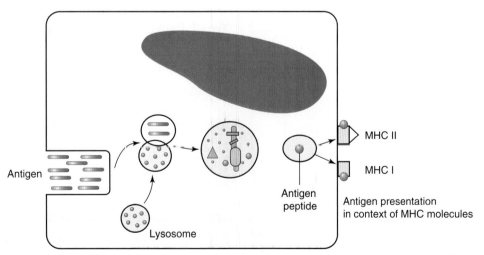

Fig. 8.3 Antigen processing and presentation. Antigen undergoes hydrolytic cleavage within antigen-presenting cells. The resultant oligopeptides are loaded on antigen-binding grooves of major histocompatibility complex (MHC) molecules and are expressed at the cell surface. (From Flint PW, Haughey BH, Lund V, et al. *Cummings Otolaryngology—Head and Neck Surgery*. 7th ed. Philadelphia, PA: Elsevier, 2021, Fig. 35.3.)

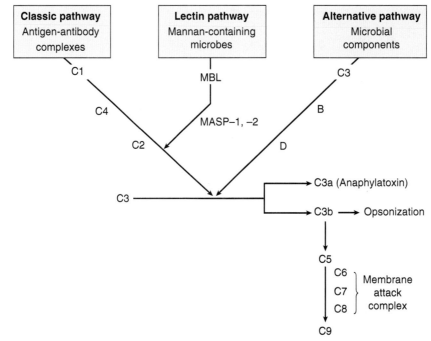

Fig. 8.4 Complement pathways. Three pathways of the complement system. *B*, Factor B; *D*, factor D; *MASP*, MBL-associated serine proteases; *MBL*, mannan-binding lectin. (From Flint PW, Haughey BH, Lund V, et al. *Cummings Otolaryngology—Head and Neck Surgery.* 7th ed. Philadelphia, PA: Elsevier, 2021, Fig. 35.1.)

KEY PLAYERS OF INNATE AND ADAPTIVE IMMUNITY

Cytokines (Table 8.1)

- Broad category of small proteins important in cell signaling

Chemokines (Table 8.2)

- Small proteins important in signaling chemotaxis
- Four categories: CXC, CC, CX3C, and CX

Cell Adhesion (Fig. 8.5)

- Intercellular adhesion molecule 1 (ICAM)-1
- ICAM-2
- E-selectin
- P-selectin
- Vascular cellular adhesion molecule (V-CAM)

Allergic Triggers Categories

- Inhalants
- Ingestions
- Injectables
- Contactants

Stages of Development of an Allergy

- Early response: Minutes after exposure to antigen
  - Primary mediator is histamine
  - Symptoms: Largely nasal symptoms, including rhinorrhea, sneezing, and congestion, as well as other symptoms, including tearing, wheezing, urticaria, vomiting, diarrhea
- Late response: Hours after exposure to antigen (peaks 6–9 hours after exposure)

- Mediators: Leukotrienes, eosinophils, tryptans
- Symptoms: Edema, pain, warmth, erythema

Types of Hypersensitivity (Gell and Coombs' Classification; Table 8.3)

- Type I: Immediate/anaphylaxis (IgE)
- Type II: Cytotoxic (IgG, IgM)
- Type III: Immune complex (IgG, IgM, IgA)
- Type IV: Cell mediated (T cells)

Type I: Causes of Anaphylaxis

- Inhalants
- Foods
- Drugs
- Insect stings

Type I: Anaphylaxis Symptoms

- Upper respiratory: Sneezing, itching, rhinorrhea, congestion
- Lower respiratory: Cough, bronchospasm, wheezing
- Skin: Urticarial, angioedema, itching, whealing
- Systemic: Hypotension, tachycardia, feeling of impending doom

Type I: Anaphylaxis Mechanism

- Allergen presented to T cells by APCs
- T cells signal for stimulation of B cells to produce IgE antibodies
- Cross-linking of IgE on mast cells
- Degranulation of mast cells and release of histamine and other mediators
  - Increases capillary permeability, which causes vasodilation, bronchoconstriction, tissue edema
- Release of histamine

TABLE 8.1 Cytokines

Cytokine	Cell Sources	Predominant Effects
Interleukins		
IL-1α, IL-1β functionally equivalent isoforms	Macrophages, neutrophils, epithelial and endothelial cells, monocytes, lymphocytes, keratinocytes	Fever, local inflammation, T-cell and macrophage activation; principal mediator(s) of septic shock; differentiation of TH17 cells
IL-2	Activated T cells, DCs, NK cells	Proliferation of effector T and B cells, development of Treg cells, differentiation and proliferation of NK cells
IL-3	CD4+ T cells, thymic epithelial cells, mast cells, eosinophils, macrophages, NK cells	Synergistic action in early hematopoiesis; activates and promotes recruitment of basophils and eosinophils in late allergic reactions
IL-4	TH2 cells, mast cells, basophils, NK T cells, eosinophils, γ/δ–T cells	Differentiation and growth of TH2 subset, B-cell activation, survival factor for T and B cells, isotype switch to IgE and IgG1, suppression of TH1 cells, growth factor for mast cells
IL-5	Activated TH2 cells and mast cells, NK cells, NK T cells, eosinophils	Eosinophil survival, differentiation, and chemotaxis, differentiation and function of myeloid cells, remodeling and wound healing
IL-6	T cells, mononuclear phagocytes, vascular endothelial cells, fibroblasts	T- and B-cell growth and differentiation, acute-phase protein production by the liver
IL-7	Stromal cells in bone marrow and thymus, B cells, monocytes, macrophages, epithelial cells, keratinocytes, DCs	Growth of pre–B cells and pre–T cells, synthesis induction of inflammatory mediators in monocytes
IL-8, CXC chemokine	Activated mononuclear phagocytes, fibroblasts, and endothelial cells	Chemoattractant for neutrophils, NK cells, T cells, basophils, eosinophils; promotes neutrophil inflammatory responses, mobilization of hematopoietic stem cells
IL-9	TH2 cells, TH9 cells, mast cells, eosinophils	T cell and mast cell growth factor, inhibition of TH1 cytokines, proliferation of CD8 + T cells and mast cells, IgE production, chemokine and mucus production in bronchial epithelial cells
IL-10	T cells, B cells, monocytes, macrophages, DCs	Important in innate and adaptive immunity, immunosuppression
IL-11	Stromal cells: fibroblasts, epithelial cells, endothelial cells, vascular smooth muscle cells, synoviocytes, osteoblasts	Growth factor for myeloid, erythroid, and megakaryocyte progenitors; bone remodeling; protects epithelial cells and connective tissue; induction of acute-phase protein; inhibition of macrophage activity; promotion of neuronal development
IL-12	Macrophages, monocytes, neutrophils, DCs, B cells, microglia	Induces TH1 differentiation and cytotoxicity
IL-13	T cells, NK T cells, and mast cells, basophils, eosinophils	Switching to IgG4 and IgE, upregulation of CD23, MHC-II on B cells, induction of CD11b, CD11c, CD18, CD29, CD23, and MHC-II on monocytes; activation of eosinophils and mast cells, recruitment and survival of eosinophils, defense against parasitic infections
IL-14	Activated T cells	Growth factor for B cells
IL-15	Monocytes, activated CD4+ T cells, keratinocytes, skeletal muscle cells	Stimulates growth and development of NK cells; stimulates activation and proliferation of T and B cells
IL-16	T cells, mast cells, eosinophils, monocytes, DCs, fibroblasts, airway epithelial cells	Chemotaxis, modulation of T-cell response
IL-17A	TH17 cells, CD8+ T cells, NK cells, NK T cells, γ/δ–T cells, neutrophils	Induces proinflammatory cytokine and chemokine production by epithelial and endothelial cells and fibroblasts; recruitment of neutrophils
IL-17B	Neuronal cells, chondrocytes	Induces proinflammatory cytokine and chemokine production Chondrogenesis and osteogenesis
IL-17C	Immune cells under certain conditions	Induces proinflammatory cytokine and chemokine production
IL-17D	Resting B and T cells	Induces proinflammatory cytokine and chemokine production
IL-17F	TH17 cells, CD8+ T cells, NK cells, NK T cells, γ/δ–T cells, neutrophils	Induces proinflammatory cytokine and chemokine production; recruitment of neutrophils
IL-18	Macrophages, Kupffer cells, keratinocytes, osteoblasts, astrocytes, DCs	Induces IFN-γ production by T cells and NK cells; promotes TH1 or TH2 cell responses depending on cytokine milieu
IL-19	Monocytes, keratinocytes, airway epithelial cells, B cells	Unknown
IL-20	Monocytes, keratinocytes, epithelial and endothelial cells	Appears to have a role in skin development and is suspected of regulating inflammation in the skin
IL-21	T cells (predominantly TH17), NK T cells	Regulates proliferation, differentiation, apoptosis, antibody isotype balance, cytotoxic activity
IL-22	Activated T cells (predominantly TH17), NK T cells	Pathogen defense, wound healing, tissue reorganization
IL-23	Macrophages and activated dendritic cells	Stimulates production of proinflammatory IL-17 and promotes memory
IL-24	Melanocytes, T cells, monocytes	Tumor suppression
IL-25	TH2 cells, mast and epithelial cells, eosinophils and basophils from atopic individuals	Enhances allergic responses and promotes TH2 inflammation

(continued)

TABLE 8.1 Cytokines—cont'd

Cytokine	Cell Sources	Predominant Effects
IL-26	Activated T cells (predominantly TH17), NK T cells	Activates and regulates epithelial cells
IL-27	Activated DCs, macrophages, epithelial cells	Promotes development along the TH1 phenotype, suppresses the TH2 phenotype, inhibits TH17 response
IL-28 and IL-29	Monocyte-derived DCs	Induces an antiviral state in infected cells
IL-30 (p28 subunit of IL-27)	DCs, macrophages	Induces IL-12–mediated liver injury
IL-31	Activated CD4$^+$ T cells (mainly TH2) and CD8$^+$ T cells	Induces IL-6, IL-8, CXCL1, CXCL8, CC chemokine ligand 2, and CC chemokine ligand 8 production in eosinophils; upregulates chemokine mRNA expression in keratinocytes, expression of growth factors and chemokines in epithelial cells, inhibition of proliferation and apoptosis in epithelial cells
IL-32	Monocytes, macrophages, NK cells, T cells, epithelial cells	Induces TNF-α, IL-8, and IL-6 apoptosis
IL-33	Necrotic cells	Induces TH2 inflammation
IL-34	Heart, brain, spleen, liver, kidney, thymus, testes, ovary, small intestine, prostate, colon	Proliferation
IL-35	Treg cells	Proliferation of Treg cells and inhibition of TH17-cell function, suppression of inflammatory responses
IL-37	Monocytes, tonsil plasma cells, breast carcinoma cells	Suppresses proinflammatory cytokines and inhibits DC activation
IL-38	Basal cells of skin, spleen, placenta, fetal liver, thymus, proliferating B cells of tonsils	Because of its homology with other IL-1 family members, IL-38 is thought to have similar biological activity, namely, stimulation of the expression of genes associated with inflammation
TSLP	Epithelial cells	Promotes T-cell proliferation and differentiation, activates DCs to prime for TH2 cell differentiation
Interferons		
IFN-γ	T cells, NK and NK T cells, macrophages, TH1 cells, B cells	Macrophage activation, increased expression of MHC molecules and antigen-presenting components, Ig class switching, suppression of TH2 response, antiviral properties, promotes cytotoxic activity
IFN-α	Leukocytes	Antiviral, increases MHC class I expression
IFN-β	Fibroblasts	Antiviral, increases MHC class I expression
Tumor Necrosis Factor and Related Molecules		
TNF	Activated monocytes/macrophages and T, B, and NK cells	Major inflammatory mediator induced by the presence of Gram-negative bacteria and their components; potent immunoregulatory, cytotoxic, antiviral, and procoagulatory activities
LTα (previously called TNF-β)	Activated TH1, B, and NK cells	Promotes inflammation, has antiviral activity, and kills tumor cells by apoptosis
LT$\alpha\beta$	Activated TH1, B, and NK cells	Has a specialized role in secondary lymphoid organ development
OPGL	Osteoblasts, bone marrow stromal cells, activated T cells	Stimulates osteoclasts and bone resorption
BAFF	Monocytes, macrophages, dendritic cells	Survival factor required for the maturation of B cells
Transforming Growth Factor		
TGF-β	Chondrocytes, monocytes, T cells	Antiinflammatory; inhibits cell growth; induces IgA secretion by B cells; plays a role in adhesion, proliferation, differentiation, transformation, chemotaxis, and immunoregulation
Hematopoietic Growth Factors		
SCF	Stromal cells in the fetal liver, bone marrow, and thymus; in the central nervous system; and in the gut mucosa	Supports the survival and growth of the earliest hematopoietic precursors in vivo
GM-CSF	Activated T cells, macrophages, stromal cells, and endothelial cells	Stimulates growth and differentiation of myelomonocytic lineage cells, particularly dendritic cells and inflammatory leukocytes
G-CSF	Activated T cells, endothelial cells, fibroblasts, and mononuclear phagocytes	Stimulates neutrophil development and differentiation
M-CSF	Endothelial cells, fibroblasts, mononuclear phagocytes	Influences CFU-GM cells to differentiate into monocytes and macrophages in vitro

BAFF, B-lymphocyte–activating factor belonging to the TNF family; *CFU*, colony-forming unit; *CSF*, colony-stimulating factor; *DC*, dendritic cells; *G*, granulocyte; *GM*, granulocyte-macrophage; *IFN*, interferon; *Ig*, immunoglobulin; *IL*, interleukin; *LT*, lymphotoxin; *M*, macrophage; *MHC*, major histocompatibility complex; *mRNA*, messenger RNA; *NK*, natural killer; *OPGL*, osteoprotegerin ligand; *SCF*, stem cell factor; *TGF*, transforming growth factor; *TH*, helper T; *TNF*, tumor necrosis factor, *Treg*, regulatory T cells; *TSLP*, thymic stromal lymphopoietin.

From Flint PW, Haughey BH, Lund V, et al. *Cummings Otolaryngology—Head and Neck Surgery.* 7th ed. Philadelphia, PA: Elsevier, 2021, Table 35.1.

TABLE 8.2 Chemokines

Systematic Name	Common Name(s)/Ligand(s)	Target Cell(s)
CXC Chemokines		
CXCL1	GROα/MGSAα	Neutrophil
CXCL2	GROβ/MGSAβ	Neutrophil
CXCL3	GROδ/MGSAδ	Neutrophil
CXCL4	Platelet factor-4	Fibroblast
CXCL5	Epithelial neutrophil-activating peptide 78	Neutrophil
CXCL6	Granulocyte chemotactic protein 2	Neutrophil
CXCL7	Neutrophil-activating peptide 2	Neutrophil
CXCL8	IL-8	Neutrophil, basophil, T cell
CXCL9	Monokine induced by IFN-γ	Activated T cell
CXCL10	IFN-γ–inducible protein 10	Activated T cell
CXCL11	IFN-inducible T-cell α–chemoattractant	Activated T cell
CXCL12	Stromal cell–derived factor 1a/b	CD34+ bone marrow cell, T cell, dendritic cell, B cell, activated CD4 cell
CXCL13	B-cell–attracting chemokine1	Naïve B cell, activated CD4 cell
CXCL14	Breast and kidney–expressed chemokine	
CXCL15	Lungkine	
CXCL16	Small inducible cytokine B6	T cell, NK T cell
CC Chemokines		
CCL1	I-309 (a human chemokine)	Neutrophil, T cell
CCL2	MCP-1/monocyte chemotactic and activating factor/tumor-derived chemotactic factor	T cell, monocyte, basophil
CCL3	MIP-1α	Monocyte, macrophage, T cell, NK cell, basophil
CCL3L1	LD78β	
CCL4	MIP-1β	Monocyte, macrophage, T cell, NK cell, basophil
CCL5	Regulated upon activation, normal T cell–expressed and secreted (RANTES)	Monocyte, macrophage, T cell, NK cell, basophil, eosinophil, dendritic cell
CCL6	None	
CCL7	MCP-3	T cell, monocyte, eosinophil, basophil, dendritic cell
CCL8	MCP-2	T cell, monocyte, eosinophil, basophil
CCL9/10	MIP-1γ	
CCL11	Eotaxin	Eosinophil
CCL12	MCP-5	
CCL13	MCP-4	T cell, monocyte, eosinophil, basophil, dendritic cell
CCL14	HCC-1	Monocyte
CCL15	HCC-2/leukotactin 1/MIP-1δ	T cell, monocyte, dendritic cell
CCL16	HCC-4/liver-expressed chemokine	Monocyte
CCL17	Thymus- and activation-regulated chemokine	T cell, immature dendritic cell, T cell, thymocyte
CCL18	MIP-4, dendritic cell–derived CC chemokine/pulmonary and activation-regulated chemokine/activation-induced, chemokine-related molecule 1	Naïve T cell, T cell
CCL19	MIP-3β/exodus 3	Naïve T cell, mature dendritic cell, B cell
CCL20	MIP-3α/liver- and activation-regulated chemokine/exodus 1	T cell, bone marrow dendritic cell
CCL21	6Ckine/secondary lymphoid tissue chemokine/exodus 2	Naïve T cell, B cell
CCL22	Macrophage-derived chemokine-stimulated T-cell chemoattractant protein 1	Immature dendritic cell, T cell
CCL23	MPIF-1/CK 8/CK 8.1	Monocyte, T cell
CCL24	Eotaxin 2/MPIF-2	Eosinophil, basophil
CCL25	Thymus-expressed chemokine	Macrophage, thymocyte, dendritic cell
CCL26	Eotaxin 3	
CCL27	Cutaneous T-cell–activating chemokine/IL-11 receptor α-locus chemokine	T cell
CCL28	Mucosa-associated epithelial chemokine	T cell, eosinophil
XC Chemokines		
XCL1	Lymphotactin/SCM-1β/activation-induced, chemokine-related molecule	T cell, NK cell
XCL2	SCM-1β	
CXC3C Chemokine		
CXC3CL1	Fracktalkine	T cell, monocyte

CCL, CC ligand; *CK*, chemokine; *CXCL*, CXC ligand; *GRO*, growth-related oncogene; *HCC*, human CC chemokine; *IFN*, interferon; *IL*, interleukin; *MCP*, monocyte chemoattractant.
From Flint PW, Haughey BH, Lund V, et al. *Cummings Otolaryngology—Head and Neck Surgery.* 7th ed. Philadelphia, PA: Elsevier, 2021, Table 35.2.

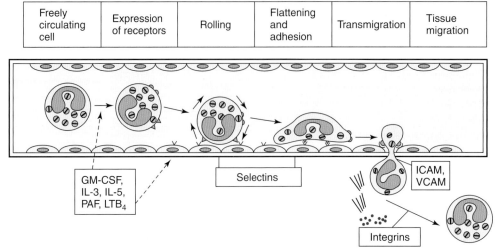

Fig. 8.5 Cellular adhesion and recruitment. *GM-CSF,* Granulocyte-macrophage colony-stimulating factor; *ICAM,* intercellular adhesion molecule; *IL,* interleukin; *LTB4,* leukotriene B4; *PAF,* platelet-activating factor; *VCAM,* vascular cellular adhesion molecule. (From Flint PW, Haughey BH, Lund VJ, et al. *Cummings Otolaryngology—Head and Neck Surgery.* 6th ed. Philadelphia, PA: Saunders; 2015, Fig. 38.4; and Mygind N, Dahl R, Pedersen S, Thestrup-Pedersen K, eds. *Essential Allergy.* 2nd ed. Oxford: Blackwell Scientific Publications: 1996.)

TABLE 8.3 Hypersensitivity Classification Schema

	Immune Reactant	Mechanism	Examples
Type I	IgE	Binding to mast cells and subsequent degranulation	Anaphylaxis, allergic rhinitis, food allergies
Type II	IgM, IgG	Antibody binding leading to complement activation	Goodpasture, autoimmune hemolytic anemia
Type III	IgM, IgG, IgA	Antigen–antibody complex deposition	Rheumatoid arthritis, poststreptococcal glomerulonephritis, systemic lupus erythematosus, serum sickness
Type IV	T cells	T-cell–mediated cytokine release "Delayed hypersensitivity"	Contact dermatitis (nickel, gold, poison oak, etc.), Type 1 diabetes mellitus, multiple sclerosis, graft rejection

Type 1: Anaphylaxis Treatment

- Epinephrine (α-1, β-1, β-2 agonist effects) is first line
  - Dosing:
    - Adults: 0.3 to 0.5 mg of 1:1000 solution
    - Children: Weight based; 0.01 mg/kg of 1:1000 solution
  - Can repeat dose every 15 to 20 minutes as needed
- Bronchodilators (albuterol)
- Antihistamines
- Glucocorticoids for late-effect symptoms

Type II: Cytotoxic Reaction Examples

- Medications: Penicillins, thiazides, cephalosporins
- Hemolytic anemia
- Transfusion reaction
- Acute graft versus host disease
- Goodpasture syndrome
- Myasthenia gravis
- Drug-induced lupus

Type II: Cytotoxic Reaction Mechanism

- IgG or IgM mediated
- Antibodies reaction with antigens on cell surface
- Activation of complement system and subsequent cell lysis

Type III: Immune Complexes Examples

- Serum sickness
- Poststreptococcal glomerulonephritis
- Rheumatoid arthritis
- Lupus
- Angioedema

Type III: Immune Complexes Mechanism

- Immune complexes form (binding of antibody to a soluble antigen)
- Complexes deposit in tissues
- Deposition triggers classical complement pathway and inflammatory reaction

Type IV: Cell-Mediated Examples

- Dermatitis
- Tuberculosis
- Sarcoidosis
- Candidiasis

Type IV: Cell-Mediated Mechanism

- Delayed hypersensitivity reaction: Takes more than 12 hours to develop
- Direct T-cell activation
- Cell-mediated inflammation

ALLERGENS

Perennial Allergens

- Mites
- Cockroaches
- Cotton particles

- Human scales
- Animal dander
- Molds
- Food allergies
  - Not responsive to traditional immunotherapy; avoidance of offending food products is treatment of choice
  - Tree nuts least likely to resolve over time (walnut, cashew, almond, pecan, brazil nut, macadamia nut, hazelnut, pistachio, pine nut)
  - Majority (80%) of reactions to eggs and milk resolve by adulthood

Seasonal Allergies

- Trees: Spring
- Grasses: Spring, Summer, and Fall
- Weeds: Summer and Fall

HISTORY AND PHYSICAL EXAM OF PATIENT WITH ALLERGIES

History

- Particular emphasis on:
  - List of medications
  - Comorbidities
- Previous operations
- Childhood history
- Family history

PHYSICAL EXAM

- Eyes: Allergic *shiners* (darkening of skin under eyes), long eyelashes, fine creases in lower eyelids
- Ears: Erythema, postauricular fissures, desquamation of external auditory canal, tympanosclerosis, tympanic membrane retraction and/or perforation, serous effusion
- Nose: Discharge, edema of turbinates, polyps, *allergic salute* (nasal tip transverse crease), excoriation of philtrum (pruritis, rhinorrhea)
- Neck: Lymphadenopathy
- Chest: Wheezing
- Pharyngeal: High, narrow arched palate, lymphoid hyperplasia, cobblestoning of posterior pharyngeal wall, hypertrophy of the lateral nasopharyngeal bands, chronic cough, edema of uvula and glottis
- Systemic: Eczema, heartburn, diarrhea, abdominal bloating, enuresis, asthma

RHINITIS

Differential Diagnosis of Rhinorrhea and Nasal Obstruction (Box 8.1)

- Allergic rhinitis
- Nonallergic rhinitis
- Nonallergic rhinitis eosinophilia syndrome
- Infectious rhinitis
- Granulomatous rhinitis
- Drug-induced rhinitis
- Rhinitis from mechanical obstruction
- Neoplastic rhinitis
- Chronic rhinitis and rhinosinusitis

ALLERGIC RHINITIS/HAY FEVER

Background and Epidemiology

- IgE-mediated inflammation of naso-ocular region due to allergens in the air
- Affects 10% to 30% of adults and 40% of children

BOX 8.1	Differential Diagnosis of Rhinorrhea and Nasal Obstruction
Allergic rhinitis	Seasonal/perennial/episodic or intermittent/persistent
Local allergic rhinitis	Negative skin/radioallergosorbent testing but positive nasal allergen challenge
Nonallergic rhinitis	• *Perennial (vasomotor):* Constant symptoms of profuse, clear rhinorrhea and nasal congestion without correlation to specific allergen exposure or signs of atopy • *Cold air–induced:* Nasal congestion and rhinorrhea upon exposure to cold, windy weather; occurs in both allergic and nonallergic individuals
Nonallergic rhinitis with eosinophilia syndrome (NARES)	Often seen in adults; characterized by eosinophilia on nasal smears and with negative test results for specific allergens
Infectious rhinitis	Bacterial, viral, fungal
Granulomatous rhinitis	Sarcoidosis, Wegener granulomatosis
Drug-Induced rhinitis	Oral contraceptives, reserpine derivatives, hydralazine hydrochloride, topical decongestants (rhinitis medicamentosa), β-blockers (eyedrops)
Rhinitis from mechanical obstruction	• *Septal deviation:* Common; might exacerbate nasal obstruction in allergic rhinitis • *Foreign body:* Unilateral purulent nasal discharge is the usual manifestation of a foreign body; resolves after removal • *Choanal atresia or stenosis:* Bilateral choanal atresia is usually diagnosed early in life, but unilateral choanal atresia or stenosis can go unnoticed for several years. It is easily diagnosed by nasal endoscopy and axial computed tomography of the midfacial skeleton • *Adenoid hypertrophy:* Common cause of nasal obstruction in children • *Others:* Encephaloceles, lacrimal duct cysts, dermoids
Neoplastic rhinitis	• *Benign:* Polyps, juvenile angiofibroma, inverted papilloma *Malignant:* Adenocarcinoma, squamous cell carcinoma, esthesioneuroblastoma, lymphoma, rhabdomyosarcoma

From Flint PW, Haughey BH, Lund V, et al. *Cummings Otolaryngology—Head and Neck Surgery.* 7th ed. Philadelphia, PA: Elsevier, 2021, Box 35.1.

Allergic Rhinitis and Asthma

- Allergic rhinitis leads to threefold increased risk of asthma
- Allergic Rhinitis and Impact on Asthma (ARIA) guidelines: Classification of allergic rhinitis as intermittent or persistent
  - Intermittent: Symptoms <4 days/week *and* <4 weeks
  - Persistent: >4 days/week *and* >4 weeks
- Rhinitis frequency and severity associated with severity of asthma

Allergic Rhinitis Common Allergens: Infants/Children

- Milk
- Eggs
- Peanuts
- Tree nuts
- Soy

- Wheat
- Dust mites
- Pet dander

Allergic Rhinitis Common Allergens: Adolescents/Adults

- Pollens
- Animal dander
- Dust Mites
- Molds
- Foods
- Latex

Pathophysiology of Allergic Rhinitis (Fig. 8.6)

- Inflammation of nasal mucous membranes
- IgE mediated to allergens (Type I)
- IgE attach to surface receptors of mast cells, leading to release of inflammatory mediators
  - Histamine, leukotrienes, cytokines, prostaglandins, platelet-activating factor

Development of Atopy

- Genetics
- Environmental exposure
- Exposure to tobacco smoke
- *Hygiene hypothesis*: Lack of exposure to certain agents, such as infectious symbiotic microorganisms, during childhood increases susceptibility later in life
- Overuse of/exposure to antibiotics

ALLERGIC RHINITIS EVALUATION

Allergic Rhinitis Diagnosis: History-Specific Questions

- Nasal, ocular, otologic, oral, facial, and skin symptoms
- Time of year, relation to wind and weather patterns, geographic location

- Present environments, for example, home, school, work, outdoors
- Family or childhood history of atopy (allergies, eczema, asthma)
- History of anaphylaxis
- Quality of life
- Past and current allergy treatments

Allergic Rhinitis Diagnosis Physical Exam

- Periorbital puffiness
- Allergic shiners
- Dennie's lines (extra creases in the lower eyelid)
- Otitis media with effusion
- Retracted tympanic membrane
- Clear rhinorrhea
- Gray/blue turbinates
- Allergic salute (transverse nasal crease)
- Adenoid facies
- Cobblestoning of pharyngeal lymphoid tissue

Allergic Rhinitis Associated Disorders

- Chronic rhinosinusitis
  - Having both conditions has greater negative quality of life impact than either alone
  - Immunotherapy does not impact polyp size but can help symptoms
- Conjunctivitis
- Asthma; *unified airway concept*
- Eczema
- Eosinophilic esophagitis
- Otitis media with effusion

Allergic Rhinitis Adjunctive Testing

- Nasal endoscopy
- Labs: Total IgE, eosinophilia
- Nasal smear
- Nasal allergen challenge
- Allergy skin testing
- In vitro allergy testing

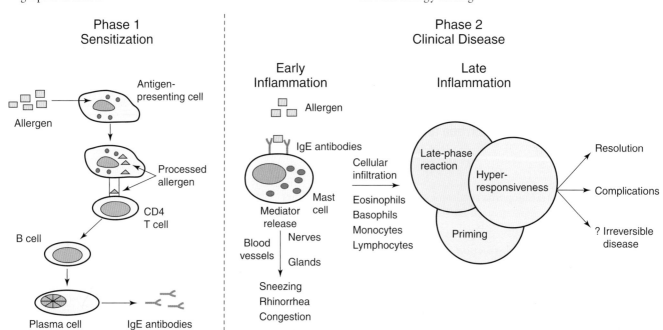

Fig. 8.6 Pathophysiology of allergic rhinitis. (From Flint PW, Haughey BH, Lund VJ, et al. *Cummings Otolaryngology—Head and Neck Surgery.* 6th ed. Philadelphia, PA: Saunders; 2015, Fig. 38.6; and Naclerio RM. Allergic rhinitis. *N Engl J Med* 1991;325:860.)

Differential Diagnosis of Allergic Rhinitis

- Infectious rhinitis
- Perennial nonallergic rhinitis
- Pollutants and irritants
- Hormonal rhinitis
- Medication-induced topical rhinitis
- Anatomical deformity
- Tumor
- Foreign body

SKIN DIAGNOSTIC TESTING

Allergic Rhinitis In Vivo Testing

- Prick test
- Intradermal test
- Skin endpoint titration (SET)/intradermal dilutional testing

Prick Test (Fig. 8.7)

- Drop of antigen placed on skin and a small-gauge needle used to penetrate into the epidermis (~1 mm) through drop of antigen
  - Negative control: Diluent for the allergen extract
  - Positive control: Histamine or codeine
- Measurement after 10 to 20 minutes
- Quantitative (size of wheal in mm) and qualitative scoring of wheal (e.g., 0–4+)
- Advantages: Rapid test, easy to perform, strong reproducibility, rare systemic reactions, not invasive, less expensive, low risk of anaphylaxis
- Disadvantages: Mostly qualitative assessment, false negatives

Intradermal Test (Fig. 8.8)

- Small-gauge needle (e.g., #26) used to inject a small amount of antigen (0.01–0.05 mL) into the superficial dermis
- Concentrations of antigens: 1:500 to 1:1000 weight/volume
- 10 to 20 minutes to allow for skin reaction

- Quantitative (size of wheal) and qualitative scoring of wheal (e.g., 0–4+)
- Advantages: Highly sensitive, moderately reproducible, allows for intradermal dilutional testing to establish starting point for immunotherapy; certain allergens such as insect stings and penicillin require this method
- Disadvantages: Poor specificity, false positives
- Contraindications: Dermatographism, areas of skin with active contact dermatitis or cellulitis

Prick Versus Intradermal Testing

- Prick: More specific
- Intradermal: More sensitive

Skin Endpoint Titration (SET)/Intradermal Dilutional Testing

- Fivefold dilution of each antigen made and placed in vials labeled 1 to 6
  - 1 cc of antigenic concentrate (1:20 weight/volume) mixed with 4 cc of inert diluent
  - First diluted preparation is referred to as the #1 dilution
  - Each dilution is subsequently diluted fivefold, for example, vial #1 is 1:100, vial #2 is 1:500, vial 3 is 1:2500, and so on.
- Vial #6 or stronger dilution is injected intradermally (Fig. 8.9)
  - Goal of creating a precise 4-mm diameter wheal in skin
- Measurement after 10 minutes
- Wheal of 7 mm or greater in diameter considered a *positive wheal response*
  - Note: 4 mm to > 5 mm wheal in 10 minutes via diffusion
  - If no response, next stronger dilution (#5) is injected
  - Absence of allergy: No positive wheal response with any concentration
- After demonstration of a first positive wheal (*endpoint*), the next stronger concentration is applied as a 4-mm diameter wheal
  - Positive second wheal is called the *confirming wheal*

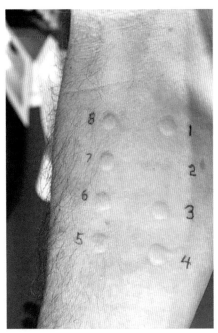

Fig. 8.7 Prick test. (From Chadwick SJ. Principles of allergy management. In: Krouse JH, Derebery MJ, Chadwick SJ, eds. *Managing the Allergic Patient*. 1st ed. Philadelphia, PA: Saunders; 2008.)

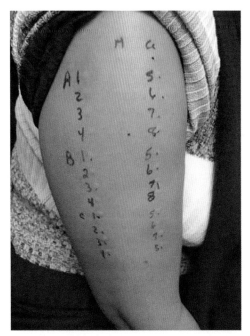

Fig. 8.8 Intradermal testing. (From Chadwick SJ. Principles of allergy management. In: Krouse JH, Derebery MJ, Chadwick SJ, eds. *Managing the Allergic Patient*. 1st ed. Philadelphia, PA: Saunders; 2008.)

- *Flash response*: A very vigorous wheal >10 mm occurs after a negative response
  - Etiology unknown but testing often stops if flash response occurs
- *Plateau response*: No progressive wheal after the endpoint of titration
- Advantages: Quantitative and qualitative, reproducible, sensitive, safe, low risk of systemic response
- Disadvantages: Decreased specificity with high concentrations of antigen, time-consuming, tester dependent, increased costs, possible false positive, current allergic medications may suppress wheal-and-flare response (e.g., antihistamines [24–36 hours], tricyclic antidepressants [4 days], steroids, theophylline)

Allergic Rhinitis In Vitro Allergy Testing

- Radioallergosorbent test (RAST)
- Serum IgE testing

Radioallergosorbent Test (RAST)

- First in vitro test for allergy
- Highly specific
- Based on detection of radioactive IgE that is added to a patient's serum and suspected allergen
- Original RAST for the quantification of IgE and diagnosis of allergy has largely been abandoned in favor of Modified RAST test (MRT), which is both specific and sensitive.
  - Examples of MRT: Radioisotope or enzyme linked
  - Classic technique:
    - Disc placed in test tube with patient's serum
    - Patient's IgE binds to disc and excess serum washed away
    - Radiolabeled anti-IgE binds to patient's IgE
    - Measure radioactivity
- Advantages: Specific, safe (no risk of anaphylaxis), useful in children or skin conditions
- Disadvantages: Lower sensitivity, fewer antigens available, can be more costly, longer time for results

In Vitro Serum Total IgE Testing

- Measurement of both total and antigen-specific serum IgE
- Helpful in those with atopic conditions or when total IgE levels are markedly elevated

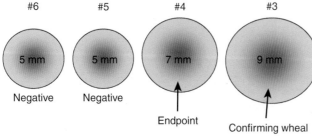

Fig. 8.9 Example of intradermal dilutional testing. Circles represent the wheal sizes 10 minutes after placing a 4-mm wheal of fivefold dilutions. The increase from 4 to 5 mm is independent of hypersensitivity and expected. The #6 dilution on the left would be placed first; if negative, then a #5 dilution is placed. In this example, the #4 dilution increases to 7 mm, which suggests a positive response (the endpoint) and the #3 dilution increases greater than or equal to 2 mm more than the #4 "confirming" the reaction. (Adapted from Haydon RC. Allergic rhinitis—current approaches to skin and in vitro testing. *Otolaryngol Clin North Am.* 2008;41(2):331–346, vii.)

- Potential utility of ratio of specific IgE to total IgE in predicting effectiveness of immunotherapy
  - High levels of specific IgE, high ratio of specific IgE to total IgE thought to predict reliable responses to immunotherapy
- Advantages: Superior safety profile, can be used in those with dermatographism or eczema, no need to stop medications prior to testing
- Disadvantages: Increased cost, longer waiting time for results

ALLERGIC RHINITIS TREATMENT

- Avoidance
- Symptomatic relief
- Diagnostic testing
- Management of severe symptoms
- Immunotherapy
- Dietary elimination
- Management of complications

Allergic Rhinitis Treatment: Avoidance

- Allergen avoidance
- HEPA (high-efficiency particulate air) filters
- Barriers: Mattress and pillow covers, pollen-rated masks

How to Decrease Allergen Exposure

- Reduce household humidity to 40% to 50%
- Wash bed linens in hot water weekly
- Remove carpets and pets from bedrooms
- Encase bedding in hypoallergenic covers
- Eliminate cockroaches
- Close windows during pollination

Allergic Rhinitis Treatment: Symptomatic Relief

- Intranasal corticosteroids (Box 8.2)
- Intranasal antihistamines
- Intranasal decongestants
- Intranasal anticholinergics
- Intranasal mast cell stabilizers
- Intranasal cromolyn sodium
- Second-generation oral antihistamines
- Oral antileukotrienes
- Systemic steroids

Mechanism of Action of Allergic Rhinitis Medications

- Antihistamines: Block binding on H_1 receptor
  - First generation: Diphenhydramine—varying degrees of anticholinergic and sedating side effects
  - Second generation: azelastine, loratadine, fexofenadine, cetirizine—less sedating side effects
- Decongestants: Act on α-adrenergic receptors of mucosa
  - Oxymetazoline, phenylephrine
  - Must be limited to short duration to avoid rhinitis medicamentosa
- Corticosteroids: Affect a wide range of cell types and mediators
  - Intranasal versus oral (systemic)
- Mast cell stabilizers (cromolyn sodium): Decrease release of mediators from degranulated mast cells
  - Must be taken prophylactically to be effective
- Anticholinergic agents: Antagonize acetylcholine at muscarinic receptors

BOX 8.2 Commonly Used Intranasal Steroid Preparations

Chemical Name	Trade Name	Formulation	Dose/Actuation	Recommended Dosage
Triamcinolone acetonide	Nasacort	Propellant, aqueous	55 µg	*2 to 5 years:* 1 spray/nostril qd (110 µg/day) *6 to 11 years:* 2 sprays/nostril qd (220 µg/day) *≥ 12 years:* 2 sprays/nostril qd (220 µg/day)
Budesonide	Rhinocort	Propellant	32 µg	*≥ 6 years:* 2 sprays/nostril qd (128 µg/day) *> 12 years:* 2 sprays/nostril qd up to 4 sprays/nostril qd (128–256 µg/day)
Flunisolide	Nasalide Nasarel	0.025% Solution	25 µg	*6 to 14 years:* 1 spray/nostril tid (150 µg/day) 2 sprays/nostril bid (200 µg/day) *≥ 14 years:* 2 sprays/nostril bid–tid (200 to 300 µg/day)
Fluticasone propionate	Flonase	0.05% Nasal spray (aqueous)	50 µg	*4 years to adolescence:* 1 spray/nostril qd (100 µg/day) *Adults:* 2 sprays/nostril qd (200 µg/day)
Mometasone furoate	Nasonex	Aqueous	50 µg	*2 to 11 years:* 1 spray/nostril qd (100 µg/day) *≥ 12 years:* 2 sprays/nostril qd (200 µg daily)
Ciclesonide	Omnaris	Suspension	50 µg	*> 6 years:* 2 sprays/nostril qd (200 µg/day)
Fluticasone furoate	Veramyst	Suspension	27.5 µg	*2 to 11 years:* 1 spray/nostril qd, can increase to 2 sprays/nostril qd (55–110 µg/day) *>11 years:* 2 sprays/nostril qd (110 µg/day)
Beclomethasone dipropionate	Qnasl	Nonaqueous aerosol	80 µg	*≥ 12 years:* 2 sprays/nostril qd (320 µg/day)
Ciclesonide	Zetonna	HFA-propelled aerosol	37 µg	*≥ 12 years:* 1 spray/nostril qd (74 µg/day)

HFA, Hydrofluoroalkane.
From Flint PW, Haughey BH, Lund V, et al. *Cummings Otolaryngology—Head and Neck Surgery.* 7th ed. Philadelphia, PA: Elsevier, 2021, Table 38.3.

- Leukotriene modifiers: Antagonize action of leukotriene receptors or inhibit 5-lipoxygenase and formation of leukotrienes
- Omalizumab: Monoclonal anti-IgE antibody

IMMUNOTHERAPY

Allergic Rhinitis Treatment: Immunotherapy

Intended for patients who have failed pharmacotherapy or desire more durable therapeutic benefit
- Subcutaneous immunotherapy (SCIT)
- Sublingual immunotherapy (SLIT)
- Specific nasal immunotherapy
- Monoclonal antibodies

Subcutaneous and Sublingual Immunotherapy Mechanisms

- Rise in serum-specific IgG
- Increased levels of IgG and IgA antibodies in nasal secretions
- Reduction in reactivity of peripheral basophils
- Reduced in vitro lymphocyte responsiveness to allergens
- Reduction in inflammatory cells in nasal mucosa and nasal secretions and a shift from the TH2 to the TH1 cytokine profile
- Suppression of the seasonal elevation of IgE antibodies

Advantages of Subcutaneous Immunotherapy

- Greater immune response/protection
- Long-term protective effect
- Affects disease process, not just symptom reduction
- Usually covered by insurance
- May be given at home in select patients (avoiding office visit)

Disadvantages of Subcutaneous Immunotherapy

- Increased risk of severe reaction
- Patient discomfort
- Often requires office visit
- Difficulty giving to young children/adolescents

Advantages of Sublingual Immunotherapy

- Ease of administration
- Avoidance of clinic visit
- Strong safety profile
- Suitable for children

Disadvantages of Sublingual Immunotherapy

- Lesser immune response than SCIT
- Longer time for clinical response
- Long-term benefit unknown
- Currently variable insurance coverage/increased patient expense

Medical Treatment Versus Subcutaneous Immunotherapy Versus Sublingual Immunotherapy

- Medical treatment/avoidance: Seasonal or episodic rhinitis
- SCIT: Perennial rhinitis
- SLIT: Seasonal and perennial allergens

Immunotherapy Indications

- Moderately severe and severe symptoms
- Allergy to allergens that cannot be treated or avoided
- Failed maximal medical therapy
- Avoid need for chronic medications
- Coexisting asthma

Immunotherapy Contraindications

- Pregnancy (initiation)
- Immunocompromised
- Unstable asthma
- Medications (beta blockers): Will not respond to epinephrine if needed in cases of anaphylaxis
- Noncompliant patients

Dosing Immunotherapy

- Starting dose
  - General principles: High enough to initiate response, low enough to prevent systemic and/or local reaction
  - Often based off of allergy diagnostic results
  - Intradermal dilutional testing: 0.05 cc of endpoint
  - RAST: 0.05 cc of endpoint minus 1 or 2 for safety in high-risk patients
- Dose escalation/maintenance dose
  - Initially weekly, then 2 to 3 weeks
  - Increase 0.05 to 0.20 cc depending on patient and time of season
  - Stop titration when evidence of clinical improvement or if excessive local or systemic reaction occurs
- Patients have variable response to immunotherapy
  - No clear biomarker to determine efficacy or endpoint of immunotherapy
  - Certain antigens (cat and dog) require higher doses to be effective

FURTHER READINGS

Adkinson N, Bochner B, Burks A, et al. *Middleton's Allergy Principles and Practice*. 8th ed. Philadelphia, PA: Elsevier; 2014.

Bunyavanich S. Allergic rhinitis. In: Sampson HA, Friedman SL, eds. Allergy and Clinical Immunology. Oxford: Wiley-Blackwell; 2015. 1st ed.

Chadwick SJ. Principles of allergy management. In: Krouse JH, Derebery MJ, Chadwick SJ, eds. *Managing the Allergic Patient*. 1st ed. Philadelphia, PA: Elsevier; 2008.

Cox DR, Wise SK, Baroody FM. Allergy and immunology of the upper airway. *Cummings Otolaryngology*. 2021;35:558–585.e9.

Golub JS, Marks SC, Pasha R. Rhinology and paranasal sinuses. In: Pasha R, Golub JS, eds. *Otolaryngology—Head and Neck Surgery: Clinical Reference Guide*. Plural Publishing; 2014.

Houck J. Immunology and allergy. In: Lee KJ, ed. *Essential Otolaryngology: Head & Neck Surgery*. New York: NY: McGraw-Hill; 2008.

James W. Mims. Allergy testing. In: Jonas J, Clark R, eds. *Bailey's Head and Neck Surgery: Otolaryngology*. 5th ed. Philadelphia, PA: Wolters Kluwer; 2014.

Khoury P, Naclerio RM. Immunology and allergy. In: Bailey BJ, Johnson JT, eds. *Head & Neck Surgery—Otolaryngology*. Philadelphia, PA: Lippincott; 2006.

Kowal J, Dubuske L. Overview of in vitro allergy tests. In: Bochner BS, Feldweg AM (eds). UpToDate. Waltham, MA. Accessed November 26, 2020. https://www.uptodate.com/contents/overview-of-in-vitro-allergy-tests?search=Overview%20of%20in%20vitro%20allergy%20tests&source=search_result&selectedTitle=1~150&usage_type=default&display_rank=1.

Krouse JH. Allergic and nonallergic rhinitis. In: Bailey BJ, Johnson JT, eds. *Head & Neck Surgery—Otolaryngology*. Philadelphia, PA: Lippincott; 2006.

Krouse JH. Introduction to allergy. In: Krouse JH, Derebery MJ, Chadwick SJ, eds. *Managing the Allergic Patient*. 1st ed. Philadelphia, PA: Elsevier; 2008.

Salamone FN, Tami TA. Acute and chronic sinusitis. In: Lawani AK, ed. *Current Diagnosis & Treatment: Otolaryngology Head and Neck Surgery*. New York, NY: McGraw-Hill Medical; 2008. Lange Series.

Shah SB, Emanuel IA. Nonallergic and allergic rhinitis. In: Lawani AK, ed. *Current Diagnosis & Treatment: Otolaryngology Head and Neck Surgery*. New York, NY: McGraw-Hill Medical; 2008. Lange Series.

9 Sleep Medicine

Elliott D. Kozin, Lauren Miller, Kevin C. Coughlin, and M. Boyd Gillespie

NORMAL SLEEP PHYSIOLOGY

Ideal Length of Sleep

- Infants: 14 to 16 hours
- Children: 9 hours
- Adults: 7 to 8 hours

Factors That Determine Sleep Length

- Genetic
- Circadian rhythm
- Voluntary control, for example, alarm clock

Sleep Architecture

- Non–rapid eye movement (NREM) sleep
  - N1, N2, N3
- Rapid eye movement (REM) sleep
  - Also known as *R sleep*
- Often a gradual transition from one stage to the next

NREM Stages of Sleep

- N1: Transition to sleep or light sleep
  - Theta activity
  - Very short duration (<10 minutes)
- N2: Sleep
  - Theta activity, K complexes, sleep spindles
  - Decreased blood pressure, brain metabolism, cardiac activity
- N3: Deep sleep
  - Slow-wave sleep

REM Sleep Stages

- Also known as *paradoxical sleep* or *active sleep*
- Often occurs 90 to 120 minutes after sleep onset and increases in length as sleep progresses
- Tonic: Parasympathically driven, no eye movements
- Phasic: Sympathetically driven, REMs, irregular cardiac and respiratory patterns, loss of peripheral muscle tone
  - Thought to be related to dream content

Aging and Sleep Stages

- Young infants and children: Increased REM and stage N3 NREM
- Elderly: Decreased stage N3 NREM

Sleep Waves and Rhythms (Table 9.1)

- Beta: 13 to 30 Hz (wakefulness)
- Alpha: 8 to 12 Hz (relaxed wakefulness)
- Theta: 4 to 8 Hz (N1 and REM)
- Delta: 1 to 4 Hz (N3)
- K complex (N2)

- Vertex sharp waves (N1)
- Sleep spindle (N2)
- Sawtooth waves (REM)

Sleep–Wake Cycles

- Homeostatic drive (Process S; increasing sleep propensity with wakefulness)
- Circadian rhythm (Process C; internal sleep–wake cycle)

Sleep Centers of the Brain

- Reticular activating system
- Hypothalamus
- Basal forebrain
- Thalamus
- Pineal gland (melatonin production)

Sleep-Related Brain Nuclei

- Locus coeruleus
- Substantia nigra
- Ventral tegmental region
- Laterodorsal tegmental nuclei
- Pedunculopontine nuclei
- Dorsal raphe nucleus

Hormones Related to Sleep Function

- Cortisol (increases during sleep)
- Thyroid-stimulating hormone (decreases during sleep)
- Growth hormone (initially increases, then decreases over the course of sleep)
- Prolactin (increases with sleep)
- Glucose/insulin (both increase with sleep)
- Hypocretins/orexins (promote wakefulness)
- Melatonin (promotes sleep)
- Leptin (elevated during sleep)
- Ghrelin (reduced during sleep)

SLEEP DISORDER CLASSIFICATION AND DEFINITIONS (TABLE 9.2)

Six Major Categories of International Classification of Sleep Disorders (ICSD)

- Insomnia: Difficulty falling and/or staying asleep
- Dyssomnias: Conditions that reduce the amount and quality of sleep
  - Obstructive sleep apnea (OSA), central sleep apnea (CSA), and more
- Central disorders of hypersomnolence
  - Narcolepsy, hypersomnia, Kleine-Levin syndrome, and more
- Circadian rhythm sleep–wake disorders
  - Delayed sleep phase, advanced sleep phase, shift work disorder, and more

TABLE 9.1 States of Sleep and Associated Brainwaves

Sleep State	Brainwave
Awake	Beta
Relaxed wakefulness	Alpha
N1	Theta, vertex waves
N2	Theta, sleep spindles, K complexes
N3	Delta, slow wave
Rapid eye movement	Beta, sawtooth waves

TABLE 9.2 Respiratory Event Definitions and Types

Respiratory Event	Definition
Apnea	A cessation of airflow for at least 10 seconds
Hypopnea	A reduction in airflow (≥30%) for at least 10 seconds with ≥4% oxyhemoglobin desaturation
	or
	a reduction in airflow (≥50%) for at least 10 seconds with ≥3% oxyhemoglobin desaturation or an electroencephalogram (EEG) arousal
Respiratory effort–related arousal	Sequence of breaths for at least 10 seconds with increasing respiratory effort or flattening of the nasal pressure waveform leading to an arousal from sleep when the sequence of breaths does not meet the criteria for an apnea or a hypopnea
Obstructive	Continued thoracoabdominal effort in the setting of partial or complete airflow cessation
Central	Lack of thoracoabdominal effort in the setting of partial or complete airflow cessation
Mixed	Respiratory event with both obstructive and central features, with mixed events generally beginning as central events and ending with thoracoabdominal effort without airflow

Based on Sleep-related breathing disorders in adults: recommendations for syndrome definition and measurement techniques in clinical research. The Report of an American Academy of Sleep Medicine Task Force. *Sleep.* 1999;22(5):667–89.

- Parasomnias: Irregular actions executed during sleep process
  - Sleepwalking, REM sleep behavior disorder, enuresis, and more
- Sleep-related movement disorders
  - Restless legs syndrome (RLS), periodic limb movement disorder, and more

DYSSOMNIAS

Definitions

Apnea

- >90% reduction of airflow by nose or mouth *and*
- 10 seconds or longer

Hypopnea (Varies Based on Laboratory)

- Decrease in airflow to ≥30% baseline *and* period of 10 seconds *and* ≥4% oxygen desaturation *or*
- Reduction in airflow (>50%) *and* period of 10 seconds *and* ≥ 3% oxygen desaturation

TABLE 9.3 Indexes of Sleep-Disordered Breathing

Index	Definition
Apnea index	Number of apneas per hour of total sleep time
Hypopnea index	Number of hypopneas per hour of total sleep time
Apneahypopnea index	Number of apneas and hypopneas per hour of total sleep time
Respiratory effort–related arousal (RERA) index	Number of RERAs per hour of total sleep time
Respiratory disturbance index	Number of apneas, hypopneas, and RERAs per hour of total sleep time
Central apnea index	Number of central apneas per hour of total sleep time
Mixed apnea index	Number of mixed apneas per hour of total sleep time

From Flint PW, Haughey BH, Lund VJ, et al. *Cummings Otolaryngology—Head and Neck Surgery.* 7th ed. Philadelphia, PA: Elsevier; 2021, Table 15.2.

Respiratory Effort–Related Arousal (RERA)

- Absence of apnea/hypopnea *and*
- 10-second or more duration of progressive negative esophageal pressure or flattening of nasal pressure waveform *and*
- EEG arousal

Indices of Apnea (Table 9.3)

- Apnea index (apneas/hour of sleep)
- Apnea hypopnea index (AHI; apneas and hypopneas/hour of sleep)
- Respiratory disturbance index (apneas and hypopneas and RERAs/hour of sleep)

Types of Apnea

- Obstructive
- Central
- Mixed

OBSTRUCTIVE SLEEP APNEA

Obstructive Sleep Apnea Spectrum

- Primary snoring
- Upper airway resistance syndrome
- Obstructive sleep apnea syndrome (OSAS)
- Overlap syndrome: OSAS and chronic obstructive pulmonary disease (COPD)
- Obesity-hypoventilation syndrome

Levels of Airway Obstruction

- Nasal cavity/nasopharynx
  - Septal deviation, turbinate hypertrophy, nasal valve collapse, nasal polyps, adenoid hypertrophy
- Oral cavity/oropharynx
  - Elongation of soft palate and uvula, palatine and lingual tonsil hypertrophy, macroglossia, retrognathia, poor upper airway muscle tone
- Hypopharynx/larynx
  - Omega-shaped epiglottis, laryngotracheal malacia or stenosis

Categories of Obstructive Sleep Apnea Based on Apnea Hypopnea Index

Adults

- Mild (5–15 events/hour)
- Moderate (15–30 events/hour)
- Severe (>30 events/hour)

SNORING

Anatomical Sites of Origin of Snoring

- Soft palate
- Tonsillar pillars
- Base of tongue
- Epiglottis/supraglottis

Nonsurgical Management of Snoring

- Weight loss
- Eliminating alcohol, tobacco, caffeine, sedatives
- Positioning while asleep
- Medically treating reflux, sinusitis, and nasal polyps
- Nasal breathing strips
- Oral appliance (Fig. 9.1)

Surgical Management of Snoring

- Septoplasty/turbinate reduction
- Palatal implants
- Radiofrequency ablation of upper airway tissue (palate, turbinate, tongue base)

UPPER AIRWAY RESISTANCE SYNDROME

Upper Airway Resistance Syndrome Diagnosis

- Excessive daytime sleepiness, AHI <5/hour and presence of RERA, often thought to be more than 50% of respiratory events
- Polysomnogram demonstrates flow limitation during sleep

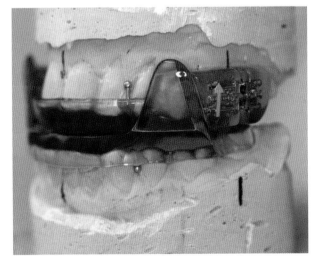

Fig. 9.1 Mandibular advancement appliance for mild to moderate sleep apnea. (From Flint PW, Haughey BH, Lund VJ, et al. *Cummings Otolaryngology—Head and Neck Surgery.* 7th ed. Philadelphia, PA: Elsevier; 2021, Fig. 15.12.)

Risk Factor for Upper Airway Resistance Syndrome

- Female gender
- Nonobese
- Younger age
- Nasal obstruction

OBSTRUCTIVE SLEEP APNEA SYNDROME

Obstructive Sleep Apnea Syndrome Diagnosis

- ≥5 respiratory events/hour *and* respiratory effort with symptoms

or

- ≥15 respiratory events/hour with respiratory effort without symptoms
  - Respiratory event: Hypopneas and apneas

Obstructive Sleep Apnea Syndrome Pathophysiology

- Upper airway collapse
- Inability for airway dilators to respond
- Decreased sensitivity of chemoreceptors
- Decreased central respiratory drive
- Defective ventilator receptors

Obstructive Sleep Apnea Syndrome Risk Factors—Basic

- Obesity
- Family history
- Anatomy (maxillary hypoplasia; retrognathia)
- Increased age
- Allergies
- Postmenopausal status
- Sedatives and alcohol
- Smoking

Obstructive Sleep Apnea Syndrome—Disease Associations

- Down syndrome
- Marfan syndrome
- Neuromuscular disorders
- Muscular dystrophy
- Kyphoscoliosis
- Amyloidosis
- Endocrine abnormalities

Clinical Consequences of Obstructive Sleep Apnea

- Sleep related
  - Daytime somnolence and fatigue, morning headache, motor vehicle accidents, poor job performance, depression, familial stress
- Cardiovascular consequences
  - Hypertension, coronary artery disease, cardiac arrhythmia, cerebrovascular accidents
- Pulmonary consequences
  - Pulmonary hypertension
  - Cor pulmonale
- Shorter life expectancy

TABLE 9.4 Medical Conditions That Cause Fatigue

Severe anemia
Endocrine dysfunction, including hypothyroidism and Addison disease
Chronic fatigue syndrome
Pulmonary disease, including asthma, emphysema, and Pickwickian syndrome
Cardiovascular disease, including congestive and left heart failure
Neoplasms, including disseminated and central nervous system lesions
Anticancer chemotherapy
Collagen vascular diseases
Chronic infections, including mononucleosis, hepatitis, and influenza
Depression and other psychiatric disorders
Malnutrition
Neurological disorders, including Parkinson disease and multiple sclerosis
Medication side effects

From Flint PW, Haughey BH, Lund VJ, et al. *Cummings Otolaryngology—Head and Neck Surgery.* 7th ed. Philadelphia, PA: Elsevier; 2021, Box 15.3.

Workup of Obstructive Sleep Apnea

- Loud nightly snoring
- Daytime sleepiness/fatigue (Table 9.4)
- Unrefreshing sleep
- History from bed partner (witnessed breathing pauses; gasps)
- Physical exam
  - Vital signs
  - Body mass index (BMI)
  - Head and neck exam
- Laboratory studies
  - Polysomnography
  - Cephalometric films
  - Oximetry
  - Thyroid and cardiac studies

Basic Sleep History

- Bedtimes
- Arousal times
- Awake times
- Body position during sleep
- Restless sleep
- Leg movements/kicking
- Alcohol or sedative use
- Caffeine intake
- Mouth breathing at night
- Menopause status

Common Physical Exam Findings of Obstructive Sleep Apnea (Table 9.5)

- Neck circumference (≥17 inches males, ≥15.5 inches females)
- Waste/hip ratio (≥0.9 male, ≥0.85 female)
- Cricomental distance (≥15 mm excludes OSA)
- Decreased maxillary and mandibular projection
- Low hanging hyoid
- Kyphosis
- Micro/retrognathia (Class II occlusion)
- Enlarged tonsils
- High arched palate
- Maxillary retrusion (Class III occlusion)
- Enlarged tongue (modified Mallampati III or IV)

TABLE 9.5 Physical Exam Findings of Obstructive Sleep Apnea

Nasal obstruction	• Septal deviation • Turbinate hypertrophy • Nasal valve collapse • Adenoid hypertrophy • Nasal tumors or polyps
Oropharyngeal obstruction	• Large soft palate • Palatine tonsillar hypertrophy • Posterior pharyngeal wall banding • Macroglossia • Large mandibular tori • Narrow skeletal arch
Hypopharyngeal obstruction	• Lateral pharyngeal wall collapse • Omega-shaped epiglottis • Hypopharyngeal tumor • Lingual tonsillar hypertrophy • Macroglossia • Retrognathia and micrognathia
Laryngeal obstruction	• True vocal cord paralysis • Laryngeal tumor
General neck obstruction	• Increased neck circumference • Redundant cervical adipose tissue
General body habitus	• Obesity • Achondroplasia • Chest wall deformity • Marfan syndrome
Cardiovascular signs	• Arterial hypertension, especially morning hypertension • Peripheral edema

From Flint PW, Haughey BH, Lund VJ, et al. *Cummings Otolaryngology—Head and Neck Surgery.* 7th ed. Philadelphia, PA: Elsevier; 2021, Box 15.4.

Tonsil Size Evaluation

- 1: 0% to 25% lateral narrowing of oropharynx (in tonsillar fossa)
- 2: 25% to 50% lateral narrowing of oropharynx (fills fossa)
- 3: 50% to 75% lateral narrowing of oropharynx (extends beyond fossa)
- 4+: >75% lateral narrowing of oropharynx (touching tonsils)

Evaluation of Maxillary Retrusion

- Frankfurt plane
- Line dropped from nasion to subnasale should be perpendicular to Frankfurt plane

Evaluation of Retrognathia

- Frankfurt plane
- Line bisecting vermillion border of the lower lip with pogonion should be perpendicular to Frankfurt plane

Mallampati Score (Fig. 9.2)

- Class I: Full view of uvula and tonsils
- Class II: Partial view of tonsils
- Class III: Soft palate edge but uvula not visible
- Class IV: Soft palate not visible

Obstructive Sleep Apnea Syndrome Diagnostic Tests

- Flexible nasopharyngolaryngoscopy
  - Evaluation of nasal, retropalatal, and retrolingual areas

- Drug-induced sleep endoscopy (DISE)
- Mueller maneuver
- Polysomnography
- Lateral cephalometric analysis
- Subjective sleep questionnaires

Drug-Induced Sleep Endoscopy

- Goal: Reproduce patterns of sleep-disordered breathing (SDB) during natural sleep
- Titrate to loss of consciousness, avoid oversedation (decreases muscle tone)
- VOTE classification (*v*elum, *o*ropharyngeal lateral walls, *t*ongue base, *e*piglottis) (Table 9.6)
  - Characterizes the directionality and severity of collapse at each subsite
  - Good intra-rater and inter-rater reliability

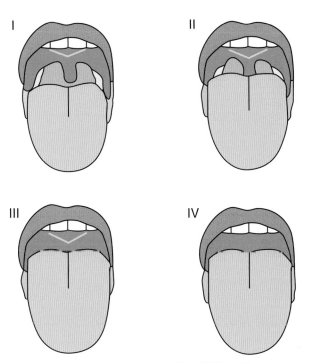

Fig. 9.2 Modified Mallampati palate position. (**I**) The entire uvula can be seen with the tongue at rest. (**II**) A partial view of the uvula is seen. (**III**) Only the soft and hard palate can be seen. (**IV**) Only the hard palate can be seen. (From Flint PW, Haughey BH, Lund VJ, et al. *Cummings Otolaryngology—Head and Neck Surgery.* 7th ed. Philadelphia, PA: Elsevier; 2021, Fig. 15.13.)

Mueller Maneuver

- Assessed in sitting or supine position while patient is awake and performing reverse Valsalva
- Assesses the degree of retropalatal and retrolingual collapse

Polysomnography Parameters

- Electroencephalogram (EEG)
- Electrooculum (EOG)
- Electromyogram (EMG)
- Electrocardiogram (EKG)
- Oronasal airflow
- Respiratory effort
- Oximetry
- Vital signs
- Snoring volume
  - Parameters that are tested depend on type of polysomnogram
    - Level I: Gold standard; minimum of seven different variables
      - Continuously attended by trained personnel
    - Level II: Same as level I but performed with a portable system setup at the patient's home
      - Unattended, no technician interventions
    - Level III: three variables, portable and unattended
      - Inadequate for diagnosis of OSA
    - Level IV: one variable, portable and unattended

Polysomnography Report (Fig. 9.3)

- Sleep latency
- Sleep efficiency
- Sleep architecture
- Types of respiratory disturbances/quantification
- Volume/presence of snoring
- Effect of position on respiratory airflow
- Effect of sleep stage on respiratory airflow
- Number/severity of the oxygen desaturation events $\geq 4\%$
- Percentage sleep time with O_2 saturation $<90\%$
- Lowest O_2 saturation level

Findings of Obstructive Sleep Apnea Syndrome on Cephalometric Imaging

- Retrognathia
- Narrowed posterior airway space (retropalatal; retroglossal)
- Increased mandibular plane to hyoid bone (low hyoid)
- Shortening of the anterior cranial base
- Elongated/thickened soft palate

TABLE 9.6 VOTE Classification for Drug-Induced Sleep Endoscopy Procedure

Structure	Degree of Obstruction	Configuration		
		Anteroposterior	**Lateral**	**Concentric**
Velum	0–2			
Oropharynx (lateral walls)	0–2	N/A		N/A
Tongue Base	0–2		N/A	N/A
Epiglottis	0–2			N/A

0–2 refers to degree of obstruction: 0, No obstruction; 1, partial obstruction; 2, complete obstruction.

N/A refers to configuration that cannot be seen for specific structure.

Adapted from Kezirian EJ, Hohenhorst W, de Vries N. Drug-induced sleep endoscopy: the VOTE classification. *Eur Arch Otorhinolaryngol.* 2011;268(8):1233–1236.

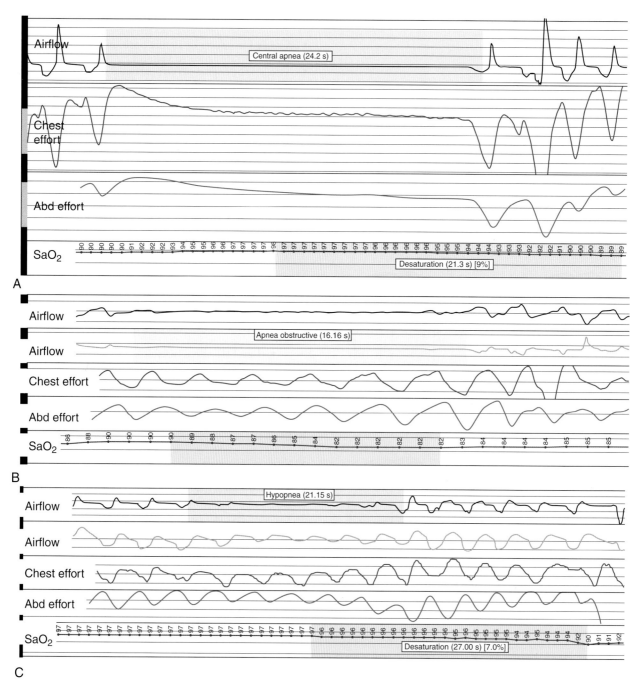

Fig. 9.3 Polysomnographic tracing of a central apnea. (**A**), obstructive apnea (**B**), and hypopnea (**C**), *Abd*, Abdominal. (From Flint PW, Haughey BH, Lund VJ, et al. *Cummings Otolaryngology—Head and Neck Surgery.* 7th ed. Philadelphia, PA: Elsevier; 2021, Fig. 15.11.)

Subjective Sleep Questionnaires

- Epworth Sleepiness Scale
- Stanford Sleepiness Scale
- Pittsburgh Sleep Quality Index

Management Sequence of Obstructive Sleep Apnea

- Can be personalized based on individual and primary source of obstruction
- Behavioral (weight loss; limit alcohol, tobacco, caffeine, and sedatives)
- Medical management (nasal blockage, reflux)

- Continuous positive airway pressure (CPAP)/bilevel positive airway pressure (BiPAP)
  - CPAP is first-line therapy for adults with moderate or severe OSA
- Oral or nasal appliances
- Mandibular repositioning
- Surgery

CPAP Compliance

- Defined as 4 hours/night for at least 5 nights a week
- Most common reason for inability to tolerate: Oral and nasal dryness

Increase CPAP Patient Compliance

- Discuss with patient beneficial effects of CPAP—has been shown to be biggest influencer of compliance
- Add humidity
- Treat nasal congestion/obstruction
- Desensitization
- Reassess mask
- Chin-strap for mouth leak
- Pressure reduction

BiPAP Indications

- Pressure support for obesity-hypoventilatory patients
- COPD
- Hypoxemic patients
- Respiratory muscle weakness
- Neurological dysfunction
- Poor CPAP compliance due to high PAP pressure ($\geq$16 cm H_2O)

CPAP/BiPAP Contraindications

- No respiratory drive
- Risk of aspiration
- Hypotension
- CSF leak
- Bullous lung disease
- Pneumocephalus
- Pneumothorax
- History of transnasal skull base surgery

Indications for Obstructive Sleep Apnea Surgery

- Loud snoring
- Poor sleep quality
- Daytime sleepiness
- Failed CPAP after 3- to 6-month trial
- Identifiable anatomical site amenable to surgical therapy

Relative Contraindications for Obstructive Sleep Apnea Surgery

- Severe obesity (BMI $\geq$40)
- Cardiopulmonary disease
- Substance abuse
- Bleeding disorder

Anatomical Locations of Surgery for Obstructive Sleep Apnea

- Nasal
- Oropharyngeal
- Hypopharyngeal
- Mandibular and midface advancement
- Tracheostomy

Nasal Surgery

- Septoplasty
- Turbinate reduction
- Polypectomy
- Nasal valve reconstruction
- Functional rhinoplasty

Oral Cavity and Oropharyngeal Surgery

- Adenotonsillectomy
- Palatal stiffening with enlargement of retropalatal space (Fig. 9.4)
- Expansion sphincter pharyngoplasty

- Partial midline glossectomy
  - Can be combined with lingualplasty, in which additional tongue tissue is removed posteriorly and laterally to the portion excised in midline glossectomy
- Tongue base reduction (radiofrequency; coblation; robotic)
  - Reduction of tongue base tissue through scar generation
- Uvulopalatopharyngoplasty (UPPP): Although most commonly performed surgical procedure for OSA, often misused as first-line surgical therapy

Steps of Uvulopalatopharyngoplasty (Fig. 9.5)

1. Remove tonsils if present
2. Incision made through anterior pillar to square edge of soft palate
3. Uvula removed and debulked at its base
4. Posterior tonsillar pillar as a flap is rotated anteriorly and sutured to the anterior pillar
5. Dorsal soft palate mucosa is advanced and sutured to the ventral mucosa, closing the uvula/soft palate incision

Hypopharyngeal Surgery

Goal: Enlarge retrolingual airway by fixing major dilators of the pharynx forward without altering dental occlusion
- Lingual tonsillectomy
- Genioglossal advancement (Fig. 9.6)
- Genioglossal suspension
- Hyoid myotomy and suspension (Fig. 9.7)
- Epiglottoplasty

Mandibular and Midface Advancement (Fig. 9.8)

- Increases the retropalatal and retrolingual airway
- Maxilla and mandible are advanced by Le Fort I maxillary and sagittal-split mandibular osteotomies

Hypoglossal Nerve Stimulation

- Implantable, pacemaker-like pulse generator with sensing lead and stimulator leads to improve neuromuscular tone of the pharynx during sleep and improve inspiratory airflow
  - Sensing lead placed between the internal and external intercostal muscles to detect respiratory effort
    - Detects inspiratory effort and coordinates electrical stimulation of hypoglossal nerve to be timed with inspiration
  - Stimulator lead implanted submentally on the hypoglossal nerve to stimulate tongue protrusion and minimize tongue retraction
    - Branches to include: Vertical and transverse intrinsic muscles, oblique and horizontal genioglossus branches
    - Branches to exclude: Styloglossus, hyoglossus
    - Neurostimulator device implanted in the right ipsilateral mid-infraclavicular region
- Indications:
  - CPAP intolerant (failed trial of CPAP)
  - BMI <32
  - Moderate to severe OSA (AHI 15–65)
    - Contraindications:
  - Circumferential concentric palatal collapse on preoperative DISE evaluation
  - Sleep apnea due to central apneas

Emergencies of Surgical Treatment of Sleep Apnea

- Intraoperative
  - Preoperative sedation resulting in airway obstruction

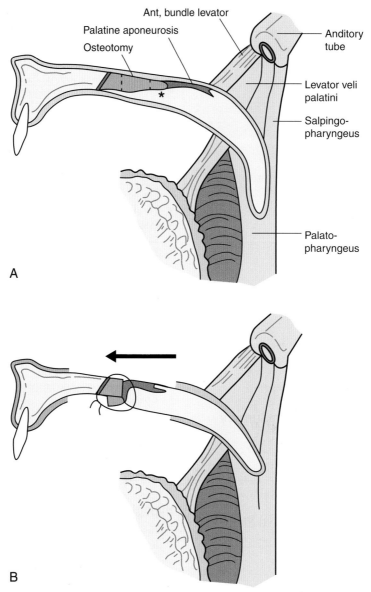

Fig. 9.4 Palatal advancement. (**A**) Drill holes are placed from the oral cavity to the nose and are anterior to bone removal (*orange*). The anterior extent of the middle flap is placed in the thinner palatal mucosa. Mucosa is thicker posteriorly. (**B**) After osteotomy, sutures are placed through the drill holes, and the bone fragment with attached tendon and ligaments is advanced. (From Woodson, BT, Robinson S, Lim HJ. Transpalatal advancement pharyngoplasty outcomes compared with uvulopalatopharygoplasty. *Otolaryngol Head Neck Surg.* 2005;133(2):211–217.)

- Inability to intubate with airway obstruction (consider awake fiberoptic)
- Premature extubation with airway obstruction (prevent with patient sitting up following commands)
- Postoperative
  - Airway obstruction due to oversedation
  - Postoperative pulmonary edema
  - Postoperative bleeding
  - Postoperative subcutaneous emphysema, pneumomediastinum, pneumothorax

Sleep Apnea in Children Pathogenesis

- Adenotonsillar hypertrophy
- Poor muscle tone
- Upper airway narrowing

Sleep Apnea in Children Signs and Symptoms

- Snoring
- Choking, gasping
- Restless sleep
- Witnessed apneas
- Enuresis
- Nonspecific findings: Chronic mouth breathing, hyponasality, dysphagia, halitosis, aggression, hyperactivity, learning disabilities

Sleep Apnea in Children Evaluation

- Physical exam
  - Nasal cavity: Masses, choanal stenosis/atresia, enlarged turbinates
  - Nasopharynx: Adenoid hypertrophy

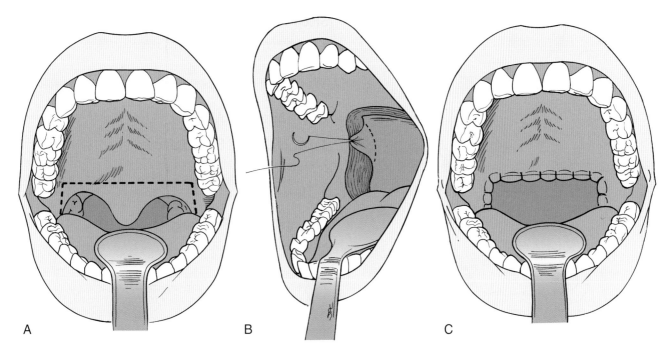

Fig. 9.5 Uvulopalatopharyngoplasty. (A) The incision along the anterior pillar meets the horizontal incision through the palate at approximately a 90-degree angle. **(B)** The mucosa of the posterior tonsillar pillar is advanced and sutured to the anterior pillar employing long-lasting absorbable sutures. The free edge of the soft palate is closed on itself employing long-lasting absorbable sutures. **(C)** The final result is a wide opening into the oropharynx. (Modified from Kent D, Schell A. Uvulopalatopharyngoplasty and related modifications (Traditional Uvulopalatopharyngoplasty, Uvulopalatal Flap, Anterior Palatoplasty). In: Myers E, Snyderman C, eds. *Operative Otolaryngology Head and Neck.* 3rd ed. Philadelphia, PA: Elsevier. 2018.)

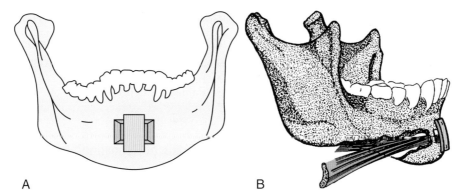

Fig. 9.6 Genioglossal advancement procedure: rectangular geniotubercle osteotomy modification. **(A)** Anterior view. The rectangular geniotubercle osteotomy modification provides tension on the genioglossus muscle with a minimal fracture risk. The geniotubercle fragment is rotated enough to allow bony overlap. A single inferiorly placed miniscrew is used to fix the fragment. **(B)** Lateral view. (From Sarber KM, Lam DJ, Ishman SE. Chapter 15: Sleep apnea and sleep disorders. In: *Cummings Otolaryngology: Head and Neck Surgery.* 7th ed. Elsevier. 2021, 215–235.)

- • Oral cavity: Macroglossia
- • Oropharynx: Obstructing tonsils
- Polysomnography (depends on particular guidelines)
- Other: Sleep questionnaires, nighttime recordings, sleep somnography (no strong data)

Categories of Obstructive Sleep Apnea Based on Apnea Hypopnea Index

Pediatrics:
- Mild (1–5 events/hour)
- Moderate (5–10 events/hour)
- Severe (>10 events/hour)

Sleep Apnea in Children Complications

- Cardiopulmonary complications
- Failure to thrive
- Poor growth
- Learning disabilities

Sleep Apnea in Children Nonsurgical Treatment

- CPAP in patients with contraindications to surgery
- Weight loss
- Treatment of other medical conditions: Nasal obstruction, asthma, reflux

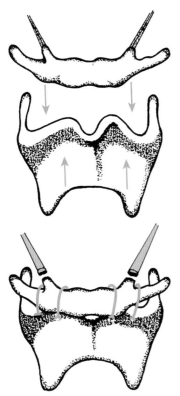

Fig. 9.7 Modified hyoid myotomy and suspension procedure. (From Sarber KM, Lam DJ, Ishman SE. Chapter 15: Sleep apnea and sleep disorders. In: *Cummings Otolaryngology: Head and Neck Surgery.* 7th ed. Elsevier. 2021, 215–235.)

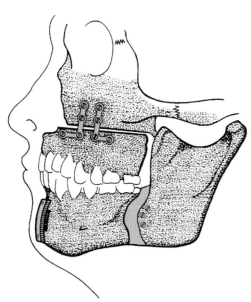

Fig. 9.8 Maxillomandibular advancement procedure. Le Fort I maxillary osteotomy with rigid plate fixation and a bilateral sagittal split mandibular osteotomy with bicortical screw fixation. The advancement is at least 10 mm. A previous genioglossal advancement is shown. (From Powell NB, Riley RW, Guilleminault C. The hypopharynx: upper airway reconstruction in obstructive sleep apnea syndrome. In: Fairbanks DNF, Fujita A, eds: *Snoring and Obstructive Sleep Apnea.* 2nd ed. New York: Raven Press; 1994, Fig. ***.)

Sleep Apnea in Children Surgical Treatment

- Adenotonsillectomy: Primary treatment for pediatric OSA as CPAP is poorly tolerated
- Less common: UPPP, upper airway radiofrequency ablation, tongue reduction, osteotomies and advancements, tracheostomy

CENTRAL SLEEP APNEA

Types of Central Sleep Apnea

- Primary CSA
- Cheyne-Stokes breathing
- High altitude CSA

Cheyne-Stokes Breathing

- Three cycles of crescendo and decrescendo breathing amplitude *and*
- Lasts 10 minutes *or*
- Associated with 5 or more central apnea or hypopneas
- Associated with heart failure (prolonged circulatory time)

Treatment of Central Sleep Apnea

- Treat underlying disorder
- CPAP
- Servo ventilator
- Triazolam
- Respiratory stimulants
- Nasal oxygen

OBESITY HYPOVENTILATION SYNDROME

Causes of Hypoventilation Syndrome

- Obesity
- Interstitial lung disease
- Pulmonary hypertension
- Sickle cell anemia
- Myxedema

Diagnosis of Hypoventilation Syndrome

- Pulmonary function tests (PFTs)
- Pulmonary artery catheterization
- Echocardiogram

Treatment of Hypoventilation Syndrome

- Treat underlying cause
- BiPAP
- Tracheotomy with nocturnal ventilation
- Weight loss

CENTRAL DISORDERS OF HYPERSOMNOLENCE

- Narcolepsy
- Idiopathic hypersomnia
- Kleine-Levin syndrome

Narcolepsy Features (Fig. 9.9)

- Excessive sleepiness, cataplexy, sleep paralysis
- Hypnagogic (imagined sensations that appear real while falling asleep) and hypnopompic (imagined sensations that appear real while awaking) hallucinations

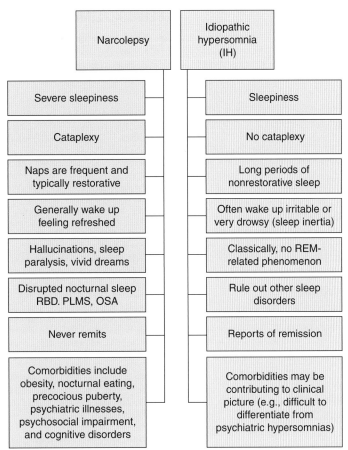

Fig. 9.9 Comparison of narcolepsy and idiopathic hypersomnia. Narcolepsy is described as a "pentad" of symptoms, including sleepiness, cataplexy, sleep paralysis, hallucinations, and disrupted nocturnal sleep. (From Kryger MH. *Atlas of Clinical Sleep Medicine.* 2nd ed. Philadelphia, PA: Elsevier. 2013.)

Kleine-Levin Syndrome Features

- Recurrent episodes of hypersomnia lasting 18 to 20 hours
  - When not sleeping, often irritable, hypersexual, aggressive
- Most commonly adolescent males

CIRCADIAN RHYTHM SLEEP–WAKE DISORDERS

- Delayed sleep phase disorder
- Advanced sleep phase disorder
- Shift work disorder

Delayed Sleep Phase Disorders

Parasomnias

Irregular actions executed during the sleep process

Non–Rapid Eye Movement Sleep

- Sleep terrors
- Somnambulism (sleepwalking)
- Confusional arousal

Rapid Eye Movement Sleep

- Nightmares
- Sleep paralysis
- REM sleep behavior disorder

Other (Not Associated With a Sleep State)

- Somniloquy (sleep talking)
- Bruxism
- Nocturnal enuresis
- Rhythmic movement disorders

REM SLEEP BEHAVIOR DISORDER

- Loss of atonia during REM sleep (movement on EMG)
  - Complex motor activity, patient acts out dreams
- Predisposing factors:
  - Male sex
  - Age >50 years old
  - Underlying neurological disease (~50% of patients have a subsequent neurodegenerative disease)
    - Parkinson disease
    - Lewy body dementia
    - Multisystem atrophy
    - Stroke

Sleep-Related Bruxism

- Sustained or phasic
- Elevation of chin EMG for >2 seconds
- Measured in masseter muscle

SLEEP-RELATED MOVEMENT DISORDERS

- Restless legs syndrome
- Periodic limb movement disorder

- Rhythmic movement disorder
- Nocturnal leg cramps

RESTLESS LEGS SYNDROME

Restless Leg Diagnosis

- Clinical diagnosis (URGE): **U**rge to move legs; **R**est makes it worse; **G**ets better with activity; **E**vening and nighttime symptoms
- Labs: Serum ferritin (low), renal function, glucose, anemia, thyroid, B_{12}, Mg, antinuclear antibody test (ANA), rheumatoid factor (RF)
- Cerebrospinal fluid (CSF) transferrin levels (low)

Restless Legs Syndrome Risk Factors

- Women and older persons
- Family history
- *BTBD9* gene

Types of Restless Legs Syndrome

- Primary: Onset in youth, familial
- Secondary: Iron deficiency (central iron deficiency causing dopamine depletion), renal failure, pregnancy, peripheral neuropathy (diabetes), medications
- Idiopathic

Medications Causing Restless Leg Syndrome

- Selective serotonin reuptake inhibitors (SSRI)
- Serotonin and norepinephrine reuptake inhibitors (SNRI)
- Tricyclic antidepressants (TCAs)
- Lithium
- Antihistamines
- Antipsychotics
- Antiemetics
- Dopamine antagonists

Treatment of Restless Legs Syndrome

- Address secondary causes
- Behavior modification
- Dopamine agonists (ropinirole; pramipexole)

PERIODIC LIMB MOVEMENT DISORDER

- Limb movement disorders
  - Similar to RLS; distinguished by strong desire to move but do not experience tingling or burning of legs
  - Common in patients with OSA

FURTHER READINGS

Bailey BJ, Johnson JT, Newlands SD. *Head & Neck Surgery—Otolaryngology*. 4th ed. Philadelphia, PA: Lippincott Williams & Wilkins; 2006.

Goldstein NA. Evaluation and management of pediatric sleep apnea. In: Flint PW, Haughey BH, Lund VJ, eds. *Cummings Otolaryngology—Head and Neck Surgery*. 7th ed. Philadelphia, PA Elsevier; 2021.

Kryger MH, Roth T, Dement WC. *Principles and Practice of Sleep Medicine*. 6th ed. Philadelphia, PA: Elsevier; 2016.

Lalwani AK. *Current Diagnosis & Treatment: Otolaryngology Head and Neck Surgery*. Lange; 2008.

Lee KJ. *Essential Otolaryngology: Head & Neck Surgery*. McGraw Hill; 2008.

Pang KE, Rotenberg B, Woodson T. *Advanced Surgical Techniques in Snoring and Obstructive Sleep Apnea*. Plural Publishing; 2013.

Pasha R. *Otolaryngology—Head and Neck Surgery Clinical Reference Guide*. San Diego, CA: Plural Publishing; 2011.

Pierce B, Brietzke SE. Non-obstructive pediatric sleep disorders. In: Flint PW, Haughey BH, Lund VJ, eds. *Cummings Otolaryngology—Head and Neck Surgery*. 7th ed. Philadelphia, PA: Elsevier; 2021.

Sarber KM, Lam DJ, Ishman SL. Sleep apnea and sleep disorders. In: Flint PW, Haughey BH, Lund VJ, eds, et al. *Cummings Otolaryngology—Head and Neck Surgery*. 7th ed. Philadelphia, PA: Elsevier; 2021.

Strollo PJ, Soose RJ, Maurer JT, et al. Upper-airway stimulation for obstructive sleep apnea. *N Engl J Med*. 2014;370(2): 139–149.

Wakefield TL, Lam DJ, Ishman SL. Sleep apnea and sleep disorders. In: Flint PW, Haughey BH, Lund VJ, eds, et al. *Cummings Otolaryngology—Head and Neck Surgery*. 6th ed. Philadelphia, PA: Elsevier; 2014.

Westerman DE. *The Concise Sleep Medicine Handbook*. GSSD Publishers; 2011.

Wetmore RF. *The Requisites in Pediatrics: Pediatric Otolaryngology*. Philadelphia, PA: Elsevier; 2007.

10 Oral and Maxillofacial Surgery

Ryan J. Smart, Srinivas M. Susarla, and Corbett A. Haas

DENTAL TERMINOLOGY

- Incisal: Refers to the biting surface of an anterior tooth (incisor and canine)
- Occlusal: Refers to the biting surface of a posterior tooth (premolar and molar)
- Apical: Toward the root tip
- Mesial: Toward the midline
- Distal: Away from the midline
- Lingual: Toward the tongue (mandibular teeth)
- Palatal: Toward the palate (maxillary teeth)
- Buccal: Toward the cheek
- Labial: Toward the lip
- Crown: Portion of the tooth covered by enamel (anatomical) or visible within the oral cavity (clinical)
- Root: Portion of the tooth covered by cementum

PEDIATRIC DENTITION

- Primary dentition (baby teeth)
- 2 incisors, 1 canine, and 2 molars in each quadrant (20 teeth total)
- No premolars
- Teeth are referenced by letter (A–T)
- Right maxillary second molar (A) → left maxillary second molar (J)
- Left mandibular second molar (K) → right mandibular second molar (T)
- Primary teeth begin to erupt around 8 months of age, with completion of the primary eruption sequence by 24 months of age

ADULT DENTITION

- Succedaneous (permanent) dentition
- 2 incisors, 1 canine, 2 premolars, and 3 molars in each quadrant (32 teeth total)
- Teeth are referenced by number (1–32)
- Right maxillary third molar (1) → left maxillary third molar (16)
- Left mandibular third molar (17) → right mandibular third molar (32)
- General ages for eruption:
  - Incisors, 6 to 9 years
  - Canines, 9 to 11 years
  - Premolars, 10 to 12 years (first) and 11 to 12 years (second)
  - Molars, 6 to 7 years (first), 11 to 13 years (second), and 17 to 20 years (third)

DENTOALVEOLAR SURGERY

Exodontia

- Understanding cross-sectional anatomy and bone density surrounding relevant tooth is of paramount importance to success
- Teeth with short, single roots, tapered toward apex and circular cross-section (maxillary central incisors, maxillary lateral incisors, mandibular premolars) can be rotated and removed easily with gentle elevation and forceps extraction

- Multi-rooted teeth, diverging roots, elongated roots, bulbous roots or teeth with dilacerated roots can be more challenging, often requiring sectioning of teeth and removal of adjacent bone
- Maxillary bone is less dense and bends in response to extraction forces, usually leaving surrounding bone intact; mandibular bone is more dense and less deforming, rendering tooth more likely to break with excessive, ill-directed forces.

Preprosthetic Surgery

- Irregular bony growths (mandibular tori, palatal tori, exostoses) and abnormally contoured alveolus require surgical correction prior to ability to wear dentures; most often done at the time of extraction of remaining teeth

Dental Implants

- Discovery of osseointegration has revolutionized the ability to replace missing teeth
- Implants can replace single missing teeth or entire arches of missing teeth
- Special attention must be paid to location of inferior alveolar nerve as well as maxillary sinus
- Bone grafting may be required to prepare site ready to receive an implant
- Zygomatic implants are available when inadequate maxillary bone present

OCCLUSION

- Overbite: Vertical overlap between incisors (normal, ~2 mm)
- Overjet: Horizontal overlap between incisors (normal, ~2 mm)
- Crossbite: Malpositioning of teeth in the horizontal plane, such that the mandibular anterior teeth are anterior to the maxillary anteriors (i.e., negative overjet) or the mandibular posterior teeth are buccal to the maxillary posterior teeth
- Open bite: Malpositioning of the teeth in the vertical plane, most commonly manifests as a gap between the incisal edges of the maxillary anterior teeth and the mandibular anterior teeth (negative overbite)
- Retrognathia: Retruded jaw position (most commonly used in reference to mandibular position)
- Prognathia: Protruded jaw position (most commonly used in reference to the mandible)
- Centric relation: Position of the mandible when the condyles are seated within the glenoid fossa in the most anterior-superior position
- Centric occlusion: Occlusion achieved with the mandibular condyles in centric relation
- Maximal intercuspal position: Best fit of teeth, independent of condylar position. May or may not coincide with centric occlusion
- Based on the relationship between the mesiobuccal cusp of the maxillary first molar to the buccal groove of the mandibular first molar

- Normal occlusion: Mesiobuccal cusp occludes with the groove, and there is a smooth arc of curvature along the dental arch, without malpositioned or rotated teeth
- Considered a malocclusion when teeth are malpositioned or rotated

MALOCCLUSION CLASSES

- Class I: The mesiobuccal cusp occludes with the mesiobuccal groove
- Class II: The mesiobuccal cusp is mesial (anterior) to the mesiobuccal groove
  - Division I: Normal incisal angulation (usually has an excessive overjet)
  - Division II: Incisors retroclined ("deep bite"—usually has a less excessive overjet and an excessive overbite)
- Class III: The mesiobuccal cusp is distal (posterior) to the mesiobuccal groove

DENTOFACIAL DEFORMITIES

- An integrated orthodontic-surgical approach is required
- Communication (patient–orthodontist–surgeon) is critical
- Characterized by the skeletal relationship between the maxilla and mandible
- Orthodontics cannot correct facial disharmony related to skeletal discrepancies but can camouflage the effects of skeletal disharmony on occlusion
- Skeletal malocclusions require skeletal correction
- Dental compensations occur naturally, may mask skeletal discrepancies, and should be addressed before surgical correction (i.e., the teeth should be decompensated before surgical correction)

SURGICAL EVALUATION OF DENTOFACIAL DEFORMITIES

- Assess pathological/etiological factors (obstructive sleep apnea, craniofacial anomalies, clefts, and maxillofacial trauma)
- Growth: Surgical correction is typically delayed until completion of skeletal growth (girls, 2–3 years after menarche; boys, ages 16–18). Completion of growth may be assessed by serial radiographic examination (e.g., hand–wrist radiographs)
- Identify the sagittal relationship between the maxilla and mandible (excessive or negative overjet, class I, class II, or class III skeletal profile)
- Identify vertical discrepancies (e.g., excessive overbite, open bite, deep bite, and gummy smile)
- Identify transverse discrepancies (crossbite and occlusal cant)

CEPHALOMETRIC EVALUATION OF DENTOFACIAL DEFORMITIES

- Allows for standardized assessment of the relationship between the skull base, maxilla, and mandible
- Establishes the anatomical basis for deformity
- For diagnostic purposes—does not dictate the type or magnitude of surgical movement (i.e., do not treat the numbers, treat the patient)
- Due to inherent limitations with two-dimensional (2D) cephalometry (image distortion, interuser variability, difficulty identifying landmarks over superimposed structures), three-dimensional (3D) cephalometric analysis is becoming more prevalent, allowing for increased attention for correction in all three planes as well as providing ability to fabricate custom hardware

AESTHETIC EVALUATION OF DENTOFACIAL DEFORMITIES

- Surgical decisions based on aesthetics (e.g., it may be better to correct a skeletal class III deformity in a male with a Le Fort I osteotomy rather than a mandibular setback to preserve a strong chin, whereas the opposite may be true in a female)
- Clinical evaluation of frontal repose and profile
- Evaluate the upper, middle, and lower facial thirds in both the horizontal and vertical planes
- Balance of proportions is the key
- Consider adjunctive treatments to obtain ideal balance, either in conjunction with orthognathic surgery or following correction of skeletal malocclusion (e.g., malar alloplastic augmentation and rhinoplasty)

COMMON DENTOFACIAL DEFORMITY DIAGNOSES

- Maxillary hypoplasia
- Maxillary hyperplasia
- Mandibular hypoplasia
- Mandibular hyperplasia
- Combination

Maxillary Hypoplasia

- May occur in the sagittal, vertical, or transverse planes
- Seen as a secondary deformity in patients with cleft lip/cleft palate
- Manifests as a concave facial profile, deficient infraorbital/perinasal regions, poor tooth show at rest/smiling, short lower facial third, deficient upper lip, and anterior or posterior crossbite
- Primary treatment is Le Fort I osteotomy
- Segmental (e.g., two- or three-piece) Le Fort I osteotomies may be performed for complex deformities
- Bone grafting may be required depending on the magnitude and direction of movement

Maxillary Excess

- Most commonly occurs in the vertical plane
- Vertical maxillary excess characterized by elongated lower facial third, narrow alar base, excessive tooth/gingival show, lip incompetence, and often with a convex facial profile
- May be associated with anterior open bite (apertognathia)
- Surgical treatment is Le Fort I osteotomy, with segmental osteotomies and bone grafting as needed

Mandibular Hypoplasia

- Class II molar/canine relationship with excessive overjet
- Manifest as a convex facial profile, retruded chin, acute labiomental fold, abnormal lip posturing, and short thyromental distance
- May be associated with syndromes/other pathology (Marfan, Pierre Robin, craniofacial microsomia, Treacher Collins, Nager, and obstructive sleep apnea)
- Primary treatment is bilateral sagittal split osteotomy (BSSO)

Mandibular Hyperplasia

- Class III molar/canine relationship with negative overjet
- Prominent lower facial third, protrusive chin, and a concave facial profile
- Surgical correction can include either Le Fort I osteotomy for advancement, BSSO for mandibular setback, or a combination of both

- Intraoral vertical ramus osteotomies of the mandible may also be used for mandibular setback but require maxillomandibular fixation

STABILITY OF ORTHOGNATHIC CORRECTION

- Relapse may occur; patients should be counseled about this
- Most important contributing factors: Jaw being moved (maxilla vs. mandible), magnitude of movement, and direction of movement
- Orthodontic factors: Inadequate decompensation, inadequate alignment of dental arches, and presurgical correction of surgical problem (e.g., transverse discrepancy)
- Surgical factors: Inaccurate condylar positioning, inadequate fixation, and condylar resorption

INNERVATION OF TEETH/GINGIVA

- Maxillary anterior teeth: Anterior-superior alveolar nerve (labial gingiva and pulp) and nasopalatine nerve (palatal gingiva)
- Maxillary premolars: Middle superior alveolar nerve (buccal gingiva and pulp) and greater palatine nerve (palatal gingiva)
- Maxillary molars: Posterior-superior alveolar nerve (buccal gingiva and pulp) and greater palatine nerve (palatal gingiva)
- Mandibular anterior teeth: Incisive nerve (labial gingiva and pulp) and lingual nerve (lingual gingiva)
- Mandibular premolars: Inferior alveolar nerve (buccal gingiva and pulp) and lingual nerve (lingual gingiva)
- Mandibular molars: Inferior alveolar nerve (pulp ± buccal gingiva), long buccal nerve (buccal gingiva), and lingual nerve (lingual gingiva)

DENTAL ANESTHESIA

- Nerve blocks are very effective for anesthetizing individual teeth or portions of the oral cavity for procedures (e.g., biopsies, tooth extraction, and arch bar placement)
- Infraorbital block: Local anesthetic deposited at the infraorbital foramen (located 5–7 mm below the inferior orbital rim, in line with the medial limbus)
- Nasopalatine block: Local anesthetic deposited at the foramen (5–7 mm posterior to the maxillary dental midline)
- Greater palatine block: Local anesthetic deposited halfway between the maxillary second molar and palatal midline (Fig. 10.1)
- Posterior-superior alveolar block: Local anesthetic deposited into the alveolar mucosa immediately above maxillary second molar, with needle oriented at a 45-degree angle to bone
- Inferior alveolar block: Local anesthetic deposited adjacent to the medial aspect of the mandibular ramus; enters the mucosa medial to the ramus, ~1 cm superior to the mandibular occlusal plane, with the needle at 45 degrees relative to the ramus
- Long buccal block: The needle is inserted into the retromolar buccal mucosa along the ascending ramus, at the level of the mandibular occlusal plane
- Maxillary anterior teeth: Infraorbital and nasopalatine blocks
- Maxillary premolars: Infraorbital and greater palatine blocks
- Maxillary molars: Posterior-superior alveolar and greater palatine blocks
- Mandibular anterior teeth: Inferior alveolar block
- Mandibular premolars: Inferior alveolar block
- Mandibular molars: Inferior alveolar block and long buccal block

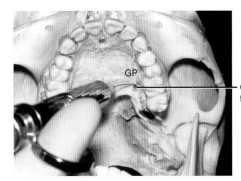

Fig. 10.1 Placement of the needle in greater palatine (GP) foramen for a greater palatine nerve lock. (From Liebgott B. The Anatomical Basis of Dentistry; 2011 Applied Anatomy. Wiley-Blackwell; 2011. ISBN-10: 0813820833. ISBN-13: 978-0813820837.)

ODONTOGENIC INFECTIONS

- May be localized or may involve one or more fascial spaces
- Mortality is most often related to airway compromise: Airway, breathing, and circulation (ABCs) first
- Polymicrobial infections (aerobic/anaerobic Gram-positive cocci and anaerobic Gram-negative rods [GNRs])
- Greater than 50% of infections are mixed aerobic/anaerobic
- Important pathogens: *Streptococcus*, *Peptostreptococcus*, *Fusobacterium*, *Prevotella*, and *Porphyromonas*
- Empiric treatment should include anaerobic coverage
- Pathogenesis: Occurs either from uncontrolled dental caries → pulpal necrosis → periapical infection that spreads into the alveolar bone or a deep periodontal pocket → periodontal infection
- Periapical infections are the most common sources
- Clinical manifestation of infection is dependent on muscle attachments (e.g., buccinator and mylohyoid)
  - Maxillary alveolar infections that erode the bone below the buccinator attachment will present with intraoral mucosal swelling (maxillary vestibular infection); those that erode above the buccinator attachment will present as infraorbital swelling
  - Mandibular alveolar infections involving the molars will often present with submandibular swelling because the roots of the molars are below the insertion of the mylohyoid; alveolar infections of the premolars and anterior teeth may present with sublingual swelling because the roots are above the mylohyoid

Treatment of Odontogenic Infections

1. ABCs first (always)—be prepared to secure emergency surgical airway as often as needed
2. Determine severity of infection
   - Fever, tachycardia, tachypnea, and hypotension
   - Trismus, dysphonia, dysphagia, inability to control secretions, and respiratory distress
   - Identify potential high-risk space involvement
3. Assess host defenses
   - Immunocompromised (steroids/chemotherapy, human immunodeficiency virus infection, diabetes, substance abuse, and malnutrition)
4. Provide surgical drainage and source control
   - Incision and drainage of all affected spaces
   - The source of the infection must be treated (i.e., tooth extraction)
5. Antibiotic treatment
   - Drainage and source control are the primary treatment
   - All infections should be cultured

- Antibiotic treatment begins empirically with penicillin or clindamycin (if penicillin allergic)
- Severe infections may necessitate additional antibiotics (e.g., piperacillin/tazobactam and metronidazole) for broader Gram-negative or anaerobic coverage
- Antibiotic therapy tailored to culture results

TEMPOROMANDIBULAR JOINT DISORDERS

1. Myofascial pain
2. Internal derangement of temporomandibular joint (TMJ)
3. Osteoarthritis
4. Rheumatoid arthritis
5. Infectious arthritis
6. Traumatic arthritis
7. TMJ ankylosis
8. Condylar hyperplasia
9. Condylar hypoplasia
10. Mandibular dislocation
11. Idiopathic condylar resorption

Myofascial Pain

- History/exam: Intermittent pain that is dull, aching, and usually unilateral; limited mouth opening, associated with headaches/earaches; tenderness to muscles of mastication; and pain that increases with function or stress
- Diagnosis: Clinical exam, panoramic radiograph to rule out condylar/mandibular pathology, reproducible "trigger points" along musculature (masseter, anterior temporalis, medial pterygoid, sternocleidomastoid)
- Treatment
  - Phase 1: Soft diet, intermittent moist heat, nonsteroidal antiinflammatory drugs (NSAIDs), and muscle relaxation; symptoms should improve within 1 month of treatment
  - Phase 2: If not better after 1 month of phase 1, bite appliance and occlusal equilibration; should improve within 1 month of treatment
  - Phase 3: Physical and relaxation therapy
  - Phase 4: Stress reduction and psychotherapy ± pain management (about 10% of patients will not respond to escalation of therapy through phase III)
  - Common etiology includes parafunctional habits (grinding, clenching, bruxism); if reported history or strong suspicion of these habits, occlusal guard and/or botulinum toxin injections can be initiated in early-phase treatment

Internal Derangement of the Temporomandibular Joint

- History/exam: Traumatic injury, parafunctional habits (tooth grinding and clenching), joint pain, joint clicking/popping/locking, and limited mouth opening
- Diagnosis: Clinical exam, panoramic radiograph or maxillofacial computed tomography (CT) to rule out condylar/mandibular pathology, magnetic resonance imaging (MRI) of the TMJ to assess articular disc positioning (static and dynamic), and arthroscopy
  - Wilkes classification:
    - I. Painless clicking, slightly forward disc that reduces on opening, and the joint contour appears normal on radiograph
    - II. Occasional painful clicking/headache, early disc deformity, and forward position
    - III. Frequent pain, joint tenderness, headache, locking, restricted motion, anterior disc, early reducing disc progresses to nonreducing, disc thickened, fibrillations, and no bone changes

- IV. Chronic pain, headache, restricted motion, nonreducing disc, and bony changes, including degeneration, osteophyte, and adhesions, but no disc perforation
- V. Variable pain, joint crepitus, painful function, anterior disc displacement, perforated disc, adhesions, and multiple degenerative changes
- Treatment
  - Clicking or popping: NSAIDs, soft diet, jaw rest, and bite appliance; consider surgical intervention (arthrocentesis, disc-plasty, or discectomy) if conservative measures fail
  - Locking: Anterior disc displacement without reduction (arthrocentesis, arthroscopic surgery, or disc-plasty); disc adhesion to articular eminence → arthrocentesis

Osteoarthritis of the Temporomandibular Joint

- History/exam: Jaw trauma, constant aching pain that increases with function, parafunctional habits, decreased mouth opening, TMJ tenderness, and joint crepitus
- Diagnosis: Clinical exam, panoramic radiograph or maxillofacial CT to assess for condylar changes (subcondylar sclerosis, condylar flattening, condylar erosion, and osteophyte formation); consider bone scan to assess for active disease process within condyles; rule out rheumatoid arthritis
- Treatment:
  - Primary: NSAIDs, soft diet, limit jaw function, bite appliance, and establish a stable occlusion
  - If no improvement after 6 months of primary treatment → TMJ arthroplasty

Rheumatoid Arthritis of the Temporomandibular Joint

- History/exam: Bilateral TMJ swelling/tenderness, dull/aching pain, TMJ stiffness—worse in the morning, limited mouth opening, history of rheumatoid disease, and anterior open bite/condylar, or retrognathia in severe cases
- Prevalent in pediatric population (juvenile idiopathic arthritis); often unilateral and can present in TMJ only; dentofacial deformity or significant asymmetry can develop as a result
- Diagnosis: Panoramic radiograph, CT scan, MRI, rheumatoid factor, antinuclear antibody, and erythrocyte sedimentation rate (ESR)
- Treatment:
  - Active disease: Medical management (NSAIDs, soft diet, moist heat, range of motion exercises, and short-term steroids); if no improvement → disease-modifying therapy, coordinated with rheumatologist; if no improvement with disease-modifying therapy → surgical intervention (arthrocentesis and synovectomy)
  - Inactive disease: Surgical correction of ankylosis, open bite, or retrognathia as needed

Infectious Arthritis of the Temporomandibular Joint

- History/exam: History of tuberculosis/syphilis/gonorrhea, associated infection in the ear/mandible/parotid gland/pharynx, fever or malaise, TMJ pain, swelling, redness, and tenderness
- Diagnosis: Clinical exam, panoramic radiograph, MRI, joint aspiration for culture and Gram stain, complete blood count (CBC) with differential, and ESR
- Treatment:
  - Empiric antibiotics (penicillin for simple infections and third-generation cephalosporin for GNRs)
  - Joint aspiration or incision and drainage
  - If there is improvement → 2 weeks of antibiotics and TMJ physical therapy once active issues are resolved

- If no improvement → change antibiotics based on cultures, consider intravenous (IV) antibiotic therapy and surgical debridement

Traumatic Arthritis of the Temporomandibular Joint

- History/exam: Trauma to mandible/TMJ, TMJ pain and tenderness, and limited motion
- Diagnosis: Panoramic radiograph ± CT scan
- Treatment: NSAIDs, intermittent moist heat, soft diet, steroid injection, and jaw rest
- If there is improvement → jaw physical therapy to prevent ankylosis
- If no improvement → arthrocentesis

Temporomandibular Joint Ankylosis

- History/exam: History of trauma or infection to the TMJ, facial asymmetry, limited to no opening; can be progressive
- Diagnosis: Panoramic radiograph, maxillofacial CT with 3D reconstructions—consider angiography if a large ankylotic mass is present with possible intimate association with internal maxillary artery or pterygoid plexus
- Treatment:
  - Pseudoankylosis (postsurgical scar, radiation fibrosis, coronoid hyperplasia, osteochondroma, untreated zygomatic arch fracture, paramandibular neoplasia, myositis ossificans, and psychogenic) → site-specific treatment
  - Ankylosis: Mechanical dilation of jaws with physical therapy or appliance (e.g., Therabite) if onset is recent; if unsuccessful or for long-standing ankylosis → surgical correction with resection of the ankylotic mass and reconstruction of the ramus-condyle unit (bone graft, distraction osteogenesis, and alloplastic reconstruction), followed by orthognathic surgery or facial aesthetic surgery to achieve facial balance
  - Coronoid hyperplasia: Does not represent true ankylosis; limited opening due to mechanical interference between elongated coronoid process and root of zygoma; occasionally, pseudoarticulation with medial zygomatic arch exists; coronoidectomy can be performed intraorally versus extraorally depending on size and baseline mouth opening

Condylar Hyperplasia

- History/exam: Facial asymmetry (usually starting in puberty), deviation of chin point away from the affected side, crossbite or open bite malocclusion, prognathic appearance, and asymmetric mandibular projection
- Diagnosis: Panoramic radiograph, anterior-posterior and lateral cephalograms, review of historical photographs to document time course and evolution of deformity, CT scan, and technetium-99 (Tc99) bone scan to assess activity and growth
- Treatment: Based on Tc99 bone scan
  - Positive bone scan: Partial condylectomy on the affected side with compensatory contralateral mandibular osteotomy, inferior-border contour correction, and possible genioplasty
  - Negative bone scan: Orthodontic treatment to address the dental component of malocclusion with subsequent orthognathic surgery and contour correction

Condylar Hypoplasia

- History/exam: History of mandibular trauma, inflammation, or radiation. Facial deformity with chin point deviation toward the affected side, micrognathia, mandibular contour asymmetry, and exaggerated antigonial notching

- Diagnosis: Clinical exam, panoramic radiograph, anterior-posterior and lateral cephalograms, and CT scan
- Treatment: Based on growth
  - Still growing: Costochondral graft or distraction osteogenesis
  - Done growing: Orthodontics → orthognathic surgery or genioplasty/contour correction

Mandibular Dislocation

- History/exam: External trauma, wide mouth opening (sudden or prolonged), joint subluxation, muscular disease, and open lock
- Diagnosis: Clinical exam and panoramic radiograph or CT scan
- Treatment: Based on time course
  - Acute: Manual reduction and immobilization (intermaxillary fixation or head wrap for 5–7 days)
  - Chronic: Manual reduction under general anesthesia; if unsuccessful → manual reduction with angle traction wires; if unsuccessful → temporalis myotomy, if unsuccessful → subcondylar osteotomy or condylectomy

Idiopathic Condylar Resorption

- History/exam: History of orthodontic treatment or orthognathic surgery, female predilection (age 15–35 years, "Cheerleader" syndrome), class II skeletal profile, class II malocclusion, high mandibular plane angle, and anterior open bite
- Diagnosis: Clinical exam, panoramic radiograph, CT scan, and rule out rheumatoid arthritis, scleroderma, and other autoimmune processes
- Treatment: Based on Tc99 bone scan (Fig. 10.2)
  - Positive scan: Delay treatment until scan is negative
  - Negative scan: Orthognathic surgery ± condylectomy with TMJ reconstruction

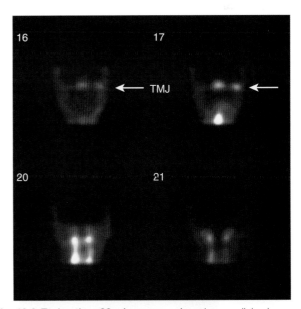

Fig. 10.2 Technetium-99m bone scan. A nuclear medicine bone scan evaluates metabolic activity in the condyles. The bone scan is sensitive to increased activity, and it serves as a guide for determining the stability of the asymmetry. (From Farrell BB, Tucker MR. Mandibular asymmetry: diagnosis and treatment considerations. In: Bagheri SC, Bell RB, Khan HA, eds. *Current Therapy in Oral and Maxillofacial Surgery.* Philadelphia, PA: Saunders; 2012:671–684, Fig. 80.8.)

COMMON ODONTOGENIC CYSTS AND TUMORS

1. Radicular (periapical) cyst
2. Dentigerous cyst
3. Residual cyst
4. Lateral periodontal cyst
5. Eruption cyst
6. Traumatic bone cyst
7. Odontogenic keratocyst (OKC)
8. Calcifying epithelial odontogenic tumor (CEOT; Pindborg tumor)
9. Clear cell odontogenic carcinoma (clear cell odontogenic tumor)
10. Adenomatoid odontogenic tumor
11. Odontogenic myxoma
12. Calcifying odontogenic cyst (Gorlin cyst)
13. Ameloblastoma
14. Ameloblastic carcinoma
15. Ameloblastic fibroma
16. Ameloblastic fibro-odontoma
17. Odontoma

Radicular (Periapical) Cyst

- Round or oval lesion that arises from residual odontogenic epithelium and nonvital pulp
- Treatment: Enucleation of cyst, endodontic treatment, or extraction of tooth

Dentigerous Cyst (Fig. 10.3)

- Develops in relationship to the crown of the erupting tooth
- Unilocular or multilocular
- Most common in the third molar and maxillary canine regions
- Treatment: Removal of the impacted tooth and enucleation or decompression of the cyst

Residual Cyst

- Persistent cyst after the tooth is removed
- Treatment: Enucleation

Lateral Periodontal Cyst

- Interradicular lesion that develops from epithelial rests in periodontal ligament
- Commonly located in the mandibular canine and premolar regions and maxillary lateral incisor regions
- Treatment: Enucleation

Eruption Cyst

- Dentigerous cyst that is associated with an erupting tooth
- Treatment: Excision of overlying soft tissue and exposure of tooth

Traumatic Bone Cyst

- Mandibular lesion of unknown etiology
- Usually found in asymptomatic patients <25 years of age
- Not a true cyst because the bony cavity is typically not epithelium lined
- Aspiration is necessary to rule out other possible diagnoses (hemorrhagic bone cyst and arteriovenous malformation [AVM])
- The area can be explored surgically to confirm the diagnosis
- Serial radiographs are used for follow-up

Odontogenic Keratocyst (Also Known as Keratocystic Odontogenic Tumor) (Fig. 10.4)

- Differentiated from other odontogenic cysts because it has an orthokeratinized lining
- Mandible > maxilla
- Up to 90% recurrence rate with simple enucleation, 30% with enucleation and peripheral ostectomy, and 2% with resection
- Multiple OKCs are seen in nevoid basal cell carcinoma syndrome
- Treatment is based on size, accessibility, and surgical morbidity
  - Small, accessible cyst: Enucleation and curettage with peripheral ostectomy ± cryotherapy

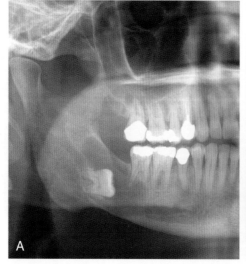
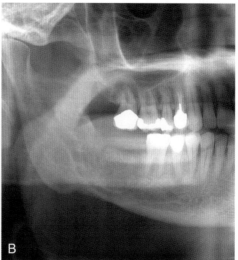

Fig. 10.3 Dentigerous cyst radiograph. Note that the lesion surrounds a tooth, and radiographic margins begin at the cement-enamel junction. (**A**) Dentigerous cyst. (**B**) Bone regeneration after removal of the dentigerous cyst. (From Marx RE. Jaw cysts, benign odontogenic tumors of the jaws, and fibro-osseous diseases. In: Bagheri SC, Bell RB, Khan HA, eds. *Current Therapy in Oral and Maxillofacial Surgery*. Philadelphia, PA: Saunders; 2012:390–410, Fig. 50.2.)

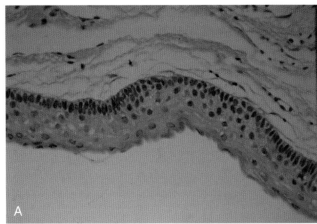

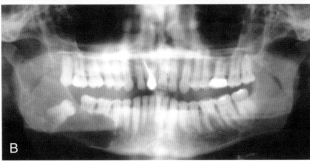

Fig. 10.4 Keratocystic odontogenic tumor radiograph and histology. (A) Histological appearance of a typical keratocystic odontogenic tumor showing a tumor lining five to six cells in thickness, with parakeratinization and polarization of the basal layer. (H & E; original magnification ×40.) **(B)** Panoramic radiograph showing a large radiolucent lesion in the right posterior mandible with an associated impacted third molar. The lesion has also resulted in resorption of the adjacent second and first molar roots and extends into the condyle. Biopsy showed keratocystic odontogenic tumor.) (A, From Pogrel MA. Keratocystic odontogenic tumor. In: Bagheri SC, Bell RB, Khan HA, eds. *Current Therapy in Oral and Maxillofacial Surgery*. Philadelphia, PA: Saunders; 2012:380–383, Fig. 48.1. B, From Marx RE. Jaw cysts, benign odontogenic tumors of the jaws, and fibro-osseous diseases. In: Baghori SC, Boll RB, Khan HA, eds. *Current Therapy in Oral and Maxillofacial Surgery*. Philadelphia, PA: Saunders; 2012:390–410, Fig. 50.4.)

- Large, inaccessible cyst: Decompression—once decompressed, may be amenable to enucleation
- More recent literature supports enucleation and curettage with peripheral ostectomy followed by the adjuvant use of 5-fluorouracil (5-FU) topical application for 24 hours; reported recurrence rates are much lower
- Recurrent/invasive cyst: Previously required en bloc/segmental resection but now can be treated with topical 5-FU in attempt to spare large resection

Calcifying Epithelial Odontogenic Tumor (Pindborg Tumor) (Fig. 10.5)

- Wide age distribution, but peak incidence is in the fifth decade
- Molar area of mandible > maxilla
- "Driven snow" opacity, can be radiolucent; cortical expansion with "soap bubble appearance"
- Histology: Liesegang rings (concentric calcified ring) and amyloid-like protein
- Treatment: Unencapsulated tumor, thus, resection with 1-cm margins decreases recurrence

Clear Cell Odontogenic Carcinoma (Clear Cell Odontogenic Tumor)

- Rare but predominant in women in their sixth and seventh decades of life
- 3:1 female to male predilection
- Low-grade malignancy from odontogenic epithelium
- Mandible is most commonly affected
- Large cells with clear cytoplasm histologically (similar to renal cell carcinoma)
- Treatment: Wide local excision with 1-cm margins

Adenomatoid Odontogenic Tumor

- "2/3" tumor: 2/3 occur in young females; 2/3 are in the anterior maxilla (canine area); and 2/3 are associated with an unerupted tooth
- Can form a sclerotic border on a radiograph
- Histologically, the tumor is encapsulated with gland-like "rosettes," which are small, duct-like structures
- Treatment: Enucleation

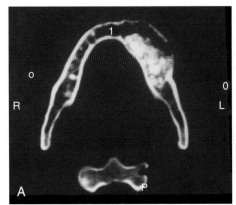

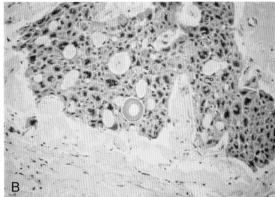

Fig. 10.5 Calcifying epithelial odontogenic tumor (CEOT). (A) The CEOT (Pindborg tumor) will present as a mixed radiolucent-radiopaque expansile mass. **(B)** The unique histopathology of a CEOT shows large epithelial cells with large bizarre nuclei and prominent intercellular bridges. There is also amyloid and some dystrophic calcifications. (H & E; original magnification ×2.) (From Marx RE. Jaw cysts, benign odontogenic tumors of the jaws, and fibro-osseous diseases. In: Bagheri SC, Bell RB, Khan HA, eds. *Current Therapy in Oral and Maxillofacial Surgery*. Philadelphia, PA: Saunders; 2012:390–410, Fig. 50.36.)

Odontogenic Myxoma

- Mandible > maxilla
- Predilection for children and young adults, although it can be seen in older adults
- Shows a characteristic trabecular pattern on radiography owing to preservation of medullary bony trabeculae
- Histologically, this is a hypocellular tumor that overproduces glycosaminoglycan ground substance (mixoid substance) and can look like a normal dental papilla or follicle
- These are unencapsulated; thus, the treatment is resection with 1-cm margins to avoid recurrence

Calcifying Odontogenic Cyst (Gorlin Cyst) (Fig. 10.6)

- Mandible is more common than maxilla
- No age predilection
- Clinically, the only ondontogenic cyst that produces opacifications on radiographs
- Histologically similar to ameloblastomas with peripheral palisading nuclei with reverse polarity; different in that they contain ghost cells (eosinophilic, glassy, and no nucleus)
- Treatment: Enucleation

Ameloblastoma (Fig. 10.7)

- Most common in patients 30 to 50 years of age
- Typically asymptomatic but can become very large and disfiguring
- Usually benign, but can be life-threatening when large
- Treatment is based on type
  - Clinical subtypes:
    - Unicystic: Mural ameloblastoma, unilocular cysts, and tumor is just in the lumen or wall of the cyst; 10% recurrence if truly unicystic and small; pathologist needs entire surgical specimen to diagnose as mural; unicystic ameloblastomas can be treated with enucleation and curettage versus resection
    - Solid or multicystic ameloblastomas require excision with tumor-free margins (at least 1-cm bone margin)
    - Malignant ameloblastoma: Benign ameloblastoma that has spread to extragnathic site (most common location is the lung); rare (some authors think that the spread is due not to true metastatic potential but rather to pieces of large tumors spreading by bulk shedding)

Ameloblastic Carcinoma

- Very rare
- Behaves clinically as an aggressive malignancy with early metastasis to the lung and brain
- Histologically similar to ameloblastoma but with markers of malignancy such as nuclear pleomorphism and mitotic figures

Ameloblastic Fibroma

- Occurs in the posterior mandible of children and young adults
- Radiolucent lesions; histologically, appear as cords of odontogenic epithelium with abundant cellular connective tissue
- Some consider these to be precursor lesions to odontomas
- Treatment: Enucleation

Ameloblastic Fibro-Odontoma

- Similar pathologically and epidemiologically to ameloblastic fibroma, but the epithelium is more mature and forms tooth product
- Results in a mixed radiopaque/radiolucent lesion clinically
- Treatment: Enucleation

Odontoma

- Similar pathologically and epidemiologically to ameloblastic fibromas and ameloblastic fibro-odontomas
- Appear on radiograph as either amorphous mixed-density lesions or like balls of tiny teeth
- Subtypes:
  - Complex odontomas (Fig. 10.8) consist of a haphazard arrangement of tooth product
  - Compound odontomas (Fig. 10.9) consist of a more organized arrangement of tooth product and, thus, resemble tiny teeth
- Treatment: Enucleation

FIBRO-OSSEOUS LESIONS

1. Fibrous dysplasia
2. Cherubism
3. Ossifying fibroma

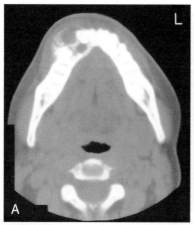
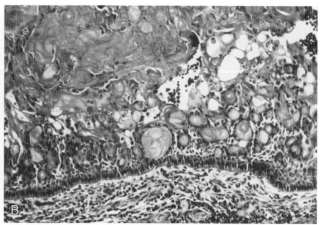

Fig. 10.6 Calcifying odontogenic cyst (Gorlin cyst). (**A**) A calcified odontogenic cyst with expansion and radiopacities. (**B**) A calcified odontogenic cyst may show keratinized and calcified areas within the lining, as well as clear "ghost" cells. (H & E; original magnification ×10.) (From Marx RE. Jaw cysts, benign odontogenic tumors of the jaws, and fibro-osseous diseases. In: Bagheri SC, Bell RB, Khan HA, eds. *Current Therapy in Oral and Maxillofacial Surgery*. Philadelphia, PA: Saunders; 2012:390–410, Fig. 50.10.)

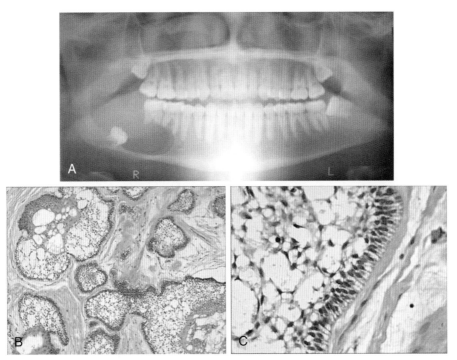

Fig. 10.7 Ameloblastoma radiograph and histology. (A) Large unilocular radiolucency of the posterior right mandible with displacement of the third molar to the inferior border and resorption of adjacent molar roots. **(B)** Ameloblastoma (follicular variant). Numerous neoplastic odontogenic islands featuring peripheral columnar cells with reverse polarization surrounding central zone of cells resembling stellate reticulum. **(C)** Higher magnification that shows the reverse polarization of the peripheral columnar cells. (From Kademani D, Junck DM. Contemporary treatment of ameloblastoma. In: Bagheri SC, Bell RB, Khan HA, eds. *Current Therapy in Oral and Maxillofacial Surgery*. Philadelphia, PA: Saunders; 2012: 384–390, Figs. 49.9 and 49.4.)

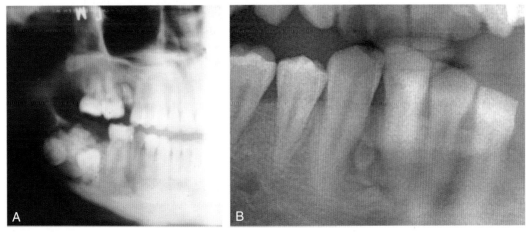

Fig. 10.8 Complex odontoma. (A) A complex odontoma presents as a diffuse radiopacity. **(B)** A compound odontoma presents with the appearance of small, toothlike structures. (From Marx RE. Jaw cysts, benign odontogenic tumors of the jaws, and fibro-osseous diseases. In: Bagheri SC, Bell RB, Khan HA, eds. *Current Therapy in Oral and Maxillofacial Surgery*. Philadelphia, PA: Saunders; 2012:390–410, Fig. 50.38.)

4. Osteoblastoma
5. Periapical cemental dysplasia
6. Cemento-osseous dysplasia

Fibrous Dysplasia

- Pathophysiology
  - Result of a mutation in the *GNAS-1* gene during embryogenesis—the effect is pleiotropic
  - If occurring early in embryogenesis → polyostotic (café au lait spots, endocrinopathy: McCune-Albright syndrome)
  - If it occurs late in embryogenesis → polyostotic (café au lait spots, no endocrinopathy: Jaffe-Lichtenstein syndrome) or monostotic (craniofacial fibrous dysplasia)
- Histological features
  - Woven bone without osteoblastic rimming
  - Bone trabeculae are not connected and can form curvilinear shapes → "Chinese script" writing
  - Findings are not seen in all specimens or even uniformly throughout a single lesion
  - Diagnosis is often made based on the history and physical exam along with radiographic adjuncts

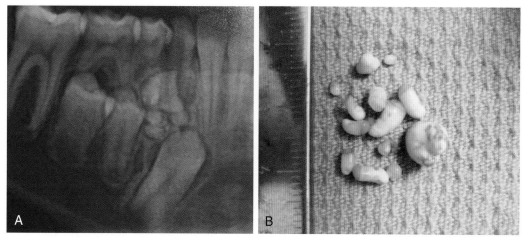

Fig. 10.9 Compound odontoma. (A) Radiograph of odontoma. **(B)** Odontoma after enucleation. (From Abramowicz S, Padwa BL. Pediatric head and neck tumors: benign lesions. In: Bagheri SC, Bell RB, Khan HA, eds. *Current Therapy in Oral and Maxillofacial Surgery.* Philadelphia, PA: Saunders; 2012:813–820, Fig. 92.2.)

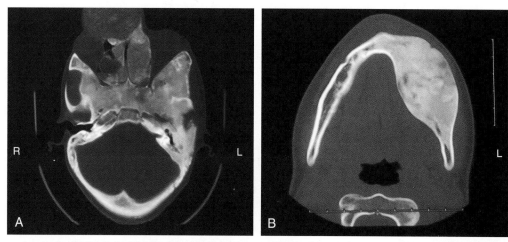

Fig. 10.10 Fibrous dysplasia. (A) Craniofacial fibrous dysplasia involves contiguous bones of the face and/or base of skull. **(B)** Monostotic fibrous dysplasia involves a single bone with a fusiform, poorly demarcated, ground-glass appearance. (From Marx RE. Jaw cysts, benign odontogenic tumors of the jaws, and fibro-osseous diseases. In: Bagheri SC, Bell RB, Khan HA, eds. *Current Therapy in Oral and Maxillofacial Surgery.* Philadelphia, PA: Saunders; 2012:390–410, Fig. 50.41.)

- Clinical features
  - Maxilla > mandible
  - Orbit can also be affected, leading to vision loss
  - Cranial neuropathies associated with foraminal narrowing
  - Painless swelling occurring during the first 2 decades of life
  - Functional deficits related to cranial neuropathies
  - Pain may occur during periods of growth or hormonal changes (e.g., pregnancy)
  - Disease usually stable after age 25
- Diagnosis
  - Radiographic changes: May be a multilocular radiolucency with cortical thinning or a mixed "ground glass" appearance (classical appearance) (Fig. 10.10)
  - Markers for metabolic bone disease (calcium, phosphate, alkaline phosphatase, calcitonin, and parathyroid hormone) are usually normal
  - Skin should be examined for pigmentation changes (café au lait spots)
  - Endocrine workup should be initiated to identify endocrinopathy

- Treatment
  - Biopsy for diagnosis (clinical diagnosis, but confirmatory biopsy)
  - Contour resection → in minor cases, should be delayed until after puberty to avoid recurrence and need for further operation
  - Contour resection → in severe cases should be undertaken to prevent sequelae of nasal obstruction, impingement on orbital contents, or cranial neuropathy
  - Therapeutic radiation is not recommended → high rate of sarcomatous transformation

Cherubism

- Pathophysiology
  - Autosomal-dominant trait with 50% to 70% penetrance in females and 100% penetrance in males; has three clinical variations
    - Type I affects only the ramus and angle of the mandible bilaterally

- Type II involves the ramus, angle, and body of the mandible bilaterally to the mental foramen
- Type III involves both the maxilla and mandible; gives the patient the appearance of an upward gaze; taken together with the symmetric facial expansion, these individuals resemble cherubs depicted in Renaissance art
- Clinical features
  - Usually first apparent by age 3; expansion is slow and progresses until adolescence
  - In some cases, the expansion involutes; in others, it is incomplete
- Diagnosis
  - Radiographs show bilateral multilocular radiolucencies (Fig. 10.11)
  - Histologically, these lesions resemble giant cell lesions consisting of vascular fibrous tissue with variable numbers of multinucleated giant cells
- Treatment
  - Observation in most cases and contour resection in patients who do not achieve spontaneous remission
  - The lesions are highly vascular; thus, the surgeon should be prepared for intraoperative bleeding

Ossifying Fibroma

- Clinical features
  - Considered a variant of fibrous dysplasia
  - Appears as a localized, painless swelling
  - The mandible is affected more frequently compared with the maxilla
  - Occurs in the third and fourth decades of life but can occur in children and adolescents
- Diagnosis
  - On radiographs, these are well-defined radiolucent lesions with increasing radiopacity and less distinct borders as they mature (Fig. 10.12)

- Histologically similar to fibrous dysplasia but ossifying fibromas have more distinct borders
- Treatment
  - Enucleation is easily performed because these lesions are well encapsulated

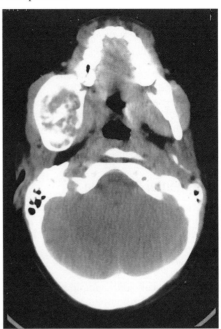

Fig. 10.12 Ossifying fibroma. An ossifying fibroma will appear radiographically as a spherical or oval expansion with an expanded but identifiable cortex. (From Marx RE. Jaw cysts, benign odontogenic tumors of the jaws, and fibro-osseous diseases. In: Bagheri SC, Bell RB, Khan HA, eds. *Current Therapy in Oral and Maxillofacial Surgery.* Philadelphia, PA: Saunders; 2012:390–410, Fig. 50.43.)

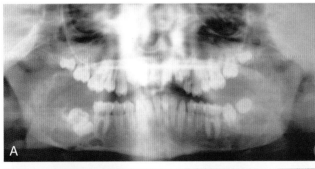

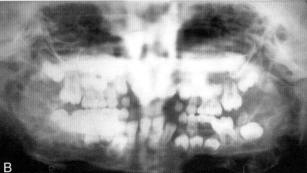

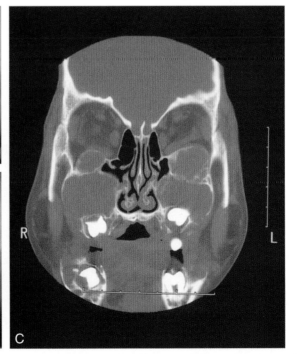

Fig. 10.11 Cherubism. (A) Type I cherubism is limited to the ramus and posterior mandible. **(B)** Type II cherubism involves the bilateral mandible to the mental foramen and the posterior maxilla. **(C)** The eyes turned toward the heavens in type III cherubism is due to expansion of the maxillary bone's contribution to the orbital floor. (From Marx RE. Jaw cysts, benign odontogenic tumors of the jaws, and fibro-osseous diseases. In: Bagheri SC, Bell RB, Khan HA, eds. *Current Therapy in Oral and Maxillofacial Surgery.* Philadelphia, PA: Saunders; 2012:390–410, Fig. 50.45.)

Osteoblastoma

- Clinical features
  - Most commonly seen in the vertebral column, long bones, and sacrum
  - A rare disease of the craniofacial skeleton
- Diagnosis
  - Presents as a chronic swelling with ongoing dull pain
  - These lesions occur in ages 5 to 22 years, with a slight male predominance
  - Radiographically appearing as radiolucent lesions with areas of mineralization
  - Histological examination reveals mineralized material with sheets of irregular trabeculae surrounded by scattered multinucleated osteoclast-like cells
- Treatment
  - En bloc resection because of a propensity to recur

Periapical Cemental Dysplasia

- Clinical features
  - Most commonly seen in middle-aged African women
  - Usually incidental findings on intraoral radiographs or panoramic radiography during routine exam
  - Asymptomatic lesions
- Diagnosis
  - Based on clinical and radiographic findings where lesions are mixed radiolucent-radiopaque or completely radiopaque lesions along the roots of the anterior teeth (Fig. 10.13)
  - Treatment: Observation

Cemento-osseous Dysplasia

- Clinical features
  - Similar presentation and demographic predilection as periapical cemental dysplasia but can affect teeth and alveolar bone, not limited to the mandibular anterior teeth

- Diagnosis
  - Based on clinical and radiographic findings as in periapical cemental dysplasia but can be seen in any part of the jaw
- Treatment
  - Observation

VASCULAR MALFORMATIONS (TABLE 10.1)

Slow-Flow Malformations

Capillary—also known as "port-wine stain"
- Clinical features
  - Equal sex predilection and 0.3% birth prevalence; enlarged postcapillary venules because of decreased density of precapillary neuromodulation; lesions occur along the trigeminal nerve distribution; Sturge-Weber syndrome consists of capillary malformation and leptomeningeal vascular anomalies
- Diagnosis
  - Lesion is present at birth and blanches with pressure, with possible enlargement of underlying soft or hard tissue; MRI and Doppler ultrasound (US) are adjuncts in identifying other associated vascular anomalies deep near the superficial lesion
- Treatment
  - Consists of pulsed-dye light amplification by stimulated emission of radiation (LASER) for the malformation and surgical correction of the underlying surgical deformity

TABLE 10.1 Outdated and Current Terms for Circulatory Malformations

Outdated Term	Correct Term
Port-wine stain, capillary hemangioma	Capillary malformation
Lymphangioma, cystic hygroma	Lymphatic malformation
Cavernous hemangioma	Venous malformation

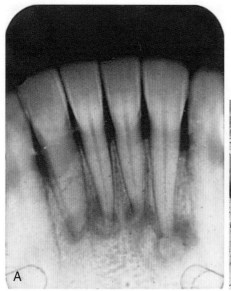
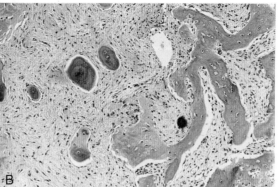

Fig. 10.13 Periapical cemental dysplasia. (A) Periapical cemental dysplasia occurs in the anterior mandible with radiolucencies and radiopacities at the apex of the incisor teeth, usually in an adult of black African descent. **(B)** Histopathology of a periapical cemental dysplasia will show a stromal proliferation of periodontal ligament fibroblasts and islands of bone/cementum. (H & E; original magnification ×4.) (From Marx RE. Jaw cysts, benign odontogenic tumors of the jaws, and fibro-osseous diseases. In: Bagheri SC, Bell RB, Khan HA, eds. *Current Therapy in Oral and Maxillofacial Surgery*. Philadelphia, PA: Saunders; 2012:390–410, Fig. 50.48.)

Venous Malformation

- Background
  - Autosomal-dominant mutation of *TIE2/TEK* gene; chromosome 9p21-22; 95% are sporadic with an incidence of 1:10,000; 40% occur in the head and neck
- Clinical features
  - Blue, soft, compressible mass; Valsalva causes engorgement; phleboliths and intralesional thrombosis can result in pain; histology shows dilated vascular channels with normal endothelium
- Diagnosis
  - Physical exam with MRI using pre- and postcontrast T1 and T2 images with fat suppression show hyperintensity on T2; phleboliths and thrombi appear as signal voids; plain film or CT may show skeletal deformity
- Management
  - Intralesional coagulation of large malformations can precipitate disseminated intravascular coagulopathy. Check coagulation. Daily aspirin therapy prophylaxis against phlebolith formation and intralesional injection of absolute ethanol (large lesions) or 1% sodium tetradecyl sulfate (smaller lesions) can result in sclerosis and shrinkage

Lymphatic Malformation

- Background
  - Associated with *VEGFR3* mutations; incidence is unknown; histology shows lymphatic spaces walled with eosinophilic and protein-rich fluid; microcystic or macrocystic based on radiographic appearance; large cervicofacial lymphatic malformations can be detected prenatally via US and necessitate surgical airway management at birth (ex utero intrapartum treatment procedure)
- Clinical features
  - Swelling; overlying skin can be normal or have a blue hue; intralesional hemorrhage can cause the vesicles to appear dark red; dermal involvement can cause skin to pucker. Lesions are soft, noncompressible, and result in underlying skeletal enlargement, mandibular overgrowth, malocclusion, and macroglossia
- Diagnosis
  - Physical exam and MRI: Malformations are hyperintense on T2-weighted MRI and hypointense on T1-weighted sequences. Macrocystic lesions can have fluid-fluid levels with large cystic space; microcystic malformations are less well defined and appear as T2 intense infiltrative lesions
- Treatment
  - Macrocystic malformations are treated with sclerosing agents such as a compound of ethanol, doxycycline, bleomycin, and sodium tetradecyl sulfate. OK-432 (killed strain of Group A *Streptococcus pyogenes*) in penicillin suspension is used outside of the United States. Microcystic lesions require surgical excision

HIGH-FLOW MALFORMATIONS

Arteriovenous Malformations

- Clinical features
  - Less common overall, pure arterial malformations are exceedingly rare; 1.5:1 female predilection; associated with Rendu-Osler-Weber syndrome; head and neck involvement is usually intracranial followed by cheek, ear, nose, mandible, and then maxilla. Histologically, arteries and veins communicate without intervening capillary beds
    - A staging system has been formulated, consisting of four stages of progression:
      I. Quiescent: Warm pink lesion
      II. Expansion: An enlarging warm pink lesion with pulsation, thrill, bruit, and tortuous veins
      III. Destruction: Physical exam stigmata of a stage II lesion with overlying skin or mucosa changes, ulceration, tissue necrosis, bleeding, and pain
      IV. Decompensation: All of the findings in stage III but with cardiovascular failure
- Diagnosis
  - CT is useful for demonstrating bone destruction, and MRI is useful in assessing the extent of the lesion within the surrounding soft tissues. Doppler US is commonly used to assess the high-flow nature of the lesion
- Treatment
  - Consists of a combined approach of superselective arterial embolization to obliterate the feeding vessels of the AVM nidus followed by surgical excision of the nidus within 2 to 3 days to avoid re-formation of feeder vessels

FURTHER READINGS

Flynn TR. What are the antibiotics of choice for odontogenic infections, and how long should the treatment course last? *Oral Maxillofac Surg Clin North Am.* 2011;23(4):519–536. v–vi.

Greene AK. Current concepts of vascular anomalies. *J Craniofac Surg.* Jan 2012;23(1):220–224.

Kaban LB. *Pediatric Oral and Maxillofacial Surgery.* Philadelphia, PA: Saunders; 1990.

Ledderhof NJ, Caminiti MF, Bradle G, Lam DK. Topical 5-fluorouracil is a novel targeted therapy for the keratocystic odontogenic tumor. *J Oral Maxillofac Surg.* 2017;75(3):514–524.

Lone PK, Nisar AW, Janbaz ZA, Bibi M, Kour A. Topical 5-fluorouracil application in management of odontogenic keratocysts. *J Oral Biol Craniofac Res.* 2020;10(4):404–406.

Marx RE, Stern D. *Oral and Maxillofacial Pathology: A Rationale for Diagnosis and Treatment.* 2nd ed. Hanover Park, IL: Quintessence; 2012.

Nelson SJ. *Wheeler's Dental Anatomy, Physiology, and Occlusion.* 10th ed. St. Louis, MO: Saunders Elsevier; 2015.

Neville BW. *Oral and Maxillofacial Pathology.* 4th ed. St. Louis, MO: Saunders Elsevier; 2015.

Wilkes CH. Internal derangements of the temporomandibular joint (pathological variations). *Arch Otolaryngol Head Neck Surg.* 1989;115:469–477.

11 Head and Neck Pathology

Amir Afrogheh, William C. Faquin, and Peter M. Sadow

PREFACE

This chapter is a practical, image-based review of common head and neck lesions encountered in routine pathology practice. Included are over 100 histological images, along with legends that succinctly summarize the key histomorphological features. In some cases, the legends are expanded to provide a brief description of the pathological entities and their histological mimics. We focus on practical pathology for the practicing general otolaryngologist; unusual and rare entities are not included. The majority of images are of standard hematoxylin and eosin (H & E)–stained slides. Some special stains—including methenamine silver stain for fungal organisms, immunohistochemical stains, and in situ hybridization—highlight unique findings. This chapter is structured roughly according to the anatomical regions within the head and neck: oral cavity and oropharynx, osseous jaw, larynx and hypopharynx, nose, paranasal sinuses and nasopharynx, ear, and thyroid and parathyroid glands, with salivary gland lesions separately illustrated. Each section is then arranged into the following themes: nonneoplastic lesions (including infectious, reactive, inflammatory, and hamartomatous lesions), benign tumors, and malignant tumors. This compilation of images should serve as a useful resource for otorhinolaryngology trainees as well as a basic reference for those in practice.

ORAL CAVITY AND OROPHARYNX

Developmental Lesions

- Nasopalatine duct cyst (Fig. 11.1)

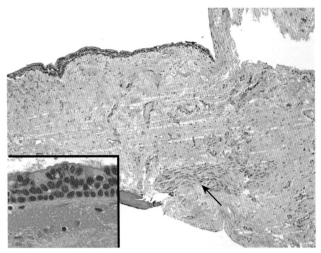

Fig. 11.1 Nasopalatine duct cyst, 200×. The cyst is lined by a ciliated pseudostratified cuboidal to the low columnar epithelium (inset lower left, 400×) with underlying fibroconnective tissue and a prominent nerve (*arrow*). Nasopalatine duct cysts originate from embryonic remnants of the nasopalatine ducts. Although nonodontogenic, when lined by squamous epithelium, the cyst may resemble a periapical (radicular) cyst. Clinical and radiographic information combined with pathology are essential in arriving at the correct diagnosis.

Reactive and Nonneoplastic Lesions

- Fibroepithelial polyp (Fig. 11.2)
- Lobular capillary hemangioma (pyogenic granuloma) (Fig. 11.3)

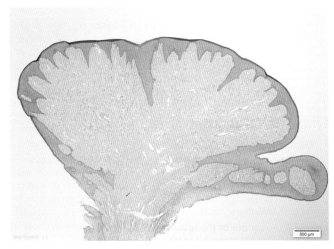

Fig. 11.2 Fibroepithelial polyp (fibroma), 20×. The polyp is lined by an acanthotic, stratified squamous epithelium with a dense fibrovascular tissue stroma. Fibroepithelial polyps are common in the oral cavity, frequently occurring in areas that are prone to trauma, such as the tongue, buccal mucosa, and lower lip. They may be referred to as "irritation" or "bite" fibromas.

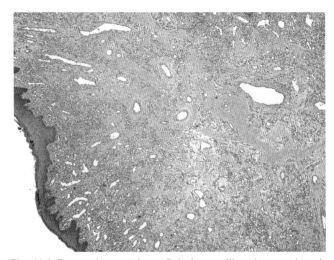

Fig. 11.3 Pyogenic granuloma (lobular capillary hemangioma), 40×. The image shows proliferation of small capillary-sized blood vessels in a lobular arrangement with a central small ectatic feeder vessel in each lobule and an inflammatory background. Lobular capillary hemangioma is a common lesion of the oral cavity. When pyogenic granulomas occur during pregnancy, they are commonly referred to as *pregnancy epulis* or *granuloma gravidarum*.

- Mucocele (Fig. 11.4)
- Reactive lymphoid follicular hyperplasia (Fig. 11.5)
- Necrotizing sialometaplasia (Figs. 11.6 and 11.7)

Vascular Malformation

- Lymphangioma (Fig. 11.8)

Infections

- Candidiasis (Fig. 11.9)
- Granulomatous inflammation (Fig. 11.10)

- Tuberculosis (Fig. 11.11)
- Histoplasmosis (Fig. 11.12)

Benign Tumors

- Granular cell tumor (Fig. 11.13)
- Lipoma (Fig. 11.14)
- Spindle cell lipoma (Fig. 11.15)

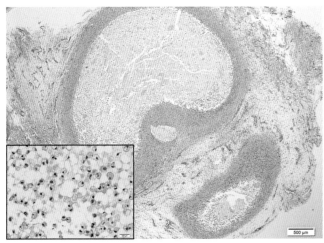

Fig. 11.4 Mucocele of the lower lip, 20×. The image shows extravasated mucin surrounded by a wall of granulation tissue and as such, mucoceles are pseudocysts (lacking an epithelial cyst lining). The mucin (which appears gray/pink in color) contains abundant histiocytes with mucin in their cytoplasm (muciphages) (inset lower left, 400×). Mucoceles are commonly seen in the lower lip because of bite injury to the minor salivary gland ducts. Mucoceles that arise from the sublingual glands push up into the floor of the mouth, forming a noticeable smooth cystic mass, termed ranula.

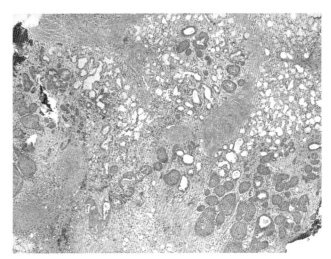

Fig. 11.6 Necrotizing sialometaplasia, 20×. The image shows squamous metaplasia of the minor salivary gland ducts in a lobular arrangement. A few open ducts are present; however, many have been obliterated by the squamous metaplastic process. A moderate chronic inflammatory cell infiltrate is seen in the background with marked atrophy and destruction of the minor salivary gland acini (see also Fig. 11.7).

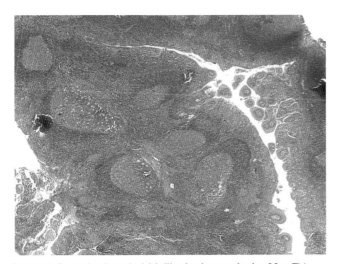

Fig. 11.5 Reactive lymphoid follicular hyperplasia, 20×. This hyperplastic tonsil shows a lymphoid-rich stroma with prominent germinal centers, including tingible-body macrophages. When clinically worrisome, ancillary studies—such as flow cytometry, immunohistochemistry (IHC), and molecular testing for clonal gene rearrangements—are essential to exclude a neoplasia (including lymphoma).

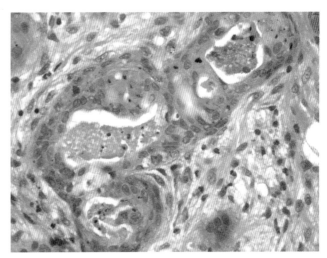

Fig. 11.7 Necrotizing sialometaplasia, 400×. Necrotic debris and neutrophils are seen within the lumens of the metaplastic ducts. The metaplastic ductal cells are crowded and show nuclear hyperchromasia. The lesion may mimic squamous cell carcinoma (SCC) in small biopsy specimens, in which the lobular arrangement of the cells is difficult to appreciate. Necrotizing sialometaplasia presents as an ulcerative lesion of the hard palate and may clinically simulate a carcinoma. However, these lesions usually lack the marked nuclear atypia and increased mitoses seen in SCC.

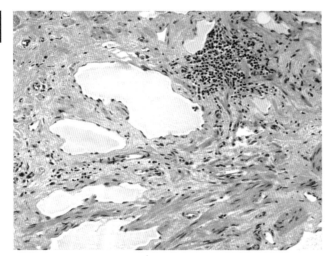

Fig. 11.8 Lymphangioma, 200×. The image shows large dilated lymphatic vessels lined by a flat, inconspicuous layer of bland endothelial cells. The lymphatic channels contain a pale proteinaceous material (lymph). A dense collection of lymphocytes is seen in the stroma surrounding the vessels. Lymphangiomas are generally seen in the head and neck region of newborns and are treated surgically.

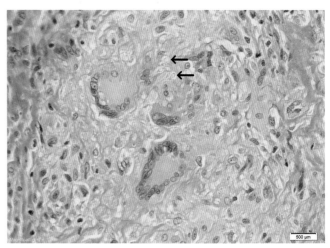

Fig. 11.10 Granulomatous inflammation, 200×. The image shows a granuloma consisting of epithelioid histiocytes with elongated, curved nuclei, multinucleated giant cells, and peripheral small lymphocytes. Spherical fungal organisms are present (*arrows*). The differential diagnosis of granulomatous inflammation is broad and includes a wide range of bacterial (e.g., tuberculosis), fungal (e.g., histoplasmosis), immunological (e.g., sarcoidosis, Crohn disease) and neoplastic conditions (e.g., Hodgkin lymphoma). (Image courtesy of Prof. Johann Schneider, University of Stellenbosch.)

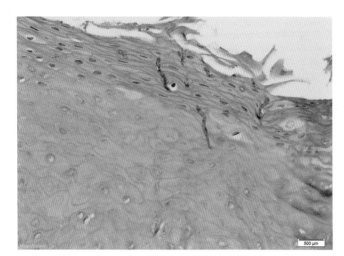

Fig. 11.9 Candidiasis (Periodic Acid Schiff), 200×. Thickened parakeratotic squamous epithelium containing numerous non-septate hyphae and spore forms, consistent with Candida spp. Although not present in this image, some degree of epithelial infiltration with neutrophils is often seen.

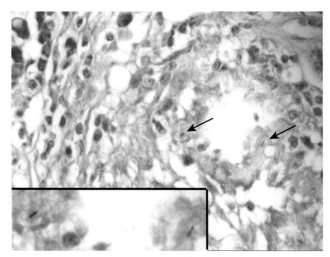

Fig. 11.11 Tuberculosis (Ziehl-Neelsen stain), 200×. The image shows acid-fast bacilli (indicated by *arrows* in the image and magnified in the inset lower left). Oral tuberculosis usually presents as an atypical area of ulceration in the oral cavity and may clinically resemble a malignancy. It results from direct inoculation of acid-fast bacilli into the oral tissues.

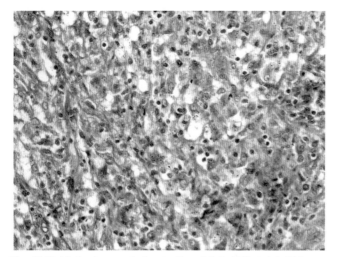

Fig. 11.12 Histoplasmosis (periodic acid–Schiff stain), 200×. The foamy macrophages possess numerous small fungal spores (1–4 μm) in their cytoplasm, surrounded by clear halos.

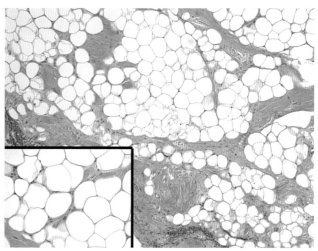

Fig. 11.14 Lipoma, 100×. The image shows lobules of mature adipose tissue separated by thick bands of fibrous tissue. The adipocytes are univacuolated with their slender hyperchromatic nuclei located at the periphery of the cell, often not apparent (inset lower left, 400×). Nuclear atypia or marked variation in size might raise the possibility of liposarcoma. Lipomas are usually solitary lesions in adults that commonly involve the oral cavity and the larynx. The degree of cellularity and fibrosis is location dependent.

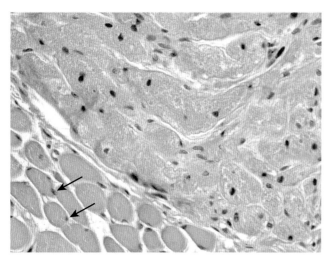

Fig. 11.13 Granular cell tumor of the tongue, 200×. Cytologically bland large polygonal cells with abundant granular, oncocytic (pink) cytoplasm and centrally located small, dark nuclei. In this image, the granular cells abut skeletal muscle cells (*arrows*). Note the similarity between the two cell types, distinguished by the circumscription of the granular cell tumor with granular, pink fluffy cytoplasm and the skeletal muscle with a glassy/striated cytoplasm. The granular cells react strongly and diffusely with antibodies to S100 protein and are thought to be of Schwannian origin.

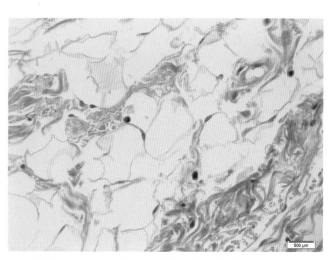

Fig. 11.15 Spindle cell lipoma, 400×. Spindled fibroblasts, shredded collagen fibers, mast cells, myxoid change, and mature adipocytes characterize this variant of lipoma, commonly seen in the oral cavity.

Epithelial Precursor Lesions

- Mild epithelial dysplasia (Fig. 11.16)
- Severe epithelial dysplasia/carcinoma in situ (Fig. 11.17)
- Verrucous hyperplasia (Fig. 11.18)

Malignant Epithelial Lesions

- Verrucous carcinoma (Fig. 11.19)
- Keratinizing squamous cell carcinoma (Figs. 11.20 and 11.21)
- Basaloid squamous cell carcinoma (Fig. 11.22)
- Adenosquamous carcinoma (Fig. 11.23)

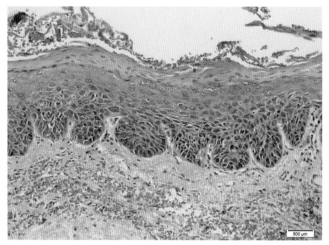

Fig. 11.16 Mild epithelial dysplasia, 200×. The epithelium shows drop-shaped rete processes and loss of nuclear polarization. Cytologically, there is nuclear hyperchromasia and prominent nucleoli. The architectural and cytological features are confined to the lower one-third of the epithelium.

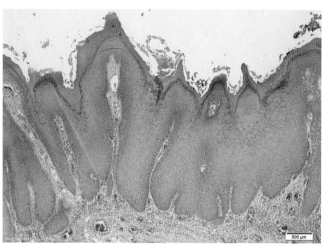

Fig. 11.18 Verrucous hyperplasia, 20×. Although the rete processes appear elongated, they are relatively uniform and do not appear deeper than the surrounding normal epithelium. The lesion lacks significant cytological atypia. Verrucous hyperplasia is seen in the oral cavity, often in the setting of proliferative verrucous leukoplakia. It has a high recurrence rate and may transform into verrucous carcinoma or invasive squamous cell carcinoma. The word *verrucous* reflects the warty appearance of these lesions with pointy, spire-like architecture.

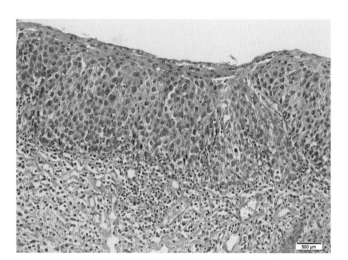

Fig. 11.17 Severe epithelial dysplasia/carcinoma in situ, 200×. There is full-thickness, marked nuclear atypia and pleomorphism, with suprabasilar mitoses and disordered maturation of cells.

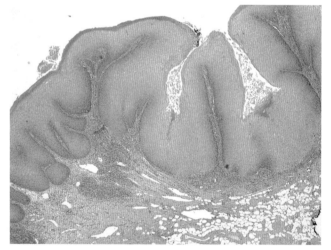

Fig. 11.19 Verrucous carcinoma, 20×. Large and broad rete processes push deeply into the submucosa in broad, pushing nests. The folded and thickened epithelium shows marked surface keratinization. A dense chronic inflammatory response may be seen at the advancing front of the lesion, and there is no epithelial atypia. Small and superficial biopsies can create diagnostic difficulties because the base of the lesion may not be visualized.

- Nonkeratinizing squamous cell carcinoma (Fig. 11.24)
- Immunohistochemistry for p16 (Fig. 11.25)

Malignant Mesenchymal Tumors

- Kaposi sarcoma (Fig. 11.26)

Immune-Mediated Lesions

- Pemphigus vulgaris (Fig. 11.27)
- Pemphigoid (Fig. 11.28)
- Lichen planus (Fig. 11.29)
- Sjögren syndrome (Fig. 11.30)

Lesions of the Osseous Jaw

- Osteomyelitis (Fig. 11.31)
- Osteoradionecrosis (Fig. 11.32)
- Central giant cell granuloma (Fig. 11.33)
- Osteoma (Fig. 11.34)

- Osteosarcoma (Fig. 11.35)
- Fibrous dysplasia (Fig. 11.36)
- Ossifying fibroma (Fig. 11.37)

SELECTED ODONTOGENIC CYSTS AND TUMORS

Odontogenic Cysts

- Periapical (radicular) cyst (Fig. 11.38)
- Dentigerous cyst (Fig. 11.39)

Benign Epithelial Odontogenic Tumors

- Solid/multicystic ameloblastoma (Fig. 11.40)
- Calcifying epithelial odontogenic tumor (Fig. 11.41)
- Adenomatoid odontogenic tumor (Fig. 11.42)
- Keratocystic odontogenic tumor (Fig. 11.43)

Benign Mixed Epithelial Tumors

- Odontoma (Fig. 11.44)

Benign Mesenchymal Odontogenic Tumors

- Odontogenic myxoma (Fig. 11.45)

LARYNX AND HYPOPHARYNX

Nonneoplastic Lesions

- Contact ulcer of the larynx (Fig. 11.46)
- Vocal cord polyp (Fig. 11.47)

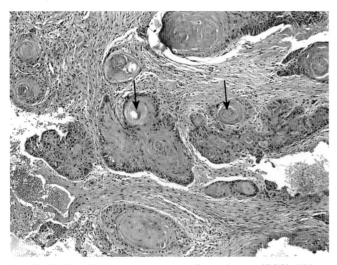

Fig. 11.20 Keratinizing squamous cell carcinoma (SCC), 200×. The image shows a well-differentiated SCC with abundant intralesional keratinization, forming keratin pearls (*arrows*).

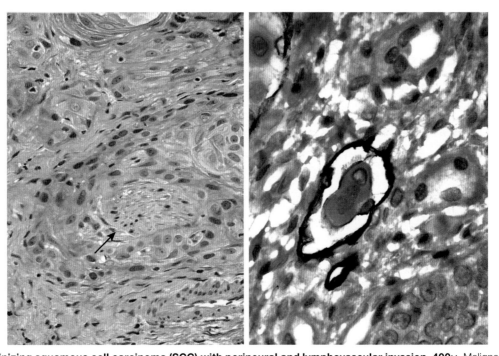

Fig. 11.21 Keratinizing squamous cell carcinoma (SCC) with perineural and lymphovascular invasion, 400×. Malignant squamous cells surround a peripheral nerve (*arrow*, left image). Malignant squamous cells in a lymphatic vessel (right image, D2-40 immunohistochemistry). Perineural invasion and lymphovascular invasion are frequently observed in SCCs.

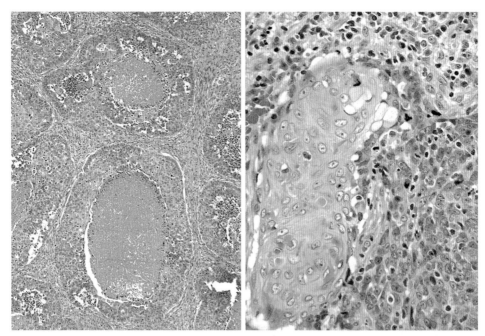

Fig. 11.22 Basaloid squamous cell carcinoma (BSCC). Islands of atypical basaloid cells (the term *basaloid* means that the cells show a high nuclear-to-cytoplasmic ratio with small, dense hyperchromatic nuclei, similar to basal epithelial cells) with central areas of necrosis (comedo-type necrosis; left image, 100×). Most BSCCs show focal areas of high-grade surface dysplasia or keratinizing SCC (right image, 400×). Correctly diagnosing a BSCC can be challenging in small biopsies. The differential diagnosis includes other basaloid lesions, such as adenoid cystic carcinoma (ADCC), salivary duct carcinoma, and nonkeratinizing, human papillomavirus–related SCC.

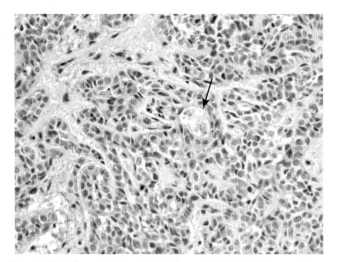

Fig. 11.23 Adenosquamous carcinoma, 200×. The image shows a squamous cell carcinoma with areas of true glandular differentiation (*arrow*). Adenosquamous carcinomas often behave aggressively.

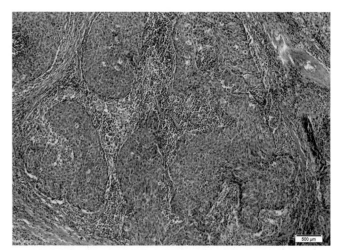

Fig. 11.24 Nonkeratinizing oropharyngeal squamous cell carcinoma, 200×. The tumour exhibits lobulated growth with nests of non keratinizing squamous cells with basaloid features and intraluminal necrosis associated with a dense lymphoid stroma. Most oropharyngeal cases with this appearance are positive for high-risk (HR) HPV subtypes. They are most frequently found in the base of tongue and palatine tonsils, and careful attention may be needed to distinguish these malignant nests of non keratinizing squamous cell carcinoma from the surrounding lymphoid stroma.

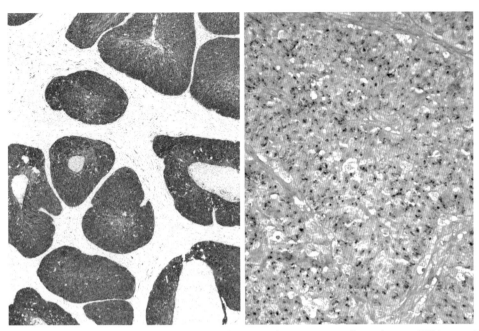

Fig. 11.25 Human papillomavirus-related nonkeratinizing oropharyngeal squamous cell carcinoma. P16 immunohistochemistry (IHC) and in situ hybridization (ISH) for high-risk human papillomavirus (HR-HPV). Strong cytoplasmic and nuclear staining for P16 (image left, 200×). P16 IHC is a sensitive but nonspecific screening test for HR-HPV. More than 70% of the tumor cells should be positive for this antibody. P16-positive tumors are further evaluated for the presence of HR-HPV by polymerase chain reaction or ISH. The image on the right shows punctate positivity for HR-HPV (ISH, 400×).

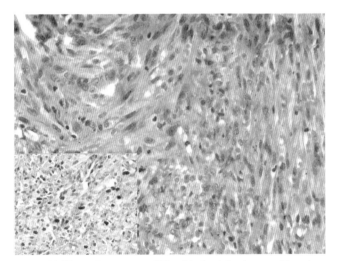

Fig. 11.26 Kaposi sarcoma, 400×. Moderately pleomorphic spindled cells surround slit-like vascular channels with extravasation of red blood cells. Nuclear reactivity with antibodies to human herpesvirus 8 is seen in most Kaposi sarcomas (inset lower left, 200×).

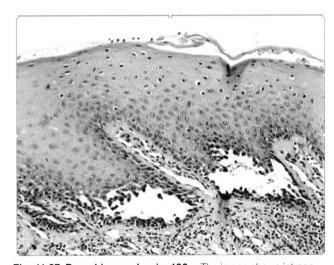

Fig. 11.27 Pemphigus vulgaris, 100×. The image shows intraepithelial vesicles. The basal layer is intact. Pemphigus vulgaris is an autoimmune vesiculobullous disease. The immunoglobulin G antibodies directed against the interepithelial desmosomes cause squamous cells to lose cohesion (acantholysis).

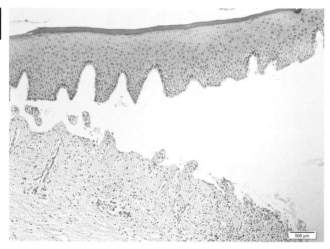

Fig. 11.28 Pemphigoid, 200×. A sub-basilar cleft is observed. Pemphigoid is an autoimmune vesiculobullous disease with antibodies directed against basement membrane antigens that connect the epithelial cells to the basement membrane.

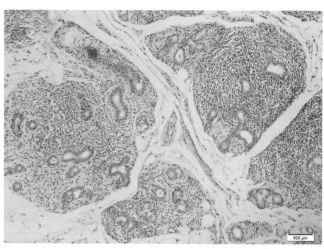

Fig. 11.30 Sjögren syndrome. Lip biopsy, 200×. The image shows a multifocal dense lymphoid infiltrate within the parenchyma of the minor salivary glands. More than 50 lymphocytes are seen in one focus. Sjögren syndrome is a systemic autoimmune disease associated with a focus score of greater than or equal to 1 per 4 mm². Patients may present with SICCA syndrome, including dry eyes and dry mouth. The diagnosis is a clinical diagnosis that may be supported by pathological findings, generally by biopsy of non-bite line minor salivary gland tissue.

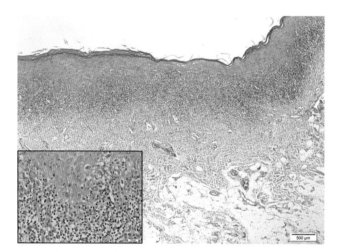

Fig. 11.29 Lichen planus, 100×. A dense band-like lymphocytic infiltrate is seen at the epithelial-stromal interface, with associated hydropic (vacuolar) degeneration of basal keratinocytes and apoptotic bodies (inset, lower left 400×). The histological features of lichen planus can be mimicked by a number of conditions, which include lichenoid contact reactions, lichenoid drug eruptions, chronic graft versus host disease, and lupus erythematosus. Careful clinicopathological correlation is essential at arriving at the correct diagnosis. (Image courtesy of Prof. Jos Hille, University of the Western Cape.)

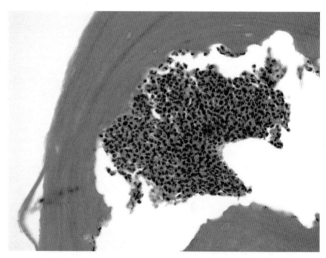

Fig. 11.31 Osteomyelitis, 400×. The marrow space contains a dense collection of neutrophils. The surrounding nonvital bone shows loss of osteocytes from the lacunae and peripheral "moth-eaten" areas of resorption (an attempt by the osteoclasts to remove the dead bone). Osteomyelitis commonly involves the mandible and is associated with trauma or spread of infection from an odontogenic focus.

Benign Epithelial Tumors

- Laryngeal papilloma (Fig. 11.48)
- In situ hybridization for human papillomavirus (HPV) (Fig. 11.49)

Malignant Epithelial Tumors

- Squamous cell carcinoma of the larynx with thyroid cartilage invasion (Fig. 11.50)
- Papillary squamous cell carcinoma (Fig. 11.51)
- Spindle cell (sarcomatoid) carcinoma (Fig. 11.52)

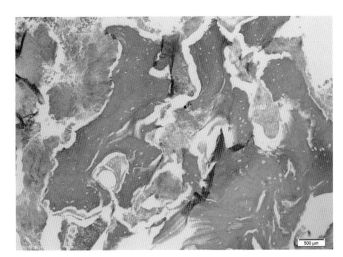

Fig. 11.32 Osteoradionecrosis, 40×. Necrotic bone with loss of osteocytes from the lacunae and peripheral ragged areas of resorption. The dead bone is surrounded by basophilic bacterial colonies consistent with *Actinomyces* spp. The diagnosis of osteoradionecrosis requires history of prior irradiation because the histological picture is identical to osteomyelitis of bacterial origin.

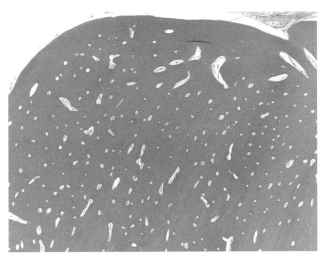

Fig. 11.34 Osteoma, 20×. The lesion is well circumscribed and consists of dense, mature cortical bone. Osteomas are histologically classified into compact (cortical) and spongy (trabecular) types. Multiple osteomas are seen in the setting of Gardner syndrome, an autosomal-dominant disorder characterized by gastrointestinal (GI) polyps and skin and soft-tissue tumors. The GI polyps have a 100% risk of undergoing malignant transformation.

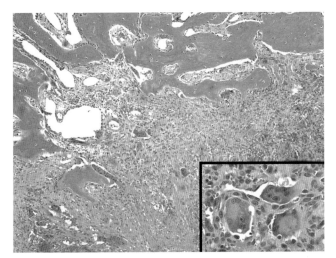

Fig. 11.33 Central giant cell lesion (giant cell reparative granuloma), 40×. Plump cytologically bland spindled cells, osteoclast-like multinucleated giant cells, and extravasated red blood cells (inset lower right, 400×). Reactive bone is seen at the advancing front of the lesion. These are commonly seen in young adults and frequently involve the mandible. Before a diagnosis of central giant cell lesion is rendered, other entities with identical histology should be excluded. These include the brown tumor of hyperparathyroidism, cherubism, aneurysmal bone cyst, and peripheral giant cell granuloma.

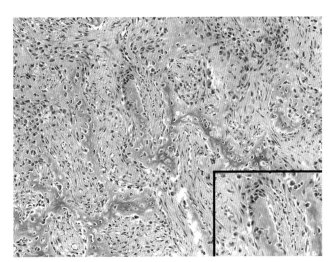

Fig. 11.35 Osteosarcoma, osteoblastic type, 100×. Atypical osteoblasts with lace-like areas of osteoid (malignant bone) deposition. A few malignant osteoblasts are entrapped within the osteoid (inset lower right, 400×). Osteosarcoma is the most common primary malignancy of bone. In the head and neck, osteosarcomas commonly arise in the mandible and may present as rapidly enlarging painful lesions with loose teeth. Tumors may show extensive fibroblastic or chondroblastic differentiation.

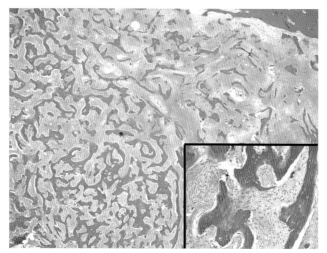

Fig. 11.36 Fibrous dysplasia, 20×. Fibrous stroma and irregular trabeculae of bone that are said to resemble Chinese characters. The bony trabeculae lack osteoblastic rimming (inset lower right, 400×). Fibrous dysplasia is a developmental fibro-osseous lesion with mutations involving the *GNAS-1* gene. It can be monostotic (involving a single bone only) or polyostotic. The polyostotic form can be associated with endocrine disorders, most commonly precocious puberty.

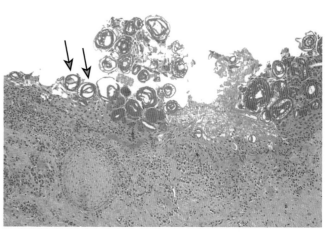

Fig. 11.38 Periapical (radicular) cyst, 100×. The cyst is lined by stratified squamous epithelium with Rushton (hyaline) bodies (eosinophilic curved glassy structures, *arrows*). A dense chronic inflammatory cell infiltrate is seen immediately beneath the cyst lining. The periapical cyst is an inflammatory odontogenic cyst, seen at the apex of a non vital tooth.

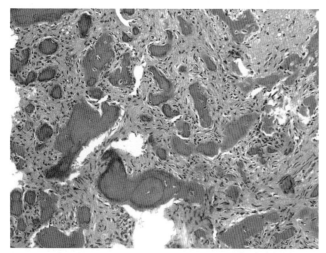

Fig. 11.37 Ossifying fibroma, 100×. The image shows dense fibrous tissue, short trabeculae of bone, and numerous rounded psammomatoid (calcified psammoma body-like) deposits. Ossifying fibroma is a neoplastic fibro-osseous lesion. All fibro-osseous lesions (fibrous dysplasia, osseous dysplasia, and ossifying fibroma) share similar histology and require clinical and radiological correlation.

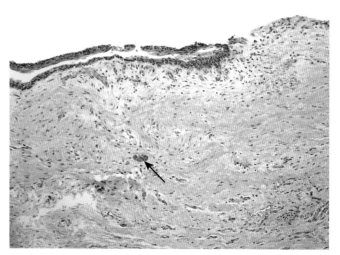

Fig. 11.39 Dentigerous cyst, 100×. The cyst is lined by a thin epithelium that resembles the reduced enamel epithelium of a developing tooth. Small islands of odontogenic epithelium (*arrow*) are sometimes seen in the connective tissue wall of the cyst. A dentigerous cyst is a developmental odontogenic cyst and is associated with the crown of an unerupted tooth.

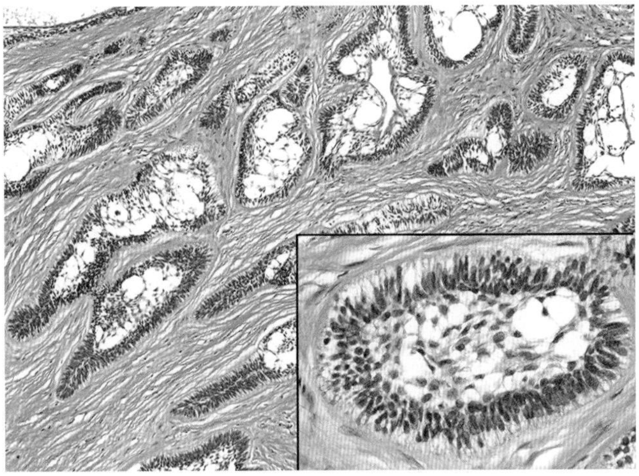

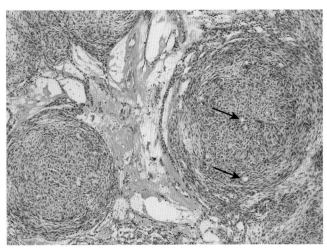

Fig. 11.40 Solid/multicystic ameloblastoma, 100×. The tumor shows a follicular growth pattern. The follicles are bordered by ameloblast-like cells with reverse nuclear polarity (inset lower right, 400×). The center-most areas often demonstrate cystic degeneration and are characterized by loosely connected cells, stellate reticulum-like cells. The stellate cells may display squamous (acanthomatous), granular, or basal cell differentiation.

Fig. 11.42 Adenomatoid odontogenic tumor, 100×. Solid nests of spindle-shaped epithelial cells. The solid nests contain duct-like structures (rosettes) lined by a single row of columnar epithelial cells (*arrows*). Adenomatoid odontogenic tumor is considered to be a hamartoma rather than a true neoplasm. It is commonly seen in the anterior segments of the jaw and usually surrounds the crown of an unerupted tooth.

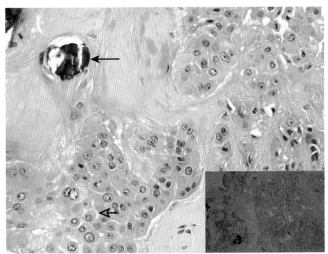

Fig. 11.41 Calcifying epithelial odontogenic tumor, 200×. Rounded squamoid (squamous-like) cells with dense eosinophilic cytoplasm, hyperchromatic, moderately pleomorphic nuclei, and prominent nucleoli. Intercellular bridges are clearly visible (*arrow*). The cells surround globules of pale acellular eosinophilic material (amyloid) with a focus of calcification (*arrow*). The amyloid demonstrates an apple-green birefringence when viewed under polarized light (inset lower right, 40×).

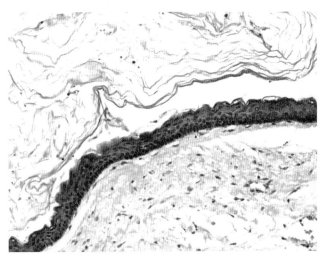

Fig. 11.43 Odontogenic keratocyst, 200×. The cyst is lined by a thin squamous epithelium with a distinct palisaded basal layer and a superficial corrugated layer of parakeratin. The lumen contains abundant laminated keratin. Multiple odontogenic keratocysts occur in the setting of Gorlin (nevoid basal cell carcinoma) syndrome, an autosomal-dominant disorder associated with mutation of the *PTCH1* gene.

Neuroendocrine Carcinoma

- Poorly differentiated neuroendocrine carcinoma (small cell carcinoma) (Fig. 11.53)

Mesenchymal Tumors

- Low-grade chondrosarcoma (Fig. 11.54)

NOSE, PARANASAL SINUSES, AND NASOPHARYNX

Inflammatory and Infectious Lesions

- Chronic rhinosinusitis (Fig. 11.55)
- Allergic fungal sinusitis (Fig. 11.56)
- Invasive fungal sinusitis (Fig. 11.57)
- Inflammatory nasal polyp (Fig. 11.58)
- Rhinosporidiosis (Fig. 11.59)

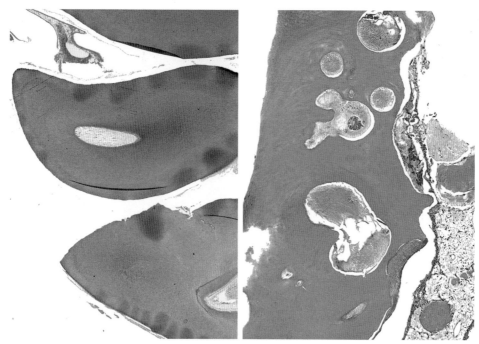

Fig. 11.44 Compound odontoma. Formation of two miniature tooth-like structures (odontoids) (left image, 40×). Odontomas are considered to be hamartomatous rather than truly neoplastic. There are two forms: compound odontoma and complex odontoma. When complex, they are composed of a disorganized mass of mineralized material with no resemblance to a tooth (image right, 100×).

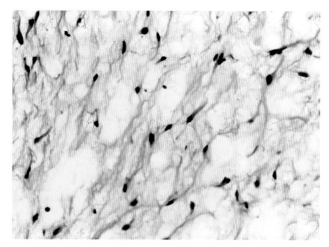

Fig. 11.45 Odontogenic myxoma, 400×. The tumor is relatively hypocellular and consists of bland spindle-shaped cells suspended in a myxoid stroma.

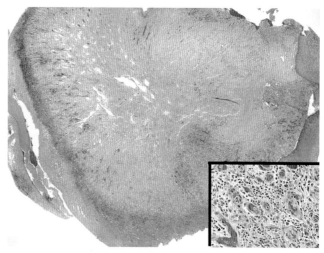

Fig. 11.46 Contact ulcer of the larynx (contact granuloma), 20×. Polypoid lesion with surface ulceration. The majority of the lesion consists of granulation tissue with vessels arranged in radial spokes (inset lower right, 400×). Contact ulcers form in response to mechanical or chemical trauma.

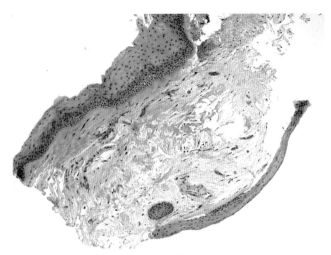

Fig. 11.47 Vocal cord polyp, 40×. Polypoid squamous tissue with an underlying myxoid stroma. The stroma may be hyalinized or hemorrhagic with fibrin. Depending on the chronicity of the lesion, more chronic changes such as ossification or atypical stromal fibroblasts may be seen in longer-standing lesions.

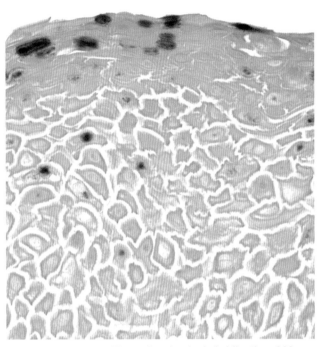

Fig. 11.49 Human papillomavirus in situ hybridization, 200×. Laryngeal papillomas are caused by infection of the mucosa with human papillomavirus types 6 or 11.

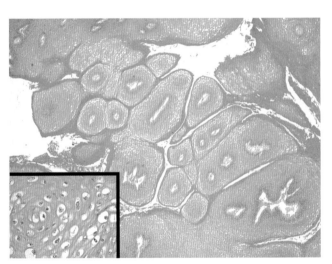

Fig. 11.48 Laryngeal papilloma, 20×. Exophytic projections of keratinizing squamous epithelium with fibrovascular cores. Koilocytes, human papillomavirus (HPV)–induced cytopathic changes, are seen in the superficial layers of the epithelium (inset lower left, 400×). They may be binucleated and contain clear cytoplasm and wrinkled, or raisinoid, nuclei. Papillomas are caused by low-risk HPV type 6 or 11. Squamous papillomas of the larynx may be solitary or multiple. Multiple lesions (laryngeal papillomatosis) are more common in young patients. Squamous papillomas are benign and do not generally transform to carcinoma.

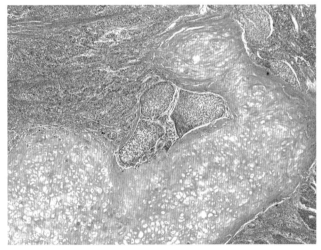

Fig. 11.50 Squamous cell carcinoma (SCC) of the larynx, 40×. The image shows invasion of the thyroid cartilage by moderately differentiated islands of SCC.

Hamartomatous and Heterotopic Lesions

- Nasal glial heterotopia (Fig. 11.60)
- Dermoid cyst (Fig. 11.61)
- Respiratory epithelial adenomatoid hamartoma (Fig. 11.62)

Epithelial and Neuroepithelial Tumors

- Inverted papilloma (inverted papilloma, Schneiderian type; Fig. 11.63)
- Schneiderian carcinoma (nonkeratinizing sinonasal carcinoma) (Fig. 11.64)
- Nasopharyngeal carcinoma (Fig. 11.65)
- Sinonasal undifferentiated carcinoma (SNUC; Fig. 11.66)
- Sinonasal adenocarcinoma, intestinal type (ITAC; Fig. 11.67)
- Olfactory neuroblastoma (esthesioneuroblastoma; Fig. 11.68)
- Sinonasal meningioma (Fig. 11.69)

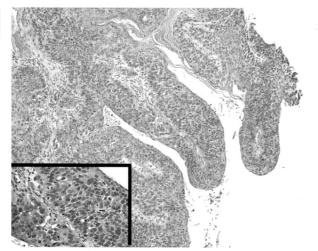

Fig. 11.51 Papillary squamous cell carcinoma (SCC), 40×. The tumor is exophytic and has a papillary architecture, reminiscent of squamous papilloma. However, the papillary fronds are covered by severely stratified squamous epithelium (inset lower left, 400×). This uncommon variant of SCC is most often seen in the larynx, oropharynx, and sinonasal tract. In some cases, it is associated with high-risk human papillomavirus infection.

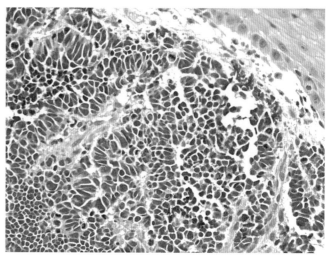

Fig. 11.53 Small cell carcinoma or poorly differentiated neuroendocrine carcinoma, 200×. Small cell carcinoma located beneath the normal-appearing epithelium. The cytomorphological features are similar to those of pulmonary small cell carcinomas, with nuclear molding, granular chromatin, frequent mitoses, and apoptotic bodies. They are most commonly seen in middle-aged to elderly men and carry a dismal prognosis. The diagnosis is confirmed by immunohistochemical demonstration of neuroendocrine differentiation using markers such as synaptophysin.

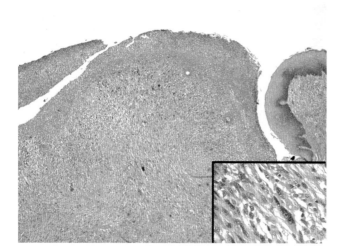

Fig. 11.52 Spindle cell (sarcomatoid) squamous cell carcinoma (SCC), 20×. The tumor has a polypoid appearance with surface ulceration, and it contains highly atypical spindled cells in a fascicular arrangement (inset lower right, 400×). Spindle cell SCCs often show foci of squamous differentiation or surface dysplasia. When absent, a definitive diagnosis can be difficult to obtain, and the differential diagnosis includes sarcoma and spindle cell melanoma. In such cases, ancillary testing may be of some assistance, but additional clinical information may be crucial.

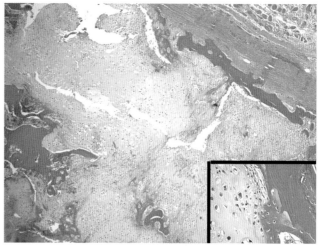

Fig. 11.54 Well-differentiated (low-grade) chondrosarcoma of the thyroid cartilage, 20×. The tumor is composed of well-formed hyaline cartilage. In comparison with normal cartilage, the tumor is more cellular, with nuclear pleomorphism and hyperchromasia (inset lower right, 400×). Binucleated chondrocytes are frequently observed in laryngeal chondrosarcomas (not shown). Low-grade tumors share similar morphology with chondromas and are essentially diagnosed based on their infiltrative growth pattern.

Malignant Lymphoid and Melanocytic Lesions

- Natural killer/T-cell lymphoma, nasal type (Fig. 11.70)
- Sinonasal melanoma (Fig. 11.71)

Mesenchymal Lesions

- Angiofibroma (Fig. 11.72)
- Glomangiopericytoma (Fig. 11.73)
- Chordoma (Fig. 11.74)
- Rhabdomyosarcoma (Figs. 11.75 and 11.76)

Immune-Mediated Lesions

- Wegener granulomatosis (Figs. 11.77 and 11.78)

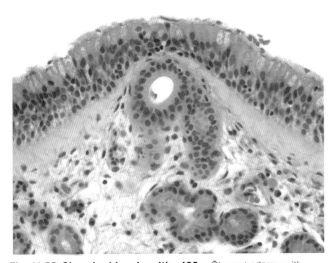

Fig. 11.55 Chronic rhinosinusitis, 400×. Stromal edema with chronic inflammatory cells. The chronic nature of the disease is marked by subepithelial hyalinization.

SALIVARY GLANDS

Vascular Malformation

- Hemangioma (Fig. 11.79)

Inflammatory and Lymphoid Lesions

- Lymphoepithelial cyst (Fig. 11.80)
- Mucosa-associated lymphoid tissue lymphoma (Fig. 11.81)
- Chronic sclerosing sialadenitis associated with IgG4 disease (Mikulicz disease) (Fig. 11.82)

Benign Tumors

- Pleomorphic adenoma (Fig. 11.83)
- Basal cell adenoma (Fig. 11.84)
- Warthin tumor (Fig. 11.85)

Malignant Tumors

- Adenoid cystic carcinoma (Fig. 11.86)
- Polymorphous low-grade adenocarcinoma (Fig. 11.87)
- Mucoepidermoid carcinoma (Fig. 11.88)
- Mucoepidermoid carcinoma (mucicarmine stain) (Fig. 11.89)
- Acinic cell carcinoma (Figs. 11.90 and 11.91)
- Epithelial-myoepithelial carcinoma (Fig. 11.92)
- Carcinoma ex-pleomorphic adenoma (Fig. 11.93)
- Salivary duct carcinoma (Fig. 11.94)

EAR

External Ear

- Branchial cleft cyst (Fig. 11.95)
- Chondrodermatitis nodularis chronicus helicis (Fig. 11.96)
- Basal cell carcinoma (Fig. 11.97)
- Ceruminous adenoma (Fig. 11.98)

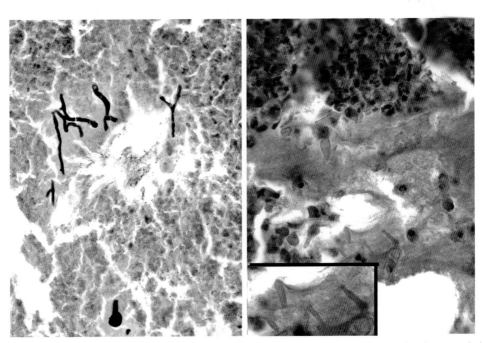

Fig. 11.56 Allergic fungal sinusitis. Abundant mucus with numerous entrapped eosinophils and Charcot-Leyden crystals (allergic mucus; right image, 200×). The silver stain shows occasional fungal hyphae (left image, 400×).

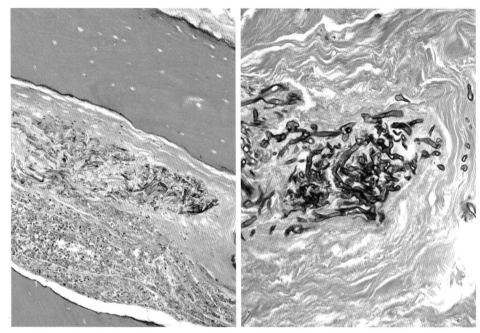

Fig. 11.57 Invasive fungal sinusitis. Fragments of nonvital bone adjacent to a necrotic marrow cavity containing granular debris, neutrophils, and thick nonseptate fungal hyphae, consistent with Mucor (left, 100×). Thick nonseptate fungal hyphae are seen within the lumen of a blood vessel (methenamine silver stain, right, 400×). Vascular invasion is often associated with necrosis, hemorrhage, and inflammation. The condition is generally seen in immunocompromised patients (e.g., in the setting of diabetes, human immunodeficiency virus [HIV] or lymphoid malignancies), often caused by fungi of the order Mucorales (e.g., Rhizopus and Mucor).

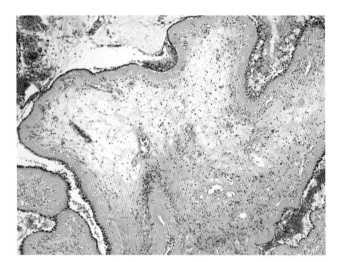

Fig. 11.58 Inflammatory nasal polyp, 40×. The polyp is lined by respiratory epithelium, with marked subepithelial hyalinization and stromal edema with an inflammatory background.

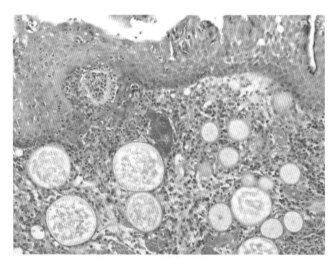

Fig. 11.59 Rhinosporidiosis, 200×. Thick-walled, rounded, variably sized cyst-like structures (sporangia) (10–200 μm in diameter), filled with small spores. Rhinosporidiosis is caused by the fungus *Rhinosporidium seeberi* and is endemic to South India and Sri Lanka. The disease usually presents as a unilateral polypoid lesion.

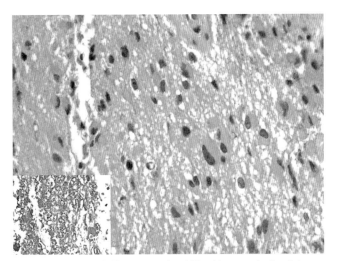

Fig. 11.60 Nasal glial heterotopia, 400×. Nonneoplastic glial tissue found within the nasal cavity separate from the central nervous system. The glial tissue can be difficult to appreciate on hematoxylin and eosin sections. Immunostaining with antibodies to S100 protein or glial fibrillary acidic protein can be helpful in identifying the glial component (inset lower left, 400×).

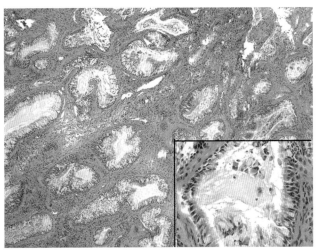

Fig. 11.62 Respiratory epithelial adenomatoid hamartoma, 40×. Numerous glandular structures lined by ciliated columnar cells and occasional mucus cells (inset lower right, 400×). The glands contain mucus. The stroma exhibits dense chronic inflammation. Clinically, the lesions are polypoid and usually involve the posterior nasal septum.

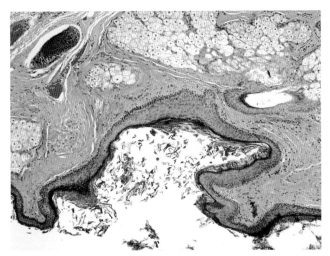

Fig. 11.61 Dermoid cyst, 100×. The cyst is lined by keratin, producing squamous epithelium with a prominent granular cell layer. The cyst wall contains hair follicles and sebaceous glands. Dermoid cysts are usually midline cysts and occur in a number of locations within the head and neck region. They contain ectodermal and mesodermal elements. Nasal dermoids are often seen at the dorsum of the nose.

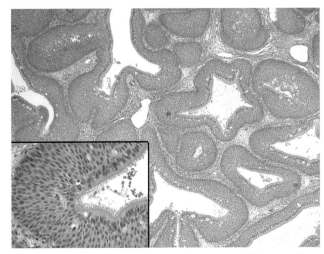

Fig. 11.63 Inverted papilloma, 40×. The tumor exhibits an endophytic growth with islands of transitional-type epithelium containing occasional mucus cells and small collections of neutrophils. Respiratory cells overlie the transitional epithelium (inset lower left, 400×). A distinct basal layer is observed, and there is rarely atypia

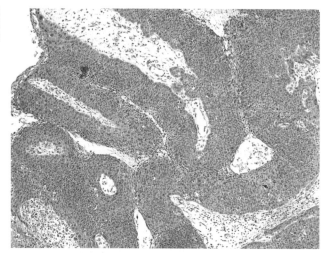

Fig. 11.64 Sinonasal squamous cell carcinoma, nonkeratinizing type (Schneiderian carcinoma), 100×. The tumor shows a plexiform or ribbon-like growth pattern and full-thickness severe epithelial atypia, and it lacks keratinization. Tumors may be positive for high-risk human papillomavirus.

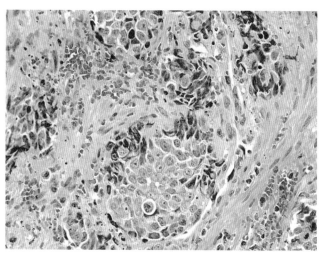

Fig. 11.66 Sinonasal undifferentiated carcinoma (SNUC), 400×. Nests of undifferentiated medium-sized to large-sized cells. The hyperchromatic nuclei are round to oval shaped and pleomorphic, and they show prominent nucleoli. SNUC is a rare, highly aggressive malignancy arising in the sinonasal tract. Patients usually present with signs and symptoms secondary to local invasion (e.g., proptosis, pain, anosmia, and diplopia). Because many tumors in this region appear histologically similar, the diagnosis of SNUC, a diagnosis of exclusion, is generally conferred following a battery of immunohistochemical stains.

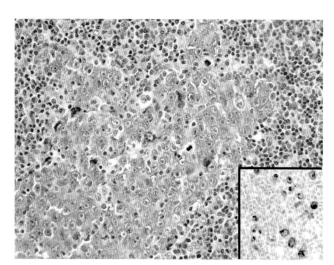

Fig. 11.65 Nasopharyngeal carcinoma, nonkeratinizing types, 400×. An island of undifferentiated cells with indistinct cell borders (syncytial pattern) associated with dense lymphoid stroma. The tumor cells have large nuclei with open chromatin and prominent nucleoli. Almost all nonkeratinizing nasopharyngeal carcinomas are radiosensitive and Epstein-Barr early mRNA (EBER)–positive (inset lower right, 400×).

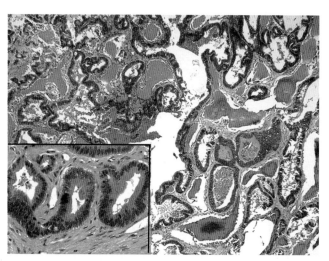

Fig. 11.67 Intestinal-type sinonasal adenocarcinoma, 40×. The tumor has a papillary-tubular architecture, similar to the pattern seen in many colorectal adenocarcinomas (inset, 400×). Glands are lined by tall columnar cells with elongated hyperchromatic nuclei that appear stratified. Intestinal-type adenocarcinomas have been linked to exposure to hardwood and dust particles and show an exceptionally high recurrence rate (here shown infiltrating bone).

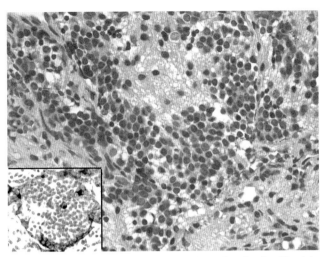

Fig. 11.68 Olfactory neuroblastoma, 400×. Small cells with minimal cytoplasm are suspended in an eosinophilic fibrillary background. The nuclei are monomorphic and round, with fine granular chromatin. Prominent nucleoli and mitotic figures are not seen. Immunostaining with S100 protein is confined to the slender sustentacular (supporting) cells that surround the groups of neoplastic cells (inset lower left, 400×). Olfactory neuroblastomas develop in the upper nasal cavity in the region of the olfactory epithelium near the cribriform plate.

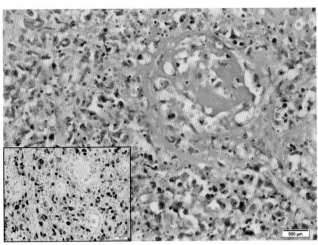

Fig. 11.70 Extranodal NK/T-cell lymphoma, nasal type, 400×. The image shows a blood vessel surrounded and invaded by atypical lymphoid cells with irregular nuclear contours (angiocentricity and angioinvasion). Positive ISH for EBER is seen with this extranodal NK/T-cell lymphoma (inset lower left, 400×). NK/T-cell lymphomas usually present as midline destructive lesions. NK/T-cell lymphoma is an aggressive malignancy that carries a poor prognosis.

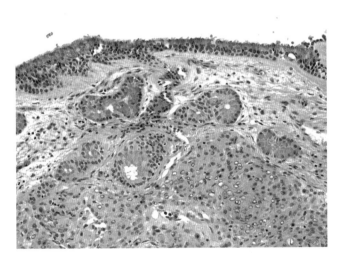

Fig. 11.69 Sinonasal meningioma, 100×. Whorled nodules of bland spindled cells are seen within the nasal mucosa. The spindled cells have abundant eosinophilic cytoplasm and oval nuclei with intranuclear pseudoinclusions. Sinonasal meningiomas are rare and usually involve the nasal cavity and paranasal sinuses.

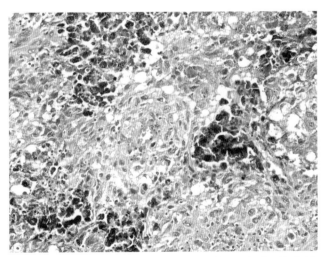

Fig. 11.71 Sinonasal melanoma, 200×. Highly atypical epithelioid and spindled cells with abundant intracytoplasmic melanin pigment (*dark-brown*). Sinonasal melanomas arise from melanocytes resident within the nasal epithelium. Clinically, they may present as a nasal polyp. Unlike skin melanomas, the depth of invasion does not correlate with biological behavior. Immunohistochemical stains for S-100, HMB-45, and other markers are used to confirm the diagnosis, but often MiTF is the most useful.

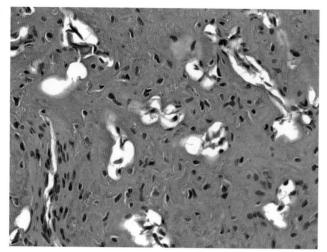

Fig. 11.72 Angiofibroma, 400×. The tumor is composed of variably sized blood vessels and moderately cellular fibrous tissue, with bland spindled cells. Angiofibromas predominantly affect male adolescents, arise from the posterior lateral nasal wall, and often present with nasal obstruction and epistaxis. Patients with familial adenomatous polyposis are more likely to have angiofibromas, suggesting that mutations of the *APC* gene may be involved in the pathogenesis of these lesions.

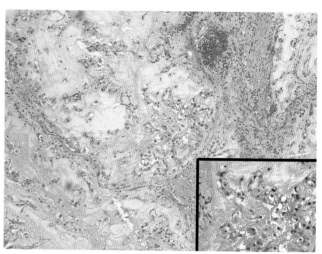

Fig. 11.74 Chordoma, 40×. Lobules of myxoid material containing characteristic vacuolated (physaliferous) cells (inset lower right, 400×). Chordomas are believed to be of notochordal origin. In the head and neck, they develop in the skull base and may extend to involve the nasopharynx, nasal cavity, paranasal sinuses, or maxilla secondarily.

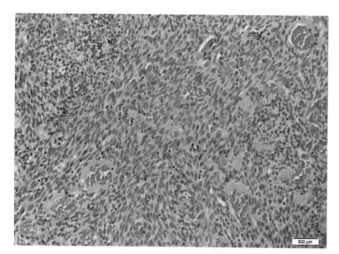

Fig. 11.73 Glomangiopericytoma, 200×. Sheet-like arrangement of monotonous rounded cells without distinct cell borders (syncytial pattern). The cells surround irregular vascular structures. In some areas, the cells are spindled, and they demonstrate a fascicular growth (upper right and lower left). Glomangiopericytomas arise within the nasal cavity or paranasal sinuses and show a smooth muscle phenotype. This is a benign lesion usually cured by excision but on rare occasions can exhibit aggressive behavior.

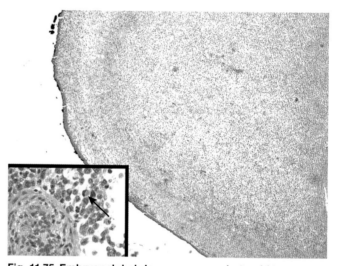

Fig. 11.75 Embryonal rhabdomyosarcoma, botryoid type, 400×. The tumor presents as a nasal polyp, covered with respiratory-type epithelium. The polyp contains a solid growth of small blue cells with minimal cytoplasm that are concentrated at the periphery of the polyp, immediately beneath the epithelium (cambium layer). A cell with abundant eosinophilic cytoplasm, a "differentiating" rhabdomyoblast, is seen in a background of cells with little cytoplasm (*arrow*, inset lower left).

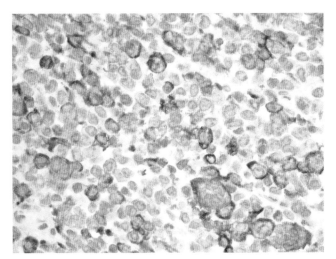

Fig. 11.76 Embryonal rhabdomyosarcoma, desmin immuno-histochemistry, 400×. Embryonal rhabdomyosarcomas are more common in children, and they display skeletal muscle differentiation. Tumor cells are positive for antibodies to muscle-specific proteins: desmin, myogenin, myoglobin, and myo-D1, with the latter three being more specific for skeletal muscle differentiation.

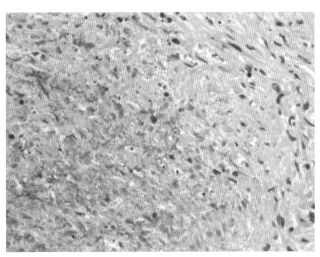

Fig. 11.78 Wegener granulomatosis, 400×. A characteristic feature is fibrinoid/granular degeneration of collagen.

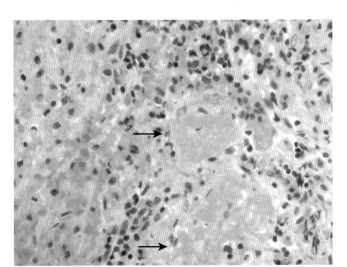

Fig. 11.77 Wegener granulomatosis (granulomatosis with polyangitis), 400×. The walls of the blood vessels seen in this image are largely destroyed by the inflammatory process (*arrows*). This is an immune-mediated systemic vasculitic process, and patients often have elevated serum antineutrophil cytoplasmic antibodies (C-ANCA).

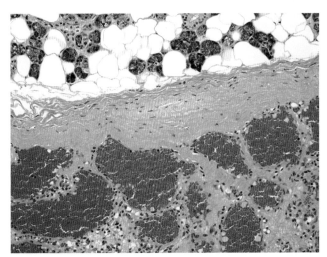

Fig. 11.79 Hemangioma of the parotid gland, 200×. The image shows benign parotid tissue and densely packed blood-filled vascular channels. Hemangiomas are generally classified into capillary and cavernous types depending on the size of the blood vessels.

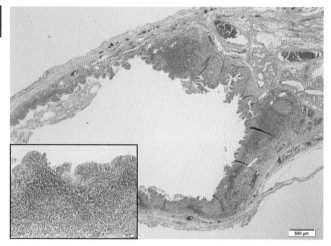

Fig. 11.80 Lymphoepithelial cyst, 40×. The cyst is lined by ciliated epithelium (inset lower left, 400x). Dense lymphoid tissue with lymphoid follicles is seen directly beneath the epithelial lining. A separate and distinct pattern of multiple small lymphoepithelial cysts is a widely recognized cause of parotid swelling in HIV-infected patients.

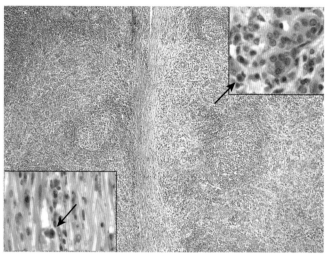

Fig. 11.82 Immunoglobulin G4 (IgG4)–related sialadenitis. This low-power image shows marked cellular fibrosis and chronic inflammation with follicle formation and loss of submandibular gland acini. The residual ducts (inset upper right) and the fibrotic areas (inset lower left, 40×) show an increased number of plasma cells (*arrows*, 400×). The plasma cells show strong cytoplasmic staining with IgG4 antibody. The lesion formerly referred to as *chronic sclerosing sialadenitis* (*Kuttner tumor*) was treated by excision. IgG4-related sialadenitis is a systemic immune-mediated disease that responds to corticosteroid therapy.

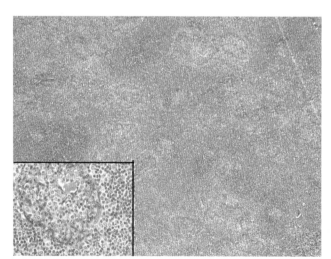

Fig. 11.81 Extranodal marginal zone lymphoma, 20×. Destruction of the parotid gland architecture by a diffuse lymphoid infiltrate. The lymphoepithelial islands (consisting of neoplastic lymphoid cells and metaplastic parotid gland ducts) are widely separated by the neoplastic lymphoid infiltrate. The inset shows an epithelial island being surrounded and infiltrated by malignant lymphoid cells with pale cytoplasm and small irregular, folded nuclei (400×). The tumors occur more frequently in older women and in patients with a prior history of Sjögren syndrome.

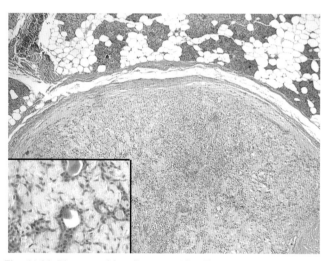

Fig. 11.83 Pleomorphic adenoma, 40×. The tumor is well circumscribed by a fibrous capsule and is sharply demarcated from the adjacent parotid gland tissue. The tumor consists of a combination of myoepithelial cells and small ducts within a chondromyxoid stroma (inset lower left, 400×). The myoepithelial cells can be spindled, epithelioid, plasmacytoid, or have clear cytoplasm. Pleomorphic adenoma is the most common benign salivary gland tumor.

Middle Ear

- Otic polyp (Fig. 11.99)
- Cholesteatoma (Fig. 11.100)
- Encephalocele (Fig. 11.101)
- Middle ear adenoma/carcinoid (Fig. 11.102)
- Paraganglioma (Fig. 11.103)

Inner Ear

- Vestibular schwannoma (Fig. 11.104)

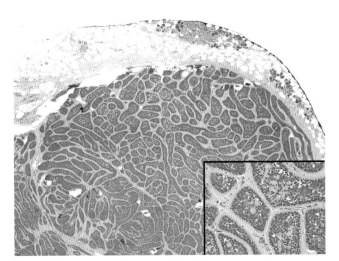

Fig. 11.84 Basal cell adenoma, 20×. The tumor is well circum-scribed and is composed of variably shaped nests of cytologically bland basaloid cells arranged in a "jigsaw puzzle" pattern. The tumor cell nests are surrounded by an acellular eosinophilic basement-mem-brane-like material (inset lower right, 400×). Nuclear palisading is noted at the periphery of tumor cell nests. Basal cell adenomas are primarily distinguished from basal cell adenocarcinomas by their lack of invasion.

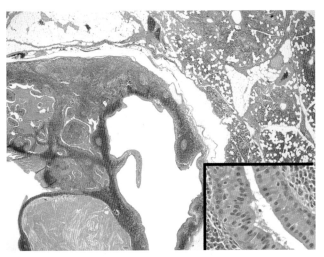

Fig. 11.85 Warthin tumor, 40×. A papillary projection can be seen protruding into a cystic space. The papillary projections are lined by a double layer of cuboidal to columnar oncocytic epithelial cells, with ample pink, granular cytoplasm and nuclei with a central, prominent nucleolus and an underlying lymphoid stroma (inset lower right, 400×). This pattern is very characteristic of this tumor.

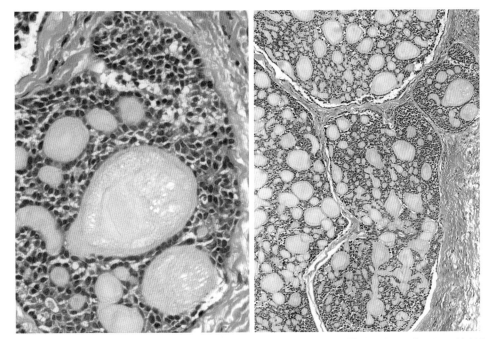

Fig. 11.86 Adenoid cystic carcinoma (ADCC), 40×. ADCCs typically show a cribriform, or "Swiss cheese," pattern (right image). The neo-plastic myoepithelial cells, with their hyperchromatic small angulated nuclei, surround rounded spaces containing acid mucopolysaccharidoses (left image, 200×). ADCC is the second most common malignant neoplasm of the seromucinous glands of the upper aerodigestive tract. They are often painful lesions because of their frequent perineural invasion. The disease follows a protracted course, with poor long-term survival.

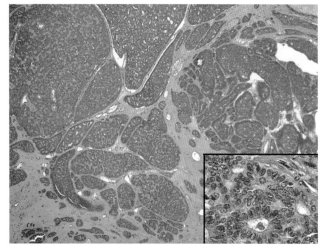

Fig. 11.87 Polymorphous adenocarcinoma, 20×. The tumor shows polymorphous growth with solid, cribriform, and tubular architectural growth patterns. Despite the architectural diversity, individual tumor cells are monomorphic, displaying bland round-to-oval nuclei with vesicular chromatin and inconspicuous nucleoli (inset lower right, 400×). The tumor occurs almost exclusively in minor salivary glands and most commonly involves the junction of the hard and soft palate in middle-aged women.

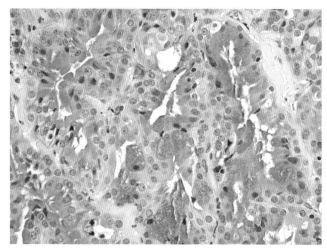

Fig. 11.89 Mucoepidermoid carcinoma, mucicarmine stain, 400×. A mucicarmine stain is used to highlight goblet-shaped mucus cells containing intracellular mucin in mucoepidermoid carcinoma.

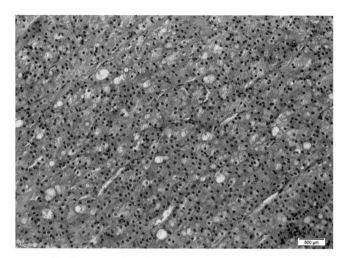

Fig. 11.90 Acinic cell carcinoma, 200×. The tumour exhibits distinct acinar differentiation, with neoplastic acinar cells having numerous blue-purple cytoplasmic zymogen secretory granules. Acinic cell carcinomas closely recapitulate the acinar tissue of a normal salivary gland, however a normal lobular pattern is not found within the tumour, an important clue to the diagnosis.

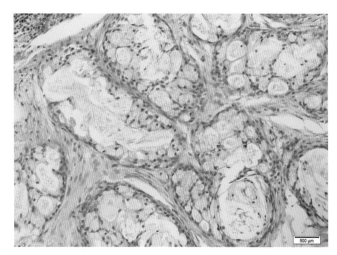

Fig. 11.88 Mucoepidermoid carcinoma, low grade, 200×. The image shows nests with abundant neoplastic mucocytes with few basaloid intermediate cells. High grade mucoepidermoid carcinomas usually demonstrate an abundance of squamoid cells (not seen here), and histologically mimic a squamous cell carcinoma. Mucoepidermoid carcinoma is the most common salivary gland malignancy in both children and adults. A majority of cases show a characteristic chromosomal translocation t (11;19) (q21;p13), leading to the MECT1/MAML2 fusion protein.

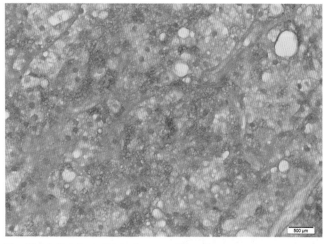

Fig. 11.91 Acinic cell carcinoma, 400×. The cytoplasmic zymogen granules are periodic acid Schiff positive and diastase resistant.

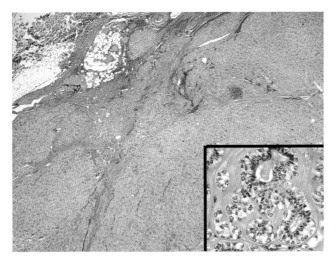

Fig. 11.92 Epithelial-myoepithelial carcinoma, 20×. The tumor is invasive and shows tubular growth. The tubules are lined by an inner layer of eosinophilic ductal cells and an outer layer of myoepithelial cells that exhibit abundant clear cytoplasm and large round eccentrically located nuclei with prominent nucleoli (inset lower right, 400×).

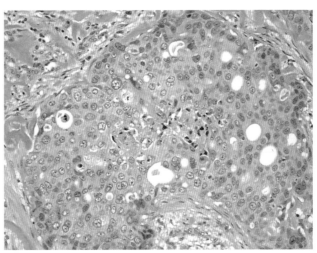

Fig. 11.94 Salivary duct carcinoma, 400×. Salivary duct carcinomas are histologically similar to infiltrating ductal carcinomas of the breast. The image shows a nest of tumor cells with comedo-type necrosis and rounded cystic spaces. The cells have abundant eosinophilic cytoplasm and exhibit large pleomorphic round nuclei with prominent nucleoli. Salivary duct carcinomas are high-grade malignancies that most commonly involve the parotid glands of elderly men.

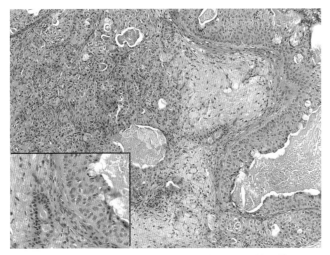

Fig. 11.93 Carcinoma ex-pleomorphic adenoma, 20×. The image shows a mixture of pleomorphic adenoma with chondromyxoid stroma and benign glandular elements, along with highly atypical glands of a carcinoma (in this case, a mucoepidermoid carcinoma; inset lower left, 400×). The type of carcinoma developing in a pleomorphic adenoma is not always classifiable (carcinoma, not otherwise specified) and is often high grade. Salivary duct carcinoma is the most common malignant component. Carcinoma ex-pleomorphic adenoma is further classified into in situ, minimally invasive, and invasive.

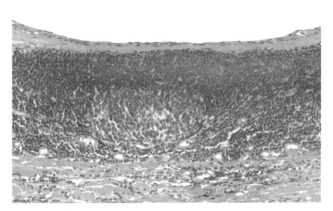

Fig. 11.95 Branchial cleft cyst, 200×. The cyst is lined by a thin and flattened squamous epithelium that overlies a dense lymphoid infiltrate with lymphoid follicles. First branchial cleft cysts are usually seen anterior to the tragus and sometimes contain cartilage.

THYROID AND PARATHYROID GLANDS

Nonneoplastic Lesions

- Thyroglossal duct cyst (Fig. 11.105)
- Hashimoto thyroiditis (Fig. 11.106)
- Graves disease (Fig. 11.107)

Benign Thyroid Tumors

- Follicular adenoma (Fig. 11.108)

Malignant Thyroid Tumors

- Papillary thyroid carcinoma, classical type (Fig. 11.109)
- Papillary thyroid carcinoma, follicular variant (Fig. 11.110)
- Papillary thyroid carcinoma, tall-cell variant (Fig. 11.111)
- Papillary thyroid carcinoma, diffuse sclerosing variant (Fig. 11.112)
- Follicular carcinoma (Fig. 11.113)
- Oncocytic (Hurthle cell) carcinoma (Fig. 11.114)

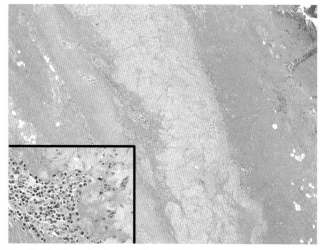

Fig. 11.96 Chondrodermatitis nodularis helicis, 20×. A chronic inflammatory cell infiltrate extends from the skin surface and surrounds the auricular cartilage. The inflammatory cell infiltrate consists predominantly of plasma cells (inset lower left, 400×).

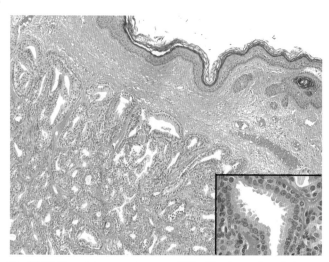

Fig. 11.98 Ceruminous adenoma, 100×. The tumor is well circumscribed, and it shows solid proliferation of cystically dilated glandular structures. The glands are lined by an inner layer of eosinophilic ductal cells that exhibit apical snouting (apocrine differentiation) and an outer layer of basal cells that rest on a thick acellular hyalinized basement membrane (inset lower right, 100×).

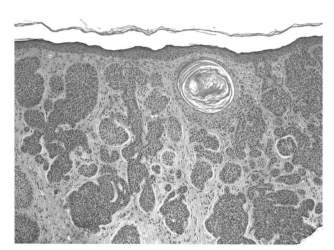

Fig. 11.97 Basal cell carcinoma, 100×. Nests of basaloid cells with peripheral clefting. Nuclear palisading is seen at the periphery of the nests. The tumor is focally attached to the overlying epidermis (upper right). (Courtesy Michelle Forestall Lee, MGH.)

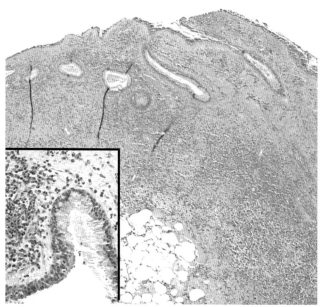

Fig. 11.99 Otic polyp, 40×. The polyp contains granulation tissue, small blood vessels, lymphocytes, and plasma cells. The epithelium covering the polyp may be squamous or columnar (inset lower left, 400×). Otic polyps are usually secondary to otitis media.

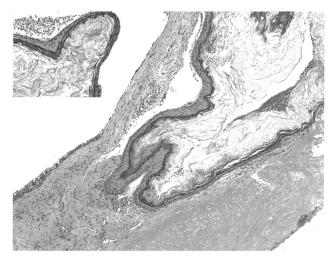

Fig. 11.100 Cholesteatoma. The cholesteatoma is an outpouching of the squamous epithelium on or near the tympanic membrane into the middle ear mucosa, similar to an epidermal inclusion cyst (lower right, 40x). It is composed of keratin debris and stratified squamous epithelium (inset upper left, 400x). Although histologically benign, cholesteatomas are often aggressive and destructive, eroding middle ear ossicles.

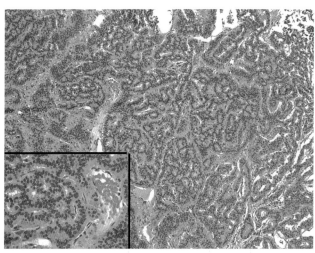

Fig. 11.102 Middle ear adenoma/carcinoid, 40x. Orderly trabeculae of eosinophilic cells with ovoid nuclei. Glandular spaces are readily observed. The nuclei exhibit fine granular chromatin ("salt and pepper") characteristics of neuroendocrine tumors (inset lower left, 200x).

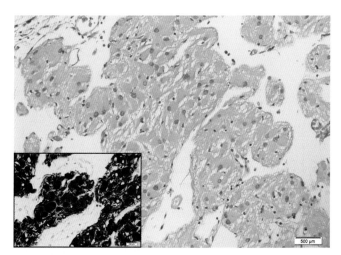

Fig. 11.101 Middle ear encephalocele, 400x. The image shows gemistocytes (reactive astrocytes). An encephalocele is a herniation of brain tissue into the middle ear covered by meninges. The gemistocytes are positive for GFAP (inset lower left, 400x). They arise because of a bony defect in the skull or can be secondary to trauma or surgical intervention.

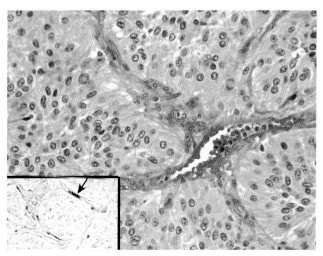

Fig. 11.103 Paraganglioma, 400x. Well-developed nests of epithelioid cells (Zellballen arrangement), surround delicate vascular channels. The round-to-ovoid nuclei exhibit fine granular chromatin and small nucleoli. Supporting the cell nests are the inconspicuous sustentacular cells, best appreciated with S100 immunostain (arrow, inset lower left, 400x). Paragangliomas are negative for epithelial markers such as keratin, helping to distinguish them from neuroendocrine carcinomas.

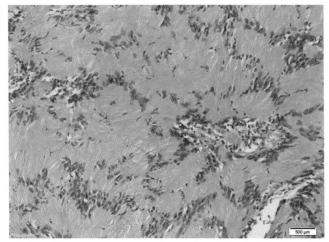

Fig. 11.104 Vestibular schwannoma, 400×. The neoplastic spindled Schwann cells exhibit slender wavy or buckled nuclei with nuclear palisading forming Verocay bodies. Vestibular Schwannomas arise from the eighth cranial nerve. Unilateral lesions are commonly seen in adults, whereas bilateral lesions frequently occur in younger patients with neurofibromatosis type 2. (Image courtesy of Dr. Johan Opperman, University of the Western Cape.)

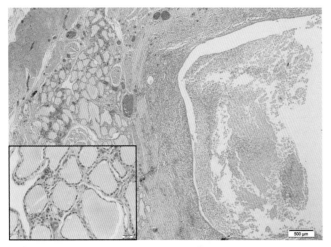

Fig. 11.105 Thyroglossal duct cyst, 100×. The cyst is lined by ciliated, cuboidal, or squamous epithelium. Skeletal muscle and thyroid follicles are seen in the connective tissue wall of the cyst (inset lower left, 400×). Thyroglossal duct cysts present as midline neck masses that are closely associated with the hyoid bone. Lesions move vertically upon swallowing.

- Poorly differentiated carcinoma (Fig. 11.115)
- Medullary thyroid carcinoma (Fig. 11.116)
- Anaplastic thyroid carcinoma (Fig. 11.117)

Parathyroid

- Parathyroid adenoma (Fig. 11.118)
- Parathyroid carcinoma (Fig. 11.119)

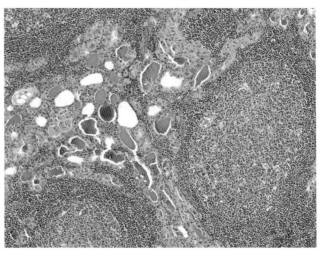

Fig. 11.106 Hashimoto thyroiditis, 200×. The follicular cells show oncocytic features and are surrounded by a dense lymphoid stroma with prominent lymphoid follicles.

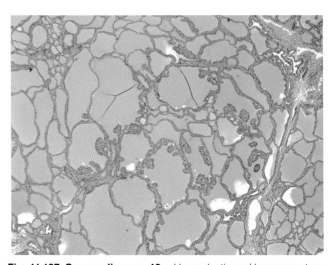

Fig. 11.107 Graves disease, 40×. Hyperplastic and hypersecretory thyroid tissue with irregularly shaped thyroid follicles. Small, poorly formed papillary projections extend into the irregular thyroid follicles.

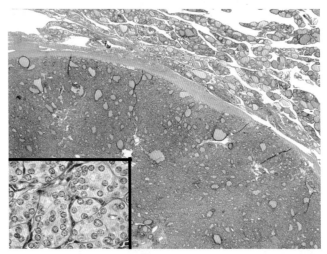

Fig. 11.108 Follicular adenoma, 20×. A well-defined capsule separates the tumor from the surrounding thyroid gland. There is no evidence of invasion. The follicular epithelial cells are arranged in small follicles (inset lower left, 400×). The follicular cells have uniform small round nuclei with fine granular chromatin and small inconspicuous nucleoli.

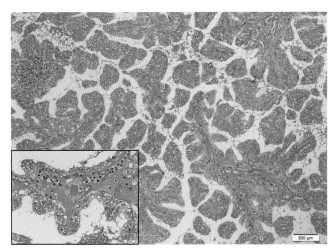

Fig. 11.109 Papillary thyroid carcinoma, classic type, 200×.
Well-formed papillae with fibrovascular cores. The papillary structures are lined by cells that show characteristic enlarged pale overlapping nuclei with grooves and pseudoinclusions (inset lower left, 400×).

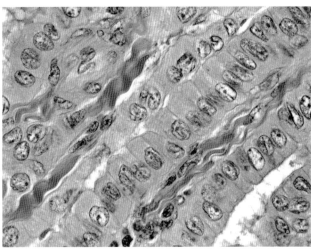

Fig. 11.111 Papillary thyroid carcinoma, tall-cell variant, 400×.
Papillary carcinomas that demonstrate a predominance of tall columnar cells, whose height is at least 2 to 3 times their width, are termed *tall-cell variants*. The columnar cells in this image are tightly packed, and they show pronounced nuclear features of papillary carcinoma. Note the nuclear grooves and irregular nuclear membranes. The tall-cell variant has typically been associated with a more advanced stage at presentation than classical papillary carcinomas, but patients generally still have a very favorable outcome.

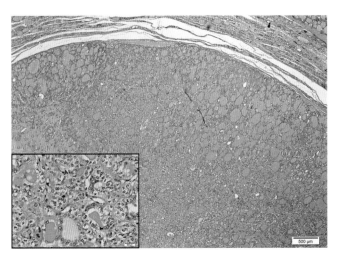

Fig. 11.110 Non-invasive follicular thyroid neoplasm with papillary-like nuclear features (NIFTP), 40×. The lesion is well circumscribed and consists of microfollicles. The microfollicles are lined by follicular cells that exhibit papillary thyroid carcinoma nuclei (enlarged pale overlapping nuclei with grooves) (inset lower left, 400×). By definition NIFTPs lack foci of capsular and vascular invasion, and papillary structures are not a feature. NIFTP carries an excellent prognosis similar to a follicular adenoma.

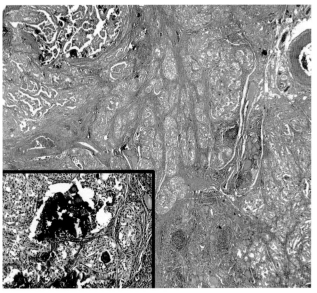

Fig. 11.112 Papillary thyroid carcinoma, diffuse sclerosing variant, 20×. Extensive fibrotic areas separate the tumor cell nests in this papillary thyroid carcinoma variant. They often arise in a background that shows marked lymphocytic thyroiditis, as is seen here. Numerous psammoma bodies are present (inset lower right, 200×). These lesions typically occupy an entire lobe of the thyroid or the entirety of the gland with no discrete mass noted grossly or by imaging.

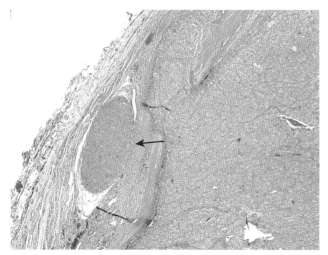

Fig. 11.113 Follicular carcinoma, 100×. This follicular neoplasm has a thick capsule, penetrated by tumor cells with mushrooming capsular invasion. Additionally, tumor cells penetrate a thick-walled vein in the lesional capsule (angioinvasion, *arrow*).

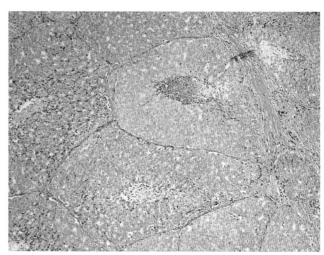

Fig. 11.115 Poorly differentiated thyroid carcinoma, 100×. In this image, nests of tumor cells with small round hyperchromatic nuclei are separated by thin bands of fibrous tissue (insular growth pattern). Comedo-type necrosis is seen as a small, well-defined focus located in the center of solid nests or insulae.

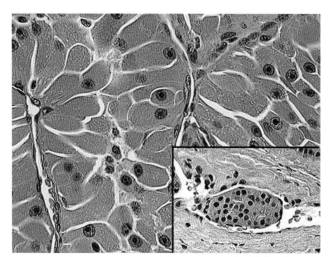

Fig. 11.114 Follicular thyroid carcinoma, oncocytic (Hurthle cell) type, 400×. A follicular carcinoma of the thyroid and yet the cells have abundant granular cytoplasm and round to oval nuclei with prominent nucleoli (oncocytes). As in other follicular carcinomas, the diagnosis of malignancy requires the identification of capsular and/or vascular invasion. In this case, the tumor invaded a blood vessel within the capsule (inset lower right, 400×).

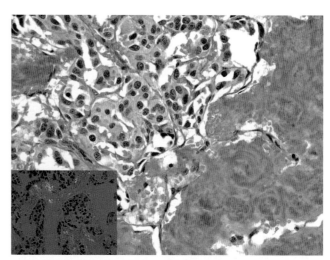

Fig. 11.116 Medullary thyroid carcinoma, 400×. Nests of plasmacytoid cells associated with an acellular eosinophilic material (amyloid). The cells have round, eccentrically located nuclei with granular chromatin. The amyloid has an apple-green birefringence when stained with Congo red and viewed under polarized light (inset lower left, 200×). Medullary thyroid carcinoma is a malignant neoplasm of parafollicular C cells.

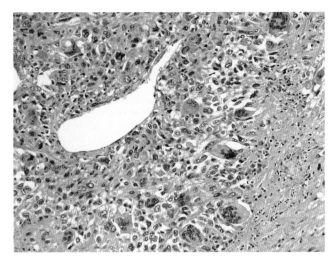

Fig. 11.117 Undifferentiated (anaplastic) thyroid carcinoma, 400×. Atypical spindle cells surround a residual vascular channel. Tumor giant cells demonstrate multiple large hyperchromatic nuclei with prominent nucleoli. Necrosis is present (*right*), and there are often several atypical mitotic figures (not shown).

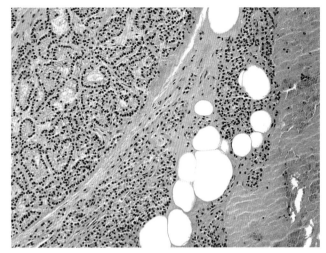

Fig. 11.118 Parathyroid adenoma, 200×. A thin capsule separates the adenoma from the surrounding normal parathyroid tissue. The adenoma is devoid of intercellular (stromal) fat. Parathyroid adenomas can be multiple. Multiple parathyroid adenomas may be seen in patients with multiple endocrine neoplasia type 1 syndrome.

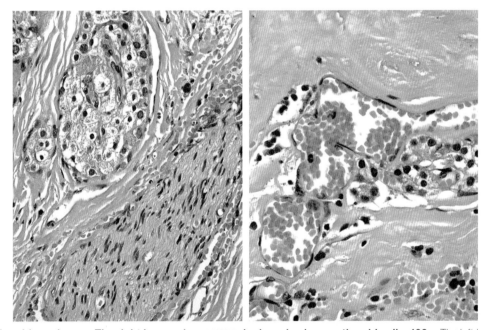

Fig. 11.119 Parathyroid carcinoma. The right image shows vascular invasion by parathyroid cells, 400×. The left image shows a nest of parathyroid cells extending into a vessel located close to a nerve (*arrow*), 400×. The diagnosis of parathyroid carcinoma is difficult to make and often occurs after the development of metastatic disease.

ACKNOWLEDGMENTS

The authors wish to thank Stephen Conley, director of the Massachusetts General Hospital Pathology Photo Laboratory, for photo editorial assistance.

SUGGESTED READINGS

Bamba R, Sweiss NJ, Langerman AJ, Taxy JB, Blair EA. The minor salivary gland biopsy as a diagnostic tool for Sjögren syndrome. *Laryngoscope.* 2009;119(10):1922–1926.

Barnes L. Intestinal-type adenocarcinoma of the nasal cavity and paranasal sinuses. *Am J Surg Pathol.* 1986;10(3):192–202.

Barnes L, Eveson JW, Reichart P, Sidransky D. *World Health Organization Classification of Tumours. Pathology and Genetics of Head and Neck Tumours.* Lyon: IARC; 2005.

Batsakis JG, el-Naggar AK. Rhinoscleroma and rhinosporidiosis. *Ann Otol Rhinol Laryngol.* 1992;101(10):879–882.

Bishop JA, Lewis JS Jr. Rocco JW, Faquin WC. HPV-related squamous cell carcinoma of the head and neck: an update on testing in routine pathology practice. *Semin Diagn Pathol.* 2015;32(5):344–351.

Cancer Genome Atlas Research Network Integrated genomic characterization of papillary thyroid carcinoma. *Cell.* 2014;159(3):676–690.

Deshpande V. IgG4 related disease of the head and neck. *Head Neck Pathol.* 2015;9(1):24–31.

El-Mofty SK, Patil S. Human papillomavirus (HPV)–related oropharyngeal nonkeratinizing squamous cell carcinoma: characterization of a distinct phenotype. *Oral Surg Oral Med Oral Pathol Oral Radiol Endod.* 2006;101(3):339–345.

Furlong MA, Fanburg-Smith JC, Childers EL. Lipoma of the oral and maxillofacial region: site and subclassification of 125 cases. *Oral Surg Oral Med Oral Pathol Oral Radiol Endod.* 2004;98(4):441–450.

Gomes CC, Diniz MG, Gomez RS. Review of the molecular pathogenesis of the odontogenic keratocyst. *Oral Oncol.* 2009;45(12):1011–1014.

Guertl B, Beham A, Zechner R, Stammberger H, Hoefler G. Nasopharyngeal angiofibroma: an APC-gene-associated tumor? *Hum Pathol.* 2000;31(11):1411–1413.

Kanavaros P, Lescs MC, Brière J, et al. Nasal T-cell lymphoma: a clinicopathologic entity associated with peculiar phenotype and with Epstein-Barr virus. *Blood.* 1993;81(10):2688–2695.

Lin BM, Wang H, D'Souza G, et al. Long-term prognosis and risk factors among patients with HPV-associated oropharyngeal squamous cell carcinoma. *Cancer.* 2013;119(19):3462–3471.

Mazur MT, Shultz JJ, Myers JL. Granular cell tumor. Immunohistochemical analysis of 21 benign tumors and one malignant tumor. *Arch Pathol Lab Med.* 1990;114(7):692–696.

Muzyka BC, Epifanio RN, Mazur MT, et al. Update on oral fungal infections. *Dent Clin North Am.* 2013;57:561–581.

Scully C, Carrozzo M. Oral mucosal disease: lichen planus. *Br J Oral Maxillofac Surg.* 2008;46(1):15–21.

Scully C, Lo Muzio L. Oral mucosal diseases: mucous membrane pemphigoid. *Br J Oral Maxillofac Surg.* 2008;46(5):358–366.

Scully C, Mignogna M. Oral mucosal disease: pemphigus. *Br J Oral Maxillofac Surg.* 2008;46(4):272–277.

Seethala RR, Dacic S, Cieply K, Kelly LM, Nikiforova MN. A reappraisal of the MECT1/MAML2 translocation in salivary mucoepidermoid carcinomas. *Am J Surg Pathol.* 2010;34(8):1106–1121.

Shear M, Speight P. *Cysts of the Oral and Maxillofacial Regions.* 4th ed. Oxford: Wiley-Blackwell; 2007.

Slootweg PJ. Odontogenic tumours—an update. *Curr Diagn Pathol.* 2006;12(1):54–65.

Tabareau-Delalande F, Collin C, Gomez-Brouchet A, et al. Diagnostic value of investigating GNAS mutations in fibro-osseous lesions: a retrospective study of 91 cases of fibrous dysplasia and 40 other fibro-osseous lesions. *Mod Pathol.* 2013;26(7):911–921.

Triantafillidou K, Venetis G, Karakinaris G, Iordanidis F. Ossifying fibroma of the jaws: a clinical study of 14 cases and review of the literature. *Oral Surg Oral Med Oral Pathol Oral Radiol.* 2012;114(2):193–199.

van der Waal I. Potentially malignant disorders of the oral and oropharyngeal mucosa; terminology, classification and present concepts of management. *Oral Oncol.* 2009;45(4-5):317–323.

Voz ML, Aström AK, Kas K, Mark J, Stenman G, Van de Ven WJ. The recurrent translocation t(5;8)(p13;q12) in pleomorphic adenomas results in upregulation of PLAG1 gene expression under control of the LIFR promoter. *Format Oncogene.* 1998;16(11):1409–1416.

West RB, Kong C, Clarke N, et al. MYB expression and translocation in adenoid cystic carcinomas and other salivary gland tumors with clinicopathologic correlation. *Am J Surg Pathol.* 2011;35(1):92–99.

Williams L, Thompson LD, Seethala RR, et al. Salivary duct carcinoma: the predominance of apocrine morphology, prevalence of histologic variants, and androgen receptor expression. *Am J Surg Pathol.* 2015;39(5):705–713.

12 Head and Neck Radiology

Anandh G. Rajamohan and John L. Go

TEMPORAL BONE

Case 1: Mondini Malformation (Fig. 12.1)

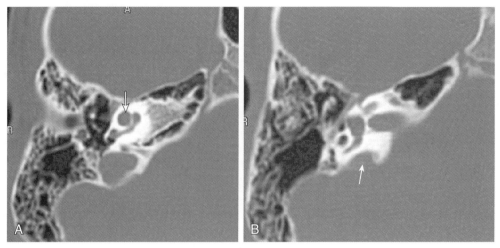

Fig. 12.1 Mondini malformation. (A) Axial computed tomography (CT) image demonstrates incomplete partitioning of the middle and apical turn of the right cochlea with deficient modiolus (*arrow*). **(B)** Axial CT one slice superior demonstrates an enlarged vestibular aqueduct (*arrow*).

Imaging findings: A congenital malformation of the cochlea with a well-formed basal turn and incomplete partitioning of the middle and apical turns. In addition, modiolar deficiency is present with loss of the normal "Christmas tree" appearance of the modiolus and spiral lamina on the axial images. The normal 2½ turns are absent, with >1½ turns of the

cochlea present. There may also be enlargement of the vestibular aqueduct because of dilatation of the endolymphatic duct and sac.

Differential diagnosis: Cochlear dysplasia (<1½ turns of the cochlea) or branchial–oto-renal syndrome (elongation of the basal turn and small middle and apical turns of the cochlea).

Case 2: Cholesterol Granuloma (Fig. 12.2)

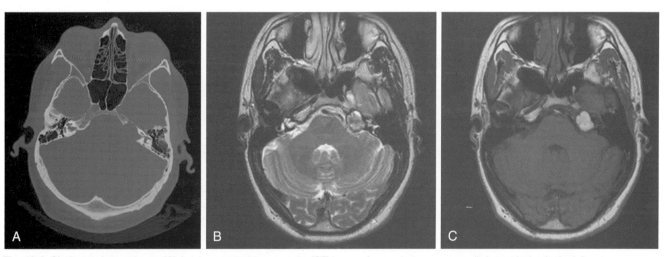

Fig. 12.2 Cholesterol granuloma. (A) Axial computed tomography (CT) image demonstrates an expansile lucent lesion in the left petrous apex. **(B)** The lesion is heterogeneous but predominantly increased in signal on T2-weighted imaging. **(C)** There is also T1-weighted hyperintensity characteristic of the cholesterol crystals and hemorrhagic material within a cholesterol granuloma. Postcontrast imaging does not play a significant role in the diagnosis as cholesterol granulomas do not intrinsically enhance.

Imaging findings: Expansile unilocular cystic lesion most commonly present in the petrous apex. These lesions may also occur in the mastoid portion of temporal bone and in the middle ear cavity.

Computed tomography (CT): Well-circumscribed unilocular expansile lesion with sclerotic smooth margin, sharp zone of transition, and most commonly posterior to the horizontal aspect of the petrous internal carotid artery.

Magnetic resonance imaging (MRI): Classically, these lesions are hyperintense on both T1- and T2-weighted images and do not demonstrate enhancement or diffusion abnormality.

Differential diagnosis: Petrous apex mucocele, petrous cephalocele, or congenital epidermoid.

Case 3: Otospongiosis (Fig. 12.3)

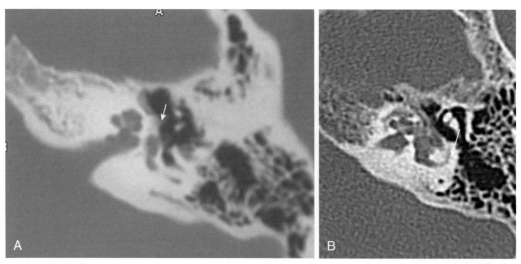

Fig. 12.3 Otospongiosis. (A) Spongiotic plaque (*arrow*) with mildly lucent bone is seen at the level of the fissula ante fenestram to the oval window on CT temporal bone. This is the fenestral form of otospongiosis. **(B)** Retrofenestral otospongiosis is seen in another patient with a characteristic "double ring" of lucency (*arrow*) around the cochlea.

Imaging findings: Otospongiosis (OS), or otosclerosis, is an osteodysplasia associated with the petrous temporal bone and is a common CT imaging diagnosis in a setting of conductive hearing loss. The two types of OS are the fenestral and retrofenestral forms. The fenesteral form occurs at the fissula ante fenestram, located in the prevestibular region anterior to the oval window. Due to the presence of plaque formation in the fenestral form, this may extend posteriorly onto the oval window and cause stapes fixation. The retrofenestral form represents the presence of rarefied lucent bone, which occurs around the otic capsule and results in sensorineural hearing loss. The retrofenestral form most commonly

occurs in conjunction with the fenestral form whereas the fenestral form may be present in isolation. Rarely, the retrofenestral form has been described without the fenestral form present.

CT: In the early phase, spongiotic bone or a plaque appearing ground-glass density or mildly lucent develops at the fissula ante fenestram. In the retrofenestral type, lucent bone can be seen around the cochlea focally or circumferentially, creating a "double ring" sign. Later-stage disease shows sclerotic change in the bone.

Differential diagnosis: Osteogenesis imperfecta and secondary syphilis involving the petrous temporal bone.

Case 4: External Auditory Canal Atresia (Fig. 12.4)

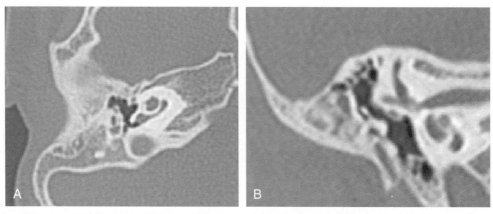

Fig. 12.4 External auditory canal (EAC) atresia. (A) A bony plate is seen replacing the right EAC on this axial CT image. The bone is solid without pneumatization. **(B)** Coronal CT in the same patient again shows absence of the right EAC and low tegmen. The malleus is fused to the atresia plate in this patient as well.

Imaging findings: Hypoplastic or absent pinna and absence of the external auditory canal (EAC). The EAC is located posterior and superior to the condylar fossa. The atresia plate may or may not be pneumatized. The middle ear cleft, measured from the medial aspect of the atresia plate to the cochlear plate, normally should measure >3 mm; <3 mm is not amenable to surgical repair. The position of the middle cranial fossa relative to the atresia plate may be of importance. A low-lying middle cranial fossa relative to the atresia plate should be noted. The ossicular chain is typically abnormal. The manubrium should be partially fused to the atresia plate. Malleoincudal or incudostapedial fusion may be present. Assess ossicles for their integrity. The stapes superstructure is perhaps the most important structure to identify. In addition, determine the presence of the oval and round windows. The facial nerve may take an anomalous course. The vertical/mastoid segment should be identified and is typically in an anterior location. The position of this segment relative to the oval window on coronal images should be determined. If at the level of the oval window on coronal images, the patient may not be amenable to surgery.

Differential diagnosis: None

Case 5: Cholesteatoma (Fig. 12.5)

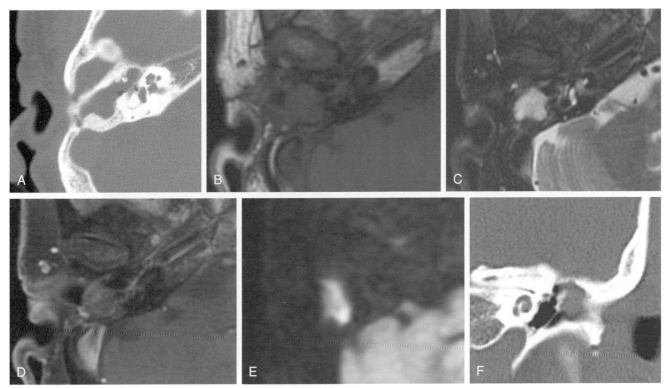

Fig. 12.5 Cholesteatoma. (A) There is opacification of the right middle ear cavity at the level of the epitympanum extending to the aditus ad antrum and the mastoid antrum with expansile features as shown on axial computed tomography (CT). Note the absence of the body and short process of the incus. **(B)** On magnetic resonance imaging (MRI), the T1-weighted axial image without contrast shows hypointense material in the mastoid antrum, aditus ad antrum, and epitympanum corresponding to the CT image. **(C)** The material in the middle ear cavity and mastoid air cells as well as the adjacent chronic otitis media are both hyperintense on T2-weighted and are indistinguishable. **(D)** There is no enhancement of this material on the postcontrast T1-weighted image. Minimal enhancement along the periphery is typical of minimal adjacent chronic otitis media. **(E)** The axial diffusion weighted image confirms that the nonenhancing material was cholesteatoma with reduced diffusion. **(F)** In another patient, coronal CT demonstrates a mass in the left Prussak space, with erosion of the scutum consistent with a pars flaccida–type cholesteatoma.

Imaging findings: Representing keratinized squamous epithelium forming mass-like tissue, these lesions are destructive in nature, causing ossicular/bony erosion, a hallmark of these lesions. Cholesteatomas may be congenital or acquired. The congenital type most commonly occurs at the petrous apex. The second most common location is in the attic of the epitympanum. Cholesteatomas in this location are often congenital in origin. The acquired cholesteatomas include the pars flaccida and pars tensa types. The pars flaccida type is located in the Prussak space, which is found between the head of the malleus and the scutum, and, classically, causes erosions of the scutum. The pars tensa type occurs in the middle ear cavity away from the Prussak space.

CT: Soft-tissue mass in the middle ear cavity causing bony or ossicular erosion. A small early cholesteatoma may not demonstrate bony/ossicular erosion. Soft-tissue mass in the Prussak space will cause blunting or erosion of the scutum. At the petrous apex, these lesions will cause bony erosion of the petrous apex.

MRI: All cholesteatomas demonstrate hypointense signal intensity on T1-weighted images, hyperintense signal intensity on T2-weighted images, and no enhancement. All cholesteatomas demonstrate restricted diffusion on the diffusion-weighted images.

Differential diagnosis: Middle ear cavity mass—glomus tympanicum tumor, schwannoma, or middle ear cavity adenoma/adenocarcinoma.

Petrous apex: Cholesterol granuloma, petrous apex mucocele, and petrous apex cephalocele.

Case 6: Endolymphatic Sac Tumor (Fig. 12.6)

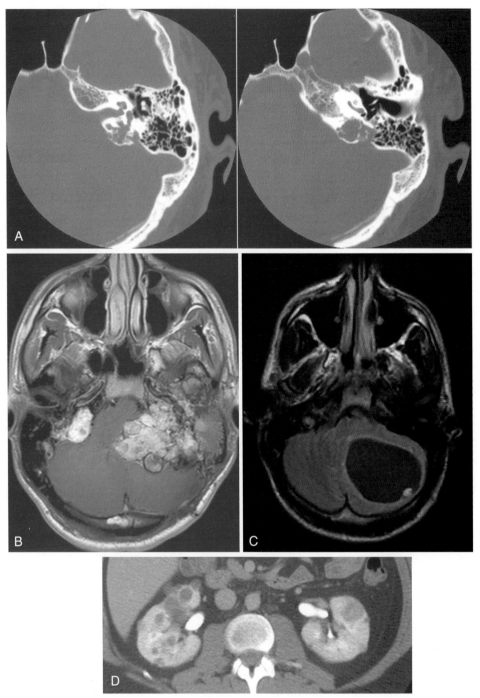

Fig. 12.6 Endolymphatic sac tumor. (A) Computed tomography (CT) temporal bone images show a multicystic lucent lesion along the vestibular aqueduct. **(B)** In an another patient with bilateral endolymphatic sac tumors, postcontrast T1-weighted magnetic resonance imaging shows bilateral cystic and solid masses. **(C)** Evaluation for other tumors can help suggest the presence of Von Hippel-Lindau prior to formal genetic testing. T2-FLAIR (fluid attenuated inversion recovery) image of a patient with endolymphatic sac tumor shows a hemangioblastoma in the left cerebellum. **(D)** CT images of the abdomen and pelvis with contrast in another patient with endolymphatic sac tumor shows multiple renal cysts and potential renal cell carcinomas highly suggestive of Von Hippel-Lindau syndrome.

Imaging findings: Endolymphatic sac tumors (ELST) arise from the endolymphatic sac in the vestibular aqueduct. The operculum of the vestibular aqueduct opens along the posterior aspect of the petrous pyramid and is located lateral and separate to the internal auditory canal. Identifying the anatomical center of the mass can be critical in making the diagnosis as these lesions can be locally destructive. Histologically, these tumors are papillary cystadenomas. These tumors may occur sporadically but more commonly occur in the setting of Von Hippel-Lindau (VHL) syndrome where they may be found unilaterally or bilaterally.

CT: CT is often helpful to assess the anatomy of the temporal bone and recognize that the mass arises retrolabyrinthine from the posterior aspect of the petrous pyramid at the site of the vestibular aqueduct. ELSTs are commonly complex masses with both solid and cystic components showing lytic or destructive osseous change intermixed with enhancing tissue.

MRI: The cystic components of these lesions are classically hyperintense in T1-weighted signal intensity due to the presence of blood products, cholesterol clefts, and proteinaceous material. These masses demonstrate varying degrees of enhancement.

Case 7: Gradenigo Syndrome/Petrous Apicitis (Fig. 12.7)

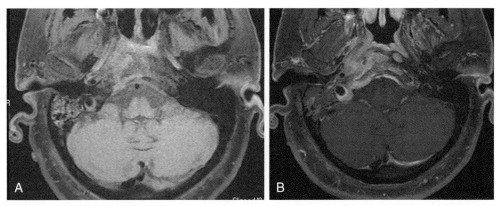

Fig. 12.7 Gradenigo syndrome/petrous apicitis. (A) Axial noncontrast T1-weighted image with fat saturation demonstrates abnormal intermediate signal intensity and infiltrative change at the right nasopharynx, petrous apex, and adjacent clivus extending intracranially to the dura. Involvement of the prevertebral musculature below the skull base is also present. Concurrent mastoid airspace disease is also seen. **(B)** Postcontrast T1-weighted axial image demonstrates enhancement in this region consistent with an infectious or inflammatory process. This enhancement approaches the right carotid canal and jugular foramen. Involvement more superiorly (not pictured) extended to the right Meckel cave and Dorello canal around the trigeminal and abducens nerves, respectively, causing the classic Gradenigo syndrome presentation.

Imaging findings: Opacification of the petrous apex air cells with destructive change and inflammatory enhancement of the petrous apex, skull base, and adjacent dura.

CT: Opacification of the petrous apex air cells with erosion or permeative change of the adjacent bone. Gradenigo syndrome classically consists of the triad of otorrhea, periorbital pain (involvement of the trigeminal nerve), and diplopia (involvement of the abducens nerve).

MRI: Opacification of the petrous apex air cells, which may demonstrate variable signal intensity on T1- and T2-weighted

images because of the presence of exudate/proteinaceous material. Postcontrast images demonstrate enhancement of the mucosa of the petrous air cells, as well as exuberant dural enhancement around the petrous apex. Adjacent cranial nerve enhancement may also be seen.

Differential diagnosis: Tumor of the petrous apex, such as metastatic disease.

Case 8: Vascular Loop Compression (Fig. 12.8)

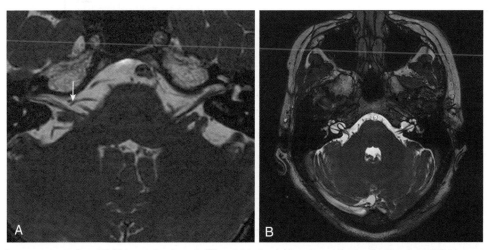

Fig. 12.8 Vascular loop compression. (A) Thin-section heavily T2-weighted axial imaging at the level of the right VII/VIII nerve complex demonstrates a vessel representing the right anterior inferior cerebellar artery (AICA) displacing the cisternal segment of the nerve complex posteriorly (*arrow*). **(B)** In another patient presenting with right hemifacial spasm, we see the right AICA loop extend beyond the midpoint of the right internal auditory canal.

Imaging findings: Most common vessel is the anterior inferior cerebellar artery (AICA), although a high-riding posterior inferior cerebellar artery or vertebral artery may also be the cause. The vessel may impinge at the root entry zone of the seventh/eighth nerve complex at the level of the brainstem. The vessel may displace the cisternal segment of the nerve or it may extend into the internal auditory canal (IAC) in cases of AICA loop. If the AICA loop extends laterally past the mid-point of the IAC, vascular loop compression may be present because of the lack of space within the IAC. Though veins may also be a causative agent, the pulsatile motion of the artery is suspected as the more common cause of the symptoms.

MRI: Thin-section heavily T2-weighted images are used to determine the relationship of the vascular loop to the nerve complex. Axial as well as reformatted images along the long and short axis of the nerve complex should be examined. The source images from a magnetic resonance angiography (MRA) of the head may also be of utility to determine whether there is arterial or venous compression.

Case 9: Facial Neuritis (Fig. 12.9)

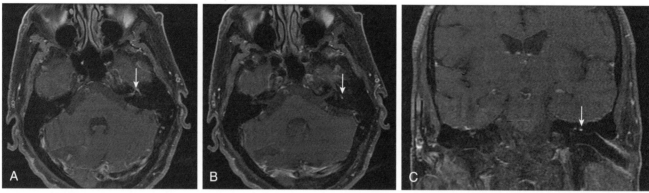

Fig. 12.9 Facial neuritis. (A) On axial postcontrast T1-weighted imaging with fat suppression, there is abnormal enhancement of the left facial nerve from the labyrinthine segment to the geniculate ganglion to the tympanic segment (*arrow*). **(B)** Increased enhancement of the left facial nerve extends to the mastoid segment (*arrow*). **(C)** Coronal images show the asymmetric nature of the left facial nerve enhancement (*arrow*) compared with the right.

Imaging findings: In the normal facial nerve, any segment of the intratemporal facial nerve may have enhancement except for the labyrinthine segment. The most common area of normal facial nerve enhancement is the geniculate fossa. The mastoid segment is the second most common area of potentially normal intratemporal enhancement. The canalicular segment of the facial nerve should not enhance. In facial neuritis, there is asymmetric and increased enhancement of the facial nerve compared with the normal opposite side. In Bell palsy, there is fusiform enhancement of all segments of the intratemporal facial nerve. Enhancement of the main trunk of the facial nerve below the skull base may also be seen.

CT: Typically negative.

MRI: Asymmetric and increased enhancement of the facial nerve on the affected side compared with the opposite asymptomatic side. In Bell palsy, there is fusiform enhancement and enlargement of the intratemporal facial nerve. Facial neuritis may also manifest as enhancement of the canalicular segment or enhancement of the fundal aspect of the IAC. IAC enhancement in neuritis tends to be indistinct or have a brush-like pattern on postcontrast images.

Differential diagnosis: Facial schwannoma, perineural spread of tumor, metastatic disease, tuberculosis, granulomatous disease, or Guillain-Barré syndrome.

Case 10: Vestibular Schwannoma (Fig. 12.10)

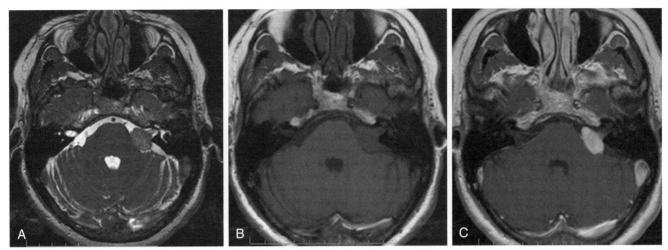

Fig. 12.10 Vestibular schwannoma. (A) Axial thin-section heavily T2-weighted image shows an extra-axial mass in the left cerebellopontine angle. **(B)** The lesion is lower in signal intensity on T1-weighted imaging than the adjacent brain parenchyma. **(C)** Postcontrast T1-weighted imaging demonstrates avid enhancement of the lesion with an ice cream cone–like appearance characteristic of vestibular schwannoma. There is no visible dural tail, a finding more typical for meningioma.

Imaging findings: These are the most common tumors to develop in the IAC/CPA (cerebellopontine angle) cistern. Originating from the vestibular component of the vestibulocochlear nerve, these masses arise at the Schwann cell–glial cell interface. Small lesions are seen within the IAC. The relationship to the crista falciformis is somewhat important to determine before surgery. As these lesions grow, they extend concentrically outward and have a classic "ice cream cone" appearance in the IAC/CPA cistern. Points to determine are the relationship of the mass to the brainstem as well as to the space remaining in the fundal area of the IAC. Schwannomas follow the nerve of origin; if there is penetration into the otic capsule, this should be into the vestibule for vestibular schwannoma. Penetration of the cochlea indicates the presence of cochlear schwannoma. Extension into the facial canal indicates a facial schwannoma.

CT: Used to determine bony remodeling. CT may be negative for small lesions. Larger lesions may demonstrate expansion of the IAC, blunting of the porous acousticus, or remodeling of the otic capsule if penetration has occurred.

MRI: These masses are classically hypointense on T1-weighted images and isointense or heterogeneously hyperintense on T2-weighted images, and they demonstrate heterogeneous, moderate to avid enhancement on postcontrast images. Lesions usually do not restrict on diffusion-weighted images. Local mass effect is seen on the brainstem if large, but because of the slow growing nature of these lesions, there are no signal changes of the adjacent brain parenchyma.

Differential diagnosis: Other schwannomas (facial/cochlear), meningioma, metastatic disease, lymphoma, tuberculoma, or granulomatous disease.

Case 11: Cerebellopontine Angle Meningioma (Fig. 12.11)

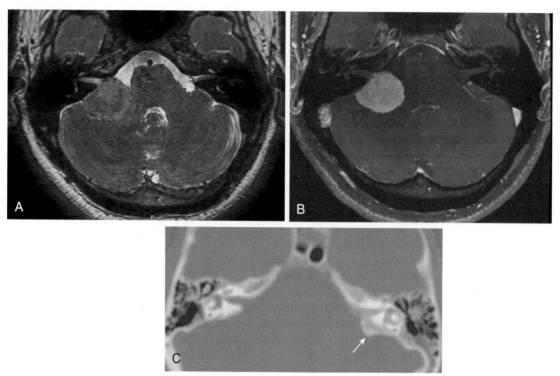

Fig. 12.11 Cerebellopontine angle (CPA) meningioma. (**A**) A right CPA mass is seen on heavily T2-weighted images. It does not enter the internal auditory canal and shows a hemispherical shape. (**B**) Postcontrast T1-weighted magnetic resonance imaging confirms lack of internal auditory canal extension, and the meningioma can be seen growing along the dura more posteriorly. There is an obtuse angle of the meningioma relative to the temporal bone along the posterior margin of the mass. (**C**) In a different patient with CPA meningioma, computed tomography shows hyperostosis (*arrow*) characteristic of meningioma and not seen with schwannoma. (From Flint PW, Haughey BH, Lund VJ, et al. *Cummings Otolaryngology—Head and Neck Surgery.* 6th ed. Philadelphia, PA: Saunders; 2015.)

Imaging findings: Magnetic resonance (MR) and CT are imaging modalities that allow for differentiation of these tumors from other CPA lesions, such as acoustic neuromas. These tumors represent 3% of tumors at this location. Unlike acoustic neuromas, 60% of CPA meningiomas extend to the middle fossa. Meningiomas are typically hemispheric because of the attachments to the posterior petrous wall. A dural tail is often visualized.

MRI: On MRI, meningiomas are variable on T2-weighted images and isointense or slightly hypointense on T1-weighted images. Surface-flow voids may be present, and calcifications and cystic foci cause heterogeneity on MR images of meningiomas.

CT: Approximately two-thirds are hyperintense relative to the brain. Unlike acoustic neuromas, meningiomas are homogeneous and occasionally calcified. They show homogeneous enhancement to contrast. Hyperostosis of adjacent bone is infrequent but characteristic of meningiomas.

Differential diagnosis: Acoustic neuroma or epidermoid.

Case 12: Facial Hemangioma (Fig. 12.12)

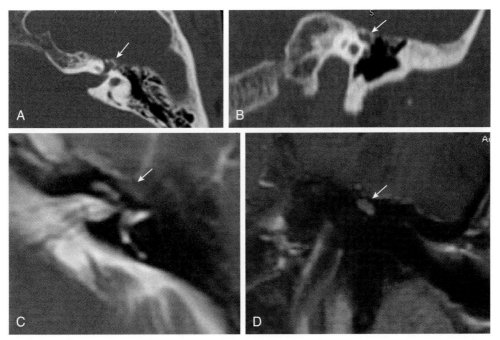

Fig. 12.12 Facial hemangioma. (A) Axial computed tomography (CT) at the level of the anterior genu of the left facial nerve canal demonstrates a bony lesion involving the geniculate segment (*arrow*). **(B)** Coronal CT shows a lucent well-circumscribed structure superior to and involving the facial nerve canal (*arrow*). **(C)** This lesion is relatively hypointense in signal intensity on T2-weighted imaging and not fluid containing (*arrow*). **(D)** Postcontrast coronal T1-weighted image demonstrates moderate enhancement of this mass (*arrow*).

Imaging findings: These lesions are not true tumors; rather, they represent venous vascular malformations. They are classically associated with the facial nerve and most commonly occur at the geniculate fossa. Another less common location is the IAC. Unlike facial schwannoma, patients develop facial nerve symptoms early in the course of the disease process and early surgical intervention is often required.

CT: As these lesions arise from the adjacent bone, bony proliferation with spicules of bone is seen on CT, which is why these lesions are also termed *ossifying hemangiomas*. The lesions may demonstrate the presence of phleboliths;

therefore, calcifications in the IAC should suggest a venous vascular malformation.

MRI: These lesions are typically hypointense on T1-weighted images and markedly hyperintense on T2-weighted images. On the T2-weighted images, focal areas of signal drop-off may be seen, which may represent phleboliths. On postcontrast images, the lesions demonstrate variable patterns of enhancement, from minimal to avid enhancement.

Differential diagnosis: Facial schwannoma or perineural spread of tumor.

Case 13: Superior Semicircular Canal Dehiscence (Fig. 12.13)

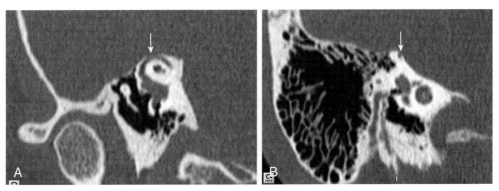

Fig. 12.13 Superior canal dehiscence. (A) Poschl view of the superior semicircular canal on computed tomography of the temporal bone reveals a defect associated with the roof of the superior semicircular canal (*arrow*). **(B)** Stenver plane also demonstrates a defect associated with the roof of the superior semicircular canal (*arrow*).

Imaging findings: Bony defect associated with the superior semicircular canal is best demonstrated on high-resolution CT. Patients with this abnormality present with Tullio phenomenon, which is vertigo in response to loud sounds. In addition, rotatory nystagmus, also called *oscillopsia*, may be present. These findings are the result of the "third window phenomenon" with abnormal processing of the aberrant fluid wave within the perilymph.

High-resolution CT best demonstrates the defect of the superior semicircular canal on both sagittal and coronal images. Multiplanar reformatting of the temporal bone may also be performed in the Stenver and Poschl plane.

Differential diagnosis: Petrous apex mucocele, petrous cephalocele, or congenital epidermoid.

SKULL BASE

Case 14: Jugular Foramen Meningioma (Fig. 12.14)

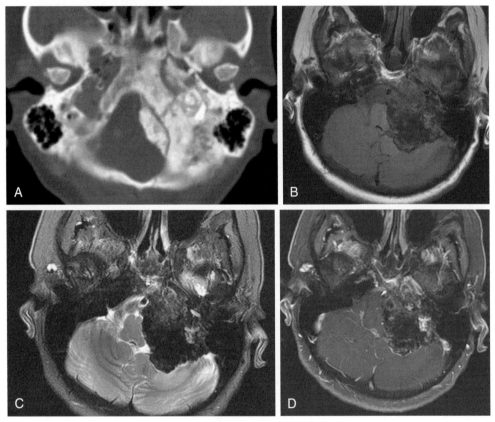

Fig. 12.14 Jugular foramen meningioma. (A) There is extensive hyperostosis and bone proliferation at the level of the left jugular foramen without destructive changes. **(B)** Axial T1-weighted image demonstrates bony expansion of the lateral skull base with isointense to hypointense signal relative to the brain. **(C)** Axial T2-weighted image also demonstrates hypointense signal with mass effect of the meningioma on the adjacent medulla and left cerebellum. **(D)** Postcontrast T1-weighted axial image demonstrates mild enhancement of this lesion as the majority is heavily calcified. The extensive hyperostosis is typical for meningiomas in this location.

Imaging findings: Arising from meningothelial rests within the dura, these masses induce a markedly proliferative hyperostosis of bone. There may be expansion of the jugular foramen, and additional foramina of the skull base may be involved. Both intracranial and extracranial extension of the meningioma above and below the skull base may be present.

CT: Soft-tissue mass at the level of the jugular foramen with the presence of bony hyperostosis around the jugular foramen.

MRI: Typically isointense to the gray matter cortex on both T1- and T2-weighted images. These masses demonstrate homogeneous avid enhancement on postcontrast images. A dural tail is typically associated with these masses. One-third of the lesions demonstrate diffusion restriction on diffusion-weighted images.

Differential diagnosis: Jugular foramen schwannoma, glomus jugulare tumor, metastatic disease, lymphoma, or plasmacytoma.

Case 15: Glomus Jugulare Tumor (Fig. 12.15)

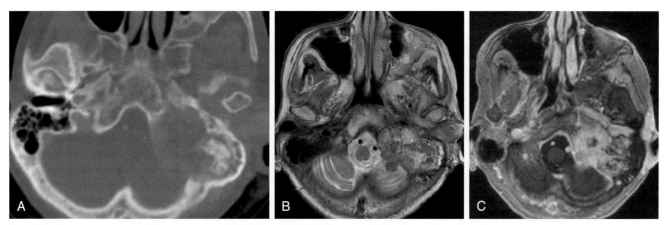

Fig. 12.15 Glomus jugulare. (**A**) There is a destructive left temporal bone mass that extends from the petrous apex to the left jugular foramen and surrounding mastoid air cells on this axial CT image. (**B**) The mass is primarily hyperintense on axial T2-weighted imaging with smaller internal areas of hypointensity ("salt and pepper") suggesting flow voids typical of paraganglioma. (**C**) The mass shows primarily avid enhancement on the postcontrast T1-weighted imaging.

Imaging findings: Arising from the glomus bodies at the dome of the jugular foramen, glomus jugular tumors are paragangliomas with permeative change and destruction of the adjacent bone.

CT: Soft-tissue mass that demonstrates avid enhancement with associated destruction and permeative change of the adjacent bone. Superior extension of this mass may destroy the jugular plate with extension of the mass into the middle ear cavity.

MRI: "Salt-and-pepper" appearance on both T1- and T2-weighted images. On T1-weighted images, these lesions are hypointense with focal areas of hyperintense signal, which may represent hemorrhage. On T2-weighted images, these lesions are hyperintense with focal areas of signal drop-off representing the presence of arterial vessels within the lesion. On postcontrast images, these lesions demonstrate avid heterogeneous enhancement.

Nuclear medicine: These masses show radiotracer uptake on an octreotide scan.

Differential diagnosis: Jugular foramen schwannoma, meningioma, lymphoma, plasmacytoma, or metastatic disease.

Case 16: Jugular Foramen Schwannoma (Fig. 12.16)

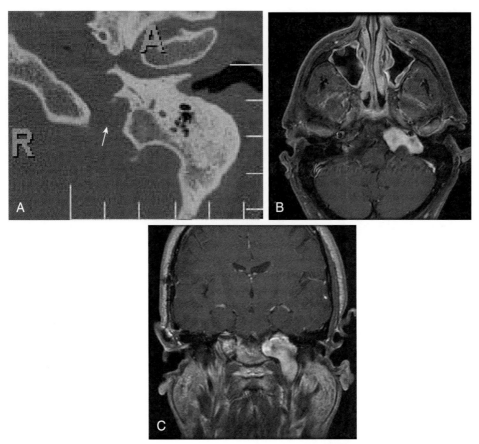

Fig. 12.16 Jugular foramen schwannoma. (**A**) CT axial image of the lateral skull base demonstrates smooth expansile remodeling and enlargement of the left jugular foramen (*arrow*) without frank destruction. (**B**) On a different patient also with jugular foramen schwannoma, a well-circumscribed mass also smoothly enlarges the left jugular foramen with solid enhancement on postcontrast T1-weighted imaging. (**C**) On coronal postcontrast T1-weighted sequence, the schwannoma can be seen exiting the skull base into the carotid space of the upper neck.

Imaging findings: These masses arise from cranial nerves IX to XI, most commonly the vagus nerve (X). The lesions present as a soft-tissue mass with expansion and smooth remodeling of the jugular foramen.

CT: Soft-tissue mass, which demonstrates moderate to avid heterogeneous enhancement. There is smooth remodeling of the jugular foramen with sclerotic margins and a sharp zone of transition.

MRI: Typically hypointense on T1-weighted images, heterogeneously hyperintense on T2-weighted images, and demonstrating heterogeneous moderate to avid enhancement on postcontrast images.

Differential diagnosis: Jugular foramen meningioma, glomus jugulare tumor, metastatic disease, lymphoma, or plasmacytoma.

Case 17: Chondrosarcoma (Fig. 12.17)

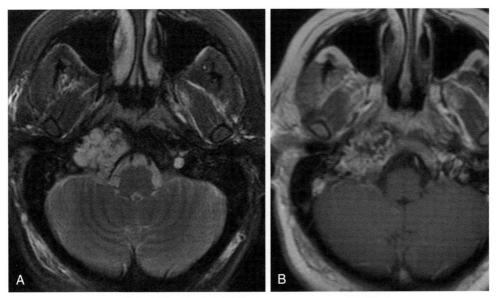

Fig. 12.17 Chondrosarcoma of the skull base. (A) Axial T2-weighted image shows a hyperintense mass in the right petroclival region of the skull base. The T2-weighted hyperintensity is characteristic of a chondroid tumor. **(B)** Patchy enhancement is present on axial postcontrast T1-weighted imaging. Note the off-midline location of this mass, which is more typical for chondrosarcoma than for chordoma.

Imaging findings: These tumors arise from the chondroid elements of the central skull base; the most common location is the petro-occipital fissure between the anterior basiocciput of the clivus and the petrous temporal bone. A second common location is a midline mass at the spheno-occipital synchondrosis between the basisphenoid and the anterior basiocciput.

CT: Typically an off-midline lesion at the central skull base centered at the petro-occipital fissure with adjacent erosion and permeative change of the adjacent bone. Punctate calcifications may be present and represent chondroid calcifications. As these lesions extend superiorly to involve the petrous temporal bone,

they classically displace the horizontal petrous internal carotid artery superiorly and anteriorly.

MRI: These lesions are hypointense on T1-weighted images and markedly hyperintense on T2-weighted images with low-signal-intensity foci, which may represent calcifications. These lesions demonstrate variable patterns of enhancement. On MRA, there is superior and anterior displacement of the horizontal petrous internal carotid artery.

Differential diagnosis: Typically pathognomonic; however, metastatic disease, chordoma, lymphoma, and plasmacytoma may also be considered.

Case 18: Fibrous Dysplasia (Fig. 12.18)

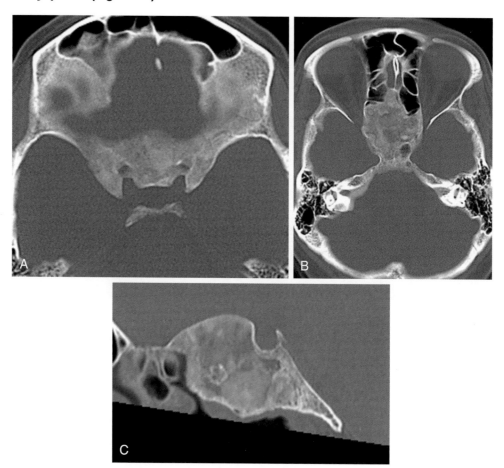

Fig. 12.18 Fibrous dysplasia. (A) Axial computed tomography (CT) image at the level of the anterior clinoid processes shows diffuse expansile change extending laterally toward the lesser sphenoid wings bilaterally. Centrally, this also involved the planum sphenoidale and tuberculum sella. **(B)** More inferiorly, this osseous change shows a "ground-glass" appearance into the sphenoid and posterior ethmoid sinuses. **(C)** Sagittal CT imaging again shows the changes of fibrous dysplasia in the sphenoid bone in the central skull base near the sella turcica.

Imaging findings: These lesions are developmental lesions and are not neoplastic. Representing immature bone, fibrous dysplasia has a classic "ground-glass" appearance on CT with associated bone expansion in larger lesions. A cystic form may also occur. The monostotic form is typically sporadic in etiology. Polyostotic fibrous dysplasia may be associated with McCune-Albright syndrome.

CT: Geographic bone lesion, which demonstrates "ground-glass" appearance with or without cystic change. There is no evidence of bony erosion or destruction. Larger lesions may cause neural foraminal narrowing because of mass effect and expansile change.

MRI: Hypointense on T1-weighted images and markedly hypointense on T2-weighted images. The cystic areas may be hyperintense in T2-weighted signal intensity. These lesions demonstrate moderate to avid enhancement on postcontrast images.

Differential diagnosis: CT is pathognomonic. On MRI, also consider other osteofibrous lesions or sclerotic lesions, such as metastatic disease.

Case 19: Aberrant Internal Carotid Artery (Fig. 12.19)

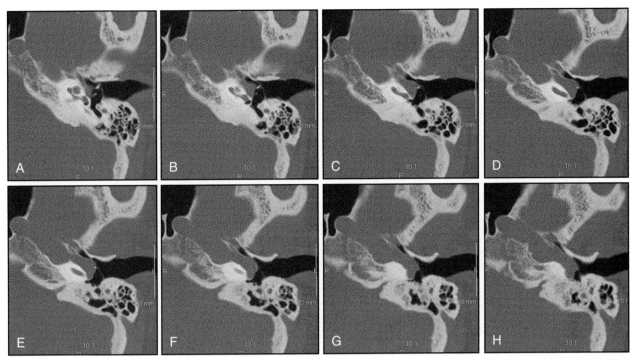

Fig. 12.19 Aberrant internal carotid artery. Consecutive axial computed tomography images progressing from superior to inferior from (**A**) to (**H**) demonstrate a structure overlying the cochlear promontory. Following the consecutive slices, note that this lesion enters the posterior genu of the petrous internal carotid artery and gives the horizontal segment of the petrous internal carotid artery an elongated appearance. Not shown is that the internal carotid artery enters the skull base at a more posterior location and turns laterally to enter the middle ear cavity.

Imaging findings: Congenital anomalous course of the internal carotid through the petrous temporal bone. The anomalous inferior cerebellar artery (ICA) enters the skull base in a posterior location and makes a hairpin loop laterally to enter the middle ear cavity. Crossing the cochlear promontory, the anomalous ICA then enters the horizontal petrous ICA canal in a lateral position with apparent elongation of the horizontal petrous ICA.

CT: Course of the aberrant ICA as just described. The vertical carotid canal is seen in a posterior location. The ICA then enters the middle ear cavity and extends into a lateralized horizontal petrous ICA canal.

MRI/MRA: Best demonstrated on MRA with course as described previously. Compression view from above on the MRA maximum intensity projection image demonstrates the posterior position of the vertical petrous ICA, the hairpin loop laterally, and the elongated horizontal petrous ICA segment.

Differential diagnosis: Pathognomonic on imaging. On physical examination, persistent stapedial artery or hypervascular tumor (glomus tumor or schwannoma).

Case 20: Persistent Stapedial Artery (Fig. 12.20)

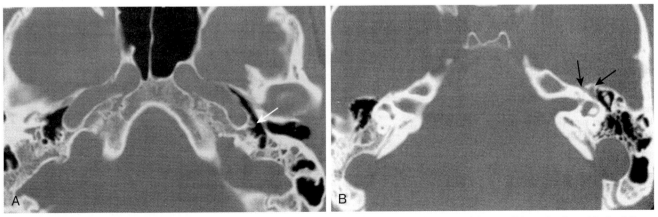

Fig. 12.20 Persistent stapedial artery. (A) There is an asymmetric structure along the posterior genu of the carotid canal adjacent to the left internal carotid artery. This represents the persistent stapedial artery (*white arrow*). (**B**) Axial computed tomography also demonstrates the classic "Y configuration" at the level of the geniculate fossa (*black arrows*). One channel represents the facial hiatus for the greater superficial petrosal nerve. The second channel represents the persistent stapedial artery, which continues as the middle meningeal artery.

Imaging findings: In most patients, this is not seen on imaging and found during surgery only. The persistent stapedial artery results from failure of regression of the embryonal stapedial artery. This vessel arises from the petrous ICA at the posterior genu, enters the middle ear cavity, and travels through the obturator foramen of the stapes. The vessel then enters the horizontal segment of the facial canal, travels anteriorly, and exits at the geniculate fossa, which may be a channel separate from the facial hiatus.

CT: Typically negative. May demonstrate a soft-tissue mass at the level of the stapes, expansion of the tympanic facial canal, and a "Y" configuration of the geniculate fossa, representing the facial hiatus for the greater superficial petrosal nerve and the channel for the persistent stapedial artery, which becomes the middle meningeal artery. The foramen spinosum in these cases is absent.

MRI/MRA: Typically normal. On MRA, may demonstrate an anomalous vessel arising from the posterior genu of the petrous internal carotid artery, which may be followed to the geniculate fossa and become the middle meningeal artery. The middle meningeal artery at the level of the foramen spinosum is absent.

Differential diagnosis: Pathognomonic on imaging. On physical examination, aberrant internal carotid artery, or hypervascular tumor (glomus tumor or schwannoma).

SINONASAL CAVITY

Case 21: Inverted Papilloma (Fig. 12.21)

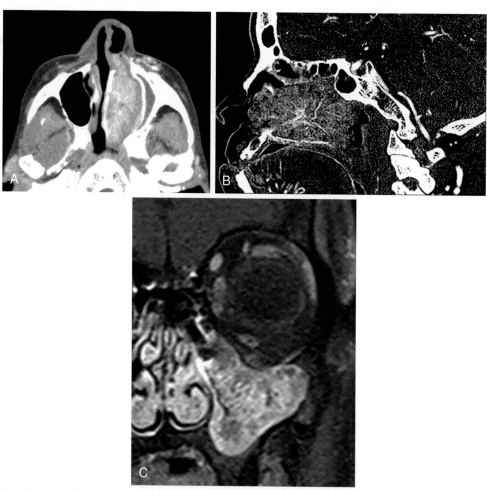

Fig. 12.21 Inverted papilloma. (A) There is a polypoid-enhancing soft-tissue mass from the left nasal cavity projecting through the left posterior choana to the nasopharynx. **(B)** On sagittal reconstruction, spiculated calcification or bony spur is seen at the origin of the inverted papilloma. **(C)** In a different patient with inverted papilloma, notice the classic cerebriform enhancement pattern on coronal postcontrast T1-weighted images.

Imaging finding: Most common type of papilloma (most common benign tumor of the sinonasal cavity) that typically arises from the lateral wall of the nasal cavity centered at the middle meatus and may extend into the antrum of the maxillary sinus.

CT: Soft-tissue mass in the nasal cavity without bone erosion or destruction. Typically centered at the level of the middle meatus and may demonstrate hyperostosis of bone, which may be the point of attachment/origin of the mass. Because of its location, this mass may cause sinus obstruction.

MRI: Alternating hyperintense and hypointense lines on T2-weighted images with curvilinear striations described as a cerebriform or convoluted pattern. Postcontrast images may show a similar cerebriform enhancement pattern with alternating hyperenhancing and hypoenhancing layers.

Differential diagnosis: Sinonasal polyp, squamous cell carcinoma, or sinonasal polyposis.

Case 22: Nasal Meningocele (Fig. 12.22)

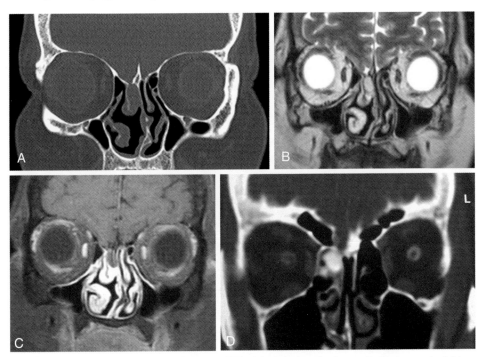

Fig. 12.22 Nasal meningocele. (A) Coronal computed tomography (CT) of the nasal cavity demonstrates a mass in right superior nasal cavity medial to the vertical strut of the middle turbinate. Note the small defect of the right cribriform plate. **(B)** Coronal T2-weighted image demonstrates this lesion to be increased in signal intensity. **(C)** Coronal postcontrast T1-weighted image demonstrates that this lesion does not enhance, consistent with a nasal meningocele. Magnetic resonance imaging also helps determine whether the brain parenchyma herniates inferiorly, the presence of encephalocele. **(D)** CT cisternogram can also be helpful in the workup, particularly if there is associated cerebrospinal fluid leak. Notice the contrast material in the subarachnoid space extending inferiorly through a defect (*arrow*) in this different patient.

Imaging findings: Nasal meningocele occurs because of a defect along the anterior skull base and herniation of the meninges containing cerebrospinal fluid (CSF) through the defect. CSF leak may be associated with meningoceles, and CT cisternogram is often helpful to anatomically define the area of leak. The most common cause is prior trauma. Dehiscence of the cribriform plate may also be a cause.

CT: Cystic lesion within the nasal cavity that extends from the anterior skull base. This lesion has a thin wall and demonstrates no enhancement. If CT cisternogram is performed, high-density contrast material with the CSF may be seen communicating from the intracranial subarachnoid compartment to the nasal cavity.

MRI: Cystic lesion isointense or hyperintense to CSF signal intensity on T1- and T2-weighted images. Because of the CSF pulsations, flow-related artifacts may be associated with a nasal meningocele, resulting in central-signal drop-off. After the administration of contrast, there is no enhancement centrally.

Differential diagnosis: Imaging is usually pathognomonic. If the defect along the anterior skull base is not seen, this lesion may be mistaken for a dermoid, epidermoid, or cystic neoplasm.

Case 23: Polyposis (Fig. 12.23)

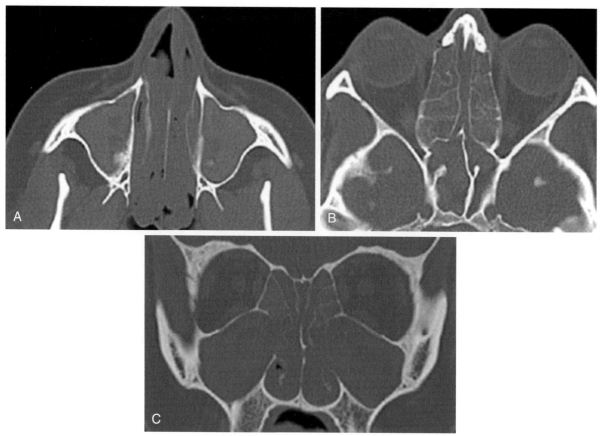

Fig. 12.23 Polyposis. (**A**) Axial computed tomography image without contrast reveals diffuse mucosal disease in the nasal cavity and visualized sinuses. There is polypoid tissue projecting through the posterior choanae. (**B**) Areas of hyperdensity are seen among the opacification indicative of inspissated secretions. Noninvasive fungal colonization in allergic sinusitis can often appear similarly. (**C**) In the coronal plane, the extensive nature of the polyposis causes near complete opacification of bilateral nasal cavities and sinuses.

Imaging findings: Polypoid masses within the nasal cavity and sinuses. There may be bony remodeling without bone erosion/destruction. Sinus opacification with or without mucocele formation may be present.

CT: Polypoid or lobulated lesions within the sinonasal cavity. These lesions are hypoattenuating in appearance, higher than CSF but lower than soft-tissue density. Sinus obstruction and mucocele formation may be present.

MRI: Peripheral rim enhancement of the sinonasal polyps is seen. Mucosal enhancement of the sinus mucosa is seen with or without fluid. Mucocele formation may also be seen.

Differential diagnosis: Squamous cell carcinoma, lymphoma, or granulomatous disease.

Case 24: Esthesioneuroblastoma (Fig. 12.24)

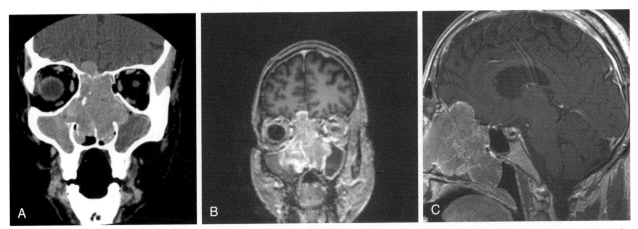

Fig. 12.24 Esthesioneuroblastoma. (A) There is an extensive lobulated soft-tissue mass involving the bilateral paranasal sinuses and nasal cavity with extension intracranially through the anterior skull base on coronal computed tomography. Calcifications are not seen in the mass in this case but have been associated with esthesioneuroblastoma along with peritumoral cyst formation. **(B)** On postcontrast T1-weighted imaging, there is relatively avid enhancement of the mass. Note the involvement of the olfactory recesses, which is characteristic for esthesioneuroblastoma. **(C)** Sagittal postcontrast T1-weighted imaging shows the intracranial and extracranial components of the mass.

Imaging findings: Arising from the olfactory nerves, this mass has often extended superiorly to the level of the cribriform plate at the time of presentation and into the subfrontal area. These are destructive tumors with associated bony erosion and permeative change. Large lesions are often shaped like a dumbbell, with the waist at the level of the anterior skull base. Macrocysts may be present at the tumor–brain interface and may be pathognomonic for this entity.

CT: Sinonasal mass in the superior half of the nasal cavity with associated bone erosion/destruction.

MRI: Hypointense on T1-weighted images, isointense to hyperintense on T2-weighted images, and heterogeneous moderate to avid enhancement on postcontrast images. These masses are diffusion positive on diffusion-weighted images. Macrocysts may be seen at the tumor–brain interface. Sinus obstruction may also be present.

Case 25: Acute Invasive Fungal Sinusitis (Fig. 12.25)

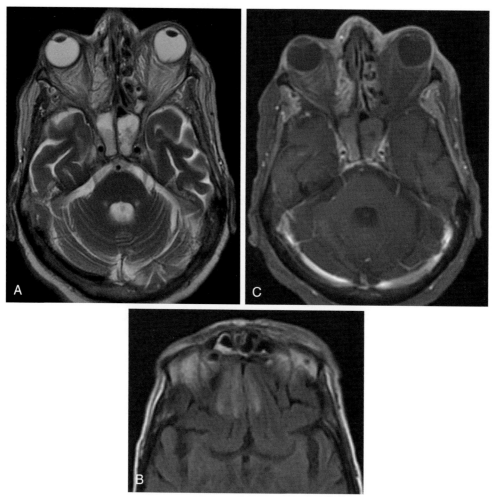

Fig. 12.25 Acute invasive fungal sinusitis. (**A**) There is sinus mucosal disease with invasive inflammatory edema in the bilateral orbits on this T2-weighted image. Note the deformity of the left globe contour. (**B**) Edema extends through the anterior skull base into the inferior frontal lobes on axial T2-FLAIR (fluid attenuated inversion recovery) imaging. (**C**) There is decreased enhancement of the soft tissues in the orbits and sinuses on postcontrast T1-weighted imaging with fat suppression. The decreased or absent enhancement is a result of tissue devascularization, a key sign of acute invasive fungal disease.

Imaging findings: Acute invasive fungal sinusitis typically occurs in the setting of uncontrolled diabetes or in immunocompromised patients. The two major fungal species associated with acute fungal sinusitis are *Mucormycosis* and *Aspergillosis*, specifically the hyphal type of these fungi, which are angioinvasive, causing a necrotizing vasculitis with vascular thrombosis and tissue necrosis. In a setting of sinus infection, aggressive fungal infections should be suspected with the presence of stranding, edema, or loss of the normal fat in the premaxillary tissue or the retromaxillary fat pad on either CT or MRI. Absence or relative lack of enhancement of the mucosal surfaces in the sinonasal cavity and surrounding tissues is the result of devascularization and is best demonstrated on postcontrast CT or MR images. Comparison of the tissue in question to normally enhancing tissue is helpful. Rapid extension into the orbit, cavernous sinuses, and intracranial compartment may occur. Thus, one should have a low threshold for obtaining an MRI with contrast to ensure a swift diagnosis, which will allow for timely surgical debridement.

Case 26: Silent Sinus Syndrome (Fig. 12.26)

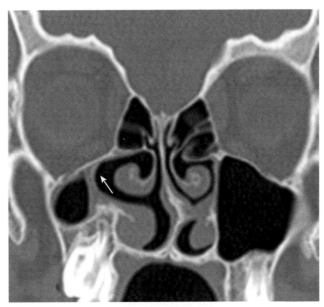

Fig. 12.26 Silent sinus syndrome. Coronal computed tomography of the sinuses shows volume loss of the right maxillary sinus with atelectasis of the uncinate process (*arrow*) obstructing the outflow. Notice the ipsilateral enlargement of the right middle meatus as the right maxillary sinus has contracted from relative negative pressure.

Imaging findings: Silent sinus syndrome shows classic imaging features of volume loss of the maxillary sinus with atelectasis of the uncinate process and chronic obstruction of the maxillary sinus drainage. Unlike in conventional maxillary sinus obstruction from mucosal disease, a pressure gradient occurs across the infundibulum, causing a net negative pressure within the maxillary sinus with outflow obstruction from the atelectatic uncinate process. This causes an inward tension on the walls of the maxillary sinus, which slowly remodel and collapse inward. The orbital floor may be pulled inferiorly, the lateral wall pulled medially, and elevation of the superior alveolar ridge superiorly, resulting in facial bony asymmetry. CT is the modality of choice for imaging with comparison to the contralateral sinus and midface a helpful way to make the diagnosis. Early detection is required, and the surgical remedy is resection of the uncinate process and opening of the maxillary sinus drainage pathway before the chronic facial bony changes occur.

Case 27: Juvenile Nasopharyngeal Angiofibroma (Fig. 12.27)

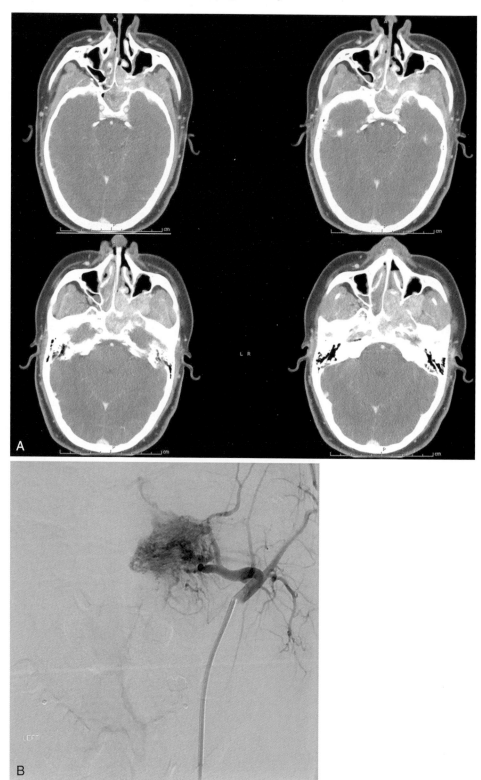

Fig. 12.27 Juvenile nasopharyngeal angiofibroma. (A) Consecutive postcontrast computed tomography images show an avidly enhancing mass arising from the left sphenopalatine foramen extending to the pterygopalatine fossa and pterygomaxillary fissure in this adolescent male presenting with epistaxis. The mass also involves the left sphenoid sinus and nasal cavity. **(B)** Digital subtraction angiography shows the hypervascular nature of the mass with multiple feeding external carotid artery branches.

Imaging findings: Juvenile nasopharyngeal angiofibromas (JNAs) are benign but locally aggressive vascular tumors most commonly occurring in the second decade of life and exclusively in males. Arising from the lateral nasopharyngeal wall at the sphenopalatine foramen, these tumors may extend into the pterygopalatine fossa and classically cause anterior bowing of the posterior wall of the maxillary sinus. CT may show that the bone is remodeled rather than frankly destroyed. On both CT and MR imaging with contrast, these masses will show features of increased vascularity and hyper-enhancement. Feeding arteries parasitized from the external carotid arteries and prominent tumor vascular blush can be seen on digital subtraction catheter angiography. Preoperative embolization of JNA may assist or complement surgical resection.

PHARYNX

Case 28: Tornwaldt Cyst (Fig. 12.28)

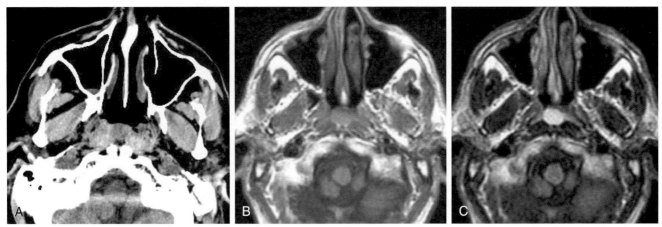

Fig. 12.28 Tornwaldt cyst. (**A**) Axial computed tomography at the level of the nasopharynx demonstrates a midline cystic lesion in the posterior superior aspect of the nasopharynx. (**B**) T1-weighted axial image at the level of the nasopharynx demonstrates the cyst to be slightly hyperintense relative to muscle signal intensity. (**C**) T2-FLAIR (fluid attenuated inversion recovery) axial image demonstrates the cyst to be homogeneously hyperintense in signal intensity.

Imaging findings: A pseudocyst found in the superior posterior aspect of the midline nasopharynx and related to closure of the Tornwaldt diverticulum. Represents the site at which the embryonic notochord and endoderm of the primitive pharynx came in contact.

CT: Midline cystic lesion of the superior posterior nasopharynx. Typically demonstrates no enhancement or minimal wall enhancement unless infected.

MRI: Variable signal intensity because of the presence of proteinaceous material on T1- and T2-weighted images.

Differential diagnosis: Mucous retention cyst, adenoidal cyst from minor salivary gland, benign mixed tumor, or nasopharyngeal carcinoma.

Case 29: Oropharyngeal Lymphoma (Fig. 12.29)

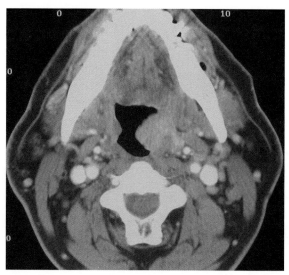

Fig. 12.29 Oropharyngeal lymphoma. Postcontrast axial computed tomography (CT) at the level of the oropharynx demonstrates a bulky mildly enhancing mass in the left tonsillar fossa. This may be difficult to distinguish from squamous cell carcinoma on CT imaging alone. Assessment of the lymph nodes in the neck and diffusion weighted imaging on MRI may help but often may not be definitive for differentiating lymphoma from squamous cell carcinoma.

Imaging findings: Waldeyer ring, comprising the adenoids, palatine and lingual tonsils, and the posterior margin of the soft palate, is the most common location for the extranodal form of lymphoma. Separating squamous cell carcinoma from lymphoma may be difficult on CT imaging and easier on MRI. Lymphoma is isointense to muscle signal intensity on T1-weighted images, isointense to mildly hyperintense on T2-weighted images, and demonstrating moderate to avid enhancement. The nodal disease is typically well circumscribed without extracapsular extension or cystic change. This may also be diffusion positive on diffusion-weighted images.

Case 30: Oropharyngeal Squamous Cell Carcinoma (Fig. 12.30)

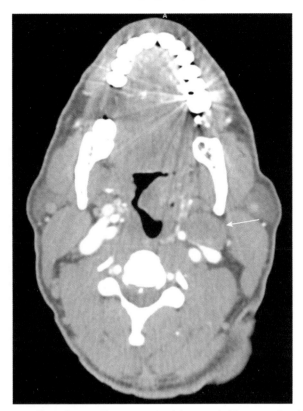

Fig. 12.30 Oropharyngeal (OP) squamous cell carcinoma. Postcontrast axial computed tomography at the level of the oropharynx demonstrates a mass in the left tonsillar fossa. An enlarged pathological lymph node is seen in level IIA station on the left (*arrow*) in this patient with human papillomavirus–related OP squamous cell carcinoma.

Imaging findings: Unilateral tonsillar enlargement and presence of a neck mass in level II is usually pathognomonic for oropharyngeal squamous cell carcinoma. This may be difficult to distinguish from lymphoma as described previously. Some imaging findings that may be useful are the presence of extracapsular extension within the lymphadenopathy as well as cystic change or necrosis. On MRI, squamous cell cancer is mildly hyperintense on T2-weighted images and is not diffusion positive.

Case 31: Subglottic Stenosis and Tracheal Stenosis (Fig. 12.31)

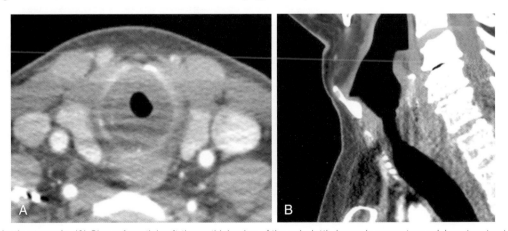

Fig. 12.31 Subglottic stenosis. (**A**) Circumferential soft-tissue thickening of the subglottic larynx is present on axial postcontrast computed tomography of the neck. (**B**) In the sagittal plane, the resulting focal narrowing of the airway can be appreciated.

Imaging findings: Typically caused by prolonged intubation and associated pressure necrosis of the mucosa related to the balloon of the endotracheal tube with subsequent scar formation; obstructive granulation and scar tissue in the subglottic region or trachea can lead to dyspnea. Greater than 25% narrowing of the airway results in dyspnea.

CT/MRI: CT without contrast is sufficient to make a radiological diagnosis. The mucosal surface of the subglottic region and trachea are not seen on CT. Any soft tissue identified is abnormal. The percentage of stenosis is determined by degree of patency relative to the normal lumen size.

Differential diagnosis: Granulomatous disease, papilloma, or squamous cell cancer.

Case 32: True Vocal Fold Paralysis (Fig. 12.32)

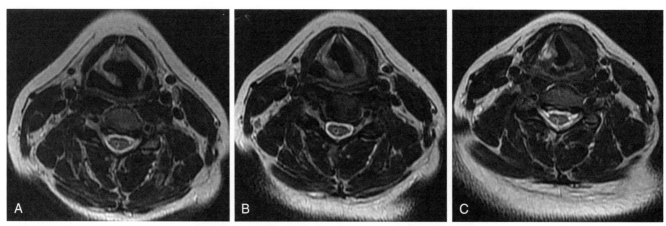

Fig. 12.32 True vocal fold paralysis. (A) Axial T2-weighted imaging of the cervical spine was done on a patient who had extensive injury to the right medulla and cervical spinal cord causing true vocal fold paralysis. Notice the enlargement of the right piriform sinus compared with the left. **(B)** The right aryepiglottic fold is turned inward. **(C)** The right true vocal fold is medialized and shows fatty atrophy with T2-weighted hyperintensity from chronic denervation and paralysis.

Imaging findings: True vocal fold paralysis may be divided into acute, subacute, and chronic forms. In acute vocal fold paralysis, the true vocal fold is medialized and may be identified on both CT and MRI. In subacute true vocal fold paralysis, the true vocal fold begins to lose volume without loss of the normal density on CT. This diagnosis is made on MRI of the larynx, which demonstrates hyperintense signal intensity of the affected true vocal fold on T2-weighted images. In chronic true vocal fold paralysis, there is lateralization of the true vocal fold with fatty replacement, which is well demonstrated on both CT and MRI.

Imaging on CT or MR should extend from the skull base to the level of the pulmonary artery to encompass the jugular foramen and the course of the vagus nerve and recurrent laryngeal nerve.

Differential diagnosis: Glottic squamous cell carcinoma.

Case 33: Laryngeal Chondrosarcoma (Fig. 12.33)

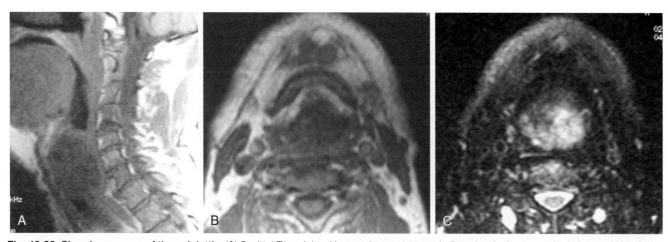

Fig. 12.33 Chondrosarcoma of the epiglottis. (A) Sagittal T1-weighted image demonstrates a bulky mass in the supraglottic larynx. Note that this mass is predominantly hypointense compared with the mucosa elsewhere. **(B)** T1-weighted axial image demonstrates the large mass filling the supraglottic larynx. **(C)** T2-weighted axial image with fat suppression demonstrates that this lesion is markedly hyperintense consistent with chondroid matrix with the low-signal-intensity foci representing calcifications.

Imaging findings: The cartilaginous portions of the larynx include the epiglottis, arytenoid, cricoid, and thyroid cartilage. These are the sites for laryngeal chondrosarcoma, a rare malignancy of the larynx.

CT: Soft-tissue mass centered on one of the cartilaginous structures of the larynx. Calcifications may be present. This mass may demonstrate variable patterns of enhancement.

MRI: Hypointense on T1-weighted images, markedly hyperintense on T2-weighted images with foci of signal drop-off, which may represent calcifications. Variable degree of enhancement on postcontrast studies.

Differential diagnosis: Laryngeal squamous cell carcinoma, lymphoma, or granulomatous disease.

Case 34: Nasopharyngeal Mass (Fig. 12.34)

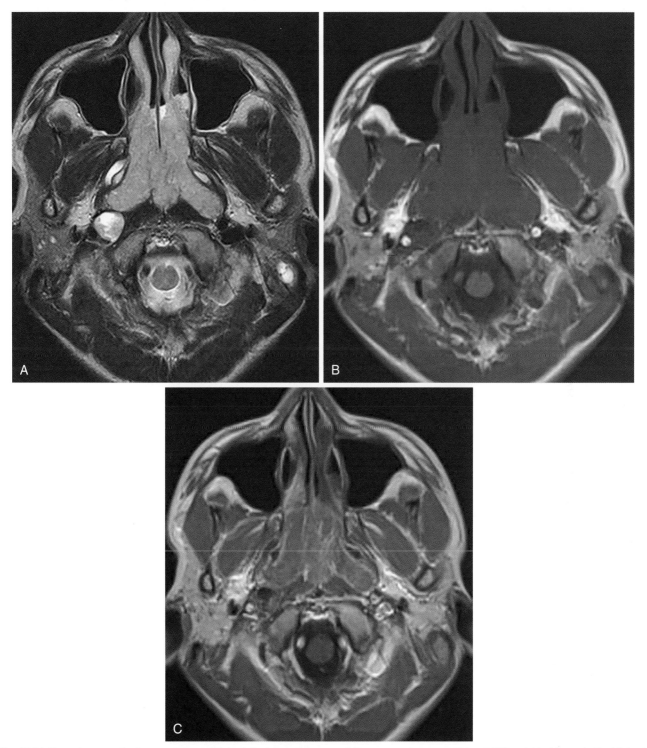

Fig. 12.34 Nasopharyngeal adenocarcinoma. (A) A relatively hyperintense soft-tissue mass is seen on this axial T2-weighted image in the bilateral nasopharynx extending through the posterior choanae into the nasal cavity. Additionally, note the right retropharyngeal and left level IIB pathological lymph nodes. **(B)** The mass appears well circumscribed and isointense to the muscle on T1-weighted imaging. **(C)** Following contrast administration, the mass shows low-grade enhancement with a somewhat peripheral pattern. This was biopsy-proven adenocarcinoma of the nasopharynx.

Imaging findings: The most common malignancies of the nasopharynx are squamous cell carcinoma and lymphoma, which comprise up to 90% of all malignancies in this location. As mentioned earlier, it may be difficult to distinguish squamous cell carcinoma and lymphoma on CT, although MRI may be useful. Lymphoma tends to be intermediate in signal intensity on T2-weighted images and is reduced in diffusion. The appearance of lymphadenopathy may also help separate these two entities as extracapsular extension and necrosis are more commonly seen in squamous cell carcinoma. Minor salivary gland malignancies may also occur in this location, including mucoepidermoid carcinoma and adenocarcinoma. For the determination of skull-base involvement, intracranial extension, and perineural spread of tumor, MR is superior to CT.

Case 35: Tonsillitis (Fig. 12.35)

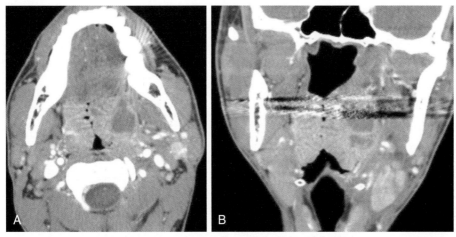

Fig. 12.35 Tonsillitis with peritonsillar abscess. (A) Postcontrast axial computed tomography (CT) images reveal enlarged bilateral palatine tonsils with a striated enhancement pattern consistent with tonsillitis. On the left, there is an adjacent rim-enhancing fluid collection consistent with peritonsillar abscess formation. **(B)** On coronal CT reconstruction, the tonsillitis with left peritonsillar abscess formation can again be seen with additional reactive left cervical lymphadenopathy.

Imaging findings: Inflammation of the tonsils may be seen as enlargement of the tonsils with a striated or striped appearance because of the presence of crypts within the tonsils. Mucosal enhancement with submucosal edema gives the inflamed tonsils this striped appearance. Edema of the muscular wall of the oropharynx may also be seen. Development of a tonsillar abscess may be seen within the tonsil or a peritonsillar abscess, which lies in the peritonsillar recess of the pharyngeal mucosal space. On CT, enhancement of the mucosal surface with submucosal edema is present. On MRI, the tonsil is hypointense on T1-weighted images and hyperintense on T2-weighted images. On postcontrast MRI, the tonsil again demonstrates a striated or striped appearance.

SALIVARY GLANDS/FLOOR OF MOUTH

Case 36: Ranula (Fig. 12.36)

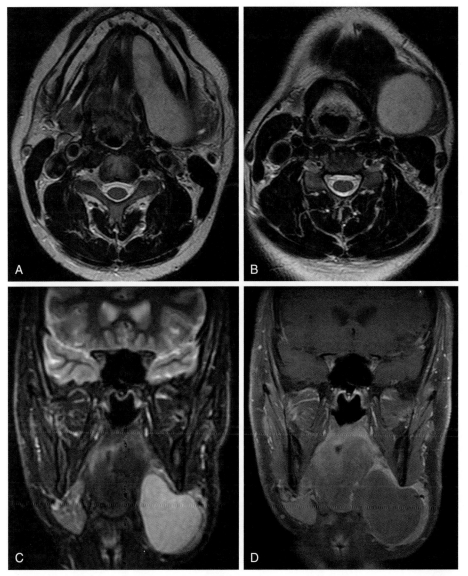

Fig. 12.36 Ranula. (**A**) Axial T2-weighted image demonstrates a lobulated hyperintense collection in the left floor of the mouth. (**B**) The collection is again seen on this axial T2-weighted image with extension inferiorly to the left submandibular space deforming the adjacent left submandibular gland. (**C**) Coronal STIR (short tau inversion recovery) imaging shows this lesion from the left sublingual space to the submandibular space, consistent with a diving or plunging ranula. (**D**) There is no enhancement of the ranula on postcontrast T1-weighted imaging given its cystic nature.

Imaging findings: A ranula is a pseudocyst of the floor of the mouth, arising from the sublingual glands or minor salivary glands. Typically midline in location, these are unilocular, well-circumscribed cystic lesions. Simple ranulas are confined to the floor of the mouth. When these extend through the mylohyoid muscle into the submental region or posteriorly and inferiorly into the submandibular space, they are called *plunging* or *diving ranulas.*

CT: Well-circumscribed unilocular cystic lesion with a thin wall, which demonstrates enhancement.

MRI: These lesions are typically hypointense on T1-weighted images and hyperintense on T2-weighted images. On postcontrast images, the wall will enhance. If proteinaceous material is present, a variable signal is seen on MRI.

Differential diagnosis: Abscess, dermoids, or epidermoid.

Case 37: Parotitis (Fig. 12.37)

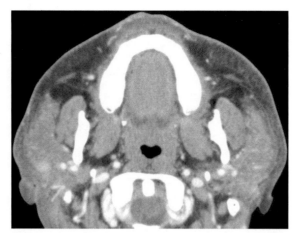

Fig. 12.37 Parotitis. Severe right facial inflammatory changes are seen centered around the right parotid gland on this axial postcontrast computed tomography image which extend into the right masticator space. An organized fluid collection has formed in the right parotid gland posterior to the angle of the mandible consistent with an abscess in this severe case of infectious right parotitis.

Imaging findings: Parotitis is sialadenitis of the parotid gland. The earliest finding is increased size and attenuation of the parotid gland. The parenchyma may demonstrate stranding or reticulation. Thickening of the capsule of the gland may be seen. Associated stranding of the adjacent fat, thickening of the skin, and abscess formation may be present. The draining salivary (Stenson) duct should be assessed for an obstructive process such as a stone, stricture, or mass. Associated dilatation of the salivary duct with thickening and enhancement of the wall of the salivary duct is sialodochitis, or ductal sialadenitis.

Differential diagnosis: Sjögren syndrome, sialosis, lymphoma, or leukemia.

Case 38: Sialolith (Fig. 12.38)

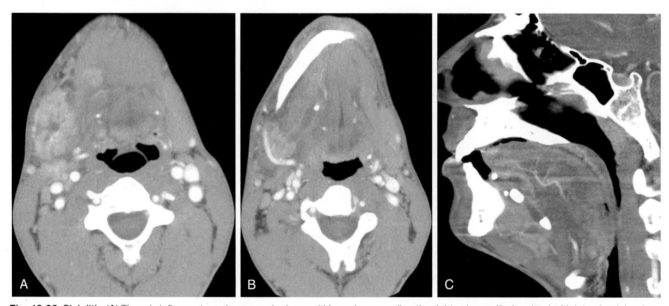

Fig. 12.38 Sialolith. (A) There is inflammatory change and edema within and surrounding the right submandibular gland with intraglandular ductal dilatation seen on this axial postcontrast computed tomography (CT) image. **(B)** The Wharton duct is dilated, and an obstructive stone can be seen within the duct. **(C)** On sagittal reconstruction of the CT images, multiple obstructive stones in the Wharton duct are evident.

Imaging findings: Stones are more commonly associated with submandibular and sublingual glands. Thin-section CT imaging is the modality of choice for evaluation. A contrast-enhanced CT is sufficient for evaluation. Stones may occur anywhere along the course of the salivary duct or in the hilum of the gland. Secondary sialadenitis or sialodochitis may be present. Plain films may be of use in the assessment of a radiodense stone.

Differential diagnosis: None

Case 39: Sjögren Syndrome (Fig. 12.39)

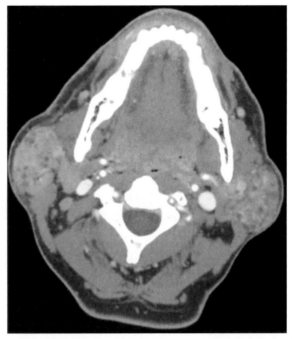

Fig. 12.39 Sjögren disease. Multiple tiny bilateral parotid cysts are seen on postcontrast axial computed tomography imaging of the neck. No calcifications or volume loss of the glands were present for the stage of disease in this patient.

Imaging findings: Chronic multisystem autoimmune process, which may involve the salivary and lacrimal glands. Involvement of the parotid glands is a common finding. The early presentation is similar to parotitis. Typically, there is bilateral involvement of the salivary glands, which rules out simple sialadenitis. In the intermediate stage, intraductal strictures within the gland causing dilatation of the acinar sacs and microcyts are present, seen as honeycombing within the gland. Benign lymphoepithelial cysts or masses are present within the parotid gland, arising from the lymphoid tissue only found in the parotid glands. Calcifications may be present. In late-stage Sjögren syndrome, involution and fatty replacement of the glands may occur. Of note, there is a 44-times increased incidence of MALT-type of lymphoma in Sjögren syndrome. A dominant enlarged mass is worrisome for lymphoma and should be evaluated.

Differential diagnosis: Chronic obstruction of a salivary duct with chronic infection, human immunodeficiency virus disease, Warthin tumors, or lymphoma.

Case 40: Pleomorphic Adenoma (Fig. 12.40)

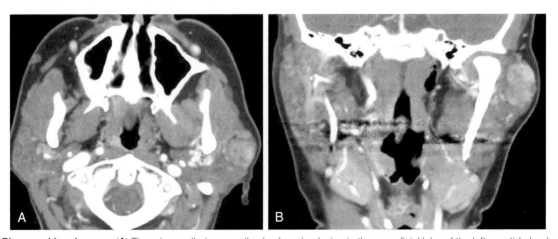

Fig. 12.40 Pleomorphic adenoma. (A) There is a well-circumscribed enhancing lesion in the superficial lobe of the left parotid gland on this postcontrast computed tomography (CT) image. **(B)** Coronal CT again demonstrates the well-circumscribed borders of the mass.

Imaging findings: Pleomorphic adenoma is the most common benign tumor of salivary gland origin. Well-circumscribed, heterogeneously moderate to avid enhancement is present. These lesions may demonstrate cystic change, calcification, and hemorrhage. The borders of the lesion are the best sign to determine benign from malignant salivary gland tumor. Benign tumors demonstrate well-marginated, sharp borders without stranding in the adjacent salivary parenchyma. Lack of facial paralysis for a parotid lesion is also useful. On MRI, the lesions are typically hyperintense on T2-weighted images and do not restrict on diffusion-weighted imaging.

Differential diagnosis: Warthin tumor, lymphadenopathy in the parotid gland, nerve sheath tumor, or malignant tumor (adenoid cystic carcinoma, mucoepidermoid carcinoma, lymphoma).

Case 41: Mucoepidermoid Carcinoma (Fig. 12.41)

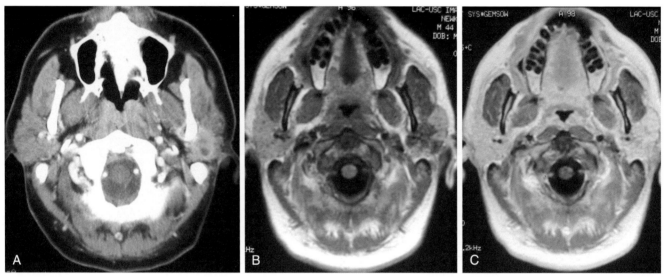

Fig. 12.41 Mucoepidermoid carcinoma. (A) Postcontrast computed tomography (CT) demonstrates a complex mass with both solid and cystic components in the superficial lobe of the left parotid gland posterior to the ramus of the mandible. Note the ill-defined margins of the mass. **(B)** T1-weighted axial image demonstrates the mass is isointense to muscle signal intensity. The ill-defined borders of the lesion are again seen compared with the parotid signal intensity. The borders of the lesion are better appreciated on the CT study. **(C)** Postcontrast axial image demonstrates enhancement of the lesion and the surrounding parotid tissue with poor delineation of the two.

Imaging findings: The most common parotid malignancy and second most common in the remaining salivary glands. Ill-defined borders and associated pathological nodes are present though low-grade mucoepidermoid tumors may demonstrate a well-circumscribed border. On MRI, areas of lower signal intensity on T2-weighted images are characteristic but not pathognomonic. Perineural spread of tumor may be seen on MR imaging.

Differential diagnosis: Other malignant tumor (adenoid cystic carcinoma, acinic cell carcinoma, or lymphoma), pleomorphic adenoma, or Warthin tumor.

Case 42: Dermoid of Floor of the Mouth (Fig. 12.42)

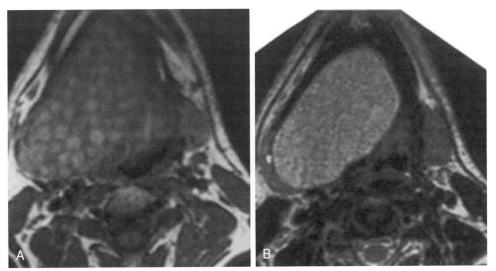

Fig. 12.42 Dermoid of the floor of the mouth. (**A**) A large mass is seen in the right-hand side of the floor of the mouth with a surrounding capsule. Note that within this lesion are numerous well-circumscribed hyperintense components representing fat globules. This is pathognomonic for a dermoid. (**B**) T2-weighted axial image demonstrates the mass to be heterogeneous with foci of hyperintensity consistent with fat.

Imaging findings: CT shows a well-circumscribed cystic lesion in the floor of the mouth. The wall is thin and may or may not enhance. Because of the presence of fat, the lesion may have lower density compared with CSF. However, dermoids and epidermoid may not be distinguishable on CT.

MRI: Because of the presence of fat, the lesion may demonstrate hyperintense signal intensity on both T1- and T2-weighted images. On occasion, fat globules may be present and have the appearance of a sack of beads, which follow fat signal intensity. On postcontrast images, no enhancement is seen.

Differential diagnosis: Epidermoid, abscess, ranula, or Ludwig angina.

NECK

Case 43: Thyroglossal Duct Cyst (Fig. 12.43)

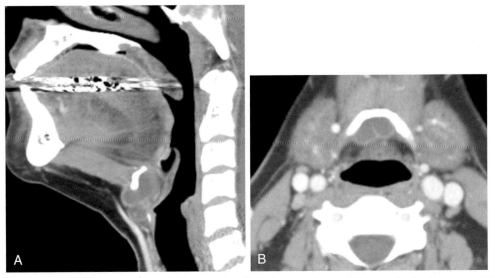

Fig. 12.43 Thyroglossal duct cyst (TGDC). (**A**) There is a lobulated cystic lesion posterior and inferior to the hyoid bone on sagittal postcontrast computed tomography images of the neck. (**B**) In the axial plane, an internal septation is evident. The location is classic for a TGDC.

Imaging findings: As they arise from the primitive thyroglossal duct, these lesions tend to be midline, especially in the suprahyoid neck. A midline cystic lesion in the base of the tongue is pathognomonic for a thyroglossal duct cyst (TGDC). However, most of these lesions are in the infrahyoid neck and may lateralize to one side, and are deep, not superficial, to the strap muscles of the neck. Noninfected TGDCs are well-circumscribed cystic lesions, unilocular, with a thin wall, which may or may not enhance. Infected TGDCs may demonstrate increased density and have thick irregular walls that mimic an abscess. At the level of the hyoid bone, these lesions are associated with the anterior, inferior, and posterior aspect of the mid-portion of the hyoid bone. Thyroid rests may be present within the TGDC, and malignancies (papillary carcinoma and squamous cell carcinoma) have been associated with these lesions, giving them a complex, aggressive appearance.

Case 44: Second Branchial Cleft Anomaly (Fig. 12.44)

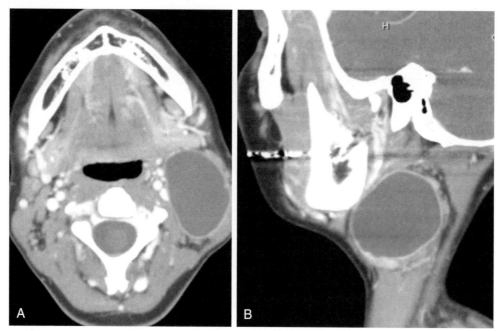

Fig. 12.44 Second branchial cleft anomaly. (A) Postcontrast computed tomography of the neck shows a cystic structure in the left neck with a thin enhancing wall deep to the sternocleidomastoid muscle and lateral to the carotid artery. **(B)** On sagittal reconstruction, the simple nature of the cyst or branchial cleft anomaly is seen with no surrounding inflammatory change or nodularity. The cyst is located near the angle of the mandible with the location diagnostic for a second branchial cleft anomaly.

Imaging findings: These are of embryological origin from the second branchial cleft. The most common location is at the angle of the mandible posterior to the submandibular gland, lateral to the carotid space, and anterior to the sternocleidomastoid muscle in the anterior cervical space. Noninfected cysts are well-circumscribed unilocular cystic lesions. The presence of septations or a solid component should raise the question of other etiologies. As all branchial cleft cysts have a sinus tract, the sinus tract for a second branchial cleft anomaly (BCA) is along the medial border and a teat sign may be present. The sinus tract is to the oropharynx. Infected cysts may demonstrate increased density on CT and variable signal on MRI, as well as a thickened irregular wall and stranding of the adjacent fat.

Differential diagnosis: Vasoformative malformation, thymic cyst, lymphadenopathy, abscess, or cystic metastatic disease.

Case 45: Third Branchial Cleft Anomaly (Fig. 12.45)

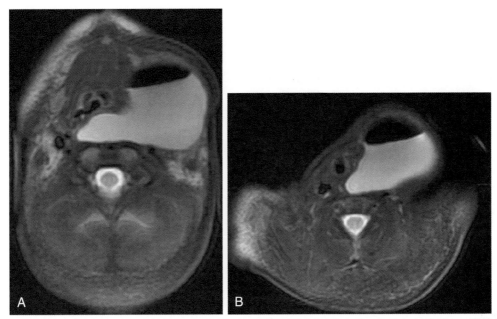

Fig. 12.45 Third branchial cleft anomaly. (A) T2-weighted axial image demonstrates a cystic lesion in the left lateral neck at the level of the hypopharynx extending medially into the retropharyngeal space. This lesion demonstrates an air-fluid level with the fluid component appearing hyperintense. **(B)** Axial image inferiorly again shows this large cystic lesion with air-fluid level. During surgery, a sinus tract was found to extend from this lesion to the apex of the piriform sinus, confirming a third branchial cleft anomaly.

Imaging findings: Arising from the third branchial cleft, these lesions are typically mistaken for an abscess in the upper posterior neck or lower anterior neck. The sinus tract for these cysts extends to the apex of the piriform sinus. CT and MRI findings are similar to the second BCA.

Differential diagnosis: Second BCA, thymic cyst, abscess, lymphadenopathy, cystic metastatic disease, or external laryngocele.

Case 46: Lymphangioma (Fig. 12.46)

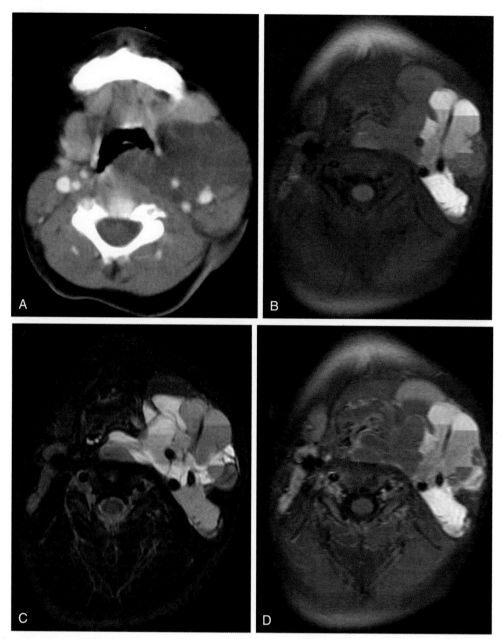

Fig. 12.46 Neck lymphangioma. (A) Postcontrast computed tomography reveals a multicystic lesion in the left lateral neck with anterior displacement of the submandibular gland. This lesion surrounds the internal jugular vein, as well as the internal and external carotid arteries with medial extension to the retropharyngeal space. **(B)** T1-weighted axial image also demonstrates that this is a multicystic lesion with fluid-fluid levels. The fluid components have varying internal signal intensity. **(C)** T2-weighted axial image also shows that the fluid components again exhibit intermediate to hyperintense signal intensity with fluid-fluid levels. **(D)** Postcontrast T1-weighted axial image demonstrates no solid enhancement. These findings in total are suggestive of a lymphangioma.

Imaging findings: A form of vasoformative malformation—a multilocular thin-walled cystic lesion that may occur anywhere in the neck where lymph nodes occur. The cysts may contain fluid, proteinaceous material, or blood products, and the walls of the cystic components may enhance. On CT, these lesions are multicystic with potential wall enhancement. On MRI, the cystic components may have variable signal intensities on T1- and T2-weighted images with fluid-fluid levels.

Differential diagnosis: Cystic metastasis, second BCA (on CT), or abscess.

Case 47: Lemierre Syndrome (Fig. 12.47)

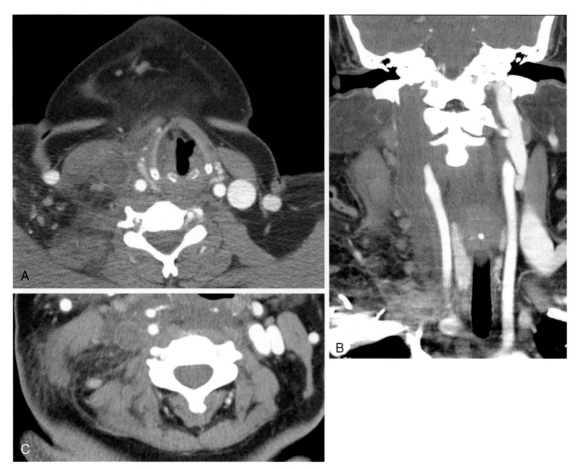

Fig. 12.47 Lemierre syndrome. (A) Acute inflammatory changes are seen in the right neck deep to the sternocleidomastoid muscle in the carotid space centered around a thrombosed right internal jugular vein on this postcontrast computed tomography (CT). Reactive right cervical lymph nodes are present. **(B)** On coronal CT reconstructions, thrombophlebitis of the right internal jugular vein is nicely shown with adjacent fat stranding and reactive lymphadenopathy. **(C)** Concurrent retropharyngeal abscess is present.

Imaging findings: The imaging findings in Lemierre syndrome are thrombophlebitis of the internal jugular vein and presence of a retropharyngeal (RP) abscess. The most common organism is *Fusobacterium necrophorum*, although *Staphylococcus* and *Streptococcus* are also known causative agents. Because of the thrombophlebitis, the patient may go on to pulmonary thromboembolic disease. On CT, thrombosis of the internal jugular vein with thickening of the wall and stranding of the adjacent fat is present. An RP abscess or fluid collection is also present.

CASE 48: Retropharyngeal Abscess (FIG. 12.48)

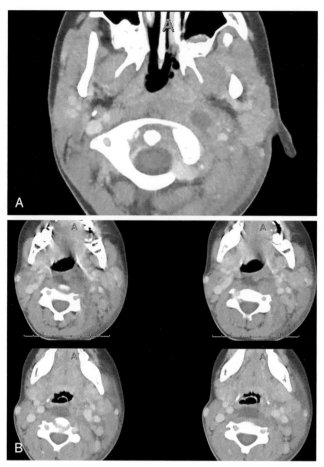

Fig. 12.48 Retropharyngeal abscess. (A) Postcontrast axial computed tomography (CT) demonstrates a suppurative left retropharyngeal lymph node in this child presenting with a sore throat. **(B)** Additional serial CT images more inferiorly show fluid collection in the retropharyngeal space without discrete rim enhancement. This was surgically drained and shown to be an abscess.

Imaging findings: RP abscess manifests as fluid or inflammatory material in the retropharyngeal space (RPS) replacing the normal thin layer of fat with other infectious changes in the neck typically present, such as suppurative lymphadenitis from oropharyngitis or tonsillitis. RP abscess most commonly occurs in the pediatric population when the lymphatic channels draining the oropharynx are patent with direct spread to the RP lymph nodes. Necrosis within infected RP lymph nodes leads to rupture of the lymph node capsule and extension of infection within the RPS. The RPS (along with danger space more posteriorly) serves as a conduit from the skull base to the mediastinum, which may result in skull base osteomyelitis or mediastinitis, making timely diagnosis and treatment critical. Due to the lack of vascularity within the RPS, RP abscess may not demonstrate peripheral or rim enhancement on postcontrast CT or MRI, a finding unique to abscess in this location. Loculated fluid collections within the RPS in particular are suggestive of an RP abscess. Diffusion weighted imaging on MRI may be helpful to distinguish abscess from simple edema as the contents of the abscess may show reduced diffusion or decreased free water motion, suggesting viscous or thick material.

Case 49: Squamous Cell Carcinoma of the Larynx (Fig. 12.49)

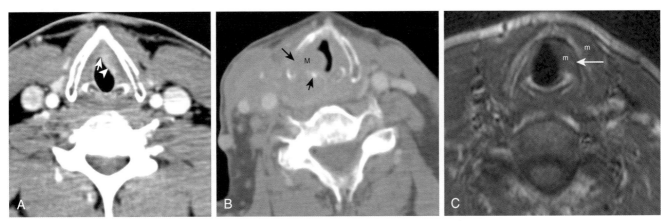

Fig. 12.49 Squamous cell carcinoma of the larynx. (A) This axial postcontrast computed tomography (CT) shows a tumor of the left true vocal cord (*arrowhead*) with mild expansile change and enhancement that extends anteriorly to involve the anterior commissure (*arrow*). **(B)** In another patient with laryngeal squamous cell carcinoma, CT shows a right laryngeal soft-tissue mass (*M*) that destroys both the right thyroid cartilage ala (*long arrow*) and the posterior right cricoid cartilage (*short arrow*). **(C)** In a third patient, T1-weighted magnetic resonance imaging shows thyroid cartilage invasion (*arrow*). A glottic carcinoma (*m*) extends through the left lamina of the thyroid cartilage. (From Flint PW, Haughey BH, Lund VJ, et al. *Cummings Otolaryngology—Head and Neck Surgery.* 6th ed. Philadelphia, PA: Saunders; 2015.)

Imaging findings: CT and MRI are excellent methods for evaluating the subsite involvement in squamous cell carcinoma of the larynx and determining the presence or extent of cartilage invasion for staging. True vocal fold paralysis and disease extension beyond the larynx may also be suggested on the basis of both CT and MRI.

Cartilage involvement of laryngeal squamous cell carcinoma may manifest as sclerotic change, erosion, destruction, or soft-tissue extension through the cartilage on CT. MRI is more sensitive but less specific than CT for detection of cartilage involvement. Increased T2-weighted signal on fat suppressed images and contrast enhancement, particularly when the signal intensity is similar to the primary tumor, may indicate carcinoma invasion into the cartilage. More recent studies have also suggested that diffusion-weighted imaging may be helpful in detecting cartilage invasion.

Differential diagnosis: Papilloma, laryngocele, hemangioma, or salivary gland neoplasm.

Case 50: Carotid Body Tumor (Fig. 12.50)

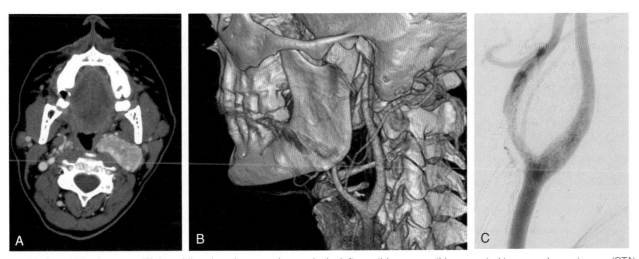

Fig. 12.50 Carotid body tumor. (A) An avidly enhancing mass is seen in the left carotid space on this computed tomography angiogram (CTA) of the neck with the contrast bolus in a mixed arterial to venous phase. **(B)** A 3-dimensional reconstruction of the left carotid bifurcation from the CTA shows the classic splaying of the internal and external carotid arteries caused by the carotid body tumor. **(C)** This finding was confirmed on digital subtraction catheter angiography.

Imaging findings: A carotid body tumor is a paraganglioma that occurs in the crotch between the origins of the internal and external carotid arteries, splaying them apart.

MRI: MRI demonstrates classic flow voids and the characteristic salt-and-pepper appearance. An isolated carotid body tumor can be differentiated from an isolated glomus vagale tumor by anterior displacement of both the internal and external carotid in the case of a glomus vagale tumor.

Angiography: Selective carotid angiography can be used both for diagnostic and for preoperative embolization.

Differential diagnosis: Glomus vagale, glomus jugulare, vagal schwannoma, or lymphadenopathy.

FURTHER READINGS

Abdel Razek AAK. Imaging of connective tissue diseases of the head and neck. *Neuroradiol J.* 2016;29(3):222–230.

Abdel Razek AAK, Mukherji S. Imaging of sialadenitis. *Neuroradiol J.* 2017;30(3):205–215. https://doi.org/10.1177/1971400916682752.

Abdel Razek AAK, Mukherji SK. Imaging of minor salivary glands. *Neuroimaging Clin N Am.* 2018;28(2):295–302.

Acharya S, Naik C, Panditray S, Dany SS. Juvenile nasopharyngeal angiofibroma: a case report. *J Clin Diagn Res.* 2017;11(4):MD03–MD04.

Albadr FB. Silent sinus syndrome: interesting computed tomography and magnetic resonance imaging findings. *J Clin Imaging Sci.* 2020;10:38.

Alshuhayb Z, Alkhamis H, Aldossary M, et al. Tornwaldt nasopharyngeal cyst: case series and literature review. *Int J Surg Case Rep.* 2020;76:166–169.

Amit M, Fliss DM, Gil Z. Fibrous dysplasia of the sphenoid and skull base. *Otolaryngol Clin North Am.* 2011;44(4):891–902. vii–viii.

Andreu-Arasa VC, Sung EK, Fujita A, Saito N, Sakai O. Otosclerosis and dysplasias of the temporal bone. *Neuroimaging Clin N Am.* 2019; 29(1):29–47.

Araujo JP, Terra GTC, Cortes ARG, Hernandez A, Oliveira JX. A comparison of conventional and diffusion-weighted magnetic resonance imaging in the diagnosis of sialadenitis and pleomorphic adenoma. *Oral Surg Oral Med Oral Pathol Oral Radiol.* 2019;127(5):451–457.

Aravena C, Almeida FA, Mukhopadhyay S, et al. Idiopathic subglottic stenosis: a review. *J Thorac Dis.* 2020;12(3):1100–1111.

Aribandi M, McCoy VA, Bazan 3rd C. Imaging features of invasive and noninvasive fungal sinusitis: a review. *Radiographics.* 2007;27(5): 1283–1296.

Aydin S, Demir MG, Selek A. A giant lymphangioma on the neck. *J Craniofac Surg.* 2015;26(4):e323–e325.

Bailey H. The clinical aspect of branchial cysts. In: *Branchial Cysts and Other Essays on Surgical Subjects in the Facio-cervical Region.* London: H.K: Lewis; 1929:1–18.

Bakshi SS. Nasal meningocele. *Arch Dis Child.* 2017;102(9):845.

Batson L, Rizzolo D. Otosclerosis: an update on diagnosis and treatment. *JAAPA.* 2017;30(2):17–22.

Becker M, Zbären P, Casselman JW, Kohler R, Dulguerov P, Becker CD. Neoplastic Invasion of Laryngeal Cartilage: reassessment of criteria for diagnosis at MR imaging. *Radiology.* 2008;249:551–559.

Bhalla N, Rosenstein J, Dym H. Silent sinus syndrome: interesting clinical and radiologic findings. *J Oral Maxillofac Surg.* 2019; 77(10):2040–2043.

Bhatia KSS, King AD, Vlantis AC, Ahuja AT, Tse GM. Nasopharyngeal mucosa and adenoids: appearance at MR imaging. *Radiology.* 2012;263(2):437–443.

Cascarini L, McGurk M. Epidemiology of salivary gland infections. *Oral Maxillofac Surg Clin North Am.* 2009;21(3):353–370.

Ceylan N, Bayraktaroglu S, Alper H, et al. CT imaging of superior semicircular canal dehiscence: added value of reformatted images. *Acta Otolaryngol.* 2010;130(9):996–1001.

Chakeres DW, LaMasters DL. Paragangliomas of the temporal bone: high resolution CT studies. *Radiology.* 1984;150(3):749–753.

Chen L, Yu Z, Jiang R, Dong P, Shen B, Li Y. A case of dedifferentiated chondrosarcoma arising in the cricoid cartilage that mimicked an aneurysmal bone cyst. *Postgrad Med.* 2018;130(2):274–277.

Chin SC, Edelstein S, Chen CY, Som PM. Using CT to localize side and level of vocal cord paralysis. *AJR Am J Roentgenol.* 2003; 180(4):1165–1170.

Chittiboina P, Lonser RR. Von Hippel-Lindau disease. *Handb Clin Neurol.* 2015;132:139–156.

Chhabda S, Leger DS, Lingam RK. Imaging the facial nerve: a contemporary review of anatomy and pathology. *Eur J Radiol.* 2020; 126:108920.

Cho YT, Kim JH, Khang SK, Lee JK, Kim CJ. Chordomas and chondrosarcomas of the skull base: comparative analysis of clinical results in 30 patients. *Neurosurg Rev.* 2008;31(1):35–43.

Chong VF, Khoo JB, Fan YF. Fibrous dysplasia involving the base of the skull. *AJR Am J Roentgenol.* 2002;178(3):717–720.

Choudhri AF, Parmar HA, Morales RE, Gandhi D. Lesions of the skull base: imaging for diagnosis and treatment. *Otolaryngol Clin North Am.* 2012;45(6):1385–1404.

Chweya CM, Anzalone CL, Driscoll CLW, Lane JI, Carlson ML. For whom the Bell's toll: recurrent facial nerve paralysis, a retrospective study and systematic review of the literature. *Otol Neurotol.* 2019;40(4):517–528.

Clifton AG, Phelps PD, Brookes GB. Cholesterol granuloma of the petrous apex. *Br J Radiol.* 1990;63(753):724–726.

Contrucci RB, Sataloff RT, Myers DL. Petrous apicitis. *Ear Nose Throat J.* 1985;64(9):427–431.

Consul N, Menias CO, Lubner MG, et al. A review of viral-related malignancies and the associated imaging findings. *AJR Am J Roentgenol.* 2020;214(1):W1–W10.

Cophan DM, Popat S, Kaplan SE, Rigual N, Loree T, Hicks WL Jr. Oropharyngeal cancer: current understanding and management. *Curr Opin Otolaryngol Head Neck Surg.* 2009;17(2):88–94.

Dang L, Tu NCY, Chan EY. Current imaging tools for vestibular schwannoma. *Curr Opin Otolaryngol Head Neck Surg.* 2020;28(5): 302–307.

Datta A, Das PP, Ullah MM, Datta PG, Azad MS. Role of Computed tomography in the evaluation of nasopharyngeal mass. *Mymensingh Med J.* 2017;26(2):426–431.

Dave AV, Diaz-Marchan PJ, Lee AG. Clinical and magnetic resonance imaging features of Gradenigo syndrome. *Am J Ophthalmol.* 1997;124(4):568–570.

Di Stadio A, Dipietro L, Ralli M, et al. Loop characteristics and audio-vestibular symptoms or hemifacial spasm: is there a correlation? A multiplanar MRI study. *Eur Radiol.* 2020;30(1):99–109.

Dobre MC, Fischbein N. "Do not touch" lesions of the skull base. *J Med Imaging Radiat Oncol.* 2014;58(4):458–463.

Duggal P, Wise SK. Chapter 8: Invasive fungal rhinosinusitis. *Am J Rhinol Allergy.* 2013;27(suppl 1):S28–30.

El-Begermy MA, Mansour OI, El-Makhzangy AM, El-Gindy TS. Congenital auditory meatal atresia: a numerical review. *Ear Arch Otorhinolaryngol.* 2009;266(4):501–506.

Ewing CA, Kornblut A, Greeley C, Manz H. Presentations of thyroglossal duct cysts in adults. *Eur Arch Otorhinolaryngol.* 1999;256(3): 136–138.

Fageeh N, Manoukian J, Tewfik T, Schloss M, Williams HB, Gaskin D. Management of head and neck lymphatic malformations in children. *J Otolaryngol.* 1997;26(4):253–258.

Fiani B, Quadri SA, Cathel A, et al. Esthesioneuroblastoma: a comprehensive review of diagnosis, management, and current treatment options. *World Neurosurg.* 2019;126:194–211.

Foggia MJ, Peterson J, Maley J, Policeni B, Hoffman HT. Sialographic analysis of parotid ductal abnormalities associated with Sjogren's syndrome. *Oral Dis.* 2020;26(5):912–919.

Forli F, Lazzerini F, Auletta G, Bruschini L, Berrettini S. Enlarged vestibular aqueduct and Mondini malformation: audiological, clinical, radiologic and genetic features. *Eur Arch Otorhinolaryngol.* 2021; 278(7):2305–2312.

Friedmann DR, Grobelny B, Golfinos JG, Roland JT Jr. Nonschwannoma tumors of the cerebellopontine angle. *Otolaryngol Clin North Am.* 2015;48(3):461–475.

Friedman O, Neff BA, Willcox TO, Kenyon LC, Sataloff RT. Temporal bone hemangiomas involving the facial nerve. *Otol Neurotol.* 2002;23(5):760–766.

Friedman E, Patiño MO, Udayasankar UK. Imaging of pediatric salivary glands. *Neuroimaging Clin N Am.* 2018;28(2):209–226.

Fujimoto N, Fujii N, Nagata Y, Uenishi T, Tanaka T. Dermoid cyst with magnetic resonance image of sack-of-marbles. *Br J Dermatol.* 2008;158(2):415–417.

Gadre AK, Chole RA. The changing face of petrous apicitis—a 40-year experience. *Laryngoscope.* 2018;128(1):195–201.

Giarraputo L, Savastano S, D'Amore E, Baciliero U. Dermoid cyst of the floor of the mouth: diagnostic imaging findings. *Cureus.* 2018;10(4):e2403. https://doi.org/10.7759/cureus.2403.

Ginat DT. Imaging of benign neoplastic and nonneoplastic salivary gland tumors. *Neuroimaging Clin N Am.* 2018;28(2):159–169.

Glastonbury CM. NP carcinoma: the role of magnetic resonance imaging in diagnosis, staging, treatment, and follow-up. *Top Magn Reson Imaging.* 2007;18(4):225–235.

Gore MR. Lemierre syndrome: a meta-analysis. *Int Arch Otorhinolaryngol.* 2020;24(3):e379–e385.

Gosepath J, Mann WJ. Current concepts in therapy of chronic rhinosinusitis and nasal polyposis. *ORJ J Otorhinolaryngol Relat Spec.* 2005;67(3):125–136.

Greene AK, Rogers GF, Mulliken JB. Intraosseous "hemangiomas" are malformations and not tumors. *Plast Reconstr Surg.* 2007;119(6):1949–1950.

Griauzde J, Srinivasan A. Imaging of vascular lesions of the head and neck. *Radiol Clin North Am.* 2015;53(1):197–213.

Griauzde J, Srinivasan A. Imaging of vascular lesions of the head and neck. *Radiol Clin North Am.* 2015;53(1):197–213.

Gultekin S, Celik H, Akpek S, Oner Y, Gumus T, Tokgoz N. Vascular loops at the cerebellopontine angle: is there a correlation with tinnitus? *AJNR Am J Neuroradiol.* 2008;29(9):1746–1749.

Hamilton BE, Salzman KL, Patel N, et al. Imaging and clinical characteristics of temporal bone meningioma. *AJNR Am J Neuroradiol.* 2006;27(10):2204–2209.

Harnsberger HR, Mancuso AA, Muraki AS, et al. Branchial cleft anomalies and their mimics: computed tomographic evaluation. *Radiology.* 1984;152(3):739–748.

Hoang JK, Branstetter BF, Eastwood JD, Glastonbury CM. Multiplanar CT and MRI of collections in the retropharyngeal space: is it an abscess? *AJR Am J Roentgenol.* 2011;196(4):W426–W432.

Huisman TAGM, Schneider JFL, Kellenberger CJ, Martin-Fiori E, Willi UV, Holzmann D. Developmental nasal midline masses in children: neuroradiological evaluation. *Eur Radiol.* 2004;14(2):243–249.

Ibrahim M, Hammoud K, Maheshwari M, Pandya A. Congenital cystic lesions of the head and neck. *Neuroimaging Clin N Am.* 2011;21(3):621–639. viii.

Ikeda K, Katoh T, Ha-Kawa SK, Iwai H, Yamashita T, Tanaka Y. The usefulness of MR in establishing the diagnosis of parotid pleiomorphic adenoma. *AJNR Am J Neuroradiol.* 1996;17(3):555–559.

Ikushima I, Korogi Y, Makita O, et al. MR imaging of Tornwaldt's cysts. *AJR Am J Roentgenol.* 1999;172(6):1663–1665.

Isaacson B. Cholesterol granuloma and other petrous apex lesions. *Otolaryngol Clin North Am.* 2015;48(2):361–373.

Izumi M, Eguchi K, Ohki M. MR imaging of the parotid gland in Sjögren's syndrome: a proposal for new diagnostic criteria. *AJR Am J Roentgenol.* 1996;166(6):1483–1487.

Jackler RK, Luxford WM, House WF. Congenital malformation of the inner ear: a classification based on embryogenesis. *Laryngoscope.* 1987;97(suppl 40):2–14.

Johnson JM, Moonis G, Green GE, Carmody R, Burbank HN. Syndromes of the first and second branchial arches, part 2: syndromes. *AJNR Am J Neuroradiol.* 2011;32(2):230–237.

Joshi MJ, Provenzano MJ, Smith RJH, Sato Y, Smoker WRK. The rare third branchial cleft cyst. *AJNR Am J Neuroradiol.* 2009;30(9):1804–1806.

Kalia V, Kalra G, Kaur S, Kapoor R. CT scan as an essential tool in diagnosis of non-radiopaque sialoliths. *J Maxillofac Oral Surg.* 2015;14(suppl 1):240–244.

Kato H, Kanematsu M, Kawaguchi S, Watanabe H, Mizuta K, Aoki M. Evaluation of imaging findings differentiating extranodal non-Hodgkin's lymphoma from squamous cell carcinoma in naso- and oropharynx. *Clin Imaging.* 2013;37(4):657–663.

Kato H, Kanematsu M, Kawaguchi S, Watanabe H, Mizuta K, Aoki M. Evaluation of imaging findings differentiating extranodal non-Hodgkin's lymphoma from squamous cell carcinoma in naso- and oropharynx. *Clin Imaging.* 2013;37(4):657–663.

Kato H, Kawaguchi M, Ando T, Mizuta K, Aoki M, Matsuo M. Pleomorphic adenoma of salivary glands: common and uncommon CT and MR imaging features. *Jpn J Radiol.* 2018;36(8):463–471.

Kösling S, Plontke SK, Bartel S. Imaging of otosclerosis. *Rofo.* 2020;192(8):745–753.

Kuwada C, Mannion K, Aulino JM, Kanekar SG. Imaging of the carotid space. *Otolaryngol Clin North Am.* 2012;45(6):1273–1292.

Kuwada C, Mannion K, Aulino JM, Kanekar SG. Imaging of the carotid space. *Otolaryngol Clin North Am.* 2012;45(6):1273–1292.

Kurabayashi T, Ida M, Yasumoto M, et al. MRI of ranulas. *Neuroradiology.* 2000;42(12):917–922.

Kuwada C, Mannion K, Aulino JM, Kanekar SG. Imaging of the carotid space. *Otolaryngol Clin North Am.* 2012;45(6):1273–1292.

Langner S, Ginzkey C, Mlynski R, Weiss NM. Differentiation of retropharyngeal calcific tendinitis and retropharyngeal abscess:

a case series and review of the literature. *Eur Arch Otorhinolaryngol.* 2020;277(9):2631–2636.

Li Z, Zhang J, Yang Y, He X. Third branchial cleft cyst as a cause of hoarseness: a case report. *J Int Med Res.* 2021;49(5). 3000605211012549.

Lin ST, Tseng FY, Hsu CJ, Yeh TH, Chen YS. Thyroglossal duct cyst: a comparison between children and adults. *Am J Otolaryngol.* 2008;29(2):83–87.

Lisan Q, Laccourreye O, Bonfils P. Sinonasal inverted papilloma: from diagnosis to treatment. *Eur Ann Otorhinolaryngol Head Neck Dis.* 2016;133(5):337–341.

Lloyd KM, DelGaudio JM, Hudgins PA. Imaging of skull base cerebrospinal fluid leaks in adults. *Radiology.* 2008;248(3):725–736.

Lo WW, Solti-Bohman LG, McElveen Jr JT. Aberrant carotid artery: radiologic diagnosis with emphasis on high resolution computed tomography. *Radiographics.* 1985;5(6):985–993.

López F, Triantafyllou A, Snyderman CH, et al. Nasal juvenile angiofibroma: current perspectives with emphasis on management. *Head Neck.* 2017;39(5):1033–1045.

Lorenz RR. Adult laryngotracheal stenosis: etiology and surgical management. *Curr Opin Otolaryngol Head Neck Surg.* 2003;11(6):467–472.

Macdonald AJ, Salzman KL, Harnsberger HR, Gilbert E, Shelton C. Primary jugular foramen meningioma: imaging appearance and differentiating features. *AJR Am J Roentgenol.* 2004;182(2):373–377.

Magliocca KR, Edgar MA, Corey A, Villari CR. Dedifferentiated chondrosarcoma of the larynx: radiological, gross, microscopic and clinical features. *Ann Diagn Pathol.* 2017;30:42–46.

Mandell DL. Head and neck anomalies related to the branchial apparatus. *Otolaryngol Clin North Am.* 2000;33(6):1309–1332.

Maroldi R, Farina D, Palvarini L, Lombardi D, Tomenzoli D, Nicolai P. Magnetic resonance imaging findings of inverted papilloma: differential diagnosis with malignant sinonasal tumors. *Am J Rhinol.* 2004;18(5):305–310.

Mayer TE, Brueckmann H, Siegert R, Witt A, Weerda H. High-resolution CT of the temporal bone in dysplasia of the auricle and external auditory canal. *AJNR Am J Neuroradiol.* 1997;18(1):53–65.

McCabe R, Lee DJ, Fina M. The endoscopic management of congenital cholesteatoma. *Otolaryngol Clin North Am.* 2021;54(1):111–123.

McCann MR, Kessler AT, Bhatt AA. Emergency radiologic approach to sinus disease. *Emerg Radiol.* 2021;28(5):1003–1010.

Meyer I. Dermoid cysts (dermoids) of the floor of the mouth. *J Oral Surg (Chic) O.* 1955;8(11):1149–1164.

Moody MW, Chi DH, Mason JC, Phillips CD, Gross CW, Schlosser RJ. Tornwaldt's cyst: incidence and a case report. *Ear Nose Throat J.* 2007;86(1):45–47.

Moosa S, Fezeu F, Kesser BW, Ramesh A, Sheehan JP. Sudden unilateral hearing loss and vascular loop in the internal auditory canal: case report and review of literature. *J Radiosurg SBRT.* 2015;3(3):247–255.

Mukerji SS, Parmar HA, Gujar S, Passamani P. Intranasal meningoencephalocele presenting as a nasal polyp—a case report. *Clin Imaging.* 2011;35(4):309–311.

Mukherji SK, Fatterpekar G, Castillo M, Stone JA, Chung CJ. Imaging of congenital anomalies of the branchial apparatus. *Neuroimaging Clin N Am.* 2000;10(1):75–93.

Myssiorek D. Recurrent laryngeal nerve paralysis: anatomy and etiology. *Otolaryngol Clin North Am.* 2004;37(1):25–44.

Neelakantan A, Rana AK. Benign and malignant diseases of the clivus. *Clin Radiol.* 2014;69(12):1295–1303. https://doi.org/10.1016/j.crad.2014.07.010.

Nelson M, Roger G, Koltai PJ, et al. Congenital cholesteatoma: classification, management, and outcome. *Arch Otolaryngol Head Neck Surg.* 2002;128(7):810–814.

O'Brien CJ. Current management of benign parotid tumors—the role of limited superficial parotidectomy. *Head Neck.* 2003;25(11):946–952.

Olsen WL, Dillon WP, Kelly WM, Norman D, Brant-Zawadzki M, Newton TH. MR imaging of paragangliomas. *AJR Am J Roentgenol.* 1984;148(1):201–204.

Ow TJ, Bell D, Kupferman ME, Demonte F, Hanna EY. Esthesioneuroblastoma. *Neurosurg Clin N Am.* 2013;24(1):51–65.

Ohbayashi N, Yamada I, Yoshino N, Sasaki T. Sjögren syndrome: comparison of assessments with MR sialography and conventional sialography. *Radiology.* 1998;209(3):683–688.

Pearlman AN, Chandra RK, Chang D. Relationships between severity of chronic rhinosinusitis and nasal polyposis, asthma, and atopy. *Am J Rhinol Allergy.* 2009;23(2):145–148.

Policarpo M, Taranto F, Aina E, Aluffi PV, Pia F. Chondrosarcoma of the larynx: a case report. *Acta Otorhinolaryngol Ital.* 2008;28(1):38–41.

Politano S, Morell F, Calamari K, DeSilva B, Matrka L. Yield of imaging to evaluate unilateral vocal fold paralysis of unknown etiology. *Laryngoscope.* 2021;131(8):1840–1844.

Potsic WP, Korman SB, Samadi DS, Wetmore RF. Congenital cholesteatoma: 20 years experience at the Children's Hospital of Philadelphia. *Otolaryngol Head Neck Surg.* 2002;12(6):409–414.

Raghavan P, Mukherjee S, Phillips CD. Imaging of the facial nerve. *Neuroimaging Clin N Am.* 2009;19(3):407–425.

Rayess HM, Nissan M, Gupta A, Carron MA, Raza SN, Fribley AM. Oropharyngeal lymphoma: a US population based analysis. *Oral Oncol.* 2017;73:147–151.

Reith W, Kettner M. [Diagnosis and treatment of glomus tumors of the skull base and neck]. *Radiologe.* 2019;59(12):1051–1057.

Righini CA, Karkas A, Tourniaire R, et al. Lemierre syndrome: study of 11 cases and literature review. *Head Neck.* 2014;36(7):1044–1051.

Rodriguez DP, Orscheln ES, Koch BL. Masses of the nose, nasal cavity, and nasopharynx in children. *Radiographics.* 2017;37(6):1704–1730.

Rosa PA, Hirsch DL, Dierks EJ. Congenital neck masses. *Oral Maxillofac Surg Clin North Am.* 2008;20(3):339–352.

Sánchez MS, Corrales R. Persistent stapedial artery. *Acta Otorrinolaringol Esp.* 2015;66(5):e31.

Sanna M, Dispenza F, Mathur N, De Stefano A, De Donato G. Otoneurological management of petrous apex cholesterol granuloma. *Am J Otolaryngol.* 2009;30(6):407–414.

Sarper A, Ayten A, Eser I, Ozbudak O, Demircan A. Tracheal stenosis after tracheostomy or intubation: review with special regard to cause and management. *Tex Heart Inst J.* 2005;32(2):154–158.

Sbaihat A, Bacciu A, Pasanisi E, Sanna M. Skull base chondrosarcomas: surgical treatment and results. *Ann Otol Rhinol Laryngol.* 2013;22(12):763–770.

Schwarz D, Kabbasch C, Scheer M, Mikolajczak S, Beutner D, Luers JC. Comparative analysis of sialendoscopy, sonography, and CBCT in the detection of sialolithiasis. *Laryngoscope.* 2015;125(5):1098–1101.

Schlakman BN, Yousem DM. MR of intraparotid masses. *AJNR Am J Neuroradiol.* 1993;14(5):1173–1180.

Schuster JJ, Phillips CD, Levine PA. MR of Esthesioneuroblastoma (olfactory neuroblastoma) and appearance after craniofacial resection. *AJNR Am J Neuroradiol.* 1994;15(6):1169–1177.

Sekiya K, Watanabe M, Nadgir RN, et al. Nasopharyngeal cystic lesions: Tornwaldt and mucous retention cysts of the nasopharynx: findings on MR imaging. *J Comput Assist Tomogr.* 2014;38(1):9–13.

Sennaroglu L, Saatci I. Unpartitioned versus incompletely partitioned cochleae: radiologic differentiation. *Otol Neurotol.* 2004;25(4):520–529.

Seyed Toutounchi SJ, Eydi M, Golzari SE, Ghaffari MR, Parvizian N. Vocal cord paralysis and its etiologies: a prospective study. *J Cardiovasc Thorac Res.* 2014;6(1):47–50.

Shah GV. MR imaging of salivary glands. *Magn Reson Imaging Clin N Am.* 2002;10(4):631–662.

Silberglit R, Quint DJ, Mehta BA, Patel SC, Metes JJ, Noujaim SE. The persistent stapedial artery. *AJNR Am J Neuroradiol.* 2000;21(3):572–577.

Song MH, Lee HY, Jeon JS, Lee JD, Lee HK, Lee WS. Jugular foramen schwannoma: analysis on its origin and location. *Otol Neurotol.* 2008;29(3):384–391.

Sriskandan N, Connor SEJ. The role of radiology in the diagnosis and management of vestibular schwannoma. *Clin Radiol.* 2011;66(4):357–365.

Strasilla C, Sychra V. [Imaging-based diagnosis of vestibular schwannoma]. *HNO.* 2017;65(5):373–380.

Suzumoto M, Hotomi M, Billal DS, Fujihara K, Harabuchi Y, Yamanaka N. A scoring system for management of acute pharyngo-tonsillitis in adults. *Auris Nasus Larynx.* 2009;36(3):314–320.

Swartz JD, Bazarnic ML, Naidich TP, Lowry LD, Doan HT. Aberrant internal carotid artery lying within the middle ear. High resolution CT diagnosis and differential diagnosis. *Neuroradiology.* 1985;27(4):322–326.

Taha MS, Hassan O, Amir M, Taha T, Riad MA. Diffusion-weighted MRI in diagnosing thyroid cartilage invasion in laryngeal carcinoma. *Eur Arch Otorhinolaryngol.* 2014;271:2511–2516.

Tan GC, Stalling M, Al-Rawabdeh S, Kahwash BM, Alkhoury RF, Kahwash SB. The spectrum of pathological findings of tonsils in children: a clinicopathological review. *Malays J Pathol.* 2018;40(1):11–26.

Tanitame K, Konishi H. Thyroglossal duct cyst. *N Engl J Med.* 2019;380(26):2563.

Tewfik TL, Al Garni M. Tonsillopharyngitis: clinical highlights. *J Otolaryngol.* 2005;34(suppl 1):S45–S49.

Thomas AJ, Wiggins RH, Gurgel RK. Nonparaganglioma jugular foramen tumors. *Otolaryngol Clin North Am.* 2015;48(2):343–359.

Tolisano AM, Lin K, Isaacson B. Jugular foramen meningioma. *Otol Neurotol.* 2018;39(3):e222–e223. https://doi.org/10.1097/MAO.0000000000001709.

Touska P, Juliano AFY. Temporal bone tumors: an imaging update. *Neuroimaging Clin N Am.* 2019;29(1):145–172.

Valentino M, Quiligotti C, Carone L. Branchial cleft cyst. *J Ultrasound.* 2013;16(1):17–20.

Vieira F, Allen SM, Stocks RMS, Thompson JW. Deep neck infection. *Otolaryngol Clin North Am.* 2008;41(3):459–483. vii.

Walkty A, Embil J. Lemierre's syndrome. *N Engl J Med.* 2019;380(12):e16.

Wang Q, Chen H, Zhou S. Chondrosarcoma of the larynx: report of two cases and review of the literature. *Int J Clin Exp Pathol.* 2015;8(2):2068–2073.

Wei YT, Jiang S, Cen Y. Fibrous dysplasia of skull. *J Craniofac Surg.* 2010;21(2). 538–452.

Wick CC, Manzoor NF, Semaan MT, Megerian CA. Endolymphatic sac tumors. *Otolaryngol Clin North Am.* 2015;48(2):317–330.

Wilson MA, Hillman TA, Wiggins RH, Shelton C. Jugular foramen schwannomas: diagnosis, management, and outcomes. *Laryngoscope.* 2005;115(8):1486–1492.

Yilmaz T, Bilgen C, Savas R, Alper H. Persistent stapedial artery: MR angiographic and CT findings. *AJNR Am J Neuroradiol.* 2003;24(6):1133–1135.

Yousem DM, Fellows DW, Kennedy DW, Bolger WE, Kashima H, Zinreich SJ. Inverted papilloma: evaluation with MR imaging. *Radiology.* 1992;185(2):501–505.

Yousem DM, Kraut MA, Chalian AA. Major salivary gland imaging. *Radiology.* 2000;216(1):19–29.

Yu T, Xu YK, Li L, et al. Esthesioneuroblastoma methods of intracranial extension: CT and MR imaging findings. *Neuroradiology.* 2009;51(12):841–850.

Yue Y, Jin Y, Yang B, Yuan H, Li J, Wang Z. Retrospective case series of the imaging findings of facial nerve hemangioma. *Eur Arch Otorhinolaryngol.* 2015;272(9):2497–2503.

Zadvinskis DP, Benson MT, Kerr HH, et al. Congenital malformations of the cervicothoracic lymphatic system: embryology and pathogenesis. *Radiographics.* 1992;12(6):1175–1189.

Zaghi S, Alonso J, Orestes M, Kadin N, Hsu W, Berke G. Idiopathic subglottic stenosis: a comparison of tracheal size. *Ann Otol Rhinol Laryngol.* 2016;125(8):622–626.

Zhang CX, Liang L, Zhang B, et al. Imaging anatomy of Waldeyer's ring and PET/CT and MRI findings of oropharyngeal non-Hodgkin's lymphoma. *Asian Pac J Cancer Prev.* 2015;16(8):3333–3338.

Zhou G, Gopen Q, Poe DS. Clinical and diagnostic characterization of canal dehiscence syndrome: a great otologic mimicker. *Otol Neurotol.* 2007;28(7):920–926.

INDEX

Note: Page numbers followed by "f" indicate figures, "t" indicate tables, and "b" indicate boxes.